Textbook of Renal Disease

Dedication

To the memory of Adam Linton whose energy, perceptive intelligence, humour and dedication to renal medicine and the wider realm of appropriate medical care inspired his friends and colleagues.

For Churchill Livingstone:

Publisher: Michael Parkinson
Project Editor: Dilys Jones
Copy Editor: Ruth Swan
Project Controller: Nancy Arnott
Sales Promotion Executive: Maria O'Connor

Textbook of Renal Disease

Edited by

Judith A. Whitworth DSc MD PhD MB BS FRACP
Professor of Medicine, University of New South Wales at St George
Hospital, Kogarah, Sydney, Australia

J. R. Lawrence AO MB BS FRACP FACP (Hon) FRCPE
Professor of Medicine, University of Sydney at Concord Hospital,
Concord, New South Wales, Australia

Foreword by
Priscilla Kincaid-Smith DSc MD FRCP FRACP FRCPA
Professor Emeritus, University of Melbourne; Director of Nephrology, Epworth Hospital,
Richmond, Victoria, Australia

SECOND EDITION

CHURCHILL LIVINGSTONE
EDINBURGH LONDON MADRID MELBOURNE NEW YORK AND TOKYO 1994

CHURCHILL LIVINGSTONE
Medical Division of Longman Group Limited

Distributed in the United States of America by Churchill
Livingstone Inc., 650 Avenue of the Americas, New York, N.Y.
10011, and by associated companies, branches and
representatives throughout the world.

© Longman Group Limited 1987, 1994

First edition 1987
Second edition 1994

ISBN 0-443-04786-3

British Library Cataloguing in Publication Data
A catalogue record for this book is available from the British Library.

Library of Congress Cataloging in Publication Data
A catalog record for this book is available from the Library of Congress.

The
publisher's
policy is to use
paper manufactured
from sustainable forests

Produced by Longman Singapore Publishers (Pte) Ltd.
Printed in Singapore

Contents

Contributors

W. R. Adam MB BS FRACP
Executive Director and Director of the Renal Unit, Heidelberg Repatriation General Hospital; Professorial Associate, University of Melbourne, Victoria, Australia

R. C. Atkins MB BS MSc DSc FRACP
Professor of Medicine and Director of Nephrology, Monash Medical Centre, Melbourne, Victoria, Australia

Ross R. Bailey MD FRACP FRCP
Department of Nephrology, Christchurch Hospital, Christchurch, New Zealand

G. J. Becker MD FRACP
Professor and Director of Nephrology, The Royal Melbourne Hospital and Melbourne University, Melbourne, Victoria, Australia

W. M. Bennett MD
Professor of Medicine and Pharmacology, Oregon Health Sciences University; Co-Head, Division of Nephrology, Hypertension and Clinical Pharmacology, Portland, Oregon, USA

M. A. Brown MB BS FRACP MD
Associate Professor of Medicine and Renal Physician, St George Hospital and University of New South Wales, Sydney, Australia

J. R. Chapman MD(Camb) MRCP FRACP
Director, Renal Unit, Westmead Hospital, Westmead; Director, Tissue Typing Laboratory, Red Cross Blood Transfusion Service, Sydney; Clinical Senior Lecturer, University of Sydney, New South Wales, Australia

J. A. Charlesworth MD BS FRACP
Associate Professor of Renal Medicine, Prince Henry Hospital, Little Bay and University of New South Wales, Sydney, Australia

A. R. Clarkson MD FRCPE
Director, Renal Unit, Royal Adelaide Hospital; Clinical Associate Professor, Department of Medicine, University of Adelaide, South Australia, Australia

J. K. Dawborn MB BS(Melbourne) PhD(London) FRACP
Professorial Associate, University of Melbourne and Department of Medicine, Austin Hospital, Heidelberg, Victoria, Australia

Karen A. Douek MD
Fellow in Nephrology, Oregon Health Sciences University, Portland, USA

G. Duggin MB BS FRACP
Clinical Associate Professor of Medicine and Pharmacology, Royal Prince Alfred Hospital, Camperdown, New South Wales, Australia

B. T. Emmerson MD PhD FRACP
Professor of Medicine and Head, Department of Medicine, The University of Queensland, Princess Alexandra Hospital, Brisbane, Queensland, Australia

Z. H. Endre BSc(Med) MB BS PhD FRACP
Associate Professor, Reader in Medicine, Department of Medicine, University of Queensland; Consultant Nephrologist and Consultant General Physician, Royal Brisbane Hospital, Brisbane, Queensland, Australia

M. J. Field MD BS BSc(Hons) FRACP
Associate Professor of Medicine, University of
Sydney at Concord Hospital, Concord, New
South Wales, Australia

Eileen D. M. Gallery MD FRACP
Clinical Professor of Medicine, Clinical
Professor of Obstetrics and Gynecology,
University of Sydney; Senior Staff Specialist in
Nephrology, Royal North Shore Hospital;
Visiting Medical Officer, Mater Misericordiae
Hospital, Sydney, New South Wales, Australia

Ákos Z. Györy MB BS MD DSc FRACP
Professor of Medicine, University of Sydney at
Royal North Shore Hospital, Sydney, New
South Wales, Australia

David C. H. Harris MD (Syd) BS FRACP
Senior Lecturer in Medicine, University of
Sydney; Nephrologist, Westmead Hospital,
Westmead and Blacktown Hospital, Blacktown,
New South Wales, Australia

S. R. Holdsworth MD BS PhD FRACP
Professor of Medicine, Monash University
Department of Medicine (Personal Chair);
Head, Clinical Nephrology Section, Monash
Medical Centre, Clayton, Victoria, Australia

C. I. Johnston MB BS FRACP
Chairman, Department of Medicine,
University of Melbourne, Austin and
Repatriation Hospitals, Melbourne, Victoria,
Australia

J. R. Lawrence AO MB BS FRACP FACP(Hon)
FRCPE
Professor of Medicine, University of Sydney at
Concord Hospital, Concord, New South Wales,
Australia

Kevin L. Lynn MB ChB FRACP
Head, Department of Nephrology, Christchurch
Hospital, Christchurch, New Zealand

G. J. Macdonald MD FRCP FRACP
Professor of Medicine, University of New South
Wales; Chairman, Department of Nephrology,
Prince Henry Hospital, Little Bay, New South
Wales, Australia

T. M. J. Maling MD FRACR FRCR
Radiologist, Department of Radiology,
Christchurch Hospital; Clinical Lecturer in
Radiology and Chairman, University
Department of Radiology, Christchurch School
of Medicine, Christchurch, New Zealand

V. R. Marshall MB BS MD FRACS
Professor and Head of Department, The
Flinders University of South Australia; Senior
Director of Urology, The Flinders Medical
Centre, Australia

T. H. Mathew MB BS FRACP
Director, Renal Unit, The Queen Elizabeth
Hospital, Woodville South; Clinical Senior
Lecturer, Department of Medicine, University
of Adelaide, Australia

T. O. Morgan BSc(Med) MB BS MD FRACP
Professor and Head of Physiology, University of
Melbourne; Head, Hypertension Clinic,
Repatriation Hospital, Heidelberg, Victoria,
Australia

R. S. Nanra MB BS FRACP
Senior Staff Nephrologist, John Hunter Hospital;
Clinical Associate Professor of Medicine,
University of Newcastle, New South Wales,
Australia

P. A. Phillips MB BS(Adelaide) DPhil(Oxford) FRACP
Senior Lecturer, University of Melbourne,
Department of Medicine, Austin Hospital,
Heidelberg, Victoria, Australia

R. A. Robson MB ChB BPharm FRACP PhD
Senior Lecturer, Department of Medicine,
Christchurch School of Medicine, University of
Otago, New Zealand

L. P. Roy MB BS BSc(Med) FRACP
Head, Department of Nephrology, Royal
Alexandra Hospital for Children, Camperdown,
Sydney; Clinical Associate Professor, University
of Sydney, New South Wales, Australia

G. B. Ryan MD PhD FRCPA FRACP
Professor of Anatomy and Dean of the Faculty
of Medicine, University of Melbourne, Victoria,
Australia

A. G. R. Sheil MB BS MA(Oxon) BSc (Oxon) FRCS FRACS FALS Hon FRCS(Eng)
Professor, Deparment of Surgery, Royal Prince Alfred Hospital, University of Sydney, New South Wales, Australia

Visith Sitprija MD PhD FACP FRCP FRACP
Professor and Chairman, Department of Medicine, Faculty of Medicine, Chulalongkorn University Medical School, Bangkok, Thailand

J. H. Stewart MB ChB FRACP FRCP (Lond)
Professor in Medicine and Associate Dean, Western Clinical School, University of Sydney; Consultant Nephrologist, Nepean Hospital, New South Wales, Australia

A. C. Thomas MB BS BSc MSc PhD FRCPath FRCPA
Senior Specialist in Tissue Pathology, Institute of Medical and Veterinary Science; Honorary Senior Hospital Consultant, Royal Adelaide Hospital; Clinical Senior Lecturer, Department of Pathology, School of Medicine, University of Adelaide, Adelaide, South Australia, Australia

N. M. Thomson MB BS FRACP MD
Professor of Medicine, Monash University at Alfred Hospital, Prahan, Melbourne, Victoria, Australia

D. J. Tiller MB BS FRACP
Head of Department of Renal Medicine, Royal Prince Alfred Hospital, Camperdown, Sydney; Clinical Professor of Medicine, University of Sydney, New South Wales, Australia

J. G. Turner MB ChB MD FRACP
Clinical Director of Nuclear Medicine, Christchurch Hospital, Christchurch, New Zealand

J. A. Whitworth DSc MD PhD MB BS FRACP
Professor of Medicine, University of New South Wales at St George Hospital, Kogarah, New South Wales, Australia

A. J. Woodroffe MD BS FRACP
Director, Renal Unit, Royal Adelaide Hospital; Clinical Senior Lecturer, University Department of Medicine, Royal Adelaide Hospital, Adelaide, South Australia, Australia

Foreword

As one might have anticipated from the quality of the previous edition this second edition of Whitworth and Lawrence: *Textbook of Renal Disease* is really outstanding.

The book, in the Australian tradition, has a very clear clinical focus and the authors, all but two of whom are from Australia and New Zealand, are practising clinicians who daily encounter the problems of which they write.

We have come to regard Bill Bennett, one of the overseas authors, who has written the chapter on Cystic renal disease as a surrogate Australian and Visith Sitprija also has very close ties with Australian nephrology.

From the first chapter on Renal anatomy and physiology to the last on Fluid and electrolyte disorders, it is clear that each chapter is written by an expert in the field, many of whom are internationally recognized.

The illustrations are of outstanding quality and demonstrate how close the clinician authors are to the diagnostic methods which they use, namely renal pathology and organ imaging.

If one were to single out chapters with special merit, Chapters 6 and 7 on Clinical presentation and diagnostic pathways in renal disease, written by the Editors would be my first choice, but all topics are of a uniformly high quality.

I cannot speak too highly of the way in which this volume covers the field of clinical nephrology with few wasted words but with concise and comprehensive chapters covering all important areas.

1994   P.K.-S.

Preface

The enthusiastic reception of the first edition of this textbook and the significant developments in understanding renal disease and function and end-stage renal failure management, made it important to produce a second edition. Some contributors have changed but the objectives of the book remain – enough up-to-date information in an assimilable form for trainee physicians and senior medical students. The book should be useful to all who treat patients with renal disease.

Selection of topics and data has been discriminating and there is emphasis on appropriate choice of investigative and therapeutic approaches amid the plethora of available technology and information.

We are indebted to Mrs Beverley Smith for her invaluable secretarial and administrative assistance.

Sydney 1994

J.R.L.
J.A.W.

Renal structure and function

1. Renal anatomy and physiology

M. J. Field   G. B. Ryan   T. O. Morgan

INTRODUCTION

The kidneys control the composition and volume of body fluids within narrowly defined limits by excreting unwanted substances (either produced endogenously or ingested) and regulating the excretion of essential metabolites. This is performed in association with hormones produced by endocrine glands. The regulation is precise and the kidney can adjust to major variations in intake or production of different substances. Thus a normal person can handle a daily water intake ranging from l litre to 20 litres, a sodium intake of 5–500 mmol, a potassium intake of 20–200 mmol and a protein intake of 30–150 g with no significant alteration in body composition. There are subtle but important alterations in the control systems.

The kidneys excrete a large number of substances produced by metabolism or introduced to the body and the latter may be naturally occurring or artificially manufactured. This can occur because the kidney filters a large volume of blood, reabsorbing essential constituents and leaving unwanted products behind in the urine. In addition, specific processes allow secretion of weak acids and weak bases, providing another mechanism for the excretion of unwanted products.

The kidney filters a large volume of blood each day, and from this filtrate most of the sodium chloride, bicarbonate and water is reabsorbed, together with other small, important substances, e.g. phosphate. In addition there is selective reabsorption of essential molecules like amino acids and glucose, and specific secretion of unwanted substances.

In addition to its excretory function, the kidney has a number of other important roles, such as endocrine functions related particularly to blood volume and composition, and metabolic functions — it is a major site for degradation of compounds and an important source of production of essential metabolites.

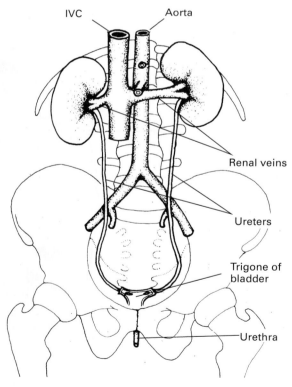

Fig. 1.1 Diagram showing the anatomical location of the kidneys, major renal blood vessels, ureters, trigone of bladder and urethra

To fulfil these multiple functions the kidney has a number of unique structures which are closely associated with particular functions.

ANATOMY OF THE KIDNEY

Each kidney lies retroperitoneally on the posterior abdominal wall in the paravertebral gutter from the 12th thoracic to the 3rd lumbar vertebra (Fig. 1.1). The right kidney is slightly lower than the left, reaching to about a fingerbreadth above the iliac crest. Each kidney is bean-shaped, measuring approximately 11 cm × 6 cm × 3 cm and weighing 120–170 g in adults. Its medial margin shows an indentation, called the renal hilus, at which are attached the renal artery, vein, lymphatics, nerves and the pelvis of the ureter. The kidney is closely surrounded by a fibrous capsule that normally strips easily from the surface. Outside the capsule is a variable amount of perirenal fat.

Posteriorly, the superior pole of the kidney is related to the diaphragm, which separates it from the pleural cavity and the 12th rib. Below the diaphragm, the kidney lies against the quadratus lumborum muscle, encroaching on the psoas major medially and the transversus abdominis aponeurosis laterally.

Anteriorly, the right kidney is related to the right adrenal gland, the liver, the duodenal loop and the right colic flexure. The left kidney is related to the left adrenal gland, stomach, spleen, pancreas, jejunum and descending colon.

Bisection of the kidney reveals the hilus, which is connected to a flattened cavity called the renal sinus. This contains fat but is mostly filled by the expanded ureteric pelvis which branches into two to four major calyces, each of which in turn branches into several minor calyces. The cut surface of the kidney is subdivided into an outer cortex and an inner medulla (Fig. 1.2). The medulla is composed of 8 to 18 conically shaped

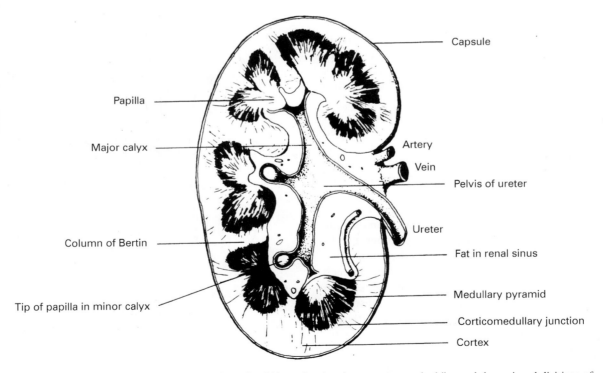

Fig. 1.2 Drawing of a longitudinal section through a kidney showing the structures at the hilus and the main subdivisions of the renal parenchyma

medullary pyramids, the base of each pyramid lying along the corticomedullary junction and its apex forming a papilla which projects into a minor calyx. The cortex forms a layer, approximately 1 cm thick in adults, on the outside of the medullary pyramids and extends between the pyramids as the columns of Bertin. Although most of the cortex shows a granular appearance (in contrast to the striated appearance of the medullary pyramids), striated elements called medullary rays radiate at intervals outwards through the cortex from the corticomedullary junction. A lobe of the kidney is composed of one medullary pyramid and its overlying cap of cortex.

The blood supply of the kidney is derived from the renal artery, which arises from the aorta at the level of the L1–L2 intervertebral disc. One or more smaller accessory renal arteries are not uncommon. The renal artery usually divides close to the hilus into an anterior division (which divides into several segmental arteries supplying the front and the upper and lower poles of the kidney) and a posterior division (which supplies the remainder of the posterior region of the kidney). On entering the renal parenchyma, these branches form the interlobar arteries that run between the medullary pyramids to the corticomedullary junction, where they turn to run along the base of the medullary pyramids to form the arcuate arteries. Branching at right angles from the arcuate arteries and radiating outwards through the cortex, midway between medullary rays, are the interlobular arteries. From these arise the afferent arterioles, each supplying a glomerular capillary tuft (see below). Each glomerular tuft is drained by an efferent arteriole. In the outer and middle cortex the efferent arterioles divide to form a peritubular capillary network. In the inner cortex the efferent arterioles give rise to multiple parallel vasa recta that dip deeply into the medullary pyramid before making a hairpin turn and returning to the corticomedullary junction. The descending and ascending vasa recta provide the vascular component of the medullary countercurrent exchange system (see later). The renal venous system follows the same pattern as the renal arteries, i.e. interlobular veins, arcuate veins, interlobar veins,

renal vein. Renal lymphatic vessels run predominantly in association with interlobular, arcuate and interlobar blood vessels and with the surface capsule. The kidney is innervated by sympathetic and parasympathetic fibres from the renal plexus.

RENAL CIRCULATION

A key to the function of the kidney is the renal circulation. The blood flow through the kidney is normally about 20–25% of cardiac output but can be readjusted dramatically. Thus, during exercise or after a meal, renal blood flow falls because of alterations in sympathetic tone. The kidney has a number of intrinsic controls which allow it to maintain its function at a relatively constant level despite major alterations in blood pressure or blood flow. These mechanisms depend on specific morphological structures and their spatial relationships to each other.

Any change in blood pressure is followed by an automatic readjustment of flow so that flow remains constant. The specific mechanism is still under debate but, as discussed later, it is probably controlled by an intrinsic system operating via the juxtaglomerular apparatus. Even if blood flow is reduced, glomerular filtration rate (GFR) tends to remain constant. This is probably also affected through the juxtaglomerular apparatus by controlling the relative tone of the afferent and efferent arterioles of the glomerulus.

The pressure along the renal circulation changes in a number of steps (Fig. 1.3). Recent work has shown that glomerular capillary pressure is about 45 mmHg, which is lower than first believed. The major sites of resistance are in the afferent and efferent arteriole. Alterations in resistance of both or either of these produce different effects. If both were increased, renal blood flow would decrease yet there may be little change in glomerular filtration pressure and GFR (see later). If the afferent arteriole is constricted, blood flow and filtration pressure will fall, thus reducing GFR. If the efferent arteriole is constricted, renal blood flow will fall, but now the glomerular pressure will rise and the effect on GFR will depend on the relative contribution of each of these to its determination. Thus the relative tone and selective constriction of

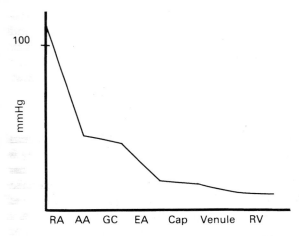

Fig. 1.3 Pressure in the different vascular segments: RA = renal artery; AA = afferent arteriole; GC = glomerular capillary; EA = efferent arteriole; Cap = capillary; RV = renal vein. Note that pressure does not fall along the glomerular capillary and that the pressure in the glomerulus is about 45 mmHg

the afferent and efferent arterioles determine renal blood flow and glomerular filtration.

THE NEPHRON

The functioning unit of the kidney is the nephron (Fig. 1.4). There are approximately one million nephrons in each human kidney. These are arranged in a complex pattern to allow integrated function. The first part of the nephron is the renal corpuscle, which is composed of circulatory and renal units and allows the ultrafiltration of blood. This is followed by the proximal convoluted tubule which reabsorbs the bulk of the filtrate and is situated in the cortex of the kidney, an area of high blood flow. The next segment is the loop of Henle, a continuation of the tubule which, due to its anatomical arrangement and the structure of its wall, allows the urine to be diluted or concentrated. The loop of Henle enters a cortical medullary ray, descends for a variable distance into the medullary pyramid and then returns to the same glomerulus from which it arose. Here, there is a unique structure composed of vascular, tubular and interstitial components, the juxtaglomerular apparatus, which is of considerable importance in the regulation of individual nephron

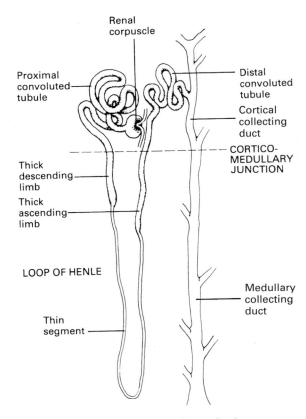

Fig. 1.4 Diagram of a nephron and the collecting system

function. The remainder of the nephron consists of a distal convoluted tubule which drains into the collecting system composed of cortical collecting tubules, which in turn unite to form cortical collecting ducts in the medullary rays. The collecting ducts flow down into the medulla and papilla, uniting to form the ducts of Bellini which discharge into the pelvis of the kidney.

Renal corpuscle

The renal corpuscle (Fig. 1.5) is composed of a tuft of anastomosing capillaries, called the glomerulus, projecting into the filling a space (named 'Bowman's space') that is in continuity with the lumen of the proximal convoluted tubule. This space is enclosed by Bowman's capsule, which consists of a basement membrane lined by flattened parietal epithelial cells. The glomerular

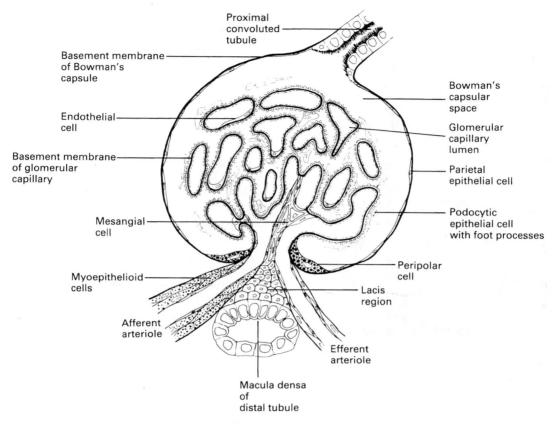

Fig. 1.5 Diagram of a renal corpuscle sectioned through the vascular pole of the glomerulus and including the juxtaglomerular apparatus

capillaries are covered by visceral (or podocytic) epithelial cells. Blood enters the vascular pole of the glomerulus via the afferent arteriole and leaves via the efferent arteriole. Within the glomerulus, the afferent arteriole divides into several primary branches which in turn give rise to several lobules of capillaries. The intercellular components of the glomerulus are (1) the glomerular capillary basement membrane and (2) the mesangial matrix. Its cellular components are (1) the endothelium, (2) mesangial cells and (3) the epithelium (Figs. 1.5–1.7).

The glomerular basement membrane is 300–350 nm thick in adult humans. It reacts positively with the periodic acid-Schiff (PAS) reagent and with silver stains. It is composed of type IV collagen (without cross-banding) and

negatively charged glycosaminoglycans, and subdivided into three layers (Fig. 1.8): an electron-dense central zone, the lamina densa, separating inner and outer paler zones; the lamina rara interna (adjacent to the endothelium); and the lamina rara externa (adjacent to the epithelial layer).

The glomerular endothelium is composed of a thin layer of cytoplasm characterized by the presence of multiple open fenestrae 50–100 nm in diameter (see Fig. 1.8). In the stalk region of the glomerulus, between the capillaries, are mesangial cells embedded in mesangial matrix (see Fig. 1.7). As well as having a supporting function, mesangial cells appear to be phagocytic and are probably contractile, possibly thereby modulating glomerular blood flow in response to vasoactive agents such as angiotensin II.

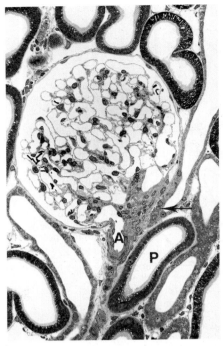

Fig. 1.6 Light micrograph of rat renal corpuscle, juxtaglomerular apparatus and cortical tubules. Note juxtaglomerular arteriole (A), proximal convoluted tubule (P) and macula densa (arrow) of distal tubule. (× 240)

Podocytic glomerular epithelial cells project elongated foot processes onto the outside of the glomerular basement membrane where they interdigitate with the foot processes from neighbouring epithelial cells (Fig. 1.9). Between the adjoining foot processes is the epithelial or filtration slit (see Fig. 1.8), at the base of which is a diaphragm with a zipper-like substructure delineating a uniform array of rectangular pores 4 × 14 nm in size.

The glomerular capillary wall acts as a sieve, allowing the passage of water and small solutes but holding back circulating macromolecules the size of albumin or larger. There has been some debate as to which of the structural components in the glomerular capillary wall are responsible for limiting the penetration of plasma proteins during normal ultrafiltration. Recent studies indicate that such macromolecules are held up at the level of the endothelial fenestrae by a functional barrier that depends critically on the maintenance of normal glomerular blood flow and a finely balanced equilibrium between convective and diffusive forces across the capillary wall. The effectiveness

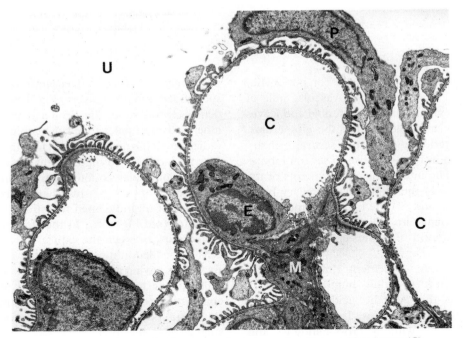

Fig. 1.7 Electron micrograph of a portion of rat glomerulus. Note capillary lumen (C), urinary space (U), endothelium (E), mesangium (M) and podocytic epithelium (P). (× 4500)

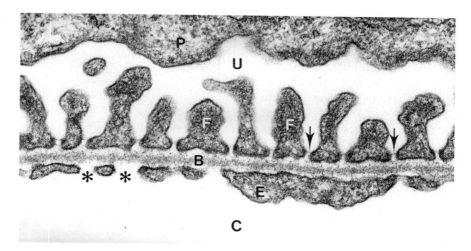

Fig. 1.8 Electron micrograph of glomerular capillary wall. Note capillary lumen (C), urinary space (U), podocytic epithelial cell body (P), foot processes (F), slit diaphragm (arrows), basement membrane (B), endothelium (E), and endothelial fenestrae (asterisks). (× 45 000)

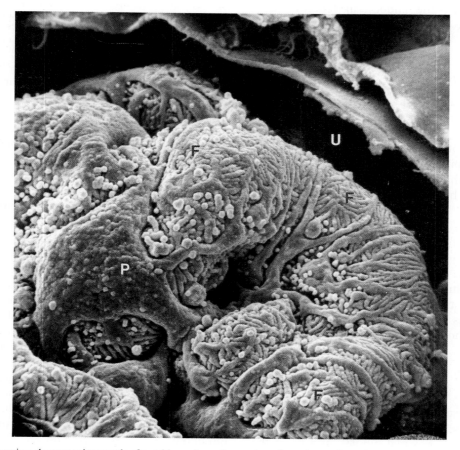

Fig. 1.9 Scanning electron micrograph of outside surface of a portion of rat glomerular tuft. Note podocytic epithelial cell body (P), interdigitating foot processes (F) and urinary space (U). (× 4500)

of this barrier is probably the result of molecular sieving phenomena at the basement membrane, possibly with the assistance of concentration-polarization effects and the presence of intrinsic anionic groups in the basement membrane. Proteinuria may result from changes in the structure and composition of the basement membrane as well as from changes in glomerular blood flow or ultrafiltration flux. It has been demonstrated that protein leakage may also occur at sites of focal loss of the epithelial layer from the outside of the basement membrane (as, for example, in patients with the nephrotic syndrome and in experimental models of proteinuria). Because the epithelial layer appears to offer the major restriction to water flux across the glomerular capillary wall, protein leakage at sites of epithelial loss may be the result of a focal 'blow-out' of ultrafiltration flux, thereby disrupting the functional barrier at the endothelial fenestrae and dragging macromolecules across the wall to the urinary space.

Glomerular filtration

Production of a cell- and protein-free ultrafiltrate of plasma is primarily dependent on the hydrostatic pressure generated by the heart, but is also influenced by other pressures operating across the glomerular capillary membrane, as well as by the properties of that membrane. These relationships are expressed by the formula

$$GFR = K_f \times P_{uf}$$

where K_f is the ultrafiltration coefficient and P_{uf} is the net ultrafiltration pressure.

The P_{uf} is itself dependent on the balance of Starling forces operating across the glomerular capillary, as shown in Figure 1.10. Thus,

$$P_{uf} = P_{gc} - (P_t + \pi_{gc})$$

where P_{gc} is hydrostatic pressure in the glomerular capillary, P_t is the hydrostatic pressure in Bowman's space (or proximal tubule), and π_{gc} is the

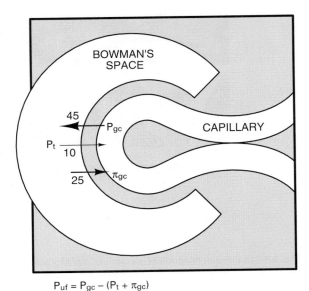

$$P_{uf} = P_{gc} - (P_t + \pi_{gc})$$

Fig. 1.10 Schematic diagram of forces acting across the glomerular capillary in the process of glomerular filtration. Symbols defined in the text. Approximate values of forces shown in mmHg

oncotic pressure in the glomerular capillary plasma.

The term π_t, the oncotic pressure in Bowman's space, is omitted since it is approximately zero as protein is not filtered across the capillary under normal conditions.

Figure 1.10 also shows the approximate values for the Starling forces relating to the dynamics of ultrafiltration, as they have been determined from experimental studies in rats. The figures given, which are those applicable at the beginning of a typical glomerular capillary, result in a relatively small net pressure available for ultrafiltration of around 10 mmHg. It should be noted that the hydrostatic pressure terms are essentially unchanged along the course of a glomerular capillary. However, as fluid filtration proceeds with retention of plasma proteins in the capillary blood, the glomerular capillary oncotic pressure term increases along the length of the capillary, thus reducing the net pressure available for ultrafiltration as a function of length along the capillary. Indeed, it is probable that a point of zero net ultrafiltration occurs ('filtration equilibrium') before the end of the glomerular capillary under normal conditions in mammals.

Although the net filtration pressure is thus relatively low, a high filtration rate is nonetheless normally obtained because of the high ultrafiltration coefficient, K_f. This term is a product of the hydraulic permeability of the membrane and the surface area available for filtration. Of these two factors, the hydraulic permeability is high and relatively constant, but variations in the surface area are probably produced under physiological circumstances by changes in the contractile state of the glomerular mesangium, as well as by changes in glomerular blood flow rate and, in pathological states, the obliterative effects of glomerular disease.

The selective permeability of the glomerular filtration barrier is probably largely due to the properties of the glomerular basement membrane (GBM). This acts to restrain the passage of plasma solutes into the filtrate on the basis of (a) molecular size (or 'effective molecular radius'): this is largely a function of molecular weight such that substances with MW > 50 000 are negligibly filtered; and (b) electrical charge, such that anions are more restrained than cations, owing to the high density of negative charges in the normal structures of the glomerular capillary wall.

Proximal convoluted tubule

The proximal convoluted tubule is the longest segment of the nephron. It is lined by a single layer of cells with a prominent brush border composed of long microvilli projecting into the lumen (Fig 1.11). The cells show an extensive system of lateral and basal processes that interdigitate with processes of adjoining cells. Basal processes contain large mitochondria oriented radially to produce a pattern of basal striations. These are cytological features of cells engaged in active reabsorption.

Approximately 180 litres of glomerular filtrate enter the proximal tubule each day, and between 65 and 80% of the sodium, chloride, potassium and water are reabsorbed. In addition there is selective reabsorption of important metabolites. In the early part of the proximal tubule there is extremely active reabsorption of glucose and amino acids. Linked to this is the reabsorption of NaCl and water (see later) and the reclamation of bicarbonate. Towards the latter part of the proximal tubule and in the pars recta, secretion of weak acids and weak bases becomes more prominent. The proximal tubule reabsorbs fluid so that the composition of the filtrate remains similar to that of plasma, but in addition it selectively reabsorbs essential metabolites. For a considerable time it has been considered that reabsorption is isotonic. However, a number of carefully controlled experiments have indicated that the reabsorbate is hypertonic and that an osmotic gradient exists between the luminal fluid and the plasma, this being greatest at the end of the proximal tubule. A unique property of the proximal tubule is its ability to adjust reabsorption rates so that the proportion of filtered salt and water reabsorbed tends to remain constant despite wide variations in flow rates ('glomerulo-tubular balance').

Loop of Henle

The outer and middle cortical nephrons give rise to short loops of Henle whereas juxtamedullary nephrons are characterized by long loops of Henle that dip deeply into the medulla before returning to the cortex (see Fig. 1.4). In the inner medulla and papilla, descending and ascending limbs of the loops of Henle are arranged in bundles in association with the collecting ducts and vasa recta, providing the morphological basis of the countercurrent system. Structurally, the loop of Henle consists of three major segments: the thick descending limb (also often called the pars recta of the proximal tubule); the thin segment (subdivided into the thin descending limb and the thin ascending limb); and the thick ascending limb (sometimes called the pars recta of the distal tubule). The cells in the thick descending limb are similar to those of the proximal convoluted tubule but with less prominent basal striations. The thin segment is relatively short in outer and middle cortical nephrons, in contrast to the very long thin segment in juxtamedullary nephrons, which typically has a long thin descending limb followed by a long thin ascending limb. The thin segment is lined by a thin squamous epithelium 1–2 μm thick.

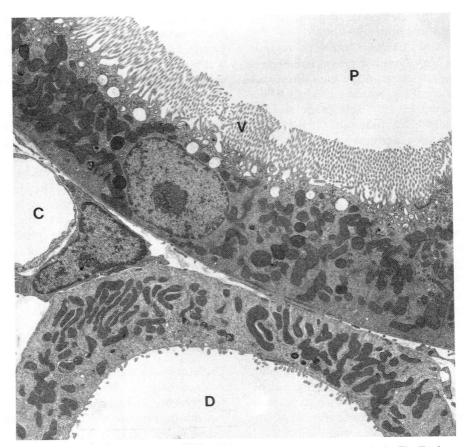

Fig. 1.11 Electron micrograph showing portions of proximal convoluted tubule (P), distal convoluted tubule (D) and intertubular capillary (C). Note microvilli (V) constituting the brush border of the proximal convoluted tubule. (× 4500)

The proximal part of the thin descending limb shows elaborate cellular interdigitations with shallow, tenuous tight junctions. More distally, its structure becomes simpler, with less elaborate cell interdigitations and longer tight junctions, presumably reflecting lower ionic permeability in this region. The thin ascending limb consists of cells with interdigitations of intermediate complexity associated with relatively shallow tight junctions. The thick ascending limb begins near the border of the inner and outer medulla and extends to the macula densa region of the distal tubule at the juxtaglomerular apparatus. The cells of the thick ascending limb are considerably thicker than those of the thin segment. They show complex interdigitations with adjoining cells, particularly in the basal region, and contain abundant mitochondria. Scattered microvilli are present in the luminal surface. Tight intercellular junctions are well developed.

Juxtaglomerular apparatus

This is a specialized structure consisting of a tubular component (the macula densa region of the distal tubule), a vascular component involving afferent and efferent arterioles, and an interstitial component (lacis or polar cushion region) which communicates with the mesangium of the glomerulus (see Fig. 1.5). The macula densa is a group of seven to eight cells on the glomerular side of the distal tubule. The cells are taller than the adjacent cells, the nuclei are close together and the intercellular spaces appear open. Mitochondria are not so plentiful. In general it is considered that these cells monitor some aspect of tubular fluid composition. The cells in the wall of the afferent and, to a lesser extent, the efferent arteriole contain cytoplasmic granules (Fig. 1.12). These cells are called epithelioid or, reflecting their medial origin, myoepithelioid cells. The degree of granularity in these cells varies according to the salt and water status of the individual, and granular cells may be found a considerable distance along the afferent arteriole. The granules contain renin but other components of the renin–angiotensin system are also found in this region. The interstitial or lacis cells are contiguous with the mesangial cells of the glomerulus, thereby providing a direct link be-

tween the juxtaglomerular apparatus and the glomerulus. Recently, an additional component of the juxtaglomerular apparatus has been described. This is the peripolar cell, which is an epithelial cell surrounding the vascular pole of the glomerulus at the junction between glomerular podocytic cells and the parietal epithelium of Bowman's capsule (Fig. 1.13). It contains many dense cytoplasmic granules, whose composition is as yet unknown. The function of the peripolar cell is not known.

The precise roles of the juxtaglomerular apparatus are not clearly understood but it is almost certainly involved in feedback control of glomerular filtration rate and blood flow (see below). In addition there are other factors controlling release of renin at this site, including baroreceptors activated by a fall in renal perfusion pressure, and a sympathetic nervous system innervation.

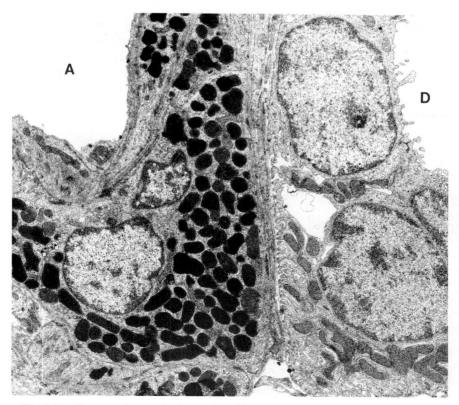

Fig. 1.12 Electron micrograph of a portion of juxtaglomerular apparatus showing multiple renin granules in myoepithelioid cells in the wall of an afferent arteriole (A), adjacent to the macula densa region of the distal tubule (D). (× 7500)

Tubuloglomerular feedback (TGF) describes the process whereby the juxtaglomerular apparatus brings about control of the glomerular filtration rate in individual nephrons in relation to the flow of tubular fluid past the macula densa. While the exact mediator(s) of this process are not precisely defined, it is clear that the signal detected at the macula densa is an increase in the sodium chloride concentration of the luminal fluid. This is in some way detected by the macula densa cells, transduced through the lacis region of the juxtaglomerular apparatus, and conveyed as a signal to the afferent arteriole which undergoes constriction, resulting in a fall of single nephron GFR to the same nephron. This mechanism thus has the effect of reducing filtration to a nephron in which tubular reabsorptive capacity is impaired or inadequate, thus preventing uncontrolled urinary loss of salt and water. This same mechanism may also contribute to the autoregulation of whole kidney GFR and renal blood flow by limiting the flow rise which would otherwise occur with an increase in renal perfusion pressure.

The exact nature of the effector signal involved in TGF is uncertain, although a number of vasoactive substances such as adenosine have been implicated. While it was formerly thought that the locally active renin–angiotensin system was the principal mediator of tubuloglomerular feedback, it is now clear that renin release from the myoepithelioid cells of the afferent arteriole is in fact triggered by a fall in distal tubular sodium concentration, rather than a rise. This mechanism of renin release may be involved in the systemic increase in renin and angiotensin occurring during volume depletion. Angiotensin II is still important in TGF, however, as it appears to play a role in modulating the sensitivity of the feedback mechanism under different conditions of extracellular fluid volume.

Distal nephron

The distal nephron commences at the macula densa. Its first segment is the distal convoluted tubule, previously defined as the segment extending from the macula densa to the first branching with another tubule. However, it is now recognized that only the early portion of this segment represents the true distal convoluted tubule, the late portion being structurally and functionally similar to the cortical collecting duct. In some

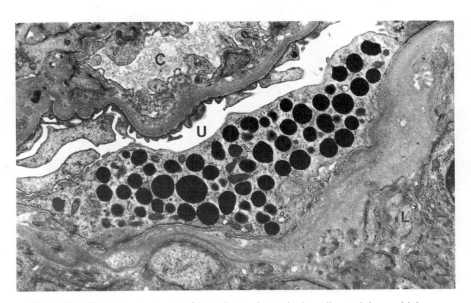

Fig. 1.13 Electron micrograph of juxtaglomerular peripolar cell containing multiple cytoplasmic granules. Note the glomerular capillary (C), urinary space (U) and juxtaglomerular lacis region L). (× 6750)

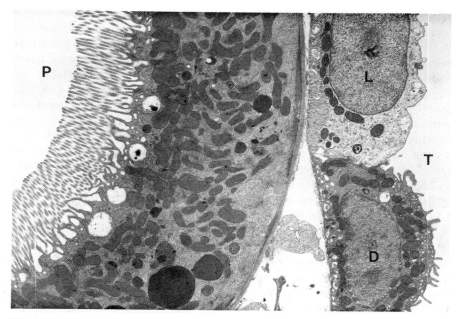

Fig. 1.14 Electron micrograph showing portions of the proximal convoluted tubule (P) and collecting tubule (T). Note the 'light' (L) and 'dark' (D) cells in the wall of the collecting tubule. (× 4500)

species, the two portions are connected by a short 'connecting tubule'.

The function of the true distal convoluted tubule appears to be limited to reabsorption of further sodium chloride as well as calcium. This segment, like the thick ascending limb, is impermeable to water. In contrast to earlier beliefs, the distal convoluted tubule appears to be relatively insensitive to both aldosterone and antidiuretic hormone.

Morphologically the distal convoluted tubule differs from the proximal convoluted tubule (see Fig. 1.11) by being composed of cells that are shorter and less acidophilic and have only few luminal microvilli. However, like the proximal convoluted tubule, it shows prominent basolateral interdigitations and prominent basal striations, although these features progressively decline as it approaches the cortical collecting tubule.

The cortical collecting tubule is composed of two types of low cuboidal cell: the principal ('light') cell with well-defined cell margins, pale cytoplasm and multiple small mitochondria; and the intercalated ('dark') cell with darker staining cytoplasm, more mitochondria packed around the

nucleus, and multiple microplicae and vesicles on the luminal surface (Fig. 1.14). The collecting tubules unite to form cortical and then medullary collecting ducts, a transition associated with a progressive increase in luminal diameter and in the height of the lining cells. There is also progressive loss of intercalated cells in the outer medulla; none are found in the larger papillary collecting ducts.

The later portion of the distal nephron, particularly the cortical collecting duct, appears to have three principal roles. Firstly, under the influence of aldosterone, it is responsible for fine regulation of sodium excretion. By active sodium reabsorption, stimulated by aldosterone, it can reduce urinary sodium concentration to as little as 1 mmol/1 in avid salt-retaining states. Secondly, it regulates excretion of potassium and hydrogen ions, both of which are secreted here. This process is intimately linked to sodium reabsorption and is also under the influence of aldosterone. Finally, it is involved in water conservation and excretion. Secretion of antidiuretic hormone (ADH) from the posterior pituitary is controlled by osmoreceptors in the hypothalamus. If the plasma osmolality is low (i.e.

if there is excess water), ADH release is suppressed and the distal nephron becomes impermeable to water; water is therefore not reabsorbed, resulting in a hypotonic urine and thus water loss in excess of solute. If water needs to be conserved, e.g. in dehydration when plasma osmolality is increased, ADH is secreted and this increases the permeability of the collecting tubule system in both cortex and medulla, causing water to be reabsorbed and a concentrated urine (see later) to be excreted.

The three components of the collecting duct, i.e. its cortical, medullary and papillary portions, have some common and some dissimilar functional properties. One very important difference is in their permeability to urea. The cortical segments are impermeable to urea while papillary segments, under the influence of ADH, are very permeable. This difference is crucial for the operation of the passive countercurrent multiplier within the papillary nephron.

CLEARANCE

Clinically, some important aspects of renal function are assessed by measuring clearance. The clearance of a substance is the apparent volume of plasma completely cleared of that substance in unit time. This is a theoretical concept because a proportion of the substance is removed from each millilitre of blood. The amount excreted by the kidney is determined by multiplying the urine flow rate (V) by the concentration of the substance in the urine (U). The plasma clearance (C) is obtained by dividing this quantity by the concentration of the substance in plasma (P).

$$C = \frac{U \times V}{P}$$

If all the blood that flows through the kidney is cleared of a certain substance, its clearance is a measure of renal plasma flow. Such a substance would need to be fully secreted by the tubules as well as freely filtered. If on the other hand a substance is filtered through the glomerulus at the same concentration as exists in plasma and is not reabsorbed or secreted, its clearance is a measure

of the glomerular filtration rate. However, the clearance of any substance excreted by the kidney can be measured, and its value in relation to GFR and renal blood flow allows interpretations to be made about its renal tubular handling. Two specific forms of clearance discussed later are osmolal clearance and free water clearance.

Glomerular filtration rate can be measured by infusing inulin (or ^{51}Cr-labelled EDTA or iothalamate), which is only excreted by glomerular filtration and appears in the initial filtrate in the same concentration as a plasma. Inulin is infused to give a constant blood level. The amount excreted per unit time is then measured and used to calculate clearance. Creatinine, a naturally occurring compound, is handled in much the same way. Approximately the same amount of creatinine is produced each day, although production varies between individuals and is greater in those with a bigger muscle mass. As glomerular filtration rate also increases with size of the person, plasma creatinine is maintained within a relatively narrow range. By measuring the amount of creatinine excreted in a set time and its plasma concentration, the glomerular filtration rate can be calculated. This is similar to the inulin clearance, the minor differences being due to different rates of creatinine release from muscles and to some secretion by the renal tubules. Creatinine clearance is required to compare function between individuals. However, as the infusion (production by muscle) of creatinine is constant for each individual and the patient is in homeostasis (i.e. excretion equals production), and the plasma creatinine is inversely related to clearance, plasma creatinine is a useful measure to determine change in renal function in an individual. Particularly in children, clearance is related to a standardized body surface area (1.73 m²).

In clinical investigative medicine the clearance of p-aminohippurate (PAH) is used to measure renal blood flow. PAH is excreted by filtration at the glomerulus and secretion by the proximal tubule. If its plasma concentration is low, all blood that passes through these structures is cleared of PAH and the clearance is a measure of plasma flow or, more correctly, the effective renal plasma flow (this is less than the total renal plasma flow, as some blood does not flow through these structures).

Clearance measurements can be made for any substance and are particularly useful for determining the half-life of drugs and to give information about how this may alter in renal disease.

TRANSPORT OF ORGANIC SOLUTES

The absorption of many organic solutes from the proximal tubular lumen occurs by 'secondary' active transport. This is illustrated in the case of *glucose* in Figure 1.15. The luminal cell membrane contains a transport protein (carrier) which has binding sites for both glucose and for sodium ions. The 'downhill' movement of sodium into the cell drives the movement of the solute against its concentration gradient into the cell, from which it can move passively (by facilitated diffusion involving countertransport with another monosaccharide species) into the peritubular capillaries across the basolateral membrane. The energy for the apical co-transport of solute with sodium thus comes indirectly from the primary active transport of sodium from the cell at the blood-facing membrane, mediated by the Na,K-ATPase ('the sodium pump').

Other substances handled in an analogous fashion include *amino acids* and *phosphate*. In the case of amino acids, at least four specific active transport systems exist, and amino acids within each group may inhibit absorption of others in that group (see box). However, the situation is more complicated than this, since subclasses of carrier molecules exist, and complex interactions between individual amino acid species and a variety of carriers are now known to occur. Some types of inherited aminoaciduria result from specific defects in the transport of one or more groups of amino acids. The resultant urinary amino acid excretory pattern depends on the specific defect involved.

A significant component of proximal phosphate reabsorption is also mediated by a specific transport process in the proximal tubule, again involving an apical membrane sodium-phosphate carrier molecule. It appears that this transport step is stimulated by Vitamin D, and inhibited by parathyroid hormone, resulting in phosphaturia under conditions of parathyroid hormone excess. It is important to note that a component of proximal phosphate reabsorption, and also the reabsorption of glucose and amino acids, is mediated by convective transport ('solvent drag') with bulk water flow across this epithelium.

A feature of the renal excretory pattern of organic solutes which undergo proximal reabsorp-

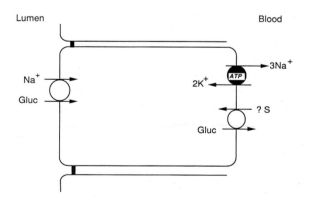

Fig. 1.15 Schematic diagram of proximal tubule cell to show the key steps involved in the transepithelial reabsorption of D-glucose. Note that exit from the cell across the blood-facing membrane is facilitated by countertransport with one or more types of monosaccharide molecule (labelled '? S')

Amino acids that share absorptive pathways

1. *Neutral*
   Alanine
   α-Aminobutyric
   Histidine
   Norvaline
   Norleucine
   Methionine
2. *Basic*
   Arginine
   Cystine
   Lysine
   Ornithine
3. *Acidic*
   Aspartic acid
   Glutaminc acid
4. *Iminoglycines*
   Glycine
   Hydroxyproline
   Proline

tion via a specific saturable carrier mechanism is that they display a characteristic 'titration' behaviour when plasma levels of the substance are raised. As shown in Figure 1.16, as plasma concentration of glucose is elevated, there comes a point (the 'threshold' level) at which glucose starts to appear in the urine, as a result of the saturation of the specific apical reabsorptive mechanism. The maximal rate at which the reabsorptive process can operate is called the transport maximum (T_m), and though characteristic of a given solute for a particular species, it is also influenced by the prevailing reabsorption rate of sodium and water, since the convective (non-carrier-mediated) transport of these solutes varies greatly with the state of general hydration.

These observations provide the basis for clinical testing for glycosuria in diabetic hyperglycaemia (where the plasma glucose concentration exceeds the threshold), and for aminoaciduria at normal plasma amino acid concentrations in the disorders involving abnormal amino acid carrier function.

Weak acids and *weak bases* constitute another general class of organic species undergoing reabsorption and/or secretion via carrier-mediated mechanisms in the proximal tubule. However, less

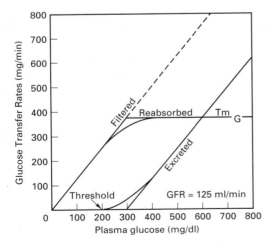

Fig. 1.16 Relationship between plasma glucose concentration and glucose transfer rates (filtration, reabsorption and secretion) during 'titration' of the renal tubules with glucose in man. TmG is the tubular maximal reabsorptive capacity for glucose

is known of the details of the transport mechanisms involved.

In broad terms, secretory mechanisms exist for organic acids (anions) and for organic bases (cations), and there is a degree of competitive inhibition within each system, though this is not absolute (see box). Para-aminohippurate serves as a prototype for the anion secreting pathway and many substances of clinical interest such as penicillins, salicylates, dyes and contrast agents appear to share this pathway. Probenecid is a drug which can be specifically used to competitively inhibit secretion of these substances, thereby raising their blood concentration (e.g. for penicillin therapy). The cationic secretory pathways transfer many endogenous mediators and transmitters, such as histamine, catecholamines, thiamine and morphine. Even less is known about the specificity, affinity and location of carrier systems on the luminal and contraluminal surfaces of the proximal tubule cells for cations than is known for anions. However in functional terms, it is clear that these secretory pathways provide a means for excreting substances which, because of a high level of protein binding, would otherwise be minimally cleared by glomerular filtration.

Uric acid is a weak acid which is of special significance since it undergoes bidirectional transport (both reabsorption and secretion) across the proximal tubule, and the net flux is clinically significant because of the potential of precipitating gout if serum uric acid levels rise. Although carrier-mediated transport contributes to both reabsorptive and secretive fluxes, an important component of reabsorption is also mediated by a relatively non-specific pathway linked to the reabsorption of salt and water. Thus if overall proximal tubular reabsorption is increased, as in volume depletion or during diuretic therapy, more urate is reabsorbed in this segment. The secretory pathway in the later part of the proximal tubule involves the weak acid secretory site referred to above, but there may also be a specific uric acid pathway. Various drugs interact with both the reabsorptive and secretive mechanisms, and the net excretory rate depends on the relative contribution of the two transport pathways, taking into

Some weak acids and weak bases actively secreted by the proximal tubule

Weak acids
  Acetazolamide
  Amiloride
  Diodrast
  Ethacrynic acid
  Frusemide
  Hippurate
  Nitrofurantoin
  p-Amino hippuric acid
  Penicillin
  Phenylbutazone
  Probenecid
  Salicylate
  Thiazide diuretics
  Triamterene
  Uric acid
Weak bases
  Dihydromorphine
  Dopamine
  Guanidine
  Histamine
  Morphine
  Neostigmine
  Procaine

Table 1.1   Drugs affecting uric acid excretion*

	Low dose		High dose	
	Increase	*Decrease*	*Increase*	*Decrease*
Chlorothiazide		X		X
Ethacrynic acid		X	XX	
Frusemide		X	XX	
Lactate				
Ketone bodies		X		XX
Phenylbutazone		X	XX	
Probenecid			XXX	
Sulphinpyrazone	X		XXX	
Salicylate		X	XX	

* The paradoxical effect by which low doses decrease excretion and high increase is due to inhibition of absorption or secretion. Diuretics interfere with transport but also alter excretion due to effect on volume status.

account the doses used and their relative affinity for the reabsorptive and secretive carriers. (Table 1.1)

SODIUM TRANSPORT AND EXCRETION

The body content of sodium located largely in the extracellular fluid compartment, is maintained within narrow limits. The kidney responds to a number of control systems and can handle a sodium intake ranging from 5 to 500 mmol daily without major alterations in body compartments. There are significant changes in a number of physiological parameters that allow these adjustments to take place.

Sodium is filtered freely at the glomerulus and its concentration in the glomerular filtrate is the same as in plasma, with minor differences due to the Gibbs Donnan equilibrium. Under physiological conditions, over 99% of the filtered sodium is reabsorbed along the tubular system, and most of the regulatory mechanisms controll-

ing sodium excretion act on these reabsorptive processes.

Proximal tubule

Some 65–80% of the filtered load of sodium is reabsorbed in the proximal tubule, and in this segment sodium, together with its accompanying anion, is transported in close linkage with the movement of water, such that the luminal fluid remains almost isotonic with plasma (see below). a number of distinct transport processes contribute to the reabsorption of sodium in this segment, and it is difficult to assess the relative contribution of each pathway. It is agreed, however, that the primary active transport step underlying all of these mechanisms is the activity of the basolateral Na,K-ATPase, as shown in Figure 1.17. Some of the other postulated contributing pathways are as follows:

(i) A limited amount of sodium crosses from the luminal fluid into the cell via co-transport with a variety of organic species, such as glucose, amino acids, and phosphate (see earlier discussion). These operate significantly only in the early proximal tubule, and contribute to the development of a small lumen-negative electrical potential difference in this segment.

(ii) The reabsorption of sodium bicarbonate, also in the earlier portions of the proximal tubule, is effected through the action of an apical membrane sodium-hydrogen exchanger, which

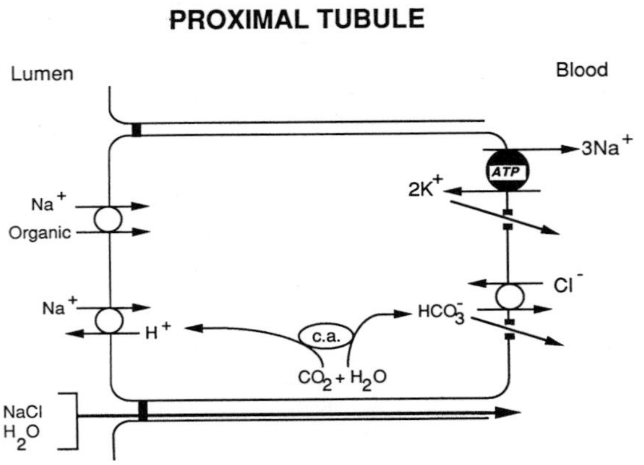

PROXIMAL TUBULE

Fig. 1.17 Schematic diagram of a proximal tubule cell to show the principal membrane transport mechanisms. In this and subsequent cell diagrams, shaded circles labelled 'ATP' denote primary active transport pumps, while open circles denote co- or counter-transport carriers not directly linked to ATP hydrolysis. 'Organic' signifies any of a number of organic solutes co-transported into the cell with the Na (e.g. glucose). c.a. refers to carbonic anhydrase

effectively removes sodium and an accompanying bicarbonate ion from the luminal filtrate and adds it to the plasma compartment. This process is dependent on the presence of the enzyme carbonic anhydrase both inside the cell and on the apical brush border membrane. Possibly 20% of proximal sodium reabsorption may take place via this mechanism.

(iii) Since luminal chloride concentration rises in the later portions of the proximal tubule as bicarbonate disappears from the luminal fluid, its outward diffusion from the lumen leads to the generation of a lumen-positive electrical potential difference. This is thought to contribute to an electrochemical driving force acting to move sodium out of the lumen, probably through the intercellular tight junctions (the 'paracellular' pathway).

(iv) An important component of transepithelial sodium movement probably occurs via 'solvent drag' by which the large transepithelial fluxes of water, particularly across the tight junctions between cells, lead to convective movement of dissolved solutes including sodium into the peritubular interstitial space and hence into the capillary circulation.

Because of the high hydraulic conductivity ('leakiness') of the proximal tubule epithelium, large fluxes of water accompany movements of sodium along this segment. However the precise mechanisms whereby this occurs have only recently been clarified.

(i) It is clear that the reabsorption of sodium proceeds at a slightly faster rate than that of water along the length of the proximal tubule. This leads to a slight but measurable fall in luminal fluid osmolality below isotonicity, thus providing an osmotic driving force for water reabsorption across the highly permeable epithelium. A further contribution to this osmotic gradient is provided by the reabsorption of organic molecules from the early part of the proximal tubule, leading to their presence in the plasma capillaries but not in the luminal fluid in the latter segments of the proximal tubule.

(ii) Tubular-capillary gradients also exist for two other physical forces in this segment. The hydrostatic pressure in the lumen exceeds that in the capillaries by a small amount, owing to the downstream resistance in the bend of the loop of Henle. In addition, an oncotic pressure differential is generated by the retention of plasma proteins in the capillary compartment and not in the lumen, thereby also contributing a physical force for water reabsorption from the lumen.

(iii) Since in the later segments of the proximal tubule bicarbonate is largely confined to the plasma compartment, while chloride is present at a higher concentration in the lumen than in the plasma, the potential for a differential osmotic effect favouring water reabsorption is generated since the reflection coefficient for bicarbonate in this epithelium is greater than that for chloride.

(iv) A theoretical concept for which there is limited experimental verification suggests that water may follow sodium across this epithelium through the lateral intercellular spaces, in which a 'standing osmotic gradient' is thought to be established through the action of sodium pumps lying along the lateral cell membrane. The existence of this mechanism is conjectural and its contribution of transepithelial water flux has not been defined.

Loop of Henle

The thick ascending limb of Henle's loop is an important site for sodium reabsorption, some 25% of the filtered load usually being reclaimed in this segment. In contrast to the proximal tubule, reabsorption of solutes in this segment is not associated with parallel water flow, since the epithelium remains water-impermeable under all conditions. The mechanism for ion reabsorption is shown in Figure 1.18. On the luminal side of the cell Na^+, K^+ and $2Cl^-$ ions bind to a carrier which translocates them across the cell membrane due to the gradient that exists for Na^+ and Cl^-. The Na^+ is actively removed from the cell in exchange for K^+ at the contraluminal membrane by Na^+/K^+ ATPase. The potassium that has accumulated in the cell exits from luminal and contraluminal surfaces by potassium channels. As the luminal membrane is impermeable to anions this gives rise to the lumen-positive p.d. The chloride in the cell may exit via Cl^- channels on the contraluminal membrane, but most leaves by a KCl co-transport carrier driven predominantly by the gradient for potassium. Thus, there is net reabsorption of Na^+, K^+ and chloride. The diuretic drug frusemide competes with chloride for the Na^+, K^+, and $2Cl^-$ co-transport carrier and exerts its effect from the luminal surface. Net reabsorption in this segment alters as increased volume is delivered. This may be due to alterations in back diffusion rather than to an alteration in intrinsic transport rate.

Reabsorption of NaCL in the thick ascending limb, coupled with relative impermeability of the membrane to water, causes the luminal fluid to become hypo-osmotic in relation to plasma. This dissociation of NaCL and water movement is the driving force for the concentration and dilution of urine (see later).

Distal tubule

The early part of the distal tubule ('distal convoluted tubule') normally reabsorbs some 5–8% of filtered sodium. Like the thick ascending limb, this tubular segment is alsways impermeable to water, so that continued sodium chloride reabsorption leads to further dilution of the urine. The mechanism of sodium absorption in this segment is shown in Figure 1.19. Sodium chloride enters the cell via an electroneutral co-transport carrier located in the apical membrane. The basolateral membrane is again the site of the Na,K-ATPase, and chloride ions leave the cell by diffusion across the basolateral membrane. This latter step is probably responsible for the lumen-positive transepithelial potential difference found, at least in the rat, in this segment. It is not known to what extent ions cross this epithelium via the intercellular route. There does not appear to be any net transepithelial transport of potassium in this seg-

THICK ASCENDING LIMB

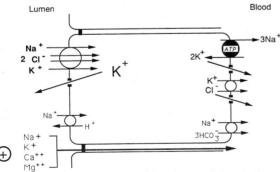

Fig. 1.18 Schematic diagram of a cell from the thick ascending limb of the loop of Henle to show the principal membrane transport mechanisms. The '+' in the lumen signifies the electrical polarity of the lumen with respect to the interstitium

EARLY DISTAL TUBULE

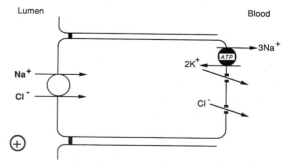

Fig. 1.19 Schematic diagram of a cell from the early part of the distal tubule to show the principal membrane transport mechanisms

ment, though it is an important site for calcium reabsorption, which tends to proceed in inverse proportion to the extent of sodium reabsorption (see later). The sodium chloride transporter in the apical membrane is the site of blocking action by thiazide drugs, leading to their natriuretic action. It is noteworthy that this tubular segment has a considerable reserve capacity to increase its reabsorption in proportion to the load of sodium chloride delivered from the loop of Henle.

The latter section of the anatomical distal tubule, sometimes called the 'initial collecting duct', has structural and functional similarities to the cortical collecting duct, described below.

Collecting duct system

The cortical collecting duct is the first part of the collecting duct system, formed where two distal tubular segments join within the cortex. It has the properties of reabsorption of sodium and some chloride, as well as secretion of potassium and hydrogen ions. Unlike the preceding two sections, this segment has a variable water permeability which is increased in the presence of antidiuretic hormone in the circulation. The cells of this segment are also sensitive to aldosterone (see below).

The mechanism of transport in this segment is shown in Figure 1.20. Sodium enters the 'princi-

pal' cell type from the luminal fluid across the apical membrane through a sodium-selective channel, and is transferred into the interstitial fluid compartment across the basolateral membrane by the Na,K-ATPase. The potassium accumulated into the cell by this pump diffuses both into the lumen across the apical membrane and back into the interstitial fluid across the basolateral membrane. However, because the cell is electrically polarized by virtue of the apical sodium diffusion potential, a lumen-negative electrical potential difference exists which favours the net diffusive movement of potassium towards the lumen, thus effecting its secretion into the urine.

The 'intercalated' cells, comprising about one third of the cells in this segment, are the site of secretion of hydrogen ions into the lumen. This is effected by a H-ATPase located in the apical membrane, the hydrogen ions being generated within these cells via the action of carbonic anhydrase. An equivalent bicarbonate ion is transferred into the interstitial fluid via a basolateral anion exchanger, as shown in Figure 1.20. The extent of acid secretion into the lumen is strongly influenced by the transepithelial potential difference, since the electrogenic hydrogen pump is sensitive to the prevailing electrical potential.

The route of reabsorptive transport of chloride across this epithelium is not certain, but is probably via a transcellular rather than a paracellular route. In quantitative terms, the sodium reabsorptive flux is electrically dissipated in approximately equal proportions by parallel reabsorption of chloride, secretion of potassium and secretion of acid. All of these processes are stimulated by aldosterone, which acts via the induction of intracellular proteins initially to enhance apical entry of sodium into the cell, but in a later phase to stimulate all steps in the transfer of sodium, potassium and hydrogen ions across this epithelium.

Regulation of renal sodium excretion

A large number of factors are involved in the control of sodium excretion by the kidney, as summarized below.

CORTICAL COLLECTING DUCT

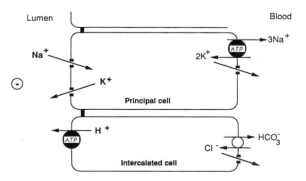

Fig. 1.20 Schematic diagram of two cell types from the late part of the distal tubule and the cortical collecting duct to show the principal membrane transport mechanisms

1. Changes in *glomerular filtration rate* are associated with parallel changes in sodium excretion, though the extent of the excretory change is reduced by parallel adjustments in proximal tubular sodium reabsorption ('glomerulotubular balance'). This is probably not an important mechanism in the day-to-day fine tuning of sodium excretion.

2. Altered *physical forces* acting around the proximal tubule may be important in states such as congestive cardiac failure and extracellular fluid volume expansion and contraction. For example, during volume depletion, there is a reduction in both glomerular filtration rate and renal plasma flow, but since efferent arteriolar constriction is relatively greater than that in the afferent arteriole, the filtration fraction rises and peritubular capillary hydrostatic and oncotic pressures change in such a way as to enhance volume reabsorption from the proximal tubule.

3. A number of *hormones* have been defined which can exert profound influences on tubular sodium handling, though the relative contribution of each hormone may vary in different physiological and pathological conditions. These hormones include both circulating and locally active substances. In the proximal tubule, angiotensin II and noradrenalin (the latter released from sympathetic nerve terminals) act to stimulate sodium reabsorption, while the incompletely characterized natriuretic hormone (probably of hypothalamic origin) acts to inhibit it. In the late distal tubule/cortical collecting duct, aldosterone is a potent stimulant of sodium reabsorption, while prostaglandins and kinins act to inhibit reabsorption at this site. In the terminal portion of the medullary collecting duct (papillary collecting duct), atrial natriuretic peptide inhibits sodium reabsorption, and this, together with its actions to enhance GFR and interfere with angiotensin II action in the proximal tubule, contributes to its powerful but short-acting natriuretic effect. Sodium transport in the thick ascending limb of Henle's loop has also been shown to be sensitive to a number of hormonal influences, but it is not certain to what extent, if any, these effects modulate the final rate of urinary sodium excretion.

It should also be mentioned that, in clinical practice, a variety of diuretic drugs act as potent modulators of tubule sodium transport. These will be discussed in further detail, though the cellular sites of action have been alluded to above.

POTASSIUM TRANSPORT AND EXCRETION

Potassium is located primarily in the cells of the body and less than 2% is in the interstitial fluid and plasma. The usual intake of potassium is 40–100 mmol/day. Potassium is lost in the faeces as well as in the urine. The kidney does not conserve potassium as efficiently as sodium and even when potassium intake is low some is still lost in urine. On the other hand, the kidney is capable of adaptation to a wide range of potassium loading, such that animals can survive acute and chronic intakes of potassium which would otherwise be lethal.

Renal handling of potassium involves free filtration at the glomerulus, followed by extensive reabsorption (up to 90% of the filtered load) along the proximal tubule and the loop of Henle (see above). The key site for adjustment of the rate of potassium excretion into the urine is the cortical collecting duct segment (including the late distal tubule) where, as described above, potassium undergoes secretion into the lumen, though the rate is extremely variable depending on the metabolic conditions.

The factors which determine the rate of potassium secretion may be divided into those acting from the peritubular (blood) side, and those acting from the luminal side of the epithelium in the late distal tubule/cortical collecting duct segment. Most important of the peritubular factors is aldosterone, particularly since it is involved in a feedback control loop via the plasma potassium concentration, small rises in which directly stimulate the zona glomerulosa cells of the adrenal cortex to secrete aldosterone. The hormone itself acts to enhance potassium secretion by principal cells of the cortical collecting duct, both via an early phase in which luminal negativity is increased due to initial stimulation of apical sodium uptake, and also in a late phase in which basolateral Na,K-ATPase activity is enhanced, accompanied by an increase in apical potassium conductance. It has also been shown, independent of the presence of aldosterone, that a rise in plasma potassium concentration acts directly to stimulate potassium secretion, and the effect of a high potassium diet is almost certainly mediated by the combination of these two factors. A further influence acting from the blood side is the acid–base status, such that alkalosis tends to stimulate potassium secretion, probably by enhancing uptake of potassium into the cell from the extracellular fluid.

Factors acting from the luminal side of the epithelium include the flow rate of urine through the potassium secretory segment, this usually being determined in physiological circumstances by the sodium delivery rate. Factors influencing the transepithelial potential difference may also alter potassium secretion via a luminal action. For example, partial replacement of filtered chloride by more impermeant anions such as bicarbonate or sulphate leads to an increase in the transepithelial potential, followed by enhanced secretion of potassium. Conversely, the action of drugs such as amiloride, which blocks the apical sodium channel in principal cells and hence depolarizes the transepithelial electrical potential, has the property of totally inhibiting potassium secretion, making such drugs useful as 'potassium-sparing' adjuncts to diuretic treatment.

The process of adaptation to increased dietary potassium appears to be achieved by both structural and functional changes. Prolonged exposure to high levels of potassium leads to marked hypertrophy of the basolateral membranes of the principal cells in the potassium-secreting segment of the distal nephron, and this has been shown to be associated with an increase in the activity of Na,K-ATPase in this segment. In addition, hyperkalaemia causes inhibition of proximal sodium reabsorption, leading to a natriuretic state with high delivery of sodium and fluid through distal nephron segments, and consequent stimulation of potassium secretion.

HYDROGEN ION TRANSPORT AND EXCRETION

The hydrogen ion concentration [H⁺] and thus the pH of the extracellular fluid is controlled by plasma buffers, the lungs (regulation of CO_2 concentration in the body), and the kidneys (excretion of acid or alkali). The pH of plasma depends on the amount of bicarbonate and carbonic acid present and can be calculated from the Henderson–Hasselbalch equation:

$$pH = pK + \log \frac{[\text{salt}]}{[\text{acid}]}$$
$$= 6.1 + \log \frac{[HCO_3^-]}{[H_2CO_3]}$$

where pK is the negative log of the dissociation constant.

The pH can thus be altered by changing the amount of HCO_3^- or H_2CO_3 in plasma. The lungs maintain carbonic acid concentration constant at between 1.3 and 1.4 mmol/l by expiration of CO_2, which is in equilibrium with H_2CO_3. The kidney controls the amount of HCO_3^- in plasma by excreting either hydrogen or bicarbonate ions. Acute acid loads are buffered by a number of other buffer systems, but long-term regulation is via the bicarbonate–carbonic acid buffer system.

Hydrogen ion secretion has two important functions: reabsorption of filtered bicarbonate in the proximal and distal tubule; and excretion of hydrogen ions in the urine and regeneration of bicarbonate. This process is essential to excrete the acid load produced by metabolism or to deal with an oral acid load.

Hydrogen ions are secreted into the proximal and distal tubule. Most of the H⁺ required for this secretion is generated from the catalysed and uncatalysed hydration of CO_2, but some is produced by another, as yet unknown, mechanism. The next step is movement of H⁺ across luminal membrane. In the proximal tubule, this is achieved via electroneutral countertransport of sodium and hydrogen ions by the apical Na-H antiporter (see Fig. 1.17). In the distal nephron segments, hydrogen secretion is largely by an electrogenic primary hydrogen-ATPase located in the apical membrane of the intercalated cells of the cortical and medullary collecting ducts (see Fig. 1.20). On entering the lumen the H^+ is trapped by HCO_3^-. In the proximal tubule, where the concentration of HCO_3^- is relatively high, the reaction is catalysed by carbonic anhydrase in the brush border. Thus there is a large secretion of H^+ which is used to reclaim filtered bicarbonate. Under normal conditions of hydration approximately 90% of the filtered bicarbonate is reabsorbed in the proximal tubule. In volume-depleted states even more bicarbonate is reabsorbed and no HCO_3^- is excreted in the urine. Thus alkalosis in a volume-depleted individual cannot be corrected by the kidney.

While bicarbonate is present in the tubular lumen, the pH of the fluid remains constant. However, when the pH drops two other buffer systems come into action. This usually happens in the distal tubule but can take place in the proximal tubule.

When the bicarbonate is utilized hydrogen ions are involved in the following reactions:

$$H^+ + HPO_4^{2-} \rightleftharpoons H_2PO_4^-$$
$$H^+ + A^- \rightleftharpoons HA$$

where HA is weak organic acid.

The hydrogen phosphate ions and various unionized weak acids are then excreted in the urine. They form the titratable acidity, which is measured by titrating the urine back to the pH of plasma. The titratable acidity depends on the extent to which the pH has been lowered but also on the amount of phosphate and organic acids available to be titrated. Parathyroid hormone inhibits phosphate reabsorption in the proximal tubule and is indirectly involved in acid–base homeostasis. In diabetic acidosis other buffer systems (e.g. hydroxybutyrate) become more important than the phosphate system. This system can handle most of the H^+ which needs to be excreted but in many circumstances its capacity is inadequate.

The other buffer system has virtually unlimited capacity. The proximal (especially) and distal tubule continuously form ammonia from glutamine by action of the enzyme glutaminase. Ammonia is highly lipid-soluble and diffuses into the blood and tubular fluid. Usually most ammonia is lost into the blood stream, as blood flow out of the kidney is approximately 1000 times the urine flow rate. However if the pH of the tubular fluid is lower than that of plasma, the NH_3 combines with H^+ to form NH_4^+ and thus the concentration gradient to the tubular fluid is greater than that to the blood and ammonia diffuses preferentially into the tubule (Fig. 1.21). As the pK of the reaction is 9.2, the reaction at the physiological pH 7.4 is heavily weighted in favour of NH_4^+ formation. Since

$$pH = 9.2 + \log \frac{NH_3}{NH_4^+}$$

the proportion of NH_3/NH_4^+ at pH 7.4 is 1:100.

At lower pH values the trapping mechanism is even more effective.

The H^+ used to reabsorb HCO_3^- causes no effective loss of hydrogen ions from the body, as H^+ is regenerated in the process of bicarbonate reabsorption. However, when H^+ is lost in the urine as titratable acid or NH_4^+ or due to a lowering of pH there is effective generation of new HCO_3^- in the cells to compensate for acidosis.

In the nephron H^+ secreted is utilized in the following ways:

$$
\begin{aligned}
H^+ + HCO_3^- &\rightarrow H_2CO_3 \rightarrow CO_2 + H_2O \\
H^+ + HPO_4^{2-} &\rightarrow H_2PO_4^- \\
H^+ + NH_3 &\rightarrow NH_4^+ \\
H^+ + \text{organic acid} &\rightarrow HA \\
H^+ &\rightarrow \text{lowering of pH}
\end{aligned}
$$

Hydrogen ions H^+ are secreted throughout the nephron but there are certain differences in the proximal and distal nephrons. Disorders at different sites cause different defects. In the proximal tubule about 5000 mmol H^+ are secreted each day but this usually makes no contribution to the final urine H^+ concentration. On the usual Western diet approximately 50–80 mmol/day is lost in the final urine as titratable acid, free H^+ and NH_4^+. The amount secreted by the distal neph-

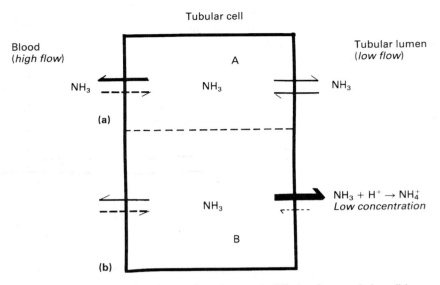

Fig. 1.21 Diagrammatic representation of ammonia diffusion from a tubular cell in two different circumstances. In (a) the pH of cell, blood and urine is the same. As blood flow is high and urine flow low, most ammonia enters the blood. In (b) the pH of the tubular fluid is low. H^+ binds to NH_3 and gives a continuous gradient favouring entry into the urine. The lower the pH the greater the effect, and ammonia in the blood moves across the cell into the urine

ron is greater than this, as some is used to reclaim bicarbonate. Paradoxically, in alkalosis due to HCO_3^- infusion more H^+ is secreted in the distal nephron than in acidosis. However, no H^+ is lost from the body. In the distal tubule, hydrogen secretion depends in part on the negative p.d. generated by sodium reabsorption and if this is inhibited H^+ secretion decreases. Potassium depletion increases H^+ secretion by an unknown cellular mechanism.

The kidney's capacity to excrete HCO_3^- and thus correct alkalosis is virtually unlimited, provided plasma volume and high renal blood flow are maintained. The capacity to excrete excess H^+ is limited and primarily related to the ability to produce ammonia. The production rate increases under conditions of chronic acidosis.

The initial control of any imbalance in acid–base status depends on the buffer systems of the plasma. This is followed by respiratory compensation through a change in ventilation rate and then by loss or regeneration of bicarbonate in the kidney.

CONCENTRATION AND DILUTION OF URINE

The ability to concentrate or dilute urine is of crucial importance for the maintenance of constant osmolality of tissue fluids and the regulation of water excretion in relation to solute and water intake. Dilution of urine is achieved by removal of NaCl from the tubular fluid in a region where the membrane is impermeable to water, i.e. in the thick ascending limb of the loop of Henle, the distal tubule, the collecting tubule and the collecting duct. The contribution of the loop of Henle is the greatest.

Concentration of urine is a complex process that depends on the same active transport process that dilutes urine. However, because of the anatomical arrangement of the nephrons and blood vessels, a countercurrent system translates the removal of sodium chloride from the ascending limb of the loop of Henle, which causes dilution, into a concentrating effect. The countercurrent system depends for its operation on (1) the anatomical arrangement of nephrons in the papilla, (2) active transport of sodium chloride out of the ascending limb, (3) countercurrent multiplication by the loop of Henle, (4) the ability of the cortical and medullary collecting ducts to respond to ADH by altering water permeability, and (5) countercurrent exchange by the blood vessels which permits the concentration gradient in the papilla to be maintained.

There are three generally accepted components to this countercurrent system. The first is an active countercurrent multiplier driven by active removal of sodium chloride from the ascending limb. This takes place primarily in the outer medulla. The second is a passive countercurrent multiplier. This depends on the same driving force as above but the concentration gradients developed for urea and the differential permeability of membranes to urea and sodium increase the concentrating ability. This is believed to occur primarily in the thin limbs of the loop of Henle in the inner medulla and papilla. The third component is the countercurrent exchanger function of the vasa recta. This does not generate or increase a gradient but permits fluid to be removed from the papilla while maintaining the high solute concentration.

Mechanism (see Fig. 1.22)

Sodium chloride without water is pumped out of the thick ascending limb into an enclosed space which has a long vertical axis. The longer this axis the greater the concentrating ability of the kidney. This transport out of a segment impermeable to water reduces osmolality in the nephron while increasing that in the space. Descending limb segments coming into this space attain equilibrium with the surrounding fluid, and as they descend down further there is a stepwise (integrated) increase in osmolality. Thus the fluid in the tubule is hypotonic while that in the papilla is hypertonic. In the absence of ADH the hypotonic fluid in the tubule passes through the cortex and medulla without attaining equilibrium with the interstitium, and a dilute urine is excreted. When ADH is present the membranes of cortical and medullary collecting systems become permeable to water and the tubular fluid initially attains

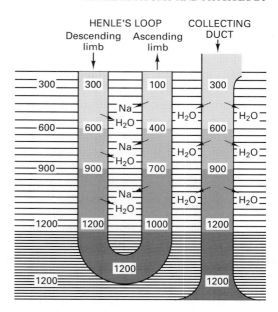

Fig. 1.22   The operation of the countercurrent multiplication of concentration in the formation of hypertonic urine (see text for explanation)

iso-osmolality with the plasma in the cortical system. Since this is achieved by removal of water, volume is markedly reduced. The small amount of urine which enters the hyperosmotic compartment (see above) attains equilibrium with that compartment but as the volume of urine is small the hyperosmolality is not dissipated but maintained.

There is no convincing evidence for active sodium chloride removal by the thin ascending limb, and a number of hypotheses have been proposed to explain the further concentration of urine in the inner medullary loops of Henle. These depend on the entry of urea into the thin limb of the loop. The cortical collecting system is impermeable to urea which thus becomes concentrated in the lumen. The papillary collecting ducts are permeable to urea and it diffuses into the interstitium and then into the ascending limb of the loop of Henle. Sodium has different permeability characteristics; it is concentrated in the descending limb of the loop of Henle by water removal and then diffuses out of the ascending limb more rapidly than urea enters. It is likely that this type of system does operate but there is conflicting evidence regarding the permeability of the descending limb of the loop of Henle.

The blood supply of the kidney has a unique arrangement into vasa recta which are highly permeable to solute and water. The descending and ascending vasa recta are arranged in bundles in conjunction with nephron elements, and small molecules are readily exchanged. Thus small molecules have difficulty entering the papilla from the circulation and small molecules produced (e.g. CO_2) or accumulated (e.g. sodium, urea) in the papilla are not removed. The papilla has a low Po_2 because of this effect and essential metabolites (e.g. glucose) enter poorly. Water is removed from the papilla by the blood vessels. Paradoxically more water needs to be removed in states of diuresis than in antidiuresis. This removal of water together with some solute will reduce the concentration of solute if it exceeds the capacity of the active transport step. If flow is increased markedly through the blood vessels, the system becomes less efficient and there may be washout of some of the gradient. The vessels are so permeable to solute that this is probably not a major determinant of concentrating ability.

Concentrating and diluting ability can be affected by a number of factors. If transport out of the thick ascending limb of the loop of Henle is prevented (e.g. by frusemide), the concentrating mechanism is destroyed but some dilution of urine can occur through transport of NaCl without water in the collecting system. If transport in the distal nephron and collecting system is inhibited, dilution capacity will be reduced but there is little effect on concentra-9ting ability.

The other factors affect primarily the ability to concentrate urine. Destruction of the tip of the papilla removes the small number of nephrons with the longest loops and thus reduces concentrating ability. There is no detectable effect on glomerular filtration rate or diluting ability, as the number of nephrons involved is very small. This occurs to various degrees in papillary necrosis due to analgesic nephropathy or other causes. Lack of response to ADH due either to absence of ADH (diabetes insipidus)

> **Factors affecting the concentrating mechanism**
> 1. *Failure to create or maintain gradient*
>   Inhibition of sodium transport in loop of Henle (e.g. by frusemide)
>   Anatomical disruption of papilla (papillary necrosis)
>   Excessive papillary blood flow
> 2. *Failure of fluid to equilibrate*
>   Absence of ADH (diabetes insipidus)
>   Resistance to ADH (circulatory inhibitors; structural defects in cell)

or impaired or altered response of the collecting system (hypokalaemia, hypercalcaemia, lithium toxicity) prevents the formation of a concentrated urine but has no effect on diluting ability. Conversely, increased water permeability due to inappropriate ADH secretion or various metabolites destroys the ability to dilute the urine but there is an associated impairment of maximal concentrating ability due to washout of some of the papillary gradient. If urea is removed or its concentration is low, the countercurrent multiplier does not function as efficiently and maximal concentrating ability is reduced. In renal failure there is a reduction in both maximum diluting ability and maximum concentrating ability. The latter may be due in part to loss of deep nephrons, but both probably relate to a high flow rate in the residual nephrons, and the presence of urea, sulphate, phosphate, etc. prevents efficient removal of sodium and water.

Two clearance terms are used and measured to provide information about the functioning of these systems. Osmolal clearance is an index of the excretion of osmoles and is calculated in a similar way to other clearances. It is constant in any individual and depends on dietary intake of electrolytes and protein (urea) which form the main constituents of the urine.

$$C_{osm} = \frac{U_{osm} \times V}{P_{osm}}$$

where U_{osm} and P_{osm} are the osmotic concentrations of urine and plasma.

The osmolal clearance does not depend on urine volume because as urine volume decreases, osmolality increases. If the solute is excreted in a volume of urine equal to the plasma cleared, i.e. if urine and plasma osmolality are equal, then there is no excretion or retention of water in excess of solute. However, if urine volume should increase and urine osmolality drop, water is lost in excess of solute. This is a positive free water clearance. If urine volume falls and osmolality rises there is a negative free water clearance and water is retained in excess of solute.

If urine osmolality is higher than that of plasma there is a positive free water clearance. The extent of free water clearance can be quantitated as follows:

$$\text{Free water clearance} = V - C_{osm}$$
$$= V \cdot \left(I - \frac{U_{osm}}{P_{osm}} \right)$$

If free water clearance is maximal this calculation gives information about the delivery of fluid to the loop of Henle. As more fluid is delivered out of the proximal tubule, the loop of Henle pumps out more NaCl. Thus if there is no removal of water or solute distally this can give quantitative information. These methods have been used to determine the site of diuretic action but the conclusions reached are not all valid and the results must be accepted cautiously.

OTHER ABSORPTIVE MECHANISMS

In addition to absorption of many substances linked to the bulk reabsorption of sodium chloride and water in the proximal tubule, there are a number of additional reabsorptive mechanisms at various sites along the nephron. Some of these act on groups of compounds while others are more specific as outlined earlier (see 'Transport of organic solutes' above). Some of these transport processes can operate in the opposite direction and cause secretion of substances from the plasma into the tubule.

Non-ionic reabsorption or secretion

This form of transport depends on the different permeability of membranes to ionized and non-ionized forms. In general, membranes are impermeable to organic anions and cations but permeable to the undissociated acid or base, as many of these are lipid-soluble. A weak acid or base produced in a kidney cell tends to diffuse into both the blood and the tubular fluid. If the pH of the tubular fluid is 7.4, equal amounts cross into the blood and the urine. However, if the pH of the urine is lower (e.g. pH 6), more of a weak base will be converted to the ionized form (B^+ and OH^-) and less of the acid (HA) will be ionized. This produces a constant high gradient for BOH to enter the urine but a lower diffusion gradient for HA so that more of this will go into the blood. A weak base in blood will distribute itself as the undissociated base across the cell and into the urine. If the pH of the urine is 6, this will continually convert BOH to $B^+ OH^-$ which will accumulate to concentrations much higher than those in the cell or plasma. If urine is acidified to pH 4.5, the concentration in urine may be 1000 times higher than in plasma. This non-active transport mechanism depends on the creation of H^+ gradients. If the pH of the urine is altered, excretion of weak acids and weak bases is modified. This mechanism is based on the lipid solubility of the undissociated weak acid or base. A particular example of this type of transport is given above for the ammonia/ammonium system.

Calcium, magnesium, lithium

Calcium is present in the plasma in three forms: ionized, non-ionized ('complexed'), and protein-bound. Only the ionized and non-ionized calcium is filtered at the glomerulus so that the Ca concentration in the ultrafiltrate is approximately 65% of the total plasma Ca concentration.

Calcium is reabsorbed at a number of nephron sites, usually in parallel to sodium reabsorption. Urinary calcium excretion thus tends to vary with urinary sodium excretion.

At the end of the proximal convoluted tubule, calcium is in slightly higher concentration in the tubular fluid than in plasma ultrafiltrate. However, about 60–70% of the filtered calcium has been reabsorbed at this point. Additional calcium is reabsorbed in the loop of Henle, and up to 8% of the filtered load is reabsorbed in the distal tubule against a concentration gradient, implying selective reabsorption in this segment. Parathyroid hormone (PTH) appears to inhibit both sodium and calcium reabsorption in the proximal tubule, to have little effect on calcium movement in the ascending limb and to increase calcium reabsorption in the distal nephron. The overall effect is to diminish calcium excretion. However, any tendency to decrease calcium excretion induced by tubular effects of PTH may be offset by increased loads of calcium presented to the kidney as a result of increased bone resorption. Vitamin D appears to increase proximal tubule reabsorption of calcium but the physiological importance is unknown.

Magnesium, although in the same group on the periodic table as calcium, is handled somewhat differently along the nephron. Like calcium, some magnesium in the plasma is protein-bound so that the ratio of glomerular ultrafiltrate to total plasma Mg^{2+} concentration is approximately 0.75. Only about 20–30% of the filtered load of Mg^{2+} is reabsorbed in the proximal tubule, the majority (50–60%) being reabsorbed in the ascending limb under the influence of PTH. The distal nephron reabsorbs some 2–10% of the filtered magnesium, apparently independent of PTH effect. Differences in the handling of calcium and magnesium along the nephron are further highlighted by the effects of diuretics on the excretion of these ions. Thiazide diuretics reduce calcium excretion, causing a tendency to hypercalcaemia, whereas they increase magnesium excretion and may cause hypomagnesaemia. The loop-acting diuretic frusemide increases both calcium and magnesium excretion while distally-acting (potassium-sparing) diuretics such as spironolactone, amiloride and triamterene decrease the excretion of both ions. Hypercalcaemia increases magnesium excretion.

Lithium is found in very low concentration in normal plasma but is used quite extensively as a therapeutic agent in psychiatric practice. Since it is reabsorbed predominantly in the proximal tubule, lithium clearance can be used as an index of proximal tubular function. Factors which increase proximal tubular reabsorption of sodium and water, e.g. volume depletion, also increase lithium reabsorption, and patients receiving lithium therapy may develop toxic symptoms.

Urea

Urea, the principal nitrogenous waste product, is excreted by the kidney. In humans there is no evidence for active transport of urea and its excretion rate is determined by filtration and subsequent reabsorption due to concentration gradients produced by water reabsorption. Urea is reabsorbed from the proximal tubule subsequent to water reabsorption but its concentration rises so that at the end of the proximal tubule it is approximately 1.5–2 times that in plasma. If water reabsorption in the proximal tubule is increased, more urea is reabsorbed. While some urea is absorbed more distally, urea excretion depends primarily on filtration and proximal tubule reabsorption.

All of the nephron segments in the papilla are permeable to urea. Urea enters the loop of Henle, where it is extensively recycled, which is important for the countercurrent system to operate effectively. The cortical segments of the distal nephron are virtually impermeable to urea and this is also important in the countercurrent system. The countercurrent system allows a large amount of urea to be excreted in a small volume.

Proteins

The glomerular membrane is a semipermeable membrane which allows passage of substances in proportion to their size and surface charge. Uncharged non-protein-bound substances of a molecular weight of less than 5000 are filtered in the same proportion as in plasma. Larger substances are retarded. Although the filtration ratio for albumin is between 0.0003 and 0.003, between 2 and 20 g are filtered each day. However, very little albumin appears in the urine. The concentration of proteins in the glomerular filtrate depends on their concentration in plasma and their filtration ratio. If tubular reabsorption of proteins is inhibited, the urine protein pattern consists predominantly of the smaller proteins.

Proteins are reabsorbed extensively in the proximal tubule by binding to an acidic phospholipid on the border. These coalesce and are absorbed by pinocytosis into the proximal tubule cytoplasm. Most peptides and proteins are then digested and destroyed by lysozymes, and the amino acids are returned to the blood stream to be reused in synthesis. The kidney is an important site of degradation of a number of peptide and protein hormones (e.g. insulin, glucagon, ACTH, parathyroid hormone, ADH). If filtration of a protein is increased, the proximal tubule reabsorbs more protein until its capacity is exceeded and proteinuria results. It should be noted that when there is a urinary protein loss of 5 g of albumin/day there may be filtration of 50 g and metabolism of 45 g by the proximal tubule. Thus the increased production rate needed to maintain plasma albumin is exceeded and hypoalbuminaemia results.

RENAL METABOLISM

The kidney is an active metabolic organ. It uses most of its energy for the active reabsorption of fluid. The cortex has an aerobic metabolism and preferentially metabolizes fatty acids to meet its energy needs. If sufficient fatty acids are provided, it forms glucose from lactate and does not utilize glucose. The papilla is different and has primarily an anaerobic metabolism due to its low oxygen tension. Its principal substrate is glucose. The mitochondria of the outer medulla appear to be able to switch from aerobic to anaerobic metabolism as the oxygen supply becomes deficient or as osmolality and sodium concentration change.

The kidney has important degradative functions and metabolizes a number of important hormones. In addition, it produces a large number of other substances. Thus it is responsible for the α-hydroxylation in the formation of $1,25(OH)_2$ cholecalciferol. Renin and angiotensin, important both in local control of renal function and in the control of the systemic circulation, are produced in the kidney as are erythropoietin and other factors that control blood formation. The kidney produces dopamine, prostaglandins and a number of other vasoactive peptides. It is not clear if these have primarily an intrarenal role or whether they make an important contribution to the circulating levels and thus have remote effects.

In most circumstances defects in renal metabolism cause little overall effect on the body's metabolism but in patients on dialysis with no renal tissue, defects may become apparent.

RECOMMENDED READING

Brenner B M, Hostletter T H, Humes H D 1978 Molecular basis of proteinuria of glomerular origin. New England Journal of Medicine 298: 826–833

Cassola A C, Giebisch G, Malnic G 1977 Mechanism and components of renal tubular acidification. Journal of Physiology 267: 601–624

de Bold A J, Borenstein H B, Veress A T, Sonnenberg H 1981 A rapid and potent natriuretic response to intravenous injection of atrial myocardial extract in rats. Life Science 28: 89–94

De Wardener H E, Clarkson E M 1985 Concept of natriuretic hormone. Physiological Review 65: 658–759

Field M J, Giebisch G H 1985 Hormonal control of renal potassium excretion. Kidney International 27: 379

Giebisch G, Berliner R W (eds) 1976 Membrane transport in the kidney. Kidney International 9: 62–230

Greger R 1985 Ion transport mechanism in thick ascending limb of Henle's Loop of mammalian kidney. Physiological Review 65: 760–796

Latta H 1973 Ultrastructure of the glomerulus and juxtaglomerular apparatus. In: Orloff J, Berliner R W (eds) Handbook of physiology, 8. Renal physiology. American Physiological Society, Washington, ch 1, p 1

Maunsbach A B 1973 Ultrastructure of the proximal tubule. In: Orloff J, Berliner R W (eds) Handbook of physiology, 8. Renal physiology. American Physiological Society, Washington, ch 2, p 31

Orloff J, Berliner R W (eds) 1973 Handbook of physiology section 8. Renal physiology. American Physiological Society, Washington

Osvaldo-Decima L 1973 Ultrastructure of the lower nephron. In: Orloff J, Berliner R W (eds) Handbook of physiology, section 8. Renal physiology. American Physiological Society, Washington, ch 3, p 81

Rector F C Jr (ed) 1972 Symposium on acid–base homeostatis. Kidney International 1: 273–389

Ryan G B 1982 Mechanisms of proteinuria. In: Jones N F, Peters D K (eds) Recent advances in renal medicine. Churchill Livingstone, Edinburgh, ch 2, p 31

Ryan G B, Coghlan J P, Scoggins B A 1979 The granulated peripolar epithelial cell: a potential secretory component of the renal juxtaglomerular complex. Nature 277: 655–656

Schafer J A 1984 Mechanisms coupling the absorption of solutes and water in the proximal tubule. Kidney International 24: 708–716

Seldin D W Giebisch G 1992 The kidney, physiology and pathophysiology, 2nd edn. Raven Press, New York

Stephenson J L 1972 Concentration of urine in a central core model of the renal counterflow system. Kidney International 2: 85–94

Sutton R A L 1983 disorders of renal calcium secretion. Kidney International 23: 665–673

2. Hormones and the kidney

P. A. Phillips   C. I. Johnston

INTRODUCTION

The kidney is an important organ for hormone physiology and pathophysiology. Not only is it the site of production of several hormones, it is also a major target organ for many, as well as being the predominant metabolic and excretory pathway for hormones, particularly the peptide hormones (Table 2.1). In some cases the kidney will play all roles, being a major site of synthesis, hormone action and degradation. It is this multiplicity of functions of the kidney that gives rise to the complex hormonal disturbances found in chronic renal failure. Loss of kidney mass produces some hormonal deficiencies (e.g. vitamin D, erythropoietin) whereas loss of excretory function produces hormone accumulation and excess (e.g. parathyroid hormone, gastrin).

Table 2.1   The kidney as an endocrine organ

---

1. *Intra-renal hormones (produced by the kidney)*
   Renin
   Kallikrein
   Prostaglandins
   Medullolipin
   1,25-dihydroxycholecalciferol (vitamin D_3)
   Erythropoietin
2. *Extra-renal hormones with kidney as major target organ*
   Aldosterone and steroids
   Vasopressin (antidiuretic hormone)
   Parathyroid hormone
   Calcitonin
   Atrial natriuretic peptide
   Catecholamines
   Endothelin
3. *Renal metabolism and excretion*
   Peptide hormones
   Conjugated steroids
   Conjugated catecholamines

INTRA-RENAL HORMONES

The kidney is the only or predominant source for at least six hormones (Table 2.1). Whereas previously renin was thought to be found only in the kidney it is now known to occur in other tissues such as blood vessels and the brain where it may play a role in blood pressure control. The relationship between intra- and extra-renal sources for all the hormones is still unclear but extra-renal renin seems to be produced locally. Whether all glandular kallikreins are identical is unresolved and the chemistry of medullolipin is also uncertain. The conversion of vitamin D_3 to the biologically active metabolite dihydroxycholecalciferol occurs exclusively in the kidney, which can thus be regarded as the source of, and a true endocrine organ for active vitamin D_3.

Renin–angiotensin system

Renin is a serine acid protease (MW 40 000) found in the juxtaglomerular apparatus of the kidney. The juxtaglomerular apparatus (JGA) consists of modified myoepithelial cells of the glomerular afferent arteriole, which contains the renin granules, in close apposition to a specialized portion of the distal convoluted tubule, the macula densa, together with intertwining lacis or matrix cells. Renin is synthesized by the myoepithelial cells as a large molecular weight precursor protein (pro-renin), undergoes post-translational processing to the active enzyme and is packaged in specialized granules and stored. It is released from the granules into the glomerular circulation and into the renal interstitium.

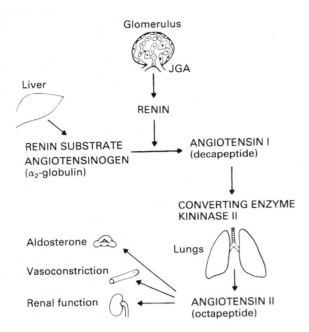

Fig. 2.1 Diagrammatic representation of the renin–angiotensin system showing the major peripheral biological actions of angiotensin. JGA — juxtaglomerular apparatus

Renin acts on a protein substrate (angiotensinogen, an α_2-globulin produced by the liver) to form the biologically inactive decapeptide angiotensin I (Fig. 2.1). The biochemical cascade is illustrated in Figure 2.2. Angiotensin I is cleaved by angiotensin-converting enzyme (ACE) to form the biologically active octapeptide angiotensin II. ACE is found in all endothelial cells, the kidney, the brain, reproductive tissues and in very high concentration in the pulmonary vasculature. Angiotensin II is then degraded by a variety of peptidases (known collectively as angiotensinases) into inactive fragments, although angiotensin III (a heptapeptide) has some biological activity.

Renin release by the kidney is increased by: reduced renal arteriolar pressure; reduced delivery of sodium or chloride in the distal convoluted tubule and macula densa; increased sympathetic nervous system activity via β_1-adrenergic receptors on the JGA; prostaglandins (especially prostacyclin); high plasma potassium via influencing sodium/chloride delivery to the JGA; and a variety of other ions and hormones (Table 2.2).

Renin secretion is inhibited by the opposite of these stimuli and negative feedback by angiotensin II and other hormones, including vasopressin and in particular by atrial natriuretic peptide.

Angiotensin II has many biological actions (Table 2.3). The most important physiological actions currently elucidated are direct vasoconstriction, stimulation of the zona glomerulosa to produce aldosterone, and regulation of renal sodium transport by the kidney. More recently all

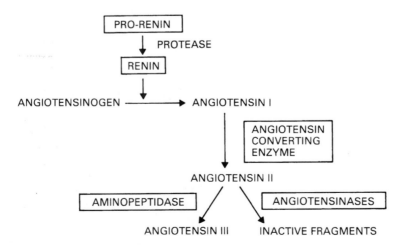

Fig. 2.2 Biochemical pathways in the renin–angiotensin system with enzymes responsible for the cascade

Table 2.2   Control of renin release from the kidney

1. Renal baroreceptor (pressure)
2. Macula densa sensor (tubular fluid)
3. Sodium, potassium and calcium ions
4. Sympathetic nervous system
5. Hormones
   Angiotensin II (negative feedback)
   Vasopressin
   Prostaglandins
   Atrial natriuretic peptide

components of the renin–angiotensin system have been found in the brain, and angiotensin can be regarded as one of the neuropeptides involved in neurotransmission. The central nervous system actions of angiotensin are thus receiving increasing attention and include influences on blood pressure, the sympathetic nervous system, thirst and vasopressin secretion and sodium appetite.

These actions are achieved by angiotensin II acting on cell membrane receptors. The main intracellular second messenger for angiotensin II is increased intracellular calcium. Two types of angiotensin II receptors have been identified on the basis of pharmacological specificity of certain antagonist compounds. The distributions and actions of the AT-1 and AT-2 receptors are currently under intensive investigation.

The renin–angiotensin–aldosterone system is fundamentally important in sodium homeostasis. With salt depletion, renin release is stimulated, angiotensin concentration increases and this in turn stimulates aldosterone production, which acts on the kidney to conserve sodium. Angiotensin furthermore causes vasoconstriction, which helps maintain blood pressure in the face of a reduced blood and extracellular fluid volume. Conversely, sodium loading inhibits the renin–angiotensin–al-

Table 2.3   Biological actions of angiotensin II

1. Vasoconstriction
2. Stimulation of aldosterone secretion
3. Renal tubular sodium reabsorption
4. Facilitation of sympathetic nerve transmission and release of catecholamines from adrenal medulla
5. Central actions
   Thirst and sodium appetite
   Vagal
   Central pressor action
   Release of vasopressin

dosterone system. In chronic renal failure, abnormalities in the renin–angiotensin system occur and contribute to the limited reserve for sodium balance displayed by patients with end-stage renal failure.

The renin–angiotensin system is also important in normal blood pressure control, and in the response to haemorrhage, diuretics and adrenal insufficiency. However, its role in the pathogenesis of essential hypertension is more controversial.

About 20% of patients with essential hypertension have suppressed renin levels but the majority of patients have normal levels. In both renovascular hypertension and some cases of hypertension with end-stage renal failure, peripheral renin and so angiotensin II levels may be high and thus contribute to the pathogenesis of hypertension.

Many factors, including drugs, are known to influence plasma renin activity (Table 2.4). These may act on the baroreceptor, the macula densa or directly on the juxtaglomerular cells. β-Blockade suppresses renin activity and ACE inhibition increases it through loss of negative feedback on renin secretion by angiotensin II. These may be important when evaluating patients — for example, when investigating renovascular hypertension.

Recently several pharmacological means have become available for blocking the renin–angiotensin system at various steps of the enzymatic cascade. Orally active renin inhibitors block the catalytic site of renin and prevent the formation of

Table 2.4   Factors influencing the plasma renin activity

Renin ↑	Renin ↓
Sodium deficiency	Sodium loading
Spironolactone	Mineralocorticoids
Diuretics	
Vasodilators	Vasoconstriction
Prostaglandins	Vasopressin
ACE inhibitors	Angiotensin
β-Adrenergic stimulation	β-Adrenergic blockade (drugs)
Isoprenaline	
Adrenaline	
Sympathetic nerve stimulation	α-Adrenergic stimulation
Calcium chelators	
Upright posture	
Renal artery stenosis	

angiotensin II. There are now several orally active ACE inhibitors (captopril, enalapril, lisinopril, perindopril, cilazapril, ramipril, quinapril) in current clinical use for the treatment of hypertension, including renal hypertension, and congestive cardiac failure. They have proved to be effective, safe and to reduce the mortality by 30% in patients with CHF. More recently specific orally active AII receptor blocking drugs have undergone clinical trials in hypertension with promising results.

Kallikrein–kinin system

Kallikreins are serine proteases (MW 24 000–40 000) found in plasma and exocrine glandular tissue. Plasma kallikrein, which is part of the blood coagulation cascade, differs from glandular kallikrein. Glandular kallikrein is found in exocrine glands (submaxillary, salivary, pancreas) and their secretions, and in the kidney and urine. It has a very similar biochemical pathway to the renin–angiotensin system (Fig. 2.3). Kallikrein acts by limited proteolysis on an α_2-globulin substrate (kininogen) to form kinins (bradykinin, lysyl bradykinin). Bradykinin is then degraded by kininase II to inactive fragments. Kininase II is now known to be identical to ACE, so that the same enzyme is responsible for activating the

vasoconstrictor angiotensin and for destroying the vasodilatory kinins. ACE inhibitors could therefore potentially lead to the accumulation of bradykinin in the body. Like renin, kallikrein is stored in an inactive zymogen form. Recent work suggests that kallikrein may be one of the activators of inactive renin.

Bradykinin has three important renal actions. It is a powerful renal vasodilator, causing an increase in renal blood flow (RBF) but only a small rise in glomerular filtration rate (GFR). There is also redistribution in blood flow, the outer cortical flow of the kidney increasing more than that in the inner medullary areas. Finally, it causes diuresis and natriuresis.

The components of the kallikrein–kinin system (KKS) have all been localized to different areas of the kidney (Fig. 2.4). Kallikrein is an ectoenzyme found on the luminal surface of the cells of the first part of the distal convoluted tubule and the first part of the collecting duct. Kininase II (ACE) has been isolated from the brush border of the proximal convoluted tubule where presumably it destroys any filtered kinins. It is also present in the glomeruli and vascular endothelium of the kidney. All components of the KKS (kallikrein, kininogen, kininases, kinins) have been found in the urine.

Bradykinin also causes increased capillary permeability, oedema and pain, and may therefore have a role in the inflammatory process and in renal immunological reactions.

The physiological role of the renal kallikrein–kinin system in the kidney is not known. It is known that renal and urinary kallikreins are inversely related to sodium balance, a low salt diet stimulating kallikrein. Kallikrein also varies directly with potassium intake, and mineralocorticoid administration increases urinary kallikrein. High levels of urinary kallikrein have been found in primary aldosteronism (Conn's syndrome) and have been used as a diagnostic test in this condition. Conversely, many patients with essential hypertension have relatively low urinary kallikrein excretion. Patients with Bartter's syndrome have very high levels of urinary kallikrein and prostaglandins. Non-steroidal anti-inflammatory agents (NSAIDs), e.g. indomethacin, which correct the hypokalaemic alkalosis found in this

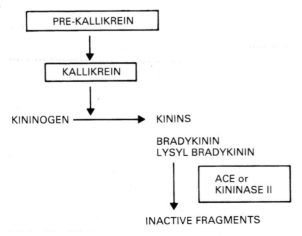

Fig. 2.3 Biochemical pathways in the kallikrein–kinin system with enzymes responsible for the cascade. ACE — angiotensin-converting enzyme

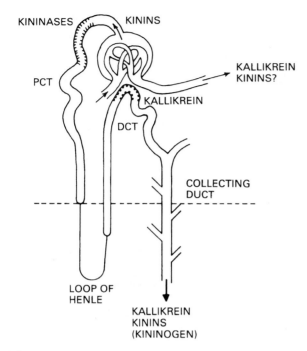

Fig. 2.4 Renal localization of the various components of the kallikrein–kinin system. All the substacnes have been found in the kidney. PCT — proximal collecting tubule; DCT — distal collecting tubule

syndrome also decrease urinary kallikrein and prostaglandins.

Renal prostaglandins and medullolipin

The kidney, like most organs, synthesizes prostaglandins (PG) from the free fatty acid precursor arachidonic acid. The kidney is capable of forming all the major prostanoid series (prostaglandin E_2, $F_{2\alpha}$, prostacyclin and thromboxane). Arachidonic acid is released from lipid membranes by phospholipase A_2. This enzyme can be stimulated by a variety of hormonal and neuronal influences. Arachidonic acid is then acted upon by a group of enzymes, cyclo-oxygenases, to form two unstable endoperoxidases (PGG_2 and PGH_2) from which the different types of prostaglandins are formed by the action of specific enzymes (Fig. 2.5).

PGE_2, the predominant renal prostaglandin, is formed by the action of an isomerase. This enzyme is found mainly in the renal medulla, and 90% of renal PGE_2 is produced in the medulla. Small amounts of $PGF_{2\alpha}$ are also formed, probably from a ketoreductase acting on PGF_2.

Prostacyclin synthetase is the enzyme responsible for forming prostaglandin I_2 (prostacyclin) from PGH_2 and thromboxane synthetase for the formation of thromboxane A_2. These enzymes are found in the glomeruli and vascular tissue in the cortex, which is the major site of production of these two prostanoids.

Whether all prostaglandins are simultaneously and continuously produced by the kidney is not known. However, it is known that synthesis of the vasoconstrictor and platelet-aggregating compound thromboxane is greatly increased by ureteral obstruction. Whether the anatomical localization of the appropriate enzymes also accounts for the distribution of the renal prostaglandins is unknown. In the medulla prostaglandins can be synthesized both by collecting ducts and by medullary interstitial cells. These specialized cells are found scattered in clumps throughout the medulla and contain lipid-staining droplets.

The prostaglandins are rapidly metabolized by the kidney: prostacyclin to the stable metabolite 6-keto-$PGF_{1\alpha}$ and thromboxane A_2 to thromboxane B_2 and other metabolites; it is unlikely that any escapes into the general circulation.

Aspirin and other non-steroidal anti-inflammatory drugs have been shown to be potent inhibitors of cyclo-oxygenase, thus blocking prostaglandin formation. This probably accounts for their anti-inflammatory action, as well as for their adverse effects on the kidney. Indomethacin can cause a fall in RBF and GFR and salt and water retention. It has been suggested that aspirin and compound analgesics may cause renal papillary necrosis and analgesic nephropathy by interfering with prostacyclin's vasodilatory effect on renal medullary flow. The effect of NSAIDs on specific cyclo-oxygenase and synthetase is dose-dependent. At low doses, thromboxane A_2 synthesis is first inhibited while prostacyclin formation continues, leading to a relatively vasodilatory, antiplatelet-aggregating state, whereas at high concentrations prostacyclin production is also inhibited.

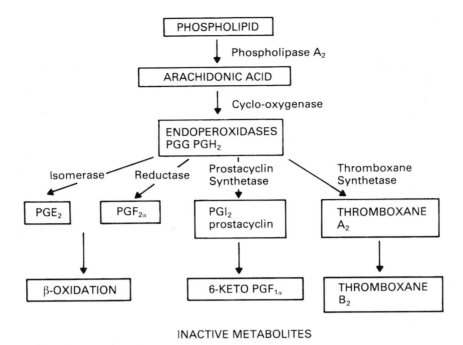

Fig. 2 5   Biosynthesis of prostaglandins. The various pathways and enzyme responsible for the major prostaglandin pathways are depicted

The renal actions of prostaglandins are multiple (Table 2.5). Under resting basal conditions prostaglandins probably exert little if any tonic influence on the kidney. However, they are effective in opposing the renal vasoconstrictor influence of angiotensin and the adrenergic nervous system, and in regulating medullary blood flow. Prostaglandins localized in the arterioles and in the glomerulus help to regulate glomerular filtration rate. Prostaglandins have been shown to be potent releasers of renin and probably act as a common transducer for a variety of stimuli to renin release. There are also inter-relationships with the kallikrein–kinin system, as bradykinin is a potent activator of phospholipase A_2 whereas some of the renal actions of bradykinin, particularly those related to renal sodium handling, are thought to involve the prostaglandins.

Prostaglandins oppose the action of vasopressin (antidiuretic hormone, ADH) in the renal collecting duct and tubules. This probably involves PGE_2, which is located in these cells and has been shown to inhibit adenylate cyclase. The increased water permeability brought about by vasopressin involves stimulation of adenylate cyclase and an increase in cyclic AMP (see below). Prostaglandin cyclo-oxygenase inhibitors all enhance ADH-stimulated water reabsorption, which probably accounts for the water retention produced by NSAIDs. The effects on renal sodium handling by prostaglandins are less clear. In general prostaglandins, when infused, lead to natriuresis and diuresis. Inhibition of prostaglandins by NSAIDs does appear to reduce the potency of loop diuretics and

Table 2.5   Renal actions of prostaglandins

1. Action on renal blood flow and distribution
2. Renal sodium excretion
3. Antagonistic to the action of vasopressin on water permeability
4. Stimulation of renin release
5. Modulation of vasoconstriction due to sympathetic nerve stimulation, catecholamines and angiotensin

other antihypertensive drugs, as well as increase blood pressure.

The renal medullary interstitial cells have also been shown to synthesize a non-prostanoid moiety called antihypertensive neutral renal lipid, medullolipin, or renal medullary vasodepressor lipid. These cells, when grown in tissue culture and transplanted to hypertensive rabbits, lower the blood pressure. Similarly, injection of medullolipin produces hypotension in experimental renal hypertension. The exact physiological functions of the renal medullary interstitial cell and medullolipin are still to be elucidated.

Vitamin D

The metabolic pathways for the formation of the bioactive metabolites of vitamin D_3 (cholecalciferol) are shown in Figure 2.6. Vitamin D_3 is formed from 7-dehydrocholesterol by the action of ultraviolet light on the skin. In addition, a signifi-

cant proportion of vitamin D_3 is obtained from the diet and gastrointestinal absorption. Approximately 80% is taken up by the liver and converted by liver microsomes to 25-hydroxyvitamin D_3 (25-OHD_3). Although this compound has some biological activity, it is not the physiologically important bioactive metabolite. The major bioactivation occurs in the kidney by the conversion of 25-OHD_3 to 1,25-dihydroxyvitamin D_3 (1,25$(OH)_2D_3$). This conversion occurs by 1α hydroxylase, found in the mitochondria of the renal cortex. 1,25-dihydroxyvitamin D_3 is the active hormone acting on the vitamin D_3 target sites in the gastrointestinal tract, the bone and the kidneys. Smaller amounts of 24,25$(OH)_2$ vitamin D and 1,24,25$(OH)_3$ vitamin D are also found. The kidney appears to be the only organ responsible for the production of 1,25-dihydroxyvitamin D_3 and can therefore be regarded as a true endocrine gland for the hormone vitamin D_3, or cholecalciferol.

The conversion to 1,25$(OH)_2D_3$ in the kidney is stimulated by low calcium and phosphate concentrations and by parathyroid hormone (PTH). 1,25-dihydroxyvitamin D_3 also exerts a negative feedback control on its own production.

The 1,25$(OH)_2D_3$ produced in the kidney plays an important physiological role in the control of calcium and phosphate metabolism by acting on specific cytoplasmic receptors which influence nuclear mRNA transcription and so specific protein synthesis. In this way it increases intestinal calcium and phosphate reabsorption, thus allowing maximal utilization of low dietary calcium. It also interacts with PTH to mobilize calcium from bone and, lastly, stimulates calcium reabsorption in the proximal tubule of the kidney. The last two actions of vitamin D depend on the presence of parathyroid hormone.

Disorders of vitamin D metabolism and action are common in renal disease (Table 2.6). In chronic renal failure the decreased ability of the diseased kidney to bioactivate 25-hydroxycholecalciferol to 1,25-dihydroxycholecalciferol is an important factor contributing to renal osteodystrophy, the secondary hyperparathyroidism and disordered divalent ion homeostasis seen in end-stage renal failure. Many of these

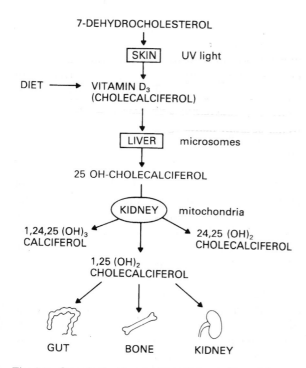

Fig. 2.6   Steps in the bioactivation of vitamin D_3 and its biological actions

Table 2.6 Clinical renal disorders associated with abnormal vitamin D metabolism and action

---

Reduced 1,25-dihydroxycholecalciferol
  Vitamin D-dependent rickets
  Chronic renal failure
  Fanconi syndrome
  Nephrotic syndrome
End-organ resistance
  Vitamin D-dependent rickets type II —'nephrogenic rickets'
Excessive 1,25-dihydroxycholecalciferol
  Hyperparathyroidism
  Sarcoidosis
  Idiopathic hypercalciuria

---

abnormalities can be corrected by administration of $1,25(OH)_2D_3$ or $1\alpha(OH)D_3$, a synthetic analogue. Some aspects of the Fanconi syndrome (abnormal tubular reabsorption of glucose, phosphate, bicarbonate and amino acids), including the metabolic bone disease, are caused by the reduced ability of the kidney to hydroxylate $25\text{-}OHD_3$. End-organ resistance to vitamin D_3 has been described as vitamin D-dependent rickets type II due to mutations in the $1,25(OH)_2D_3$ receptor, in which the kidney is unresponsive to physiological concentrations of 1,25-dihydroxyvitamin D_3. This is in contrast to vitamin D-dependent rickets type I, a rare hereditary disease caused by a deficiency of $1,25(OH)_2D_3$ due to mutations in 1α hydroxylase, which can be corrected by large doses of $1,25(OH)_2D_3$. Lastly, idiopathic hypercalcaemia is believed by some to result from renal overproduction of 1,25-dihydroxyvitamin D_3.

Erythropoietin

Erythropoietin is a glycoprotein (MW 38 000) produced by the kidney which regulates red cell development. It is produced intact, not as a prohormone. In fetal life it is produced by the liver but after birth 90% of erythropoietin is produced and released by the kidney. The exact site of production in the liver or kidney has not yet been identified. It is thought to be produced in the renal cortex — perhaps by interstitial, endothelial or glomerular cells or renal tubules. Erythropoietin production and release by the kidney is regulated primarily by the tissue oxygen concentration. Whether the renal oxygen sensor is the same cell that produces erythropoietin, or a separate cell, is also unknown. Any cause of tissue hypoxia (hypoxic or ischaemic) will stimulate erythropoietin production.

Renal erythropoietin is also stimulated by androgens (which may account for the higher haemoglobin in men), by thyroid hormone, by prostaglandins of the E series and by β-adrenergic agonists. Plasma erythropoietin has a relatively short half-life (about 3–5 hours in humans). The major catabolic organs are the liver and kidneys, where it is cleared.

Erythropoietin is the most important regulator of erythrocyte production. It acts via a specific cell surface receptor on committed erythroid stem cells inducing differentiation to erythroid precursors. It is also capable of causing release of reticulocytes into the blood.

Erythropoietin abnormalities account for several important clinical syndromes in renal disease. The anaemia of chronic renal failure provides some of the evidence for renal production of erythropoietin as production decreases as renal insufficiency worsens. However, it is not dependent on the excretory function of the kidney. Patients on maintenance dialysis with kidneys in situ generally have higher haemoglobulin levels than patients who have had a bilateral nephrectomy. Bilateral nephrectomy generally leads to further falls in erythropoietin and haemoglobin levels. Conversely, successful renal transplantation will generally elevate erythropoietin and correct the anaemia of chronic renal failure. On the other hand, successful dialysis — although correcting many of the metabolic defects of chronic renal failure — seems to have little effect on the anaemia. Recombinant erythropoietin alleviates this anaemia.

Inappropriate secondary erythrocytosis can also occur in renal ischaemia, polycystic disease, renal cell carcinoma and Bartter's syndrome. Renal cell carcinoma is the most common tumour to lead to overproduction or ectopic secretion of erythropoietin and secondary polycythaemia.

EXTRA-RENAL HORMONES ACTING ON THE KIDNEY

Many hormones act on the kidney — some in a general way like growth hormone and thyroid hormones; some in a more specific, target-directed manner, e.g. vasopressin and aldosterone; and lastly some in unknown ways, e.g. catecholamines and calcitonin. This section will deal with those hormones which have a specific and direct action and for which the kidney could be regarded as the major target organ.

Aldosterone, cortisol and mineralocorticoids

The kidney contains cytoplasmic receptors for all steroid hormones, including aldosterone, cortisol and other glucocorticoids, oestrogen, testosterone and vitamin D_3. However, the renal actions of aldosterone are the most important physiologically. Aldosterone, a mineralocorticoid synthesized in the zona glomerulosa of the adrenal gland, is stimulated by angiotensin II, ACTH and potassium ions. Its secretion rate varies with salt balance, sodium depletion stimulating aldosterone secretion.

Adrenal mineralocorticoids have three primary renal actions:

1. *Renal sodium reabsorption.* Aldosterone stimulates sodium reabsorption in exchange for potassium and hydrogen ions in the distal convoluted tubule and the collecting duct. Aldosterone thus causes anti-natriuresis and kaliuresis. This action is blocked by spironolactone, a competitive aldosterone antagonist, and by the non-competitive aldosterone antagonist amiloride.

2. *Urinary acidification.* Adrenal steroids enhance urinary acidification by modifying hydrogen ion transport (as above) and by ammoniagenesis, and both glucocorticoids and mineralocorticoids may be equally effective.

3. *Water metabolism.* Adrenal insufficiency is associated with a limited capacity for urinary dilution and concentration, and patients with Addison's disease cannot excrete free water. This is because glucocorticoids are necessary for maximal impermeability of the collecting duct to water to allow maximal water excretion (see below). Both mineralocorticoid and glucocorticoid actions appear to be involved.

In oedematous states (cirrhosis, congestive heart failure, nephrotic syndrome) associated with low 'effective' circulating blood volume the urinary sodium excretion is low and the aldosterone secretory rate high. Similarly, with low sodium diets or in the compensation to diuretic therapy, plasma renin and angiotensin as well as aldosterone increase.

Vasopressin

The major target organ for the nonapeptide, arginine vasopressin, the antidiuretic hormone, is the kidney. Vasopressin is synthesized in the hypothalamic paraventricular and supraoptic nuclei and released from the posterior pituitary gland in response to osmotic and non-osmotic stimuli. Any increase in plasma osmolality activates osmoreceptors in the brain, probably near the hypothalamus in the region adjacent to the anterior third ventricle, which stimulate the release of vasopressin. Likewise, a fall in plasma osmolality inhibits vasopressin release resulting in a water diuresis and thus a return of plasma osmolality towards normal. The plasma osmolality is thus kept within a very narrow range (270–285 mmol/kg H_2O).

There are also non-osmotic low pressure volume receptors in the atria and high pressure baroreceptors (carotid sinus and aortic arch) in the cardiovascular system that can regulate vasopressin release. These volume/pressure sensors send input to the medulla oblongata, and ascending pathways to the paraventricular and supraoptic nuclei to increase vasopressin secretion when hypovolaemia occurs. The sympathetic nervous system and other central nervous system stimuli (especially nausea and emesis) also regulate vasopressin release. If preservation of volume is threatened these can override the osmolar control of ADH release, leading to a hypo-osmolar hyponatraemic state.

The major site of the antidiuretic action of vasopressin on the kidney is the collecting duct. This passes through the renal medulla and papilla, which have a very high interstitial osmotic gradient induced by the countercurrent mechanism. The collecting ducts are normally impermeable to water, thus preventing loss of tubular fluid into the renal medullary interstitium through the high osmotic gradient. Vasopressin makes these structures permeable to water by acting on cell surface 'V$_2$' vasopressin receptors. Activation of these receptors stimulates adenylate cyclase and cyclic AMP production leading to water permeability and water reabsorption down the concentration gradient, leading to urinary concentration. The 'V$_1$' vasopressin receptor occurs on blood vessels and in the brain and is involved in the vasoconstrictor/blood pressure response to vasopressin.

Vasopressin deficiency, caused by inability to make vasopressin or destruction of the posterior pituitary, produces the clinical state of central diabetes insipidus, which is characterized by hyperosmolar hypernatraemia and the excretion of large volumes of dilute urine of low osmolality. With free access to water, water balance is maintained by drinking copious quantities of fluid. Nephrogenic diabetes insipidus, generally a hereditary disorder, but also caused by certain drug toxicity (e.g. lithium), is also characterized by copious volumes of dilute urine but it is caused by a lack of or decrease in the response of the kidney to vasopressin. The two conditions can be distinguished by measuring the urinary response to the administration of exogenous vasopressin, usually DDAVP (a synthetic analogue).

Excess vasopressin, which occurs in certain central nervous and pulmonary conditions or as the result of ectopic production from tumours, produces the syndrome of inappropriate ADH (SIADH) secretion. This is characterized by hypo-osmolar hyponatraemia with urine osmolalities disproportionately higher than the pathologically decreased plasma osmolality. To diagnose this condition it is important to ensure normal blood volume status and normal renal, adrenal and thyroid status and to ensure the patient is not taking diuretics.

Parathyroid hormone and calcitonin

Parathyroid hormone, produced by the parathyroid glands, is responsible for regulating calcium homeostasis by the body (Fig. 2.7). It does this by actions on the gut, bone and kidney. PTH undergoes extensive intracellular parathyroid post-

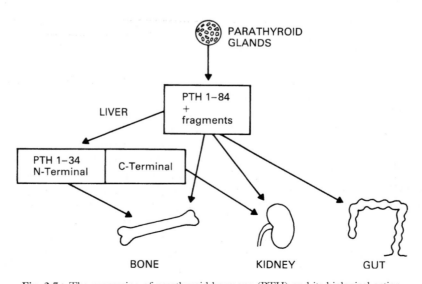

Fig. 2.7   The processing of parathyroid hormone (PTH) and its biological action

translational processing from preproPTH (115 amino acids) to proPTH (90 amino acids) to PTH (84 amino acids) as well as mainly hepatic and renal metabolism leading to two major fragments. The carboxy-terminal fragment (MW 7000) is biologically inactive but accounts for much of the immunoreactivity measured by radioimmuno-assay. Both intact PTH 1–84 and the N-terminal PTH 1–34 (MW 2500) fragment appear to be biologically active, and PTH 1–34 may be the physiologically important peptide for the hormone's action on bone. Intact PTH 1–84 and PTH 1–34 as well as carboxy-terminal degraded PTH are further metabolized and excreted by the kidney by glomerular filtration and tubular mechanisms.

PTH increases renal excretion of phosphate and bicarbonate. The phosphaturic effect is via the proximal tubule and is dependent on sodium reabsorption. These actions appear to be mediated by adenylate-cyclase coupled PTH receptors on the tubules. PTH also decreases renal clearance of calcium and magnesium ions by influencing calcium reabsorption in the proximal tubule. Lastly PTH is one of the regulators for the bioactivation of 25-hydroxycholecalciferol to 1,25-dihydroxy-cholecalciferol in the kidney.

Chronic renal failure is the commonest cause of secondary hyperparathyroidism. In chronic renal failure, immunoreactive PTH (iPTH) levels are high, mainly because of increased circulating levels of the C-fragment 1–84 of PTH. Abnormalities in PTH control and metabolism are very important in renal osteodystrophy. PTH release is stimulated in chronic renal failure by the phosphate retention and hypocalcaemia due to calcium malabsorption through low $1,25(OH)_2D_3$ levels associated with uraemia. Furthermore, chronic renal failure appears to be associated with skeletal resistance to PTH actions. Hyperparathyroidism secondary to chronic renal failure is managed by gastrointestinal phosphate-binding agents and calcium supplements, vitamin D_3 analogues and, if necessary, partial parathyroidectomy.

PTH-related peptide (PTHrp) has been identified as a major cause of hormonal hyper-calcaemia of malignancy, especially of squamous cell cancers. It is larger then PTH and has little sequence similarity to PTH except at the N-terminal end. However it does interact with the PTH receptor.

Calcitonin is a 32 amino acid peptide secreted by thyroid chief cells. It has been reported to produce natriuresis, phosphaturia and increased calcium excretion as well as its hypocalcaemic action on bone. However, the physiological renal actions of calcitonin are not yet clear. It is secreted in response to increased plasma calcium.

Calcitonin gene-related peptide (CGRP) is also transcribed from the calcitonin gene. It has cardiovascular actions and may serve as a neuro-transmitter in the central nervous system. It may also be involved in some of the renal actions of calcitonin.

Atrial natriuretic peptide (ANP)

Atrial natriuretic peptide (ANP) is a 28 amino acid circulating peptide hormone that is released from atrial myocyte granules in response to atrial stretch, usually secondary to blood volume expansion and increased atrial pressure.

PreproANP (151 amino acids) is processed within the atrial myocyte to proANP (126 amino acids) which is stored intracellularly. At the time of ANP secretion the C-terminal active ANP is cleaved and released. ANP can also be produced by myocytes in hypertrophied ventricles. ANP acts on specific membrane receptors that activate particulate guanylate cyclase with increased production of cyclic guanosine monophosphate (cGMP). Its main actions are relaxation of vascular smooth muscle with reduction of cardiac preload and increased glomerular filtration rate (GFR); natriuresis via increased GFR, inhibition of renal proximal tubule and collecting duct sodium channels and direct inhibition of adrenal cortical aldosterone biosynthesis secretion; direct inhibition of renin secretion; suppression of sympathetic activity and inhibition of thirst and vaso-pressin secretion. These actions reduce blood pressure and volume. In this way ANP acts as a counter-regulatory hormone to salt- and water-retaining hormones such as the renin–angiotensin–aldosterone system and vasopressin. ANP synthesis, secretion and plasma levels are elevated in congestive heart failure, renal failure and oedematous states.

ANP is metabolized by a specific 'clearance' receptor as well as an enzyme, neutral endopeptidase, both of which occur in abundance in the kidneys. Specific orally active endogenous inhibitors of neutral endopeptidase which reduce ANP degradation and so augment ANP actions are being investigated for the management of hypertension and heart failure and oedematous states.

Before the identification and characterization of ANP, multiple natriuretic factors were thought to exist. Endogenous digitalis-like factor is thought to be a ouabain-like compound released in response to hypervolaemia and which causes natriuresis by inhibiting $Na^+,K-ATPase$. Its exact site of synthesis, structure and physiology are as yet unclear and there may be a number of such factors.

Catecholamines

The kidney has a rich nervous innervation. Sympathetic renal adrenergic nerves innervate intrarenal blood vessels, glomeruli, efferent and afferent arterioles, the juxtaglomerular apparatus, as well as the proximal and distal tubules. The kidney has been shown to contain α_1-adrenergic receptors as well as β_1- and β_2-adrenoreceptors. The kidney is also sensitive to blood-borne endogenous adrenaline released from the adrenal medulla.

The actions of nerve stimulations and catecholamines are multiple and complex. The main well-defined actions are described below.

Renal haemodynamic

The sympathetic nervous system controls renal vascular resistance, renal blood flow and intrarenal distribution of blood flow by α-adrenergic vasoconstriction. The decrease in renal blood flow associated with haemorrhage, cardiac failure and hypertension results from increased renal sympathetic tone.

Renin secretion

Catecholamines have direct as well as indirect effects, via their influence on renal haemodynamics, on renin release from the juxtaglomerular apparatus. β-Adrenergic agonists stimulate renin release while α-adrenergic compounds inhibit renin release. These actions account for the well-known inhibition of plasma renin by the β-adrenergic blocking drugs used in the treatment of hypertension.

Renal tubular function

Catecholamines influence the reabsorption of sodium, phosphate and urea, as well as urinary concentrating ability.

Metabolic functions

As in the other tissues, catecholamines have marked effects on the metabolic functions of renal cells, increasing glucose uptake and glyconeogenesis.

Endothelin

Endothelin is a 21 amino acid peptide derived from endothelial cells throughout the vasculature, not just in the kidney. It is synthesized initially as preproendothelin (212 amino acids) which is cleaved to 'big' endothelin or proendothelin (38 amino acids) which is subsequently cleaved further to 'mature' endothelin. Its structure is well conserved across species, and similar peptides such as the sarafotoxins and apamin occur in the venom of the burrowing asp and in bee venom respectively.

Endothelin acts on specific cell surface receptors to cause a complex series of events, including activation of the phosphoinositide second messenger system and activating calcium channels to increase intracellular calcium. Although endothelin can be detected in blood, and plasma endothelin levels are increased in renal failure, myocardial infarction and shock (probably reflecting endothelial damage), its action is likely to be local or paracrine rather than as a hormone.

Its main action is potent vasoconstriction (it was initially thought to be the most potent vasoconstrictor), but other actions include: positive inotropy; stimulating secretion of vasopressin, noradrenaline, endothelial-derived relaxation factor, prostacyclin and ANP; constriction of venous, lymphatic, bronchiolar, uterine and tracheal smooth muscle; cell proliferation; and inhibition of renal renin secretion. How many of these are pharmacological or physiological are unclear.

HORMONES METABOLIZED OR CLEARED BY THE KIDNEY

The kidney is responsible for the metabolism and clearance of hormones by three general mechanisms:

1. Specific renal uptake and degradation
2. General filtration of any compound with a molecular weight less than 30 000
3. Tubular secretion.

Examples of each of these processes occur with individual hormones. PTH is specifically taken up and the C-terminal end cleaved to form an inactive fragment. Similarly, ANP is cleared by its clearance receptor and neutral endopeptidase. Some steroid hormones are specifically taken up by renal tubular cells. Most of the smaller peptide hormones (gastrin, LH, FSH) are filtered at the glomerulus and broken down by peptidases in the brush border of the proximal tubule.

Peptide hormones

Most peptide hormones with a molecular weight below 30 000 are filtered at the glomerulus. Most peptides in the glomerular ultrafiltrate are hydrolysed by the high concentration of exo- and endopeptidases found in the brush border of the proximal convoluted tubule. The resultant tri- and dipeptide amino acids are then reabsorbed by specific tubular transport processes.

Glomerular filtration and renal metabolism have been shown to play a significant role in the metabolic clearance of insulin, growth hormone, glucagon, gastrin, PTH, luteinizing hormone and follicle-stimulating hormone. In these cases renal failure leads to increases in the circulatory levels of the hormone proportional to the decrease in creatinine clearance.

However, the uraemic state is a very complex metabolic condition, and prolonged half-lives and reduced metabolic clearance rates are not the only factors responsible for the elevated peptide hormonal levels seen in chronic renal failure.

Steroids

Recently it has been realized that the kidney is also a major site of metabolism of glucocorticoids. In particular 11β-hydroxysteroid dehydrogenase (11βOHSD) is involved in the interconversion of cortisol and cortisone. This microsomal enzyme also occurs in the liver, placenta, gastrointestinal tract, prostate, muscle, lung and thyroid. 11βOHSD determines the relative amounts of cortisol/cortisone present in each tissue and hence relative degrees of glucocorticoid/mineralocorticoid activity. The direction of the 'cortisol–cortisone shuttle' varies with different tissues with a tendency towards cortisol in the liver and cortisone in the kidney. Since cortisol can bind to renal mineralocorticoid receptors and so cause sodium and water retention, congenital deficiency of 11βOHSD results in excess cortisol *within the kidney* so causing salt and water retention, hypokalaemia, hypertension and suppression of the RAS. This rare inherited condition is treated with dexamethasone so suppressing endogenous cortisol production and allowing dexamethasone to give selective replacement of glucocorticoid activity and normal activity of the RAS. Liquorice causes its renal salt and water retention by suppressing 11βOHSD activity in susceptible individuals.

The kidney is also responsible for the excretion of steroid hormones conjugated by the liver, including aldosterone, cortisol, oestrogen and testosterone.

Catecholamines

Catecholamines are taken up by renal tubular cells and some are conjugated and excreted. The kidney also excretes catecholamines conjugated at other sites.

CHRONIC RENAL FAILURE

The hormonal changes induced by chronic renal failure are many and complex. Loss of renal function can affect hormones by four major mechanisms (Table 2.7.)

1. The synthesis of intra-renal hormones may be reduced because of the reduction in renal mass consequent in chronic renal disease. The anaemia of chronic renal failure is largely due to reduced renal erythropoietin production. Likewise, the hypocalcaemia and osteomalacia are a consequence of the reduced capacity of the diseased kidney to hydroxylate 25-hydroxycholecalciferol to the bioactive 1,25-dihydroxycholecalciferol. This also affects PTH levels by removing vitamin D_3-mediated PTH suppression. Whether the hypertension seen in chronic renal failure is related to the reduced ability of the diseased kidney to produce any of the three renal vasodepressor

Table 2.7 Mechanism of hormonal disturbances in chronic renal failure

---

1. Reduced hormone production from reduced renal mass
   Erythropoietin (anaemia)
   1,25-dihydroxycholecalciferol (osteomalacia, secondary hyperparathyroidism)
2. Hormonal resistance of diseased kidney
   Sodium homeostasis — aldosterone
   Concentrating and diluting — vasopressin
   PTH regulation of vitamin D_3 hydroxylation
3. Loss of excretory and clearance function
   Prolonged half-life of peptide hormones
4. Uraemic toxins interfering with hormonal action
   Carbohydrate intolerance
   Insulin
   Hypothyroidism

---

substances (medullolipin, kallikrein, prostaglandins) is not known.

2. Hormones are less effective in the diseased kidney. For example, the limited reserve for sodium homeostasis in chronic renal failure, although due to a variety of mechanisms, including increased osmotic load, is also a result of the smaller antinatriuretic effect of aldosterone. Vasopressin likewise cannot produce maximal antidiuresis and urinary concentration. Lastly, PTH regulation of vitamin D_3 hydroxylation is probably less efficient in chronic renal failure.

3. Loss of renal excretory function will prolong the half-life of those hormones which are excreted by the kidney and reduce their metabolic clearance rate. This accounts for some of the elevation in plasma hormones during chronic renal failure and, more importantly, for the very high levels of metabolic hormonal fragments (e.g. PTH C-terminal peptide).

4. The complex changes and toxins produced by the uraemic state may interfere with hormonal actions at the target site. Some of the carbohydrate intolerance seen in chronic renal failure is due to interference with the action of insulin. Similarly, some of the hypothyroid-like metabolic changes seen in uraemia may be due to interference with the action of thyroid hormones.

In general, in established chronic renal failure most if not all of these mechanisms may operate, and the complex bone changes seen in chronic renal failure are a good example of the combined effects of the lack of vitamin D_3 giving rise to hypocalcaemia and osteomalacia, combined with osteitis fibrosa cystica caused by secondary hyperparathyroidism.

RECOMMENDED READING

De Groot L J 1989 Textbook of endocrinology, 2nd edn. Saunders, Philadelphia
Dunn M J 1983 Renal endocrinology. Williams & Wilkins, Baltimore
Goetz K L 1988 Physiology and pathophysiology of atrial peptides. American Journal of Physiology 254: E1–E15

Muirhead E E 1990 discovery of the reno-medullary system of blood pressure control. Hypertension 15: P114–116
Nayler W G 1990 The endothelins. Springer Verlag, Berlin
Stewart et al 1988 Syndrome of apparent mineralocorticoid excess: a defect in the cortisol–cortisone shuttle. Journal of Clinical Investigation 82: 340–349

3. Renal pharmacology and diuretics

G. Duggin,   M. J. Field

PART 1: PHARMACOLOGY
G. Duggin

INTRODUCTION

The kidney plays an important homeostatic role in maintaining the composition as well as the volume of body fluids. Regulation of the extra cellular composition by the kidney also affects the concentration of many drugs and their metabolites. The kidneys perform this function as a by-product of their regulation of the extra cellular fluid concentration of many endogenous end products of metabolism and also various xenobiotics encountered in foods etc.

The mechanism by which the kidney regulates the concentrations of drugs and their metabolites in the extra cellular fluid is dependant on the chemical nature of the drug or metabolite and to some extent molecular size. As a general rule the kidney excretes those drugs which have a low molecular weight and as the molecular weight of a substance increases, the greater proportion of the drug is removed via the liver and biliary system. However this is not an absolute rule and there are exceptions.

A knowledge of the way in which the kidney eliminates drugs and the mechanism by which it is achieved is often useful in making dosage adjustments during therapy. In clinical situations the likelihood of other drugs interfering with excretion can be important. Changes in renal function will also markedly alter the excretion of a drug and hence knowledge of these mech-

anisms can aid in a reliable prediction of whether either the dose or interval of the drug can be modified.

The majority of drugs excreted by the kidney appear in the glomerular filtrate and are either not reabsorbed or partially or almost completely reabsorbed by the tubular epithelial cells. Still other substances are actively secreted via the proximal tubular cells and in these circumstances the rate of clearance from plasma will exceed the rate of glomerular filtration. It is important to note that reabsorption refers to the drug being reabsorbed from the tubular fluid and ultimately into the plasma whereas secretion refers to the drug passing from plasma via the tubular epithelial cells into the tubular fluid.

MECHANISM OF RENAL EXCRETION OF DRUGS

Glomerular filtration (see Chapter 1)

The glomerulus has certain similarities to other capillary beds and filtration is subject to the physical laws that govern the transportation of fluid and permeable solutes across capillary endothelial cells and basement membranes. The glomerulus has other functions in terms of the mesangial cells and the additional barrier of the renal epithelial cells. The filtration force in the glomerulus is primarily determined by the hydrostatic pressure of the blood which is determined by the blood pressure and the oncotic pressure exerted by plasma proteins which do not diffuse through the glomerular basement membrane. This however is dependant both on the charge of the protein and the molecular size of the protein. If the molecular weight of the protein is sufficiently small it is filtered at the glomerulus, particularly if neutral with no charge on the surface or minimal charge. All the molecular constituents of blood with the exception of the medium to large molecular weight proteins and lipids and substances which are bound to these proteins will diffuse with the glomerular filtrate through the basement membranes and ultimately from the tubular fluid.

Factors which affect the glomerular filtration rate will hence affect the quantity of drug removed per unit time in the glomerular filtrate. A significant decrease in cardiac output, (in the order of 20–30% of cardiac output) will result in a decrease in glomerular filtration hence a decrease in the clearance of a drug.

A second very important factor in determining the clearance of the drug from the plasma into the glomerular ultrafiltrate is the degree of plasma protein binding, that is a percentage of the drug that is present in the plasma bound to the plasma proteins and the avidity of the binding to those proteins. The amount of protein binding has little effect on clearance when the amount bound is below approximately 80%. Thus if 20% or more of the drug is unbound in plasma water indicating that there is a smaller number of binding sites and/or that the binding is less avid the drug can diffuse with the plasma water into the glomerular filtrate. As this occurs there is a shift from the drug bound to the plasma proteins into plasma water and the dynamics are such that the binding does not become an inhibiting factor when it is below 80%. As the percentage bound increases however, the clearance is appreciably affected and with drugs such as Frusemide, which is very tightly bound to plasma proteins, usually in excess of 99%, the total plasma glomerular clearance is very low compared to the glomerular filtration rate.

Clearance from whole blood is also influenced by the amount of drug which is bound or taken up into the cellular constituents of blood. An example where there is considerable binding of drug to red cells is the immuno-suppressive agent Cyclosporin A. In excess of 50% of Cyclosporin A is present within the red cells and if the whole blood concentration is determined and the clearance calculated then the clearance is markedly less than would be anticipated because of the binding within the red cells. This phenomenon will also occur with the heavy metal, lead, as 95% of lead in blood is present within the red cells and tightly bound to proteins within the cell.

Plasma protein binding of drugs can be affected by a number of factors: the only ones of clinical importance are the presence of other drugs which displace a drug from albumin or other binding proteins within the blood. Albumin binds anionic drugs on at least three different binding sites. Drugs which are organic acids can be displaced by other organic acids, both endogenous organic acids or another anionic drug. For example fatty acids can displace drugs from plasma protein binding sites and vice versa.

Passive reabsorbtion by simple diffusion

After the glomerular filtrate is formed, the fluid flows through the three segments of the proximal tubule, S1, S2 and S3, the loop of Henle and the distal tubule collecting duct. During this entire process the tubular epithelial cells, which are highly metabolically active, reabsorb salt water and other essential organic compounds such as glucose and amino acids by an active transport process. With the extraction of water however, other organic compounds which are present in the tubular fluid increase in concentration. This increase in concentration results in the establishment of a diffusion gradient between the tubular fluid and the tubular epithelial cell and then ultimately the plasma in the peritubular capillaries. The rate of diffusion of the drug through cell membranes is the limiting factor in determining how much drug will be reabsorbed. If the drug can diffuse at the same rate through cell membranes as does water, there will be an extremely small gradient established and the concentration of the drug in the tubular fluid will be approximately equal to the concentration of the drug in plasma. If however, the rate of diffusion of the drug through cell membranes is less than that of water, then a concentration gradient will be maintained through the entire segment of the nephron but the gradient will increase progressively as it passes down the length of the nephron with the progressive extraction of water. By the time the tubular fluid reaches the collecting duct it will contain the highest concentration present in the tubular fluid with the greatest gradient to the plasma. An example is the drug Paracetamol (Acetaminophen) which is a very commonly consumed antipyretic analgesic. Paracetamol is able to pass through cell membranes at a rate less than water and hence increases in concentration in the urine. As this concentration increases there is a gradient for reabsorption. Thus the overall clearance of a drug such as Paracetamol will be less than the glomerular filtration because of reabsorption of some of the Paracetamol as it passes down the tubule.

As the concentration within the tubular fluid component to plasma is the determining factor on how much is reabsorbed, any variation on the quantity of tubular fluid present will result in a change in clearance of the Paracetamol. Thus an increase in urine flow and volume will result in a decrease in the concentration of Paracetamol present in the tubular fluid with a resulting decrease in the concentration gradient and less reabsorption of Paracetamol. The end result will be an increased rate of clearance of Paracetamol from the plasma. This does not occur however with a drug such as Ethanol, which is reabsorbed at approximately the same rate across membranes as is water. Hence the concentration of Ethanol in the urine at the end of the collecting duct will be identical to the concentration in plasma. However, one could increase the rate of clearance of Ethanol via the kidneys by increasing the urine flow rate. For example, if the renal clearance of Ethanol is 1 ml/min then increasing the urine flow rate to 10 ml/min will result in an increase in the clearance of Ethanol by a factor of 10. However it is not as practical a method for removing Ethanol from the circulation because the rate clearance of Ethanol is so low relative to the total body load of Ethanol.

Drugs which are reabsorbed by passive diffusion are those drugs without a charge in tubular fluid. They must exhibit some characteristics of solubility in cell membranes or be of a molecular size similar to water to move through membrane pores which allow water to pass rapidly through the cell membranes. Hence extremely small molecular weight compounds such as Ethanol, methanol or very lipid soluble compounds such as the thiobarbiturates or phenacetin which have very high lipid solubility have renal clearance rates equal to urine flow rates. There is a reasonable correlation between the clearance characteristics and the octanol/water partition coefficient of a drug.

Active tubular secretion and reabsorption of organic acids

Many end products of metabolism and many drug metabolites are the result of extensive oxidation which results in the production of an organic acid. Many of these metabolites are produced in the liver but other organs also have metabolic capabilities. The most common groups of organic acids are conjugated with glucuronic acid or with sulphate, less commonly taurine and glycine derivatives. An additional organic acid is the end product of glutathione conjugation and subsequent breakdown resulting in macapturic acid conjugate. Once these conjugates are formed, if the compound has a large molecular weight, it will be actively secreted in the bile. If however it is a smaller molecule, the conjugate is released into the circulation and ultimately finds its way to the kidney. The organic acid may then be filtered at the glomerulus, unless it is tightly protein bound. The organic acid will also be present in the peritubular capillaries and a series of active transport processes present on the basal cell membrane of the tubular epithelial cell actively transports it into the proximal epithelial cell. The organic acid then is secreted into the lumen of the proximal tubule again by a process of facilitated diffusion or active transport.

The transporting proteins for organic acids in the proximal tubule have yet to be clearly identified and the final number of transport proteins present in the tubular epithelium remains to be determined. However there are at least three different transport systems with differing affinities for different organic acids. A similar situation exists with active transport facilitated diffusion at the apical cell membranes.

The overall transport of some organic acids is bi-directional such that in some circumstances an organic acid may undergo transport in both directions and will result in a renal clearance less equal to or greater than the glomerular filtration rate. The renal clearance of these organic acids will usually decrease if the plasma level is increased due to the saturation of the transport system.

The active tubular secretion of some organic acids particularly those which are not protein bound is such that their rate of clearance from plasma is equal to the effective renal plasma flow. With these particular groups of organic acids there is no net tubular reabsorption and extraction of the organic acid from the plasma is virtually complete. Drugs which belong to this class are most of the penicillins and many of the cephalosporins. This accounts for the very short half lives in plasma of these drugs. More recently developed cephalosporin antibiotics have a longer half life which is a result of lower affinity or absence of affinity of the drugs for the transport binding proteins.

Differing organic acids will compete for binding proteins and this knowledge resulted in the development of the drug Probenecid which is an organic acid, which competes with penicillin for the active transport system within the proximal tubules. This results in a decrease in the transport of penicillin and hence a decrease in rate of clearance from plasma which then prolongs the half life $(t\frac{1}{2})$ of penicillin.

Still other organic acids have differing mechanisms of secretion. The compound uric acid, an end product of metabolism, undergoes both active tubular reabsorption and tubular secretion. The drug Probenecid blocks to some extent active tubular secretion and reabsorption. However the drug has a greater affinity for the reabsorptive component and this results in an increased clearance of uric acid and hence the drug Probenecid is a uricosuric agent. A further example of this is salicylate. The various metabolites of aspirin which are also organic acids such as the glucuronide and salicyluric acid and salicylate itself compete for the various transport proteins and compete also with other organic acids. The end result of these interactions is that salicylates, at low doses, and plasma concentration result in the decreased excretion of uric acid and hence an elevation in the blood urid acid level. At high doses

there is a net increase in the rate of secretion of uric acid and hence the salicylate uricosuric and lowers the blood uric acid level. The low dose level is usually in the order of 1 to 2 gm/day but at intermediate doses (2 to 4 gm/day) there is usually no effect, and at greater than 4 gm/day of salicylate is quite significantly uricosuric.

Active tubular secretion and reabsorption of organic bases

A number of drugs are organic bases which are ionised at physiological pH. Examples of organic bases commonly used as drugs are Quinine and Nicotinamide. Compounds such as these undergo active secretion into the tubular lumen. Other organic bases will compete for these transport processes. The transport processes for inorganic bases are much less clearly defined than for organic acids.

Non ionic diffusion

Drugs whose pKa is within the physiological range of urine pH, that is between pH of 4.8 and 8.2 are reabsorbed by diffusion in the non ionised state but reabsorption is prevented when the drug is ionised. The other characteristics a drug needs to be reabsorbed by this mechanism are that its non ionised form is lipid soluble and can diffuse through cell membranes. Examples of drugs in this class are phenobarbitone, Silicate and Probenecid.

An example of the phenomenon is salicylate which has a pKa of approximately 4.5. At physiological pH of plasma of 7.4 the drug will largely be in the ionised state in the tubular fluid. The tubular fluid becomes more acid as it progresses along the nephron (particularly in the distal tubular collecting duct) and the drug becomes less ionized and hence in the resulting non ionised form is able to diffuse through the cell membranes. In its ionised form the ionic charge inhibits the transport across the membrane. Thus in an acid urine salicylate will have an increased reabsorption and hence its clearance and plasma half life will be prolonged and the clearance of the compound from plasma will decrease. Conversely in an alkaline urine where the drug would be expected to be maximally ionised there will be a decrease in the reabsorption of the ionic species, and hence the clearance will be increased and the plasma half life of the drug will therefore decrease.

RENAL METABOLISM OF DRUGS

METABOLISM IN THE RENAL CORTEX

Oxidation by cytochrome p450 mixed function oxidase

The cytochrome p450 mixed function oxidases are a ubiquitous group of cytochrome p450 containing enzymes. They are present in all living systems and phylogenetically are very old. There are currently 35 different cytochrome p450 mixed function oxidases identified by molecular genetic methods and 23 of these have been identified to be present in the human liver. More will be described in the future. As yet the exact number of cytochrome p450 mixed function oxidases expressed in the kidney and in the renal cortex in particular has not been identified but research indicates that there are multiple forms present. The kidney as an organ metabolising drugs is not important in a quantitative sense, despite the fact that the kidney may contain levels of enzyme activity comparable to the liver. The very large mass of the liver results in the liver being quantitatively more important in the overall metabolism of an administered drug. However the kidney can be important in metabolism of drugs when the process of metabolism itself is involved in organ specific toxicity. The most common and notable example of this is the commonly used analgesic paracetamol, which undergoes metabolism by cytochrome p450 MFO which can produce a toxic metabolite and ultimately lead to acute renal failure.

Cytochrome p450 monoxygenases also serve physiological functions within the kidney. A cytochrome p450 mixed function oxidase present in mitochondria is responsible for the hydroxylation of 25 hydroxy cholecalciferol to the active hormone 1,25 dihydroxy cholecalciferol.

The extent of oxidative metabolism has only been investigated for a limited number of drugs. The examples are listed in Table 3.1.

Table 3.1   Drug metabolism by the kidneys

	Drug	Metabolite
Oxidation	Pethidine	Pethidine N-oxide
	Bumetanide	Hydroxybumetanide
	Paracetamol	pBenzoquinonimine
Acetylation	Sulisoxazole	N-Acetylsulfisoxazole
	PAH	N-Acetyl PAH
Deacetylation	Paracetamol	Pamino phenol
Conjugation	Paracetamol	Glucuronide, sulphate
	Salicylic acid	Salicyluric acid
Esterase	Enalapril	Enalaprilat
Reduction	Prednisone	Prednisolone
	Sulindac	Sulindac sulfide

Prostaglandin synthase

The enzyme Prostaglandin Synthase is involved in the first two steps in the generation of the prostaglandin arachadonic acid $\rightarrow PGG_2 \rightarrow PGH_2$ PG Synthone PG_2.

The first step produces an oxygen containing lipid peroxide termed PGG_2 the second step is carried out by a second active site on the enzyme which stylises the peroxide to a lipid hydroxide and in the process co-oxidises any suitable available substrate which can be a drug. The most extensively studied example is paracetamol which is oxidised to p-Benzoquinonimine which is a highly reactive radical which is responsible for the drug's toxicity.

OXIDATION BY PROSTAGLANDIN SYNTHASE

Acetylation and deacetylation

Acetylation is a relatively minor pathway of drug metabolism and deacetylation also occurs. Acetylation usually occurs on amines and results in the amine being less biologically active. Acetylation occurs with sulphonamides, para amino salicylic acid. An unusual reaction occurs within the proximal tubular cells. These cells contain a deacetylase as well as acetylase and paracetamol (an acetyl para-amino phenol) undergoes deacetylation followed by the reacetylation in a cyclical manner. This results in the no net excretion of para-amino phenol and the reaction appears to have no net metabolic gain but has considerable implications for toxicity.

Conjugation reactions

As described above, the kidney is responsible for the active secretion of many drug conjugates that are produced in the liver, particularly glucuronic acid and sulphate conjugates. In vitro studies using isolated perfused kidneys or sub cellular fractions have demonstrated that the kidney can metabolise drugs by conjugation both with enzyme UDPG transferase producing glucuronic acid derivatives and the enzyme sulphatase producing sulphate conjugates. Examples of drugs which produce conjugates are paracetamol which produces both glruconide and sulphate conjugates and salicylic acid which results in the products in the production salisuiric acid.

Reduction reactions

These are minor pathways of drug metabolism but can result in the activation or deactivation of drugs. One of the most important examples is the conversion of prednisone which is biologically inactive to prednisolone, the biologically active corticosteroid.

Esterases

The esterase group of enzymes are ubiquitous, often multi-functional and are present within the kidney. They have been demonstrated to convert the pro drug enalapril to the active drug anaprilat by splitting the ester.

METABOLISM IN THE RENAL PAPILLAE

Prostaglandin synthase

The renal papillae is regarded by many as relatively metabolically inactive. However the papillae does contain extremely high levels of activity of the enzyme prostaglandin synthase. The activity of the enzyme in the papillae is several hundred times greater than in the renal cortex or other organs and with the high availability of substrate present in the interstitial cells of the medulla is an extremely active area for metabolism. The disease analgesic nephropathy occurs as a result of the activation of drugs like Paracetamol as a co-oxidised agent in the production of prostaglandins.

While the kidney is very active in drug metabolism in a qualitative sense, in a quantitative sense the kidney is responsible for a relatively small percentage of the total metabolism of drugs. The importance of the metabolism of drugs in the kidney relates more to the potential for toxicity because of reactive intermediates generated.

DRUGS WHICH EXERT A DIRECT PHARMACOLOGICAL EFFECT ON THE KIDNEY OTHER THAN DIURETICS

Uricosuric agents

There are several drugs which have been developed as uricosuric agents in order to promote the excretion of uric acid. Two agents are occasionally used for this purpose, the first is Probenacid (see above), the second is sulfinpyrazone which is a potent inhibitor of the tubular reabsorption of uric acid. Probenicid to some extent blocks both active tubular secretion and reabsorption. However the drug has a great affinity for the reabsorptive component and this results in an increased clearance of uric acid and hence the drug Probenicid is uricosuric promoting the additional secretion of uric acid. These drugs are not commonly used today and have been largely replaced by allopurinol which inhibits the production of uric acid. They are used occasionally in those patients who have had toxic side effects caused by allopurinol.

REFERENCES

Brater D C, Sokol P P, Hall S D, McKinney T D. Renal elimination of drugs, methods and determinants. In: The kidney, physiology and pathophysiology. 2nd Edn, Raven Press, New York Ch 107, pp 3597–3628

PART 2: DIURETICS
M. J. Field

DEFINITION AND PRINCIPLES OF ACTION

A *diuretic* is a substance which increases the flow of urine. Although conceptually this may be brought about by either an increase in glomerular filtration or a reduction in tubular reabsorption, in practical terms the commonly used drugs in this class all achieve the diuretic effect by an action in the tubular system. In the great majority of cases, this is achieved by primary interference with the reabsorption of sodium, hence the term *natriuretic*. A smaller number of agents produce a pure water diuresis by specifically interfering with the process of vasopressin-mediated water reabsorption, these substances being called *aquaretics*. Use of such agents is restricted to hypo-osmolar states characterised by pathological water retention, and they will not be further discussed here.

One mechanism of interfering with tubular reabsorption in a non site-specific manner is by administration of a substance which is freely filtered but not reabsorbed by any part of the tubular system. Such substances, of which mannitol is the principal clinical example, are known as *osmotic diuretics* since they entrain fluid osmotically within the tubular lumen and thereby limit the extent of sodium reabsorption in both proximal and distal segments. The resulting diuresis is therefore abrupt and short-lived, as it depends on the maintenance of an adequate concentration of filtered solute. Mannitol, which must be given by intravenous infusion, is used to achieve short-term diuresis in conditions associated with cell swelling, such as cerebral oedema. All other diuretics in common clinical use can be given by mouth, and interfere directly with tubular sodium reabsorption, as detailed below.

Sites and mechanisms of action

Over 99% of the sodium filtered at the glomerulus is reabsorbed along the tubular system under normal circumstances. Some 65% of this reabsorption occurs in the proximal tubule, 25% in the loop of Henle (principally in its thick ascending limb), about 5–8% in the early part of the distal tubule ('distal convoluted tubule'), and 2–3% in the late distal tubule and the contiguous cortical collecting duct segment. Only about 1% of the filtered sodium load is reclaimed in the medullary part of the collecting duct system.

The available oral diuretics interfere with sodium reabsorption in one or other of these sites by interacting specifically with the mechanisms mediating sodium transport in the epithelial cells of the respective tubules. This specificity arises from the fact that different membrane transport processes are involved in sodium reabsorption at each site, as illustrated in Figure 3.1 and Table 3.2.

Table 3.2 Sites and mechanisms of action of diuretic drugs (refer to Fig. 3.1)

Site	Drug class	Representative drugs	Mechanism of action
1: Proximal tubule	Carbonic anhydrase inhibitors	Acetazolamide	Block H^+ supply to apical Na, H exchanger
2: Thick ascending limb of loop of Henle	'Loop' diuretics	Frusemide, bumetanide, ethacrynic acid[*]	Block apical Na, K, 2Cl cotransporter
3: Early distal tubule	Thiazides and related drugs	Chlorothiazide, chlorthalidone, metolazone[†]	Block apical Na, Cl cotransporter
4: Late distal tubule/ cortical collecting duct	(a) Sodium channel blockers	(a) Amiloride, triamterene	(a) Block apical Na channel
	(b) Aldosterone antagonists	(b) Spironolactone	(b) Block aldosterone receptor in cytoplasm

[*] The precise mechanism of action of ethacrynic acid has not been defined, and may not be identical to that of frusemide and bumetanide
[†] Metolazone may also have a clinically significant action on proximal tubular reabsorption

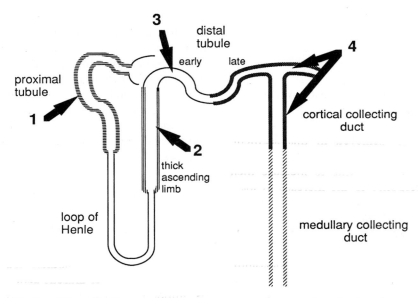

Fig. 3.1   Schematic diagram of the nephron to show the target sites of action of currently used diuretic drugs (see text for details). Representative drugs at each site are: 1, acetazolamide; 2, frusemide; 3, chlorothiazide; 4, amiloride

In general terms, these target processes are those mediating sodium entry into the tubular epithelial cell from the luminal fluid, rather than its subsequent pumping into the interstitial fluid compartment (and hence into the blood capillaries), across the basilateral membrane of the cells. This latter process is mediated in all segments by the sodium, potassium-ATPase, which is not itself the target of action of any of the available agents (inhibitors of this pump such as ouabain are not in clinical use as diuretics).

Proximal tubule

In the case of the proximal tubular cell, an inportant component of reabsorptive sodium flux is mediated via a sodium–hydrogen antiport carrier in the apical membrane of these cells, the operation of which is dependent on the generation of hydrogen ions within the cell mediated by the action of the enzyme carbonic anhydrase (for details of cellular mechanisms in this and subsequent nephron segments, *see* Chapter 1). Inhibition of this enzyme, also present in the brush border in this tubular segment, by drugs such as

acetazolamide interferes with the process of bicarbonate reabsorption and hence with the corresponding amount of sodium.

Whilst it might be expected that inhibition of proximal sodium reabsorption would yield a potentially massive diuresis, two factors limit the effectiveness of drugs like acetazolamide as clinically useful diuretics. First, only a small part of the total proximal reabsorption of sodium is mediated through the sodium hydrogen antiport, and second, sodium which escapes absorption in this segment may undergo compensatory reclamation in more distally located nephron segments. Furthermore, the metabolic acidosis generated during the action of these drugs leads to a self-limiting reduction in their effectiveness as the plasma bicarbonate falls.

Loop of Henle

The second tubular target site of diuretic action is the thick ascending limb of Henle's loop. Drugs such as **frusemide** interfere with the action of the apical cotransporter mediating entry of sodium from the luminal fluid into the cell in this segment.

The carrier in this case binds one sodium, one potassium and two chloride ions (the 'triple cotransporter'), and its inhibition leads to the loss of considerable amounts of sodium, accompanied by both potassium and chloride, into the urine. Note from Table 3.1 that the maximum extent of sodium excretion (up to 20% of the filtered load) is again somewhat less than the full extent of sodium reabsorption achieved in this segment. The reason once more relates to the capacity of more distally located segments to increase their reabsorption in response to the increase in load, thereby compensating somewhat for the primary action of the diuretic. It should also be noted that the increase in potassium excretion which accompanies this diuresis is largely related to the increased delivery of sodium into the potassium-secreting late distal tubule/cortical collecting duct site, especially as this segment is stimulated by aldosterone which is frequently elevated during diuretic therapy.

Loop-acting drugs significantly interfere with the capacity of the kidney to both concentrate and dilute the urine, since both these functions are effected in part by the thick ascending limb of the loop of Henle. This is in contrast to the capacity of proximally-acting drugs like acetazolamide to *enhance* dilution and concentration, since they deliver an increased amount of filtrate through the loop segment without themselves interfering with its action.

Early distal tubule

This is the third target site of diuretic action along the nephron, where the **thiazide** diuretics have their principal action. The tubular cells in this segment are specialised for sodium chloride reabsorption, which they achieve by uptake of sodium and chloride across the apical cell membrane via a NaCl cotransport carrier. By binding to this protein from the luminal surface, the thiazide drugs can effectively increase the maximum excretion rate of sodium by up to 6% of the filtered load. Once again, potassium excretion is enhanced during action by these drugs, not because they themselves interfere with potassium, but because they deliver increased amounts of sodium through the late distal site where sodium reabsorption is linked in part to potassium secretion. Thiazide-like drugs have no effect on urine concentration, which is related to loop of Henle function, but they do interfere with urine dilution since the early distal segment is water impermeable and normally contributes to further dilution of the luminal fluid. This explains the predisposition of patients treated with these drugs to develop hyponatraemia during periods of excessive hydration.

Late distal tubule/cortical collecting duct

Interference with sodium reabsorption in this tubular region does not lead to appreciable natriuresis or diuresis, since a relatively small fraction of the filtered sodium load is reabsorbed at this site. However diuretic action in this segment is important because the sodium reabsorption which normally does occur here is in part balanced by secretion of potassium ions and also hydrogen ions, these processes being strongly influenced by the lumen-negative transepithelial electrical potential difference generated by the movement of sodium from luminal fluid into the cell through a conductive channel in the apical membrane of the principal cell type in this segment (see Chapter 1). Drugs such as **amiloride** block this apical sodium channel, and hence lead to the loss of the transepithelial electrical potential difference, thereby indirectly inhibiting the movement of potassium and acid into the lumen. In contrast to diuretics acting in earlier tubular segments, drugs acting at this site retain rather than lose potassium from the body, and hence are called 'potassium sparing'.

This tubular segment is sensitive to the circulating steroid hormone aldosterone, which acts to enhance all the normal transport processes occurring, namely sodium reabsorption, and secretion of potassium and acid. Hence another mechanism of interference with the function of this segment is that of the aldosterone receptor-blocking agent **spironolactone**, which has similar metabolic effects to amiloride, except that it only interferes with that component of transport activity in this segment which is stimulated by aldosterone. It is of interest that this drug alone of

Table 3.3 Effects of diuretics on renal electrolyte and water excretion

Diuretic class	Na excretion[*]	K excretion	Anion excreted	Concentrating capacity	Diluting capacity
Carbonic anhydrase inhibitors	5	incr	HCO_3	incr	incr
Loop blockers	20	incr	Cl	decr	decr
Thiazides	6	incr	Cl	N	decr
K-sparers	2	decr	Cl/HCO_3	N	N

* maximum percent of filtered load of Na excreted into the urine during diuretic action; incr = increased; decr = decreased; N = no change

all the diuretics so far discussed, acts by access from the blood side of the epithelium rather than from the lumen.

While no currently available diuretics act on the medullary collecting duct component of sodium reabsorption, it is of interest that a significant part of the action of the naturally occurring substance, atrial natriuretic peptide, is thought to be via interference with sodium reabsorption at this site.

Table 3.3 summarises the effects on urinary electrolyte excretion of the four major groups of diuretic agents discussed above. The effects shown can be deduced from appreciation of the underlying tubular physiology and sites of action of the respective agents.

Chemistry and pharmacokinetics

Many of the diuretic substances mentioned above share the chemical feature of being sulphonamides, containing the $-SO_2NH_2$ grouping. This feature is common to acetazolamide and other carbonic anhyrase inhibitors, frusemide and bumetanide acting in the loop, and the thiazides as a class. This can give rise to therapeutic problems in patients who are allergic to sulphonamides but are in need of diuretic therapy. Fortunately a non-sulphonamide agent is available with action in the thick ascending limb of the loop of Henle similar to that of frusemide, namely ethacrynic acid, which is a phenoxyacetic acid derivative. All the drugs acting at the potassium secreting late distal tubular site are also non-sulphonamides, namely amiloride (a pyrazine), triamterene (a pteridine) and spironolactone (a steroid).

An important aspect of the pharmacokinetics of the diuretic drugs is that they are (with the exception of spironolactone), all weak organic acids or bases. This makes them susceptible to transport by the potent secretory carriers present in the proximal tubular epithelium, thereby increasing their plasma clearance rate and their delivery into the tubular fluid along the length of the nephron. This is important for the optimum effectiveness of these agents since all (again with the exception of spironolactone), have as target site of action, a luminal membrane transport process in a particular nephron segment. Luminal drug concentration is also increased by net water reabsorption along the length of the nephron. Proximal tubular secretion of diuretics is particularly important since most of these agents are strongly protein-bound in the plasma, which would itself lead to a very low delivery rate into the tubule by glomerular filtration alone.

Adverse effects of diuretics

Diuretic therapy is frequently complicated by a number of unwanted effects, some of which represent predictable physiological consequences of their mechanism of action, but others are of poorly understood metabolic or idiosyncratic origin.

Considering the loop-acting agents (such as frusemide) and the early distal drugs (like the thiazides) together, it would be predicted that *hypovolaemia* with associated postural hypotension and rise in plasma urea could occur with either class of diuretic, though it is encountered more frequently with frusemide being the more potent agent. A number of electrolyte disturbances may arise with frequent or prolonged use. *Hyponatraemia* may occur, and is usually mild, though in pathological states associated with high levels of circulating vasopressin or with unrestricted fluid intake, more severe falls in plasma sodium are seen. *Hypokalaemia* is perhaps the most common metabolic effect of loop and thiazidelike agents. It results largely from stimulation of late distal potassium secretion due to increased sodium and fluid delivery into this segment, but is frequently further stimulated by high circulating aldosterone levels. It is more often a problem with prolonged use of thiazides than with the shorter-acting loop agents, probably because the longer duration of action of the thiazides does not permit a compensatory phase of potassium retention by the kidney in the daily cycle.

Metabolic alkalosis also occurs with these agents due to stimulation of distal acid losses. *Hypomagnesaemia* can result either from impaired magnesium reabsorption in the loop with frusemide and related drugs, or from decreased early distal reabsorption with the thiazides. *Hyperuricaemia*, sometimes precipitating gout, can be induced by any volume-depleting agent like the diuretics, because of the compensatory increase in urate reabsorption by the proximal tubule under these conditions. Calcium is affected differently by these two classes of drugs, the loop agents promoting calcium loss and occasionally *hypocalcaemia*, while the thiazides promote calcium reabsorption along the distal tubule and can predispose to *hypercalcaemia*.

It is less well understood why the commonly used diuretic drugs cause the metabolic disturbances of *glucose intolerance* and hyperglycaemia in those predisposed to diabetes, as well as *hyperlipidaemia*, involving mild elevations in both cholesterol and triglyceride fractions. The long term significance of both of these disturbances has not been definitively established.

The adverse effects relating to the potassium-sparing agents acting in the late distal segment do not relate to sodium and volume depletion since these are not powerful natriuretic agents. However the property of retaining potassium and acid can become a problem in patients with abnormal loads of these substances, or in the presence of significant renal impairment, when *hyperkalaemia* and *metabolic acidosis* can develop.

Other complications of diuretic use are not clearly related to their physiological mechanisms of action. *Hypersensitivity reactions* are not uncommon especially with the sulphonamide group of drugs (most often the thiazides), and these can involve the kidney with interstitial nephritis, or dermatitis, vasculitis or bone marrow reactions. The thiazides are also occasionally implicated in triggering *pancreatitis* and acute *cholecystitis*. They are also associated with *impotence* in the male though the mechanisms are not clear. The loop-acting drugs are capable of causing significant *ototoxicity* by interference with electrolyte transport in the inner ear, though this is usually only seen after bolus intravenous doses. Spironolactone can induce gynaecomastia.

Combinations of diuretic drugs

Diuretics of two or more classes are sometimes given together for one of two reasons. First, it may be desired to reduce an unwanted electrolyte disturbance produced by one agent (e.g. hypokalaemia produced by a thiazide), by co-administering an agent with an opposite action (e.g. addition of amiloride to prevent losses of potassium, acid and magnesium). While there are advantages in compliance and convenience by including these drugs in a single tablet (e.g. Moduretic), the fixed ratio of component drug doses leads to loss of flexibility in adjusting the relative contributions of each.

A second reason for using combinations of diuretics is to achieve an increase in natriuresis where a state of diuretic 'resistance' has developed. This phenomenon is most often due to the development of compensatory sodium retention by tubular segments not affected by the diuretic of primary choice, e.g. enhanced proximal and distal sodium reabsorption during treatment with a loop-acting drug. Such compensation may be mediated via plasma volume depletion with its action on the proximal tubule and by hyperaldosteronism acting at the late distal segment. It follows from this that a potent diuresis might be established under these circumstances by combined use of a loop drug with a thiazide-like agent to block early distal reabsorption, and also when appropriate a potassium-sparing drug acting at the late distal segment. A special role for the thiazide-like drug metolazone has been proposed here since it appears also to have a partial inhibitory action on proximal reabsorption. Although such 'sequential nephron blockade' can achieve diuresis in otherwise intractable situations (e.g. advanced congestive heart failure), it is clearly fraught with the potential complications associated with electrolyte and fluid losses from the nephron, and should only be done with caution by experienced practitioners with hospital facilities to monitor and adjust the course of therapy.

Drug interactions

Apart from the interactions between diuretics themselves, as outlined above, a number of other pharmaceutic agents can interfere with diuretic action. Treatment with non-steroidal anti-inflammatory drugs can blunt diuretic action, since they impair prostaglandin generation within the renal medulla, which is thought to be a contributing factor in diuretic effectiveness. The secretion of diuretics by the proximal tubule can be interfered with by other drugs sharing this pathway when present in high concentrations, e.g. penicillin or probenecid. These may also result in blunted effectiveness of an administered diuretic.

Electrolyte complications can be important during co-administration of diuretics with other drugs. The effect of diuretic-induced hypokalaemia to increase the toxicity of digoxin therapy is well known. On the other hand, caution must be exercised in the use of potassium-sparing drugs like amiloride during co-administration of other potassium-retaining agents such as the ACE inhibitors, or indeed of KCl supplements themselves.

Indications and guidelines for use

These are more properly dealt with in detail by other texts, but some principles may be given here. An important group of indications is the *oedema*

disorders, such as congestive cardiac failure, cirrhosis with ascites, and the nephrotic syndrome. While a thiazide drug may be the first choice in the early stages of some of these conditions, frusemide or another loop agent is frequently required at some stage. In either case it is often rational and appropriate to co-administer a potassium-sparing drug. The oedema associated with chronic renal failure is not responsive to therapy with thiazides because of the low GFR, and high doses of loop agents are generally required. Potassium sparing agents are contraindicated in this setting.

The second major indication for diuretics is in the treatment of *hypertension*. While the advent of newer classes of potent antihypertensives has made diuretics less central for this indication than in previous decades, they still have a role in the monotherapy of many patients (especially the elderly), with mild to moderate hypertension, or in the adjunctive treatment of patients with more severe hypertension where other single agents are incompletely effective. This is particularly the case in the severe hypertension associated with renal failure, where high doses of loop drugs are needed to reduce expanded extracellular fluid volume.

There are a number of additional miscellaneous indications for diuretic use. Loop-acting drugs have a role in the treatment of *hypercalcaemia* after adequate hydration has been achieved, while the thiazides can be used to reduce calcium excretion in *idiopathic hypercalciuria*. Conditions characterised by primary or secondary *hyperaldosteronism* are well treated with spironolactone, while *glaucoma* and some cases of resistant metabolic alkalosis can be treated with acetazolamide. The thiazides have a role in the management of *nephrogenic diabetes insipidus*, while the loop-acting drugs are sometimes used together with normal saline infusions to force a diuresis in the management of some types of *poisoning*.

Some general principles may be expounded to guide the use of diuretics in all indications. First, they should be used in the *minimum dose possible* to achieve the required effect. In the case of the treatment of hypertension, this may be as little as a half or a quarter of the usually marketed tablet size, e.g. hydrochlorothiazide 12.5 mg daily. Second, diuretics should be used for as *short a period of time* as is essential for management of the underlying condition, and therapy may on occasions be intermittent (e.g. second daily) rather than given on a continuous daily basis.

Third, due attention must be given to the potential for electrolyte and metabolic *side effects* of diuretic action, and this will involve regular biochemistry checks during the period of therapy. Fourth, patients should be advised appropriately about modification of their *diet* while taking diuretic therapy. This may involve reduction of excessive salt intake, consumption of appropriate potassium and magnesium containing foods, and modest restriction of fluid intake to prevent dilutional hyponatraemia.

Finally, diuretics should *not* be used for frivolous or inappropriate indications, such as weight reduction or the control of trivial peripheral oedema, which may rebound on cessation of therapy and lead to a pattern of 'diuretic dependence' (one form of cyclical oedema).

FURTHER READING

Dirks J H, Sutton R A L 1986 Diuretics: physiology, pharmacology and clinical use. W B Saunders, Philadelphia

Field M J, Lawrence J R 1986 Complications of thiazide diuretic therapy: an update. Medical Journal of Australia 144: 641–644

Greger R, Heidland A 1992 Action and clinical use of diuretics. In: Cameron S et al (eds) Oxford textbook of clinical nephrology pp 197–223

Jacobson H R December 15 1987 Diuretics: mechanisms of action and uses. pp 129–156

Suki W N, Eknoyan G 1992 Physiology of diuretic action. In: Seldin D W, Giebisch G (eds) The kidney, physiology and pathophysiology 2nd edn Raven Press, New York pp 3629–3670

Diagnosis of renal disease

4. Renal investigative techniques

J. A. Whitworth   J. R. Lawrence

INTRODUCTION

The functions of the kidney have been reviewed in Chapter 1 and include excretion of non-volatile wastes; regulation of the volume and composition of extracellular fluid, acid–base balance, blood pressure, erythropoiesis and calcium metabolism; and metabolic activities such as gluconeogenesis.

Renal investigative techniques include those which examine the structural integrity of the kidney, such as urinalysis, microscopy, renal imaging (reviewed in Ch. 5) and renal biopsy; tests which examine renal function, including excretory function and hormone estimation; and immunological and microbiological techniques.

URINALYSIS

Urinalysis is an essential part of the physical examination. Although a negative urinalysis does not exclude renal disease, simple urinalysis together with measurement of blood pressure is a valuable method of screening for renal disease. Urinary abnormalities are an index of structural renal disease.

Ideally, the urine should be examined fresh and if possible the patient should void in front of a doctor. The colour of the urine is examined microscopically. This will show whether the urine is concentrated or dilute; whether it contains any unusual material such as gravel, stones or papillae; whether it is cloudy and offensive, as in infection, or frothy, as in the presence of proteinuria; or whether it is discoloured. Red urine commonly represents haematuria but it may also be due to a variety of other conditions, e.g. haemoglobinuria, anthocyanins (beetroot and berries), heavy urate concentration (which gives a pink urine), pyridium, phenindione, vegetable dyes used in food colouring, porphyrin, or phenolphthalein in alkaline urine. Normal urine is yellow due to the pigment urochrome. The presence of haemoglobin gives the urine the colour of port whereas urobilinogen gives a reddish-brown colour and bilirubin looks like stout. Methylene blue stains urine blue. Turbidity of urine can be due to either salts (e.g. urates, phosphates, oxalates) or pus. Lymph in the urine gives rise to a milky appearance, called chyluria, and occurs with a lympho-ureteric fistula.

Haematuria

A positive test for blood indicates free haemoglobin or myoglobin in the urine. If a positive test is obtained, the urine should be examined microscopically.

Proteinuria

Commercial 'dip-stix' are more sensitive to albumin than to other proteins. Bence Jones protein is usually not detected. A trace of protein on stick testing is usually not significant although it requires repeated observation; but if readings of one plus or higher are obtained and the proteinuria is considered clinically significant (proteinuria may occur in a variety of conditions, including fever, exercise and chronic cardiac failure), a 24-hour urine protein estimation should be performed.

Table 4.1 Distribution of haematuria and proteinuria in glomerular disease

Biopsy diagnosis	Haematuria (%)	Haematuria + proteinuria (%)
Minor glomerular lesions	26	22
Mesangial proliferative glomerulonephritis	26	23
Focal and segmental proliferative glomerulonephritis	9	16
Mesangiocapillary glomerulonephritis	3	7
Membranous glomerulonephritis	3	10
Focal and segmental hyalinosis/sclerosis	11	21

Proteinuria and haematuria

Proteinuria due to glomerular disease is very commonly accompanied by haematuria. The finding of haematuria combined with proteinuria is particularly important in the diagnosis of renal disease, although in our experience the proportion of patients with glomerulonephritis who have haematuria alone is similar to that with haematuria plus proteinuria (Table 4.1).

Glycosuria

Glycosuria commonly reflects hyperglycaemia but may occur as an isolated finding (so-called renal glycosuria) or with proximal tubular dysfunction. The renal threshold for glucose may be altered in renal disease. Glycosuria is sometimes seen in patients with nephrotic syndrome and heavy proteinuria. Conversely, in patients with diabetic nephropathy, glycosuria may disappear because of the decreased filtered load of glucose due to poor renal function.

pH

A spot estimation of urinary pH is of limited value. However, a highly alkaline urine suggests infection with urea-splitting organism (e.g. *Proteus* species), infection stones or renal tubular acidosis. A low urinary pH is sometimes a clue to the presence of uric acid stones.

Bacteriuria

'Dip-stix' incorporating a nitrite detector are used to screen for bacteriuria. These tests are of limited value, particularly in women, in whom a randomly collected urine is very frequently contaminated. In certain circumstances, however, e.g. in pregnancy or infancy, a positive finding can be a useful guide to the need for proper urine microscopy and quantitative bacteriology.

Specific gravity

Measurement of specific gravity is of limited clinical value, as it depends on the state of hydration and other factors. A fixed specific gravity is characteristic of chronic renal failure, as the kidney is unable to either concentrate or dilute the urine.

MICROSCOPY

Microscopic examination of the urine provides a valuable index of structural renal disease. It can be performed relatively simply by the practitioner in the surgery (on a fresh specimen). The urine (10 ml) is centrifuged for 5–10 min at 3000 r/min and the urinary deposit is then resuspended in the last 0.5 ml of urine. Quantitative microscopy of the resultant suspension is more accurate than simply counting cells per high-power field, and with experience is as quick.

Cells

The normal range for urinary red cells depends on the individual laboratory and is $0.8–2 \times 10^6/l$ by conventional microscopy and probably up to ten times higher when using the more sensitive phase contrast microscopy. The finding of haematuria in the past led to extensive urological examination in patients with unrecognized glomerulonephritis. Birch & Fairley (1979) have described a simple technique for differentiating glomerular from non-glomerular (lower tract) red cells. The red cells normally found in urine are typical glomerular cells and non-glomerular cells are not normally seen. Thus the finding of non-glomerular cells is an

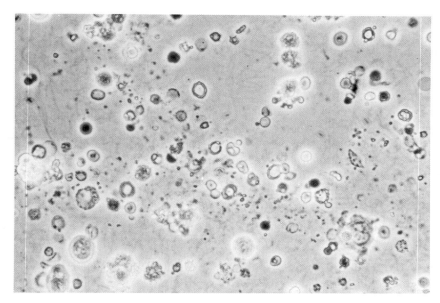

Fig. 4.1 Glomerular haematuria. (Photomicrograph kindly provided by Dr Doug Birch.)

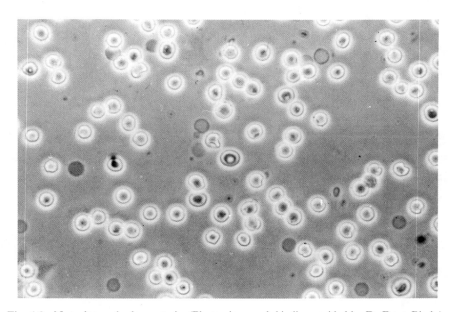

Fig. 4.2 Non-glomerular haematuria. (Photomicrograph kindly provided by Dr Doug Birch.)

indication for radiological and urological examination of the urinary tract whereas an abnormal count of glomerular red cells indicates glomerular disease. Typically, cells from the renal pelvis, ureter or bladder are all of one type, uniform in size and shape (isomorphic), whereas glomerular red cells are quite irregular in size and shape (dysmorphic) (Figs. 4.1 and 4.2).

In our laboratory less than 2×10^6 'white' cells/ l is the upper limit of normal. The commonest cause of pyuria (excluding contamination) is urinary infection. Sterile pyuria may occur in association with stones, analgesic nephropathy and a variety of other renal diseases, but the presence of sterile pyuria should always alert the practitioner to the presence of occult infection, e.g. renal tuberculosis.

Other cells seen in the urine are squamous and transitional epithelial cells and renal tubular cells.

The findings of eosinophils in the urine suggests a diagnosis of acute allergic interstitial nephritis and is valuable in the differential diagnosis of patients with acute renal failure (see Ch. 13).

Casts

Hyaline casts (Fig. 4.3) are formed from Tamm–Horsfall protein in the renal tubule. They dissolve rapidly in alkaline urine. Occasional hyaline casts may be seen in normal urine. They are increased by diuretics, fever and exercise, and are prominent in renal disease. However, granular and cellular casts indicate underlying renal parenchymal disease. Red cell casts (Fig. 4.4) are considered to indicate glomerular bleeding. The reddish tint characteristic of a red cell cast can be seen most easily on phase contrast microscopy.

White cell casts (Fig. 4.5) usually indicate pyelonephritis. Granular casts (Fig. 4.6) occur in a variety of renal diseases and may resemble red cell casts made up of haemolysed cells. Cellular casts are hyaline or granular casts containing renal tubular cells or, in acute pyelonephritis, polymorphonuclear leucocytes. In systemic lupus erythematosus a 'telescoped' sediment may be seen containing a wide range of cells and casts.

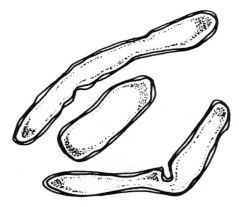

Fig. 4.3 Urinary sediment: hyaline casts

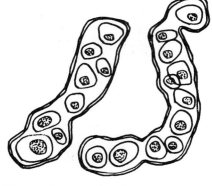

Fig. 4.5 Urinary sediment: white cell casts

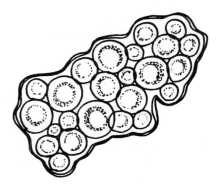

Fig. 4.4 Urinary sediment: red cell casts

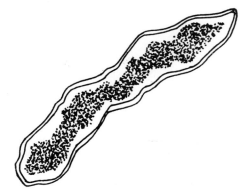

Fig. 4.6 Urinary sediment: granular cast

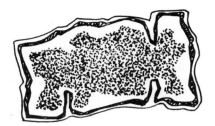

Fig. 4.7 Urinary sediment: waxy cast

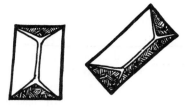

Fig. 4.8 Urinary sediment: triple phosphate crystals. Note 'coffin lid' shape

Waxy casts (Fig. 4.7) occur in chronic renal disease, and free fat globules and fat bodies are associated with some forms of glomerulonephritis and are almost universally found when proteinuria is very heavy.

Crystals

The finding of crystalluria is common but not of great diagnostic value in renal disease. Triple phosphate crystals are common, particularly in alkaline urine, and are shaped like a coffin lid (Fig. 4.8) Oxalate crystals are best seen in acid urine and resemble an envelope (Fig. 4.9). Uric acid crystals have a variety of forms, and are found in acid urine. They are seen in normal individuals as well as in those with increased uric acid excretion. The finding of hexagonal cystine crystals may identify cystinuria.

Urinary sediment in pregnancy

The urinary deposit can be very helpful in evaluating renal disease in pregnancy.

The normal red cell count in pregnancy is similar to that of the non-pregnant population and the cells are of glomerular origin. When haematuria is found in pregnancy (usually on dipstick testing), it is important to ascertain the morphology of the red cells. Non-glomerular cells indicate the presence of a stone or tumour, contamination with vaginal bleeding, or urinary tract infection. Up to 20 weeks, the finding of glomerular haematuria (frequently in association with proteinuria and/or abnormal casts) provides strong evidence for the presence of glomeru-

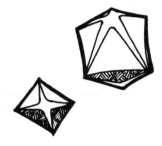

Fig. 4.9 Urinary sediment: oxalate crystals. Note 'envelope' shape

lonephritis. As term is approached, diagnosis becomes more difficult because glomerular haematuria is very common in pre eclampsia (PET). Red cell counts may be as high as 100 000 or more in PET and red cell casts may occur, but the higher the count the more likely is an underlying glomerulonephritis. There is a high incidence of free fat and hyaline casts in the urine of patients with PET.

Pyuria is a frequent but not invariable finding in urinary tract infection in pregnancy. Interpretation may be difficult, as pyuria is always present in poorly collected midstream specimens and good specimens are difficult to obtain in late pregnancy. Nucleated cells which are not leucocytes are often present and Prescott stain is invaluable in making the differentiation. Fastidious microorganisms are much commoner than conventional urinary pathogens in the urine of pregnant women, and the commonest bacterium is *Gardnerella vaginalis*. Microscopic examination of appropriate specimens (catheter specimen of urine or suprapubic bladder aspirate) frequently suggests its presence by the finding of squames covered with very small bacteria, the so-called clue cell.

QUANTITATIVE ESTIMATION OF PROTEINURIA

The normal urinary protein excretion is less than 150 mg/24 h, but the normal range may vary slightly from laboratory to laboratory. Most of the protein in normal urine migrates with the globulin fraction, and the remainder with plasma albumin. Tamm–Horsfall mucoprotein is a high molecular weight protein which migrates as an α-globulin and is excreted at a rate of about 25 mg/day. It is the major protein constituent of casts in the urine. Proteinuria (urinary protein excretion above normal) is a useful marker for underling renal disease although it can occur in the absence of renal disease (e.g. in heart failure). Conversely, the absence of proteinuria does not exclude underlying kidney disease (e.g. interstitial nephropathy). Proteinuria may occur with exercise or fever. Postural (orthostatic) proteinuria is a condition, most commonly seen in adolescents and young adults, in which proteinuria occurs in the upright but not the recumbent position. Although postural proteinuria is widely regarded as benign, it may also occur with underlying renal disease and may precede persistent proteinuria in some patients. Nonetheless, although some of these patients do have renal lesions on biopsy, the prognosis appears to be good. Persistent proteinuria clearly requires further investigation.

Paraproteins

Monoclonal proteins represent excessive quantities of normally occurring immunoglobulins. They are characterized by being strictly localized in their migration on electrophoresis. At least some monoclonal antibodies have been shown to have antibody activity, e.g. against bacterial antigens. When only light chains are synthesized Bence Jones proteinaemia and proteinuria is produced. Myeloma is discussed in Chapter 11.

Bence Jones protein

Urinary light chains have unique thermal properties. Bence Jones protein precipitates on heating at 56° and then dissolves at 100°C. As the urine cools, the Bence Jones protein again precipitates out. Sulphosalicylic acid precipitates urinary protein, including Bence Jones protein (Exton's test), and a negative sulphosalicylic acid test excludes the presence of Bence Jones proteinuria. Albustix (Ames Company) do not detect Bence Jones protein and thus a negative test does not in any way exclude Bence Jones proteinuria. The finding of a monoclonal protein in the serum requires further investigation by protein electrophoresis and immunoelectrophoresis of urine. Similarly, this is indicated in patients with multiple myeloma, amyloidosis, Waldenstrom's macroglobulinaemia and other gammopathies. The diagnosis of these diseases is discussed in Chapter 11.

RENAL BIOPSY

Renal biopsy enables histological examination of renal tissue, from which a pathological diagnosis can be made and a prognosis given. The technique was introduced by Iversen & Brun (1951) and popularized by Kark (1956).

Occasionally, e.g. in patients with a single native kidney or small kidneys, biopsy specimens are obtained by CT (computerized tomography) guidance or even open surgery under general anaesthesia, but in general renal biopsy is performed by transcutaneous puncture under local anaesthesia usually under ultrasound control.

Indications

In broad terms, renal biopsy is indicated in adults to diagnose and assess diffuse renal disease, e.g. glomerulonephritis, nephrotic syndrome, acute or chronic renal failure of unknown aetiology, and renal allograft rejection. Repeat renal biopsy is also indicated in certain circumstances to assess disease activity and response to therapy.

Precautions

Except for biopsy of the renal allograft, which is technically simpler than biopsy of a native kidney, it is essential to establish that the patient has two functioning kidneys. Although nephrectomy is a very rare complication of biopsy, the risk of closed biopsy in a single native kidney is probably sufficient to warrant an open procedure. Renal size and position should be noted.

Biopsy should only be undertaken in patients with a normal coagulation profile. We routinely check bleeding time, platelet count, prothrombin time and partial thromboplastin time. Blood pressure should be controlled before biopsy is undertaken. The nature and risks of the procedure should be carefully explained to the patient and informed consent obtained.

Procedure

Renal biopsy is a procedure for the experienced operator. Light premedication is given before the procedure, which is performed under radiological or ultrasound control to allow accurate localization of the kidney.

The patient is placed in the prone position with a bolster under the rib cage, and the renal areas are draped and prepared under sterile conditions. Local anaesthetic is injected under the skin and along the needle track, and a fine needle is gently inserted — usually aiming for 1 cm inside the outer border of the lower pole of the right kidney. The needle is advanced while the patient holds his breath in deep inspiration.

When the needle begins to swing with respiration, it is in the kidney and measurement gives the depth of the kidney. Classically the Franklin modification of the Vim–Silverman needle was used but has been replaced by disposable needles (e.g. Tru-cut®, Travenol®). The needle is advanced to the required depth while the patient holds his breath; the trochar is removed, the split needle inserted and the biopsy taken; the needles are then removed. Pressure is applied firmly to the renal area to minimize bleeding and a firm dressing is applied. The patient then lies supine for at least 4 hours, while half-hourly recordings of blood pressure and pulse rate are taken, and remains in bed for at least 24 hours. Heavy lifting, strenuous exertion and body contact sports should be avoided for 2 weeks following biopsy.

Usually cores are taken for light, immunofluorescent and electron microscopy.

Complications

The frequency of complications depends on the experience of the operator, patient factors (e.g. uraemia), the number of cores taken and the nature of the underlying disease. Bleeding is the major complication of renal biopsy.

Macroscopic haematuria occurs in about 5% of patients, may cause renal colic and/or clot retention and may require transfusion. The majority of patients settle with bed rest but occasionally embolization of a bleeding point under radiological control or surgical exploration is necessary.

Perirenal haematoma is extremely common, as judged by routine CT scanning post-biopsy, but is of clinical significance in only about 1% of patients. Occasionally, the perirenal haematoma may be infected and perirenal abscess or septicaemia may occur.

Although arteriovenous fistulae are commonly seen if renal arteriography is performed routinely post-biopsy, they are rarely of clinical significance.

RENAL FUNCTION TESTS

Glomerular filtration rate (GFR)

The concept of clearance is fundamental to an understanding of renal function tests. The clearance (C) of a substance is a measure of the volume of plasma cleared of the substance per unit time. Thus

$$C = \frac{UV}{P}$$

where U is the urinary concentration, V the urine flow rate and P the plasma concentration of the substance in question.

GFR is ideally measured by a substance which is freely filtrable, not protein-bound, not reabsorbed or secreted, and biologically inert so that it has no effect on renal function and is easily measurable. Inulin, fructose polysaccharide, is the accepted standard for measurement of GFR. Unfortunately, inulin clearance measurements are only appropriate for laboratory conditions, and in clinical practice the most widely used measurement of glomerular filtration rate is the clearance of endogenous creatinine. Clearance of creatinine approximates inulin clearance by virtue of two cancelling errors. Creatinine is not only filtered but also secreted (which would give a falsely high value for creatinine clearance), but the estimation of creatinine in plasma with conventional techniques gives a high plasma reading which cancels out the other error. The major source of error in creatinine clearance measurements is incomplete collection of urine. In our laboratory, normal creatinine clearance is 1.5–2.5 ml/s. At low GFR, creatinine clearance overestimates GFR, in contrast to inulin which underestimates it.

[51]Cr-labelled EDTA is a radionuclide handled by the kidney in a fashion comparable to inulin. Chromium-51 is a γ-emitter. The tracer is injected intravenously and serial venous samples are taken at 60 and 150 minutes post-injection for the estimation of GFR, which determines the rate at which counts fall. A single-shot technique gives similar results. This technique is most valuable in the diagnosis of minor degrees of renal impairment and is of limited value in renal failure. Other radioisotopes used to measure GFR include ^{99m}Tc-labelled DPTA (diethylene triaminepent-acetic acid) and [125]I- or ^{131}I-diatrizoate or iothalamate.

A DTPA scan provides functional information. The patient is injected with ^{99m}Tc-DTPA and multiple images of the kidneys are obtained over a 30-minute period. Immediately following injection, rapid imaging is performed to provide an assessment of arterial perfusion. Further imaging assesses glomerular function as the radiotracer behaves like inulin and is only excreted by glomerular filtration. The relative contribution of each kidney to total GFR can be accurately quantified.

In routine clinical practice, plasma creatinine is the best single guide to renal function. It depends on muscle bulk and is thus lower in children, women and the elderly, but tends to be reasonably constant in any given individual. It is relatively independent of diet, unlike plasma urea, which reflects among other things protein intake, catabolic state and hydration. In clinical practice the concentration of urea correlates with uraemic

symptoms. For example, a patient with severe renal failure and a plasma creatinine of 1.0 mmol/l may be nauseated, anorexic and lethargic with a urea of 40 mmol/l but feel well following institution of a low protein diet with the same creatinine but a urea of 20 mmol/l. The rise in plasma creatinine with a fall in GFR is hyperbolic rather than linear, so that a rapid rise occurs in late renal disease whereas earlier there may be considerable renal functional loss with very little change in creatinine. In our laboratory normal plasma creatinine is 0.05–0.11 mmol/l and urea 2.5–8.3 mmol/l. In clinical practice the modified Cockcroft–Gault formula is an adequate estimate of GFR.

In following the progression of chronic renal disease, it is useful to plot changes in glomerular filtration rate. GFR falls in a roughly linear manner in a number of chronic diseases with time, and any alteration in this curve might be an indication that a potentially reversible complication has developed, e.g. obstruction. Plasma creatinine tends to rise in a hyperbolic curve but this can be converted into a straight line by plotting the reciprocal of plasma creatinine, and this is useful in practice. The ratio of plasma urea to creatinine provides further useful information. If this is high, diuretic therapy, dehydration, profound catabolism, steroid therapy, gastrointestinal bleeding or obstruction should be considered. A low ratio is associated with a low protein diet or severe liver disease. It is important to remember that GFR increases in pregnancy so that both plasma creatinine and urea are normally low.

Effective renal plasma flow

Effective renal plasma flow, measured by ^{125}I-hippuran (sodium iodo-hippurate) or ^{131}I-hippuran (para-amino hippurate or PAH) clearance, is not widely used in clinical practice. Information on individual renal function can be very useful to the clinician, e.g. in the assessment of renal artery disease or unilateral renal disease such as hydronephrosis. Split renal function studies using bilateral ureteric catheterization are rarely used, as they are technically difficult and associated with significant morbidity. Radionuclide techniques are now widely used for this purpose to give an estimation of the relative contribution of each kidney. Renal imaging is discussed in Chapter 5.

Tubular function: urine acidification

Tests of discrete tubular functions are usually only performed in specialist units. One of the most widely performed is the urinary acidification test of Wrong and Davies, which is used when renal tubular acidosis is suspected. If the patient is acidaemic (low plasma bicarbonate), urinary pH should be 5.3 or less. In the absence of systemic acidosis, gelatin-coated ammonium chloride capsules (0.1 g/kg body weight) are given with water. Plasma electrolytes are checked to ensure that bicarbonate falls, and urine pH is measured (by pH meter) on hourly urine samples for 6 hours. The pH normally falls to 5.3 or below. The test is invalid in the presence of urea-splitting organisms which render the urine alkaline. Potassium deficiency and hypercalciuria may also impair the ability to reduce urinary pH.

Urinary concentration

Urinary concentration is tested either by fluid deprivation or administration of vasopressin (anti-diuretic hormone). In normal individuals, severe fluid deprivation will achieve a higher osmolality than vasopressin administration. For screening purposes, an early morning specimen should be tested. If the osmolality is higher than 700 mosmol/l, further investigation is unlikely to reveal a defect. Fluid deprivation is not pleasant for the patient, and can be dangerous if diuresis continues, e.g. in diabetes insipidus, or if the patient has chronic renal failure.

Injection of 5 IU vasopressin tannate in oil will normally produce a urine osmolality of 750 mmol/l or more. Secretion of antidiuretic hormone is influenced by a variety of factors, including emotion and stress, which may make interpretation difficult.

Other tests of tubular function, e.g. diluting capacity, phosphate handling, PAH (p-amino-hippuric acid) transport, are rarely used in adult clinical practice.

Aminoaciduria

Aminoaciduria is the excretion of greater than normal quantities of amino acids in the urine. Normally amino acids are freely filtered and very largely reabsorbed in the proximal convoluted tubule. Under certain pathological conditions where tubular reabsorption is defective, there is net secretion of amino acids. Aminoaciduria is evaluated by qualitative chromatography of the urine. Aminoacidurias are considered further in Chapters 17 and 26.

Urinary sodium concentration

Urinary sodium concentration should be related to total urine output as this determines total urinary sodium excretion. If urine output is high, the sodium concentration may be relatively low despite a large sodium excretion and, if urine flow is poor, the urinary sodium concentration may be high despite a low 24-hour excretion.

When the extracellular fluid volume is contracted the urinary sodium excretion should be extremely low. Diuretic therapy is a common cause of a high urinary sodium excretion in the presence of extracellular volume depletion, but in the absence of diuretics urinary sodium wastage suggests adrenal or renal insufficiency.

As discussed in Chapter 20 on acute renal failure, measurement of urinary sodium excretion is helpful in distinguishing between reversible pre-renal acute renal failure, where urinary sodium excretion is low, and established acute renal failure, where it is high.

Low urinary sodium excretion despite expansion of extracellular fluid volume occurs in a variety of oedematous conditions, e.g. the nephrotic syndrome, heart failure and cirrhosis. Disorders of water and electrolyte balance are considered in Chapter 29.

β_2-Microglobulin

This is a small protein (MW 11 800, radius 15 Å) found in serum, urine, cerebrospinal fluid, saliva, colostrum and amniotic fluid. It is removed from the blood by glomerular filtration, reabsorbed in the tubules and then catabolized. Its amino acid sequence and structure is homologous with that of the light chains of immunoglobulin and it may constitute a constant part of cell-bound HLA antigens. Although production is fairly constant, it may be increased in patients with certain malignancies, e.g. myelomatosis, or inflammatory disorders. Slightly elevated levels are found in pregnancy.

Serum β_2-microglobulin has been used as a marker for renal function, as its excretion in the urine is markedly increased in conditions associated with abnormal tubular function where glomerular filtration rate remains essentially normal, e.g. renal tubular acidosis, Wilson's disease, Fanconi's syndrome, analgesic nephropathy.

It is measured by simple radioimmunoassay. Urinary concentration is usually less than 0.1 mg/ml in healthy subjects, 0.4 mg/ml being the upper limit. Very high concentrations (up to 50 mg/ml) may be found in patients with tubular proteinuria. Urinary β_2-microglobulin is degraded by an acid urine and care must be taken to maintain a high urinary pH, preferably pH 6 or above. Urinary β_2-microglobulin has been used as a marker for nephrotoxicity and in the evaluation of new drugs.

Serum β_2-microglobulin correlates well with inulin clearance and has been regarded by some workers as more useful than serum creatinine determination for the detection of a slightly reduced glomerular filtration rate. The normal range is 0.8 to 2.4 mg/ml. In healthy subjects serum concentration increases with age, presumably due to the reduction in GFR with age, but there are no sex differences.

Urinary enzymes

Many enzymes which are present in the kidney are excreted in the urine. A variety of causes of renal damage (e.g. urinary infection, ischaemia and nephrotoxic insults) produce enzymuria. β-Glucuronidase, N-acetyl-β-glucosaminodase (NAG) and lactic dehydrogenase have all been used in this regard. The presence of catalase in the urine is used as a chemical screening test for bacteriuria. Since catalase is also present in the kidney, the test does not distinguish between infection and other causes of inflammation.

LABORATORY EVALUATION OF UROLITHIASIS

The diagnosis of urolithiasis is discussed in Chapter 19. Stone analysis is the definitive investigation and this can be done by a variety of techniques, including quantitative or qualitative chemical analysis, X-ray diffraction and infrared spectroscopy, to name a few. In Australasia, stones are always sent for section, as calcified renal papillae due to analgesic nephropathy is an important differential diagnosis of urinary calculi.

Freshly voided urine should be examined immediately for the presence of crystals. The presence of cystine crystals is diagnostic of cystinuria. In other forms of calculous disease the relationship between crystalluria and stone formation is less definite but the presence of crystals may provide a diagnostic clue.

Urinary pH may also provide a clue to the possible aetiology of calculus. An acid urine might arouse suspicion of uric acid calculi whereas a persistently alkaline urine in the absence of a urea-splitting organism might signify renal tubular acidosis.

A variety of laboratory tests may be undertaken in patients with stones, including estimation of renal function, serum calcium, phosphorus and uric acid, and in selected patients measurement of blood acid–base balance, protein electrophoresis, serum alkaline phosphatase and immunoreactive parathyroid hormone.

Dietary intake is an important determinant of urinary solute excretion. Ingestion of a wide variety of substances (e.g. calcium, phosphorus, sodium, protein, carbohydrate) can influence the excretion rate of calcium, and 24-h urinary estimations of urinary solutes such as calcium oxalate, uric acid, cystine, xanthine and others may be indicated.

Calcium and phosphorus

Measurement of serum calcium and phosphorus is useful in the investigation of patients with renal disease. Hypercalcaemia may cause renal insufficiency and is discussed in Chapter 20. Hypocalcaemia and hyperphosphataemia commonly accompany chronic renal failure and, together with alkaline phosphatase, are important in the assessment of renal osteodystrophy (see Ch. 22).

Serum uric acid

Serum uric acid is commonly elevated in renal impairment and this is discussed in Chapter 22. Measurement of serum uric acid is particularly useful in pregnancy, as it is elevated early in patients with pre eclampsia (see Ch. 25). The role of uric acid in nephrolithiasis is discussed in Chapter 19.

INVESTIGATION OF RENAL DISEASE IN PREGNANCY

Renal function in pregnancy is discussed in Chapter 25.

There are substantial increases in both renal plasma flow and glomerular filtration rate during pregnancy (of the order of 25% to 50%). Thus creatinine clearance is increased and serum creatinine and urea are decreased compared to the non-pregnant state — an important point to remember when interpreting renal function tests in pregnancy. Values which are normal in the non-pregnant women may be abnormal during pregnancy.

Aminoaciduria and glycosuria are common in pregnancy because of an increase in filtered load which is not accompanied by an appropriate increase in proximal tubular reabsorption. Uric acid is normally elevated from 12 weeks to 36 weeks. The high clearance leads to a reduction in serum uric acid concentration, and a rise in serum uric acid during pregnancy is a very valuable marker for the development of pre-eclamptic toxaemia.

MICROBIOLOGICAL TECHNIQUES

Urine collection

The diagnosis of significant bacteriuria is critically dependent on the adequacy of the urine specimen.

In males, collection of a midstream urine specimen is simple and accurate. The foreskin should be retracted and the glans gently washed. In women, a vaginal tampon is necessary to prevent contamination. The patient should wash the vulva thoroughly under vision with sterile saline and then hold the labia apart with the fingers so that the urine does not touch the skin. In both sexes the specimen should be collected with a full bladder and at least 200 ml of urine should be passed to clean the urethra before collection. A continuous stream is desirable and the patient should place the sterile container in the stream. The urine should be sent to the laboratory immediately, or refrigerated until culture facilities are available.

In a carefully collected midstream specimen, even low counts of bacteria may indicate significant infection. The commonly quoted figure of more than 10^5/ml is of particular use as an epidemiological tool. Although the likelihood of infection increases as bacterial count increases, true infection (as diagnosed by suprapubic bladder aspiration) may be present despite quite low counts of bacteria in urine. Although mixed urinary infection can occur, it is rare, and the presence of more than one organism suggests contamination of the specimen. Bacteriuria is of particular significance in infants and young children, in whom investigation of any urinary tract infection is imperative, and in pregnant women, as untreated bacteriuria in pregnancy is the forerunner of acute pyelonephritis of pregnancy.

In males with bacteriuria, particularly if the urinary tract is normal radiologically, it is important to consider the prostate as a possible source of infection. Infection can be localized to the prostate by using the three specimen technique of Stamey, provided the bladder urine has been cleared of high counts of bacteria. After voiding the first 10 ml of urine (VB1), which represents urethral flora, the patient passes about 200 ml of urine and then collects a midstream urine specimen (VB2), after which he stops voiding. The prostate is then firmly massaged and any expressed secretions are cultured. The patient then passes another 10 ml of urine (VB3), which represents prostatic flora. If the bladder urine is sterile or contains only low counts of organisms, an increase in bacterial counts in VB3 is evidence of prostatic infection.

Infection can be localized to the bladder or kidney by a variety of indirect or direct techniques but these are of limited value in clinical practice.

Culture techniques

Routine laboratories culture urine on Mac-Conkey's agar, blood agar or CLED (cysteine lactose electrolyte-deficient) agar. The finding of 'sterile pyuria' requires further investigation by cultural techniques which can grow fastidious organisms. These include anaerobic culture for anaerobes, human blood agar for *Gardnerella vaginalis*, Lowenstein–Jensen for Mycobacterium, urea-plasma agar for ureaplasmas, irradiated McCoy cells for Chlamydia. Such techniques would usually only be considered for culture of suprapubic bladder aspiration specimens.

IMMUNOLOGICAL TESTS

Although many renal diseases have an immunological basis, the current place of immunological testing in nephrology is quite limited.

Complement

The complement system can be assessed by measuring the total haemolytic complement (CH50) activity, and C3 and C4 concentrations. Measurement of other complement components may be indicated if CH50 is low, with normal C3 and C4 concentrations. A low C4 concentration indicates activation of the classic pathway, while low C3 and a normal C4 indicate alternative pathway activation.

In acute post-infectious glomerulonephritis, both classic and alternative pathways may be activated and consequently both C3 and C4 concentrations may be low. These changes are relatively short-lived and return to normal within 4–6 weeks. Failure of hypocomplementaemia to resolve within this time suggests the need for further investigation.

In 'dense deposit' or type II mesangiocapillary glomerulonephritis the alternative pathway may be activated, with a low to very low C3 but normal C4. The low C3 is a consequence of activation of the alternative pathway by C3 nephritic factor (C3 NeF). The serum contains C3 NeF and may also contain free C3d, a breakdown product of C3.

Complement concentration estimation is not useful in assessing the severity or prognosis of acute post-infectious or mesangiocapillary glomerulonephritis but may be helpful in systemic lupus erythematosus and the nephritis associated with subacute bacterial endocarditis and infected atrioventricular shunts.

Immunoglobulins

An elevated serum IgA concentration is found in 30–50% of patients with IgA nephropathy and Henoch–Schönlein disease. Elevated total IgE levels have been found in some patients with minimal lesion nephrotic syndrome and may indicate an allergic aetiology.

Paraproteinaemia is discussed in Chapter 11. The disorders most frequently associated with paraproteinaemia and renal disease are multiple myeloma, amyloid, and mixed cryoglobulinaemia. Paraproteins are best detected by serum immuno-electrophoresis. Benign monoclonal gammopathy is common in elderly patients and may present a diagnostic problem in patients with renal disease of other aetiology. Paraproteins are usually associated with a reduction in other non-paraprotein immunoglobulins, particularly in multiple myeloma. Bence Jones protein (immunoglobulin light chains) is present in the urine of 70–80% of patients with multiple myeloma and occasionally in amyloidosis. Dipstick tests for urinary protein do not detect Bence Jones protein. This can be detected by heating or by specific immunoelectrophoresis using concentrated urine.

Immune complexes

Immune complex assays have little place in the diagnosis and management of renal disease.

Cryoglobulins are immune complexes which precipitate in the cold. Mixed cryoglobulinaemia, usually secondary to a collagen vascular disease, may be associated with a severe glomerulo-nephritis.

Autoantibodies

A range of autoantibodies are detected in systemic lupus erythematosus (SLE — Ch. 9). Antinuclear factor and anti-double-stranded DNA antibody are measured commonly in nephrological practice.

The autoantibodies detected in scleroderma and mixed connective tissue disease are considered in Chapter 9. The role of ANCA — anticytoplasmic antibodies — in the diagnosis of vasculitis is considered in Chapter 9. pANCA is associated with polyarteritis and cANCA with Wegener's granulomatosis.

Anti-glomerular and anti-tubular basement membrane autoantibodies (anti-GBM and anti-TBM) are detectable by indirect immunofluores-cence on normal kidney tissue or by radioimmuno-assay.

HORMONE ESTIMATIONS

Renal hormones have been discussed in Chapter 2. Renin and aldosterone are the only renal hormones commonly measured.

Renin assays

Plasma renin concentration (PRC) measures the generation of AI (angiotensin I) from plasma renin incubated with exogenous added substrate, whereas plasma renin activity (PRA) measures generation of AI using endogenous substrate. The two measurements usually move in parallel except when renin substrate in high (e.g. in pregnancy, oestrogen therapy, Cushing's syndrome), when PRA tends to be higher than PRC. More recently immunoradiometric assays which measure renin protein have become available.

Renin is markedly affected by posture, sodium status, menstrual cycle, time of day and drugs, so that measurements without regard to these factors may not be interpretable. PRC rises on assumption of upright posture and is markedly increased by sodium or volume depletion. It is increased by the

Hypotensive drugs and renin
Drugs causing an increase in renin
Contraceptive pill
Diuretics
  Frusemide
  Ethacrynic acid
  Thiazides
Vasodilators
  Diazoxide
  Hydralazine
  Minoxidil
Drugs causing a decrease in renin
Adrenergic blockers
  Rauwolfia alkaloids
  α-Methyldopa
  Guanethedine
  β-Blockers

contraceptive pill, diuretics and vasodilators and decreased by adrenergic blockers.

Interpretation of PRC may need control of dietary sodium intake with concurrent measure-ment of 24-hour urinary sodium, but random measurement of PRC may be use in patients on uncontrolled sodium intake in certain circum-stances.

Renin in diagnosis

Plasma renin is high in some patients with chronic renal failure and severe dialysis-resistant hypertension, and may help in distinguishing patients in whom control of salt and water balance is inadequate for blood pressure control. Renin is very high in the rare condition of renin-secreting tumour, but this is a most important diagnosis to make, as it is a form of surgically correctable hypertension.

PRA (PRC) determination is a most useful screening test in patients with hypokalaemia and hypertension, as high values indicate secondary hyperaldosteronism and low values are suggestive of Conn's syndrome. It is also altered in a variety of hypertensive states.

Renin measurements are widely used in clinical practice in the assessment of patients with renovas-cular disease for surgery, Simultaneous bilateral sampling from the renal veins for PRA (PRC) following percutaneous femoral catheterization is

---

Plasma renin activity in hypertensive states

Decreased PRA

1. Primary aldosterone excess
   Adrenal adenoma
   Adrenal micronodular hyperplasia
   Indeterminate hyperaldosteronism
   Adrenocortical carcinoma
   Ovarian malignancy
   Glucocorticoid suppressible hypertension
2. Non-aldosterone mineralocorticoid excess
   17α-Hydroxylase deficiency
   IIβ-Hydroxylase deficiency
   Ovarian dysgenesis
   Deoxycorticosterone
   18-Hydroxycorticosterone
   Corticosterone
   Miscellaneous
3. Liddle's syndrome
4. Ectopic ACTH
5. Liquorice extract

Increased PRA

Accelerated hypertension
Renovascular hypertension
Phaeochromocytoma
Hyperthyroidism
Oral contraception
Renin-secreting tumours
Unilateral renal parenchymal disease, e.g.
  hydronephrosis, reflux nephropathy
Dialysis-resistant hypertension

Normal PRA

Unilateral or bilateral renal parenchymal disease
Cushing's syndrome
Phaeochromocytoma
Coarctation of the aorta

---

used in the evaluation of renal artery stenosis. A ratio greater than 1.5 between the two renal vein renin values is generally considered abnormal. An abnormal ratio is a good index of surgical curability, but false negative tests are frequent.

Evidence of suppression of renin release from the contralateral kidney is a further guide to surgical response. The diagnosis of renovascular disease is discussed in Chapter 27.

Renin is a useful marker in monitoring the adequacy of corticosteroid therapy and is often extremely high if mineralocorticoid replacement is inadequate.

Renin as a guide to therapy

It has been reported that patients with so-called 'low renin' essential hypertension (LREH) respond poorly to β-blockers whereas those with normal or high renin show a good response. This claim has been challenged by others, who found that the hypotensive effect of these drugs is not dependent on their renin-lowering effect. Patients with LREH respond favourably to diuretics but diuretics are also often effective in normal and high-renin hypertension. Converting enzyme inhibitors are particularly effective in high-renin states, although patients with low plasma renin concentrations may also respond.

Aldosterone estimation

Aldosterone concentration may be measured in plasma by radioimmunoassay, but in clinical practice 24-hour urinary aldosterone excretion is more commonly measured. As aldosterone is increased in both primary and secondary hyperaldosteronism, its measurement is usually confined to patients with hypertension, hypokalaemia, urinary potassium leak and suppressed renin.

Measurement of 1,25-dihydroxycholecalciferol is undertaken in units with special research interests.

REFERENCES AND RECOMMENDED READING

Beevers D G et al 1973 The clinical value of renin and angiotensin estimations. Kidney International 8: S181–302

Birch D F, Fairley K F 1979 Haematuria: glomerular or non-glomerular? Lancet 2: 845–846

Iversen P, Brun C 1951 Aspiration biopsy of the kidney. American Journal of Medicine 11: 324

Kark R M 1956 Needle biopsy of the kidney. Lancet 1: 51

Marks S L, Maxwell M H, Varady P D, Lupu A N, Kaufman I J 1976 Renovascular hypertension: does the renal vein ratio predict operative results? Journal of Urology 115: 365–368

Stockigt J R, Collins R D, Noakes C A, Schambelain M, Biglieri E G 1972 Renal vein renin in various forms of renal hypertension. Lancet l: 1194–1197

Whitworth J A 1981 Management of asymptomatic bacteriuria. Australian and New Zealand Journal of Medicine 11: 321–328

Wibell L, Everin P-E, Berggard I 1973 Serum α_2-microglobulin in renal disease. Nephron 10: 320–331

5. Organ imaging in urinary tract disorders

T. M. J. Maling   J. G. Turner   R. R. Bailey

During the past decade there have been rapid developments in the field of organ imaging and a variety of different imaging techniques are available for the investigation of urinary tract disorders. Many of these provide the same information. It is important that the simplest and least invasive method of imaging is employed, but this must take into account economic considerations. It may be more appropriate to perform one complex investigation rather than a series of simpler procedures which may take more time.

This chapter discusses currently available organ imaging techniques and their application in some well-defined clinical situations.

ORGAN IMAGING TECHNIQUES

Plain abdominal X-ray with or without nephrotomography

Plain abdominal radiography (KUB — *k*idney, *u*reter, *b*ladder) has a place in the diagnosis and follow-up of opaque urinary calculi. At least 80% of calculi in males and over 90% in females are sufficiently radiopaque to be evident on plain radiographs. Tomography is a valuable aid, particularly where bowel content is overlying the kidneys.

Ultrasonography

The continuing development of ultrasonography (US) has had a major impact on the investigation of patients with urinary tract disorders. A dramatic advance in instrumentation has resulted in skilled ultrasonographers readily obtaining high quality B-mode images. Further to this has been the development of duplex US instruments which superimpose doppler flow information on a standard B-mode image (Fig. 5.1). Doppler flow may be displayed with standard grey scale, or alternatively in colour, referred to as colour doppler or colour doppler imaging.

B-mode US imaging has replaced intravenous urography (IVU) as the most frequently performed imaging procedure in nephrourological practice. This turnaround is due to the ability of US to produce information about the entire urinary tract without any risk to the patient. It also has the advantage of being significantly less costly than IVU and does not require any patient preparation. US should be the first imaging procedure performed on most patients with kidney and urinary tract disorders and in many instances it will be the only one that is required.

B-mode US can demonstrate renal length, parenchymal thickness and as a consequence an assessment of nephron mass can be given (Fig. 5.2). Assessment of renal echotexture is straightforward and important. Increased echogenicity with poor differentiation between cortex and medulla is an indicator of parenchymal disease.

One of the most frequent requests made of any organ imaging service is to determine whether or not obstruction is present somewhere within the urinary tract. Chronic obstruction results in varying degrees of dilatation of the urinary tract from the calyces to the distal urethra, depending upon the site and degree of obstruction present. When dilatation occurs as a result of obstruction, it will involve the entire urinary tract above the level of obstruction. Therefore if significant chronic ob-

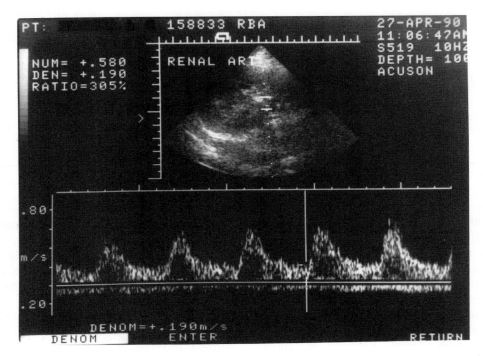

Fig. 5.1 Duplex ultrasound scanning with doppler flow beneath a B-mode scan of a renal transplant. The sample site of the doppler flow is indicated

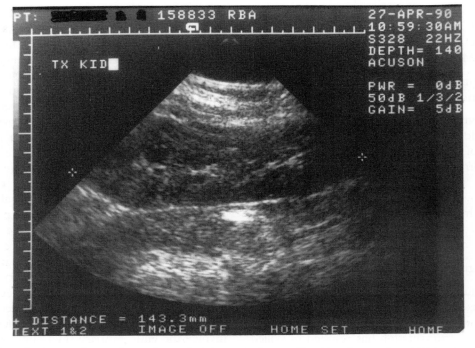

Fig. 5.2 B-mode ultrasound scan of a renal transplant demonstrating renal length and parenchymal thickness

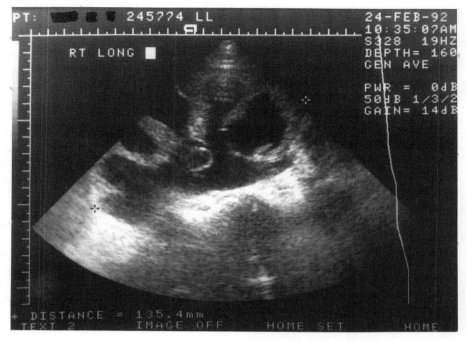

Fig. 5.3 B-mode ultrasound scan showing dilatation of the renal pelvis and collecting system indicative of significant obstruction

struction is present then dilatation of the minor calyces and the renal pelvis will occur and be readily detectable on a B-mode US scan (Fig. 5.3). This can be relied upon, except in acute obstruction, where dilatation will not occur initially, due to the intrinsic resistance provided by the ureteric wall with its elastic tissue and thick musculature. The time required for dilatation to occur varies and is not predictable. Duration of obstruction seems more important than the actual pressures attained. Whilst B-mode US scanning can be relied upon to detect chronic obstruction (hydronephrosis) it cannot define the level of the obstruction; for this further imaging with contrast medium will be necessary (Fig. 5.4).

Mass lesions of the renal parenchyma are readily detected by good quality B-mode scans as changes in the contour of the kidney or focal changes in echotexture. Solid lesions may be hyper- or hypoechoic relative to the surrounding renal parenchyma. Simple cysts are characterized as a sonolucent mass lesion with sharply defined margins and through transmission of the sound waves

(Fig. 5.5). If the characteristics of the cyst are unequivocal then no further investigation is required to establish this diagnosis.

B-mode scanning is an excellent way of examining the bladder for intrinsic lesions and for the assessment of bladder emptying. This modality, however, does not allow for an examination of the full length of the ureter, but will visualize the upper and lower portions. A further advantage of US is the ability to examine neighbouring organs and spaces. This is particularly important in the perinephric space in renal trauma and renal infections.

Doppler flow imaging of the renal vessels is increasing in frequency, particularly following transplantation where it may be used to assess the integrity of the vascular supply to the graft and to assist in the assessment of early graft dysfunction. The advent of colour doppler and its wider use will undoubtedly lead to further improvements in technology and diagnostic ability. Arteriovenous malformations of the kidney can be diagnosed with doppler flow imaging. There is experimental

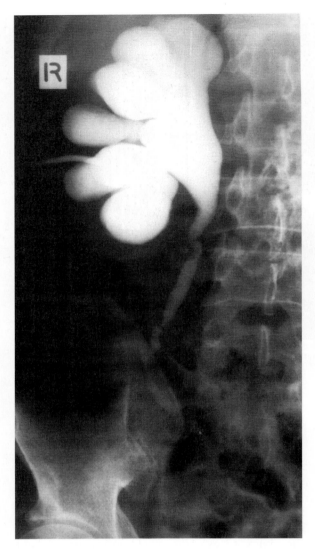

Fig. 5.4 Contrast medium injected directly into the renal pelvis through a nephrostomy tube, demonstrating the site of obstruction

evidence to suggest that colour doppler may be useful in detecting the presence of significant vesicoureteric reflux.

Intravenous urography

The improved capabilities of diagnostic US equipment have resulted in a change in the role of IVU in the investigation of the kidneys and urinary tract. It is no longer the front-line investigation, with the exception of patients presenting with renal colic or macroscopic haematuria. The other factor influencing the trend towards the greater use of US has been the development of new and more expensive contrast media.

The IVU depends on the glomerular filtration of a tri-iodinated organic compound. Recently low osmolar non-ionic media have been developed. Both these and older high osmolar ionic media are widely used, but there is an increasing and inevitable move towards the use of non-ionic, low osmolar media due to a reduced incidence of significant side effects. Unfortunately, the non-ionic low osmolar media are three to five times more expensive. The quality of the examination is little different between these two categories of contrast media and so the choice comes down to a play-off between cost and safety. The correct dose of contrast medium should be approximately 300–350 mg of iodine per kg of body weight provided that glomerular filtration is normal. A decrease in the glomerular filtration rate can be compensated for by increasing the dose, but never to above 600–700 mg of iodine per kg body weight.

The earliest phase of IVU is the nephrogram, which shows opacification of the nephron mass by the filtered contrast medium together with a small contribution from the background blood pool of contrast medium. The normal nephrogram is at its most intense when the plasma concentration of contrast medium is greatest, i.e. immediately after the injection. Interference with the normal nephrogram pattern occurs particularly in high pressure obstruction (Fig. 5.6). Historically, much was made of interpreting the different nephrogram patterns in acute renal failure. However, with the introduction of US there is now no place for IVU in acute renal failure. Other phases of IVU include opacification of the renal pelvis (pyelogram), ureters (ureterogram) and the bladder (cystogram).

IVU is usually done after thorough bowel evacuation and with the fluid intake restricted for 12 hours. If possible, diuretic therapy should be withheld on the morning of the examination. It is particularly important that patients with renal

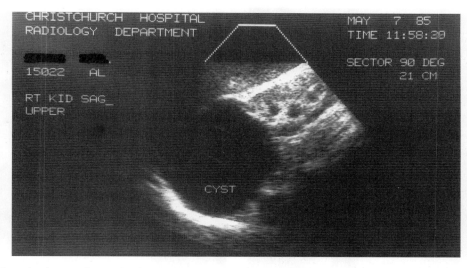

Fig. 5.5   B-mode ultrasound scan showing a sonolucent mass at the upper pole of a kidney diagnostic of a simple cyst

insufficiency are not dehydrated, as large doses of contrast in a hypovolaemic patient may cause a further deterioration in renal function. Complications after IVU are infrequent, but anaphylactoid reactions may occur. The incidence is significantly less with low osmolar non-ionic media.

Antegrade (percutaneous) pyelography

Antegrade pyelography involves the injection of contrast medium directly into the renal pelvis through a 22-gauge needle introduced under local anaesthesia and guided by either X-ray image intensification or US control (Fig. 5.4). This is a safe and simple technique for detecting the site of obstruction in the renal pelvis or ureter of a kidney where contrast excretion is poor. This approach has largely replaced retrograde pyelography.

Antegrade pyelography can be extended to allow a urodynamic assessment of the upper urinary tract. Perfusion of saline or contrast medium through a fine needle positioned in the renal pelvis will demonstrate whether significant obstruction is present (Whitaker test). Pressures are measured within the renal pelvis and bladder throughout the perfusion so that any abnormal pressure gradient (indicating obstruction) will be detected. It has been shown that an unobstructed upper urinary tract perfused at a rate of 10 ml/min should show

a pressure gradient of less than 15 cmH$_2$O. The use of contrast medium in the infusion fluid also allows visual assessment of the urinary tract.

Retrograde pyelography

During retrograde pyelography water-soluble contrast medium is injected directly into the ureter or renal pelvis through a ureteric catheter. This examination is indicated for visualization of the ureter below an obstruction.

Cystography

Voiding cystourethrography (VCU)

VCU is important in the assessment of bladder function. It is best combined with measurements of bladder pressure and urinary flow rate. The bladder is filled with a similar (but more dilute) contrast medium to that used for IVU. The contrast medium can be run in through either a urethral or suprapubic catheter. VCU with full urodynamic evaluation is essential for the complete investigation of patients with urinary incontinence.

A prerequisite for the appropriate treatment of patients with vesicoureteric reflux (VUR) is a VCU to assess the degree of reflux. There are several classifications of VUR, all of which depend on the

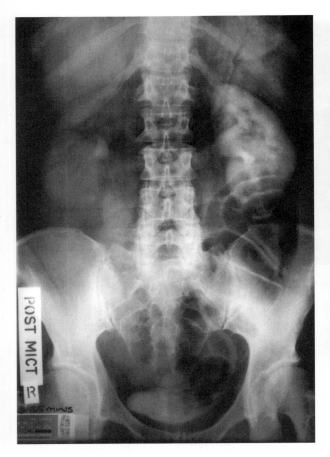

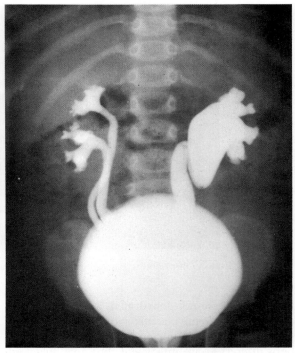

Fig. 5.7   Voiding cystourethrogram of an 8-month-old girl taken after a urinary tract infection and showing bilateral grade IV vesicoureteric reflex with widespread intrarenal reflux

Fig. 5.6   An intravenous urogram in a patient with left renal colic. The high pressure obstruction from a calculus at the vesicoureteric junction has resulted in a prolonged and denser-than-normal nephrogram on this film, taken 35 minutes after the injection of contrast medium

extent and degree of dilatation of the ureter and pelvicalycine system apparent on the VCU. Only the more severe degrees of VUR are associated with progressive renal damage. Intrarenal reflux is the retrograde passage of contrast medium along the nephron as a result of VUR (Fig. 5.7). Two factors determine whether intrarenal reflux will occur: papillary morphology and the degree of VUR. The importance of grading VUR is in separating those degrees of reflux in which intrarenal reflux will not occur from those in which it might occur if the papillary morphology is appropriate.

A workable classification is to use four grades based on the extent of ureteric filling and the degree of dilatation of the pelvicalycine system, in particular the minor calyces.

Grade I   Incomplete ureteric filling
Grade II   Complete ureteric filling but no dilatation of the ureter or pelvicalycine system
Grade III Some dilatation of the minor calyces with preservation of papillary impression (Fig. 5.8)
Grade IV   Gross dilatation with ballooning of minor calyces and loss of papillary impression (Figs 5.7, 5.8)

Intrarenal reflux never occurs with grades I and II VUR, and these degrees of reflux are not associated with progressive renal damage, see Chapter 15.

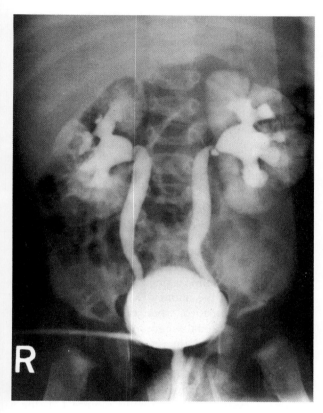

Fig. 5.8 Bilateral vesicoureteric reflux demonstrated during VCU. Note slight dilatation of the minor calyces of the right kidney but preservation of papillary impression (grade III VUR). There is grade IV VUR on the left with complete loss of the papillary impression

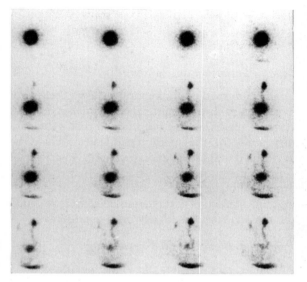

Fig. 5.9 Direct radionuclide micturating cystography. The posterior sequence (beginning top left) initially shows minor reflux on the left side and then gross reflux on the right side up into the renal pelvis. As voiding continues there is also marked reflux on the left side

More recently the classification of VUR agreed upon by the collaborators participating in the International Reflux Study in children has become widely used.

Radionuclide micturating cystography

Radionuclide micturating cystography is often preferred to VCU for the follow-up of patients with VUR. The direct method involves instillation of radioactive tracer into the bladder using suprapubic injection or urethral catheterization. The kidneys and bladder are then continuously monitored before, during and after voiding for any increase in activity from refluxing urine (Fig. 5.9). The main advantage of this radionuclide technique compared with VCU is reduced radiation exposure.

The indirect radionuclide method follows a routine intravenous injection of a radionuclide such as DTPA, when most of the activity has passed through into the bladder. Reported sensitivities for this technique vary, but are generally lower than for the direct method. It is unsuitable for children less than 3–4 years of age.

Angiography

Renal arteriography

Renal arteriography involves percutaneous catheterization of an artery (usually femoral) and advancement of the catheter under television control to a satisfactory position within the aorta or renal artery. The procedure can be performed on a day-patient basis and carries a small risk of damage to the artery at the puncture site.

Before the advent of US and computerized tomography (CT) scanning, renal arteriography was essential for the investigation of patients with a renal mass lesion, but it is now seldom required.

It is now largely confined to the investigation of renal vascular disease and persistent bleeding following trauma.

Digital subtraction angiography

Digital subtraction angiography allows the use of smaller intra-arterial catheters and smaller doses of contrast media. It had been hoped that a satisfactory study of the main renal arteries could be performed following an intravenous injection of contrast medium rather than having to use an intra-arterial catheter. The results have been disappointing and the use of intravenous injections to study the renal vessels has largely been abandoned.

Percutaneous transluminal angioplasty

Although this is not an imaging procedure, percutaneous transluminal angioplasty is intimately related to imaging. It has been shown to be an effective alternative to vascular surgery in selected patients with renovascular hypertension, including those with stenosis of a renal transplant artery. An inflatable, but non-expandable, balloon-tipped catheter is positioned so that the balloon traverses the stenotic portion of the vessel. The balloon is then inflated to a predetermined diameter and exerts a lateral force against the vessel wall. It is a relatively simple, low-risk procedure, requiring no more than 48 hours in hospital.

Renal venography

Renal venography requires catheterization of the renal veins, usually via a femoral vein. Contrast medium is injected directly into the renal vein. This investigation is most often performed in association with venous sampling for renal vein renin measurements in patients with a suspected ischaemic kidney. It is also necessary for the confirmation of renal vein thrombosis.

Computerized tomography

The impact of computerized tomography (CT) for the investigation of urinary tract disease has not been as great as in some other disciplines, simply because the alternative methods of imaging the urinary tract are so valuable and usually less expensive.

The major contribution of CT scanning, in addition to the production of axial cross-sectional images, is the increased radiographic contrast compared to conventional radiographs. This allows different types of soft tissue to be distinguished. The degree of attenuation of the X-ray beam by different tissues and media is expressed in CT or Hounsfield units (H), with water and urine having a value of approximately 0, bone + 1000 H, and air – 1000H. Normal kidney and muscle density is about 30 H, and that of fat about – 60 H. Differences of about 10 H can be readily appreciated. Intravenous contrast medium given in association with a CT scan will increase the density of perfused tissues so that the renal cortex after contrast enhancement will be approximately 60–80 H.

As it is possible to distinguish clearly the fascial planes around the kidney, CT should be the preferred examination when disease of the perirenal and pararenal spaces is suspected. CT scanning will display the retroperitoneal structures and their relationship to one another, and is therefore particularly valuable for the assessment of retroperitoneal fibrosis and lymphadenopathy.

Simple cysts do not normally require CT for diagnosis but with more complex cystic lesions the technique can occasionally provide additional information. Solid renal masses are best examined by CT and this has largely replaced angiography for the diagnosis and staging of renal tumours (Fig. 5.10.)

Obstructive uropathy is readily diagnosed by CT. However, this is more simply done by US. CT does have an important place in the examination of the patients with bilateral obstructive uropathy in whom retroperitoneal disease is suspected. Low-density or radiolucent stones on conventional radiography are easily distinguished by CT and thus there is a definite place for localized CT scanning of the ureter in patients in whom obstruction has been demonstrated by IVU but no opaque stone can be seen.

Radionuclide imaging

Renal imaging with [99m]technetium-labelled compounds can provide valuable functional informa-

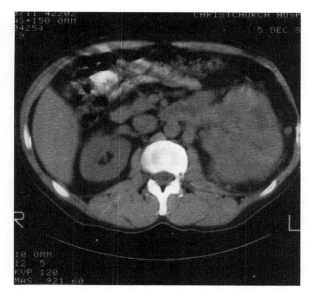

Fig. 5.10 A CT scan through the vascular pedicle of the left kidney showing marked enlargement of the kidney with replacement of normal renal tissue by a mass of heterogeneous density. There is a tongue of tumour extending in between the aorta and the superior mesenteric artery. This represents tumour 'thrombus' within the left renal vein from a primary renal cell carcinoma

tion about the urinary tract. The two procedures most commonly performed are static imaging with agents such as ^{99m}Tc-dimercaptosuccinic acid (DMSA) and dynamic imaging with ^{99m}Tc-diethylenetriamine pentaacetic acid (DTPA) or ^{99m}Tc-benzoylmercaptoacetyltriglycine (MAG3). In some centres ^{123}I-sodium iodohippurate (hippuran) is preferred.

Following intravenous injection DMSA is retained by the cells of the proximal tubules, allowing excellent scintiphotos of the functioning renal parenchyma to be obtained (Figs 5.11, 5.12). The DMSA scan is widely used to identify sites of cortical scarring in children with VUR. It may also be used to detect renal contusions and distinguish renal tumours from pseudotumours. Furthermore the computer-acquired scan allows quantification of relative function between kidneys and within a kidney.

In contrast to DMSA, the agents used for dynamic renal imaging are rapidly excreted by the kidney, either by glomerular filtration alone (DTPA) or by a combination of filtration and tubular secretion (MAG3 and hippuran). The scan is often conducted in two parts, referred to as the vascular and parenchymal studies. Following

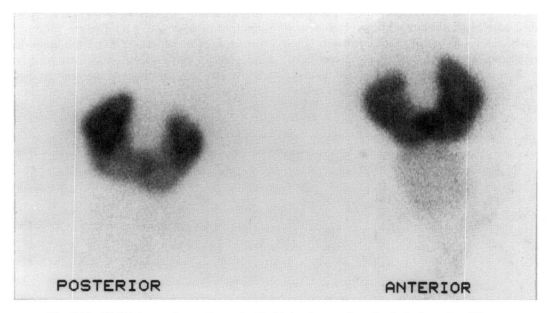

Fig. 5.11 DMSA images from a 6-month-old girl showing excellent detail of a horseshoe kidney

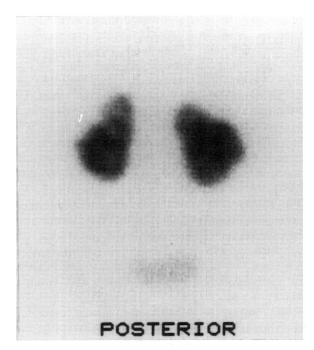

POSTERIOR

Fig. 5.12 Posterior DMSA image from a 15-month-old girl presenting with a urinary tract infection. Marked loss of function at the left upper pole due to reflux nephropathy is clearly seen. There is also focal scarring at the right upper pole

intravenous bolus injection of radiopharmaceutical the initial dynamic flow study gives a visual representation of aortic and renal perfusion (Fig. 5.13.) Various computer programs have been developed to quantitate blood flow to the kidney. The subsequent serial parenchymal images reflect kidney function and excretion (Fig. 5.14). These dynamic scans may be used to detect renal artery thrombosis or embolization and are often used to evaluate and follow up cases of obstruction. They play a very important part in distinguishing obstruction from non-obstructive dilatation. The dynamic scan performed with an angiotensin-converting enzyme inhibitor such as captopril may accurately detect functionally significant renal artery stenosis.

Renal clearance studies

Measurement of glomerular filtration rate and effective renal plasma flow

Measurements of glomerular filtration rate (GFR) by inulin and of effective renal plasma flow (ERPF) by *p*-aminohippuric acid techniques have long been recognized as the most precise indicators of renal function. Unfortunately, these procedures are time-consuming and too complex for routine diagnostic tests. However, techniques using tracer doses of radioactive pharmaceuticals have made these measurements feasible in many hospitals. They are faster and more reproducible than the endogenous creatinine clearance.

The most commonly used technique for the measurement of GFR and ERPF involves a single-shot injection with plasma sampling. The principle of these tests is that if the kidneys are the sole exit for certain substances introduced into the body, then measurement of their rate of disappearance from the body will give an estimate of the total uptake function of the kidneys. In most

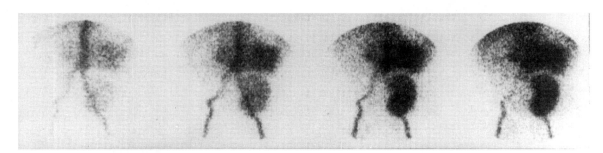

Fig. 5.13 Vascular dynamic imaging of a normally perfused and functioning renal transplant (2-second frames following intravenous bolus injection of radiopharmaceutical)

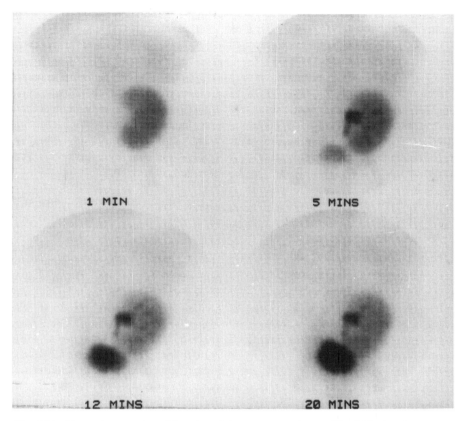

Fig. 5.14 Dynamic parenchymal imaging of the same transplant as Fig. 5.13, showing normal parenchymal uptake of DTPA, transit and excretion into the bladder

laboratories either [51]chromium-labelled ethylene-diamine tetra-acetic acid (^{51}Cr-EDTA) or ^{99m}Tc-DTPA is used for the measurement of GFR, and ^{125}I-hippuran for the measurement of ERPF. The only fundamental difference in the measurement of GFR and ERPF by the single-shot technique is the value of the extraction ratio of the compounds used. These methods have all been validated by comparison with the classic chemical methods.

Measurement of individual renal function

There are many situations in which it is valuable to establish the relative contribution of each kidney to total renal function. In the past this has been measured using bilateral ureteric catheterization. The procedure, however, requires an in-patient stay and general anaesthesia, is technically difficult and carries significant morbidity.

There is no radionuclide method which gives a precise estimate of the absolute value of individual kidney GFR or ERPF. An indirect method is generally used. Overall renal function is first determined by a single-shot technique (e.g. DTPA clearance). The relative contribution of each kidney is then calculated by measurement of relative renal uptake on a DMSA scan or on the early parenchymal uptake during a DTPA or MAG3 scan. There is also in use in some centres a 'direct' gamma camera method for measuring GFR and ERPF. The limitations of this technique for measuring differential renal function are related to the approximations used in the model for kidney tracer dynamics and the external detection of radioactivity from each kidney. Although some studies have shown good results with this gamma camera method there is still a general reservation over the accuracy and precision of the technique.

Magnetic resonance imaging

The most recent development in diagnostic imaging is magnetic resonance imaging (MRI). The principle of MRI involves excitation of nuclei of atoms such as hydrogen with radiowaves, and detection of echo radiation from these nuclei when the radio source is removed. The technique thus provides information at the cellular level and in its current stage of development gives good anatomical information and appears to have considerable potential in the physiological and metabolic assessment.

Rapid advances in MRI technology are occurring; MRI angiography is being developed and so a non-invasive method of studying the renal vessels seems likely in the near future. Where available, MRI presently contributes to the staging of malignancy in the urinary tract.

USE OF ORGAN IMAGING TECHNIQUES IN COMMON CLINICAL PROBLEMS IN NEPHROLOGY AND UROLOGY

Urinary tract infection in children

A significant number of children who develop a urinary tract infection have an underlying structural abnormality which predisposes them to infection. These abnormalities are either VUR or obstruction. Infants under 1 year of age with a urinary tract infection have a 50% chance of having an abnormality; this incidence decreases with age and by 5–10 years of age is less than 10%. The most frequently found structural abnormality is VUR.

Organ imaging is particularly important in any child with a urinary tract infection because of the incidence of significant VUR. The natural history of VUR is that it is maximal at birth and then, with bladder maturation, spontaneously improves. Grades I and II reflux almost invariably disappear by the age of 5 years. Grades III and IV reflux may persist, but are no longer associated with intrarenal reflux and thus no longer constitute a significant danger to the kidney.

If reflux nephropathy is to be prevented it is important to detect the dilating grades of VUR early in life. Any infant or child with a documented urinary tract infection should have appropriate organ imaging after treatment of the infection. The most accurate method of detecting VUR is the VCU. This examination, when performed on infants and children up to 2 years of age, is relatively simple and without risk. Beyond this age a VCU can be difficult to perform and upsetting to the child. As a result, any protocol for the investigation of children with a urinary tract infection must be a compromise.

Up until 2 years of age the investigations should include a VCU and US. The latter will exclude an underlying obstructive lesion and the VCU will detect VUR. If the findings are normal then no further imaging is required. If VUR is demonstrated then an IVU and DMSA scan should be performed to assess whether scarring is present.

In children over the age of 2 years a compromise policy can be adopted. In children over 5 years of age it is reasonable to investigate with US alone. If the examination is normal then no further imaging is required.

The difficult group consists of children aged 2–5 years. They are still in an age group where significant VUR may be present, but it is also the most difficult age group to subject to VCU. US examination is less reliable in this age group due to difficulties in obtaining the cooperation of the child. It should therefore be combined with a DMSA scan which is the single most accurate method of scar detection. An alternative and acceptable protocol to US and a DMSA scan is to undertake an IVU alone. Because the IVU demonstrates both the renal parenchyma and ureteric calibre a reliable assessment of the likelihood of the presence of significant VUR can be made and in many instances a negative VCU can be avoided.

Urinary tract infection in adults

In adults with urinary tract infection organ imaging is indicated for a recurrent clinical problem or if the patient has acute pyelonephritis. The most commonly found abnormalities are a calculus within the urinary tract or an obstructive lesion. US accompanied by a plain abdominal radiograph (KUB) is the appropriate initial investigation.

Renal papillary necrosis

The diagnosis of renal papillary necrosis can confidently be made from an IVU. The preliminary films will show some calcification in a majority of patients. This varies from fine speckled calcification in the papillary regions to a rim of dense calcification in papillary fragments.

When papillary necrosis is due to excessive analgesic intake, both kidneys are affected, with fairly symmetrical change. The kidneys are slightly smaller than normal and have a reasonably smooth outline, although centrilobar scars may occur in the later phases of the disease secondary to loss of the central nephrons in the renal lobe. The hallmark of papillary necrosis is contrast within a cavity in the papilla. This varies from a slit-like crevice to complete absence of the necrotic papilla, with only an irregular contrast-filled cavity remaining. Once the diagnosis has been established, follow-up US is valuable to exclude possible ureteric obstruction due to dislodged papillae.

Renal tuberculosis

Calcification, cavity formation and ureteric obstruction are the hallmarks of renal tuberculosis and are best diagnosed by IVU.

Renal failure

US is the investigation of choice in acute renal failure. It can also be used to exclude obstructive uropathy and to demonstrate the size and position of the kidneys before renal biopsy.

When obstruction is demonstrated antegrade pyelography can be used to demonstrate the site and nature of the obstruction. CT scanning is useful for demonstrating extrinsic obstruction from either retroperitoneal fibrosis or malignancy.

In chronic renal failure, where the kidneys are small, it may be difficult unequivocally to exclude obstruction by US and it may be necessary to proceed to high-dose IVU or occasionally retrograde pyelography.

Radionuclide studies have in the main a secondary role in the assessment of patients with renal failure.

Renal trauma

IVU is the initial investigation of choice. It is important to determine whether the renal vascular pedicle is intact. Absence of excretion by a kidney should alert the clinician to the possibility of damage to the pedicle and be followed by a dynamic radionuclide study. Renal arteriography is necessary to confirm and assess a major vascular lesion and should be performed as an emergency.

A perinephric collection of blood or urine as a result of trauma may present a clinical problem, and is best assessed by CT examination. Minor renal contusions are probably best diagnosed by a DMSA scan.

Hypertension

Rapid sequence IVU is the traditional imaging technique for detecting an ischaemic kidney. The classic features of renal artery stenosis include a reduction in renal size (but otherwise normal morphology), a slight delay in excretion on the affected side, the later appearance of an increased concentration of contrast on the affected side, and ureteric notching from collateral vessels. Unfortunately, false negative results are common, which limits the value of IVU as a screening procedure for renal artery stenosis.

IVU is also of value for demonstrating other renal lesions which may be causing the hypertension. There is a move towards US as the initial imaging procedure for suspected polycystic renal disease, reflux nephropathy or small kidneys.

Renography and other methods of computer-assisted static/dynamic renal imaging have been used to screen for renovascular hypertension, but like IVU they too have an unacceptably low predictive value. However, when captopril is given before the test these radionuclide techniques have a much improved sensitivity for detecting functionally significant renal artery stenosis. The principle is that in renal artery stenosis high angiotensin II concentrations constrict the efferent arterioles of the ischaemic nephrons and thus maintain glomerular filtration. When captopril is given this vasoconstriction is reduced and glomerular filtration falls. This will be evident in the renogram curve and may often be visible on the dynamic scintiphoto sequence. The cost efficacy of captopril renography as a screening test for detecting renal artery stenosis is, however, still uncertain.

Renal angiography is currently the only investigation generally available which will unequivocally exclude renal artery stenosis in young or uncontrolled hypertensives or when there is a strong clinical suspicion of renovascular hypertension.

The availability of percutaneous transluminal angioplasty has led to more aggressive investigation of patients with hypertension in order to detect remediable renovascular lesions. Long-term trials are necessary, however, to compare this simple new technique with conventional surgery. The initial reports and long-term follow-up are most encouraging for the treatment of fibromuscular hyperplasia, but disappointing if the stenosis is due to atherosclerosis. Re-stenosis is likely in these latter patients.

Digital subtraction angiography is almost certainly the screening procedure of choice for renovascular hypertension.

Renal mass lesions

The advent of more precise means of imaging has resulted in a higher detection rate of renal mass lesions. Simple cysts have been found in up to 50% of kidneys at autopsy, and a similar incidence has been demonstrated by both CT and US in older patients. In almost every renal mass lesion it should now be possible to make a correct diagnosis prior to, and without the need for, surgery.

The majority of mass lesions are simple cysts and are an incidental finding during the course of an investigation performed for some other reason. The US and CT appearances of a simple cyst are diagnostic in themselves, so that there is no need for further investigations. It is the lesion that is discovered on physical examination or during IVU that requires further organ imaging.

Simple renal cyst

The diagnosis of a simple renal cyst should not be made from an IVU, although it may be strongly suspected if it appears avascular and is well demarcated from the surrounding renal parenchyma. On US, a simple cyst will contain no echoes, have a sharp margin, and produce acoustic enhancement, in contrast to that part of the beam which has not traversed the cyst. If these three features are present, no further imaging is necessary (Fig. 5.5).

If the appearances are not typical of a simple cyst, it should be aspirated and the contents sent for analysis. CT scanning may provide more information in these cases.

Multiple simple cysts

Multiple simple cysts are not uncommon in the elderly. Each individual cyst will show the characteristic features of a single simple cyst. Differentiation from polycystic kidneys is not difficult as multiple simple cysts tend to be fewer and larger in size and the overall size of the kidneys is normal.

Renal pseudotumour

There are several varieties of renal pseudotumour, but the commonest are those due to a deeply situated prominent column of Bertin or to hypertrophy of a segment of a damaged kidney. In most instances the appearances are characteristic and no further imaging is required. If doubt persists, a ^{99m}Tc-DMSA scan is the best method of differentiating normally functioning renal parenchyma of a pseudotumour from a pathological mass.

Solid renal lesions

US will readily differentiate a solid lesion from a cyst, as the former will contain multiple echoes of variable intensity. CT with the use of contrast medium for enhancement will usually provide further information about the nature of a solid lesion.

Benign solid tumours are rare. An angiomyo-lipoma gives characteristically high intensity echoes on US and its fatty content is demonstrated on CT. This diagnosis can then be confirmed with angiography. Most other benign solid tumours will have to wait until surgery before their true nature can be disclosed.

Malignant renal tumours are generally obvious on US and CT. Occasionally there may be a need for angiography or aspiration biopsy. CT, how-ever, usually provides much more information, particularly with regard to the staging of the tumour.

Although advances are being made, there is no renal tumour-specific radionuclide currently in use. Radionuclide techniques, however, do permit an assessment of the function of both the contra-lateral kidney and the suspect organ, which can often be important when considering surgical intervention.

Obstructive uropathy

Acute high pressure obstruction

Patients with acute high pressure urinary tract obstruction usually present with renal colic and require urgent investigation by IVU. The high ureteric pressure resulting from the obstructing lesion (usually a calculus) produces a delay in both the nephrogram and pyelogram phases of an IVU which is proportional to the duration and intensity of the elevated intra-ureteric pressure. If the obstruction persists, contrast medium will accu-mulate within the nephrons, resulting eventually in a nephrogram of much greater intensity than normal (Fig. 5.6). The 'obstructive' nephrogram will increase in intensity as long as the obstruction persists. Eventually there will be enough contrast medium to outline the renal pelvis and ureter down to the obstructing lesion. A feature of an acute obstruction is the absence of much ureteric dilatation.

It is important to correlate the urgent IVU findings with the presence or absence of pain. Pain which is present during a normal IVU is not due to renal colic. There is rarely a place for other imaging procedures in the diagnosis of acute high pressure obstruction of the urinary tract.

Chronic low pressure obstruction

Patients with chronic low pressure obstruction tend to present with marked dilatation of the collecting system. The factors responsible for damage to renal tissue in association with obstruc-tion are not entirely clear. The number of remaining functioning nephrons determines the most effective imaging procedure.

US is the most appropriate screening test for detecting obstructive dilatation of the pelvicalyceal system. However, it may not demonstrate whether ureteric dilatation is present and thus other imaging procedures may be necessary to localize the site of obstruction. If the dilatation is severe and there is marked loss of renal parenchyma, it is preferable to undertake percutaneous pyelography. However, if the dilatation is not as marked and the renal parenchyma appears reasonably normal, then an IVU would demonstrate the level of the obstruction.

Radionuclide scanning may be useful for assess-ing the degree of obstruction and for measuring renal function in the presence of known obstruc-tion. This technique should not be used to investigate the site or aetiology of obstruction and is probably most useful for the follow-up of patients with obstructive lesions.

Non-obstructive dilatation

Non-obstructive dilatation of the upper urinary tract is often encountered as a result of VUR, previous obstruction or pregnancy, and may be demonstrated by either IVU or US. It may be possible to assess from these tests whether there is a degree of obstruction.

Computer-assisted dynamic radionuclide imag-ing combined with diuretic provocation may be used to distinguish a dilated, non-obstructive urinary system from one with a true mechanical obstruction. The principle of the technique is that if the urinary tract is dilated, but not obstructed, then by increasing the flow rate the capacity of the collecting system should become of little importance in relation to urine flow, which should be unimpeded. Conversely, a true obstruction may impede flow at high or low urine flow rates. In practice, diuresis renography has been shown to assess accurately the significance of upper urinary tract dilatation in the majority of cases. The major limitation of the technique is that patients with impaired renal function may have a poor diuretic response to frusemide.

Renal transplants

The most frequent and important use of organ imaging in renal transplant recipients is to exclude vascular or ureteric obstruction. Following surgery, these patients may also develop abnormal collections of urine, lymph, blood, or pus which are readily identified with US. If necessary, these collections can be drained under US control. US should be performed as a baseline examination as soon after transplantation as is practical. Repeated episodes of transplant rejection lead to alterations in the normal US appearance of the kidney, with a progressive reduction in the number of renal sinus echoes.

Radionuclide procedures have been widely used for assessing renal transplants. Many different computer models have been developed for quantitating transplant perfusion and cortical transit of agents like DTPA and MAG3. However, none allows accurate differentiation of the cause of renal ischaemia or transplant dysfunction. Nevertheless, serial radionuclide studies can be useful for assessing transplant progress through complications such as acute tubular necrosis and acute graft rejection. The widespread use of cyclosporin and its effect on renal function has limited the precision of these perfusion techniques for monitoring acute graft rejection.

Renal vein thrombosis

Renal vein thrombosis as a primary event occurs only in infants and young children in association with severe dehydration. They have accompanying acute renal failure, and IVU will show bilateral renal enlargement, probably a persisting and dense nephrogram, and only a faintly detectable pyelogram. Following recovery, IVU will show generalized papillary deformities more uniform and more extensive than in papillary necrosis and due to medullary necrosis.

In adults, renal vein thrombosis is often secondary to other renal disease such as membranous nephropathy or amyloidosis. In these patients, the radiological features depend on the extent of the thrombosis. If thrombosis is confined to the smaller interlobular and arcuate veins, then US and IVU findings will probably be within normal limits. Renal venography is necessary to establish the diagnosis in these patients and it is important that filling of the smaller venous radicles is adequate. This is achieved by placing the tip of the catheter as far into the main renal vein as possible and using a forceful injection of contrast medium, or combining this with an injection of 5–10 µg of adrenaline directly into the renal artery to diminish renal blood flow and so assist with retrograde filling of the smaller venous radicles. Visualization of thrombus in the smaller venous radicles establishes the diagnosis.

If the renal vein thrombosis is more extensive and involves the main venous radicles, then US and IVU findings will be abnormal. US may show an enlarged kidney with increased echogenicity, particularly within the renal vein. IVU shows generalized renal enlargement. There is probably some impairment of excretion with a poor nephrogram and pyelogram, making it difficult to discern fine detail, and poor filling of the collecting system due in part to impaired excretion and in part to compression by the swollen kidney. Vascular impressions on the upper ureter and renal pelvis may be seen; these are due to large collateral venous channels. Again the diagnosis is confirmed by renal venography, which shows filling defects within the renal vein.

CT scan will sometimes identify renal vein thrombosis.

Conclusion

Renal imaging plays a major role in the investigation of patients with urinary tract disorders but must be tailored to the individual problem. There is no single correct diagnostic approach — each problem must be analysed in turn. Care must be taken in selecting from the many imaging modalities available those most likely to establish the diagnosis and extent of the pathology. Changes in the complementary and competitive nature of imaging procedures are occurring rapidly as technology expands, and close cooperation between the clinician and imaging expert is essential to evaluate these changes and use them to their best advantage.

RECOMMENDED READING

Amis E S 1991 Contemporary uro-radiology. Radiologic Clinics of North America 29: 437–647

Becker J A, Bosniak M A, Baert A L 1992 Uroradiology update. Urologic Radiology 14: 3–33

Lang E K 1991 Radiology of the upper urinary tract. Springer-Verlag, Berlin

Raymond H W, Zweibel W J, Harnsberger H R 1991 Renal parenchymal disease. Seminars in Ultrasound, CT and MR 12: 289–374

Sherwood T, Davidson A J, Talner L B 1980 Uroradiology. Blackwell, Oxford

Strashun A 1992 Uroradiologic nuclear medicine. Urologic Radiology 14: 67–115

6. Clinical presentation

J. R. Lawrence . J. A. Whitworth

INTRODUCTION

Renal disease may be obvious, as in patients with visible haematuria, renal colic or acute anuria. Conversely, serious active renal disease may be present in the absence of symptoms. Such asymptomatic renal disease may be recognized clinically by finding protein, blood or pus in the urine. It may also be recognized by the presence of one of the concomitant metabolic or functional disturbances, such as hypertension, uraemia or anaemia.

Because renal disease is often occult, examination of fresh urine should be included as part of the routine physical examination.

The individual renal diseases are discussed later in this volume but, since there is considerable heterogeneity and overlap in clinical and pathological features and their correlations, it is useful here to consider the 'classic' syndromes and typical modes of presentation. Eleven broad categories of renal disease are included: eight propounded by Black (1972), two added by Coe (1981), and a difficult syndrome not in the preceding list. Each category has characteristic historical and physical features and laboratory findings. It is important to recognize that the various syndromes, e.g. acute nephritis, nephrotic syndrome and acute renal failure, may occur either as a result of intrinsic disease of the kidneys or as part of systemic disease (see Ch. 9).

The eleven syndromes discussed are:

1. The nephritic syndrome
2. The nephrotic syndrome
3. Asymptomatic urinary abnormality
4. Urinary tract infection
5. Acute renal failure
6. Chronic renal failure
7. Urinary tract obstruction
8. Tubulointerstitial syndromes
9. Renal calculi
10. Urological tumours
11. Haematuria/loin pain syndrome.

In this chapter only the classic syndromes are defined. In practice, there are many patients with varying combinations of clinical and pathological features which do not fit easily into one syndrome. Individual patients often illustrate the fascinating complexity of renal medicine. Just as each patient is an individual with unique characteristics, the suggested patterns are guidelines only and must be applied to the investigation and diagnosis of specific patients with care and appropriate thought.

Based on the classic patterns of disease presentation, it is possible to propose optimal pathways for diagnosis and assessment (see Ch. 7).

NEPHRITIC SYNDROME

The nephritic syndrome is characterized by haematuria, proteinuria, hypertension, oedema, oliguria and impaired excretory function. The urine may be red or, more often, brownish. Sodium retention and hypertension are characteristic but oedema is usually mild and particularly apparent as suborbital 'puffy eyes'. The increased circulating blood volume and hypertension may lead to cardiomegaly, with a pathological third heart sound at the apex and a rise in jugular venous pressure. Left ventricular failure may be manifest as pulmonary oedema, and severe hypertension may result in retinal haemorrhages or even papilloedema and other features of accelerated hypertension, including hypertensive encephalopathy.

Renal pain is not usually emphasized but a dull renal ache is not uncommon and is a feature of the acute nephritic syndrome in IgA nephropathy. Renal pain is particularly common in acute focal forms of nephritis. The swollen kidneys are tender to percussion.

If severe renal failure occurs there is usually marked oliguria. The clinical features may include mental obtundation, pericardial friction rub, twitching, hiccoughs and vomiting.

Some causes of the nephritic syndrome
Intrinsic glomerulonephritis (GN) (see Ch. 9)
Post-streptococcal GN
Other post-infectious GN
IgA nephropathy
Mesangiocapillary GN
Focal necrotizing GN
Mesangial proliferative GN
Crescentic GN
Anti-GBM GN
Hereditary/familial GN
Systemic disease
Systemic lupus erythematosus
Polyarteritis
Bacterial endocarditis
Henoch–Schönlein purpura
Haemolytic–uraemic syndrome
Acute tubulointerstitial nephritis

The nephritic syndrome in children and young adults is most likely to be due to post-streptococcal or post-infectious glomerulonephritis or to an exacerbation of IgA nephropathy. In all patients, but particularly in adults with a nephritic syndrome, the possibility of systemic disease causing nephritis, such as polyarteritis, systemic lupus erythematosus, bacterial endocarditis or Henoch–Schönlein purpura, must be considered.

The laboratory features include elevation of serum concentrations of urea and creatinine and a decreased creatinine clearance. The various immunological and bacteriological abnormalities which indicate the aetiology and pathogenesis of nephritic syndrome are described in Chapters 8 and 9.

Anaemia is usually present and is normocytic unless there is an element of intravascular coagulation or an abnormality related to underlying systemic disease.

The urine

Urinary abnormalities are critical in the diagnosis of the nephritic syndrome. Haematuria may present as a visible red or smoky-brown discoloration or be identified by impregnated dipstick testing. Microscopic examination of fresh urinary sediment reveals excess dysmorphic red cells recognized by phase contrast examination. The finding of red cell casts is particularly significant in deciding that the haematuria comes from the renal parenchyma, and they should be sought assiduously. Other casts (hyaline, cellular and granular) may also be present. Proteinuria is usually present; the amount excreted varies from 300 mg daily to the nephrotic range but is most commonly less than 3 g.

Particularly in systemic lupus erythematosus (SLE), but also in other nephritic diseases, there may be an excess of leucocytes in the urine and even white cell casts in the absence of infection. Urinary sodium tends to be low because of sodium retention. Isolated cases of active glomerulitis with an apparently normal urinary sediment have been reported.

NEPHROTIC SYNDROME

The nephrotic syndrome is the consequence of prolonged massive proteinuria, usually exceeding 3.5 g/24 hours in adults or 0.05 g/kg in children. It is characterized by usually insidious onset of massive oedema, proteinuria, hypoalbuminaemia and hyperlipidaemia.

Renal excretory failure, hypertension and haematuria are not recognized features of the nephrotic syndrome but may occur depending on the renal lesion and the aetiology of the disease. The underlying renal pathology causes increased glomerular capillary permeability to protein and when the quantity of filtered protein exceeds the reabsorptive capacity of the proximal tubule proteinuria occurs. Hypoalbuminaemia occurs because the liver is unable to compensate for the combination of loss of protein in the urine and tubular degradation of filtered protein. There is massive retention of sodium and a tendency to excessive potassium loss. Aldosterone and ADH levels are elevated. The hypoalbuminaemia and sodium retention lead to accumulation of salt and water in the tissues and spaces outside the blood vessels. Thus gross oedema and anasarca may occur. Renal excretion of urea and nitrogenous degradation products may be normal but hypovolaemia, often secondary to excessive diuretic therapy, may cause oliguric renal failure. The metabolic consequences and complications of the nephrotic syndrome relate partly to excessive losses of proteins and protein-bound substances and partly to excessive production of normal substances by the liver. One which has not been adequately explained is the hyperlipidaemia characterized by elevated concentrations of cholesterol, triglycerides and phospholipids, and corrected by infusion of sufficient albumin. There is some controversy concerning the probable deleterious vascular effects of hyperlipidaemia in the chronic nephrotic syndrome.

An important effect of the nephrotic syndrome is a tendency to hypercoagulability which leads to venous and occasionally arterial thrombosis and embolism. The described abnormalities in coagulation include increased levels of fibrinogen, decreased fibrinolytic activators, increased inhibition of fibrinolysis and increased concentrations of the coagulation factors V, VII, VIII and X. One complication, found particularly in patients with membranous nephropathy, is the development of renal vein thrombosis which is usually a secondary event but may perpetuate the nephrotic syndrome and precipitate renal failure.

There is increased susceptibility to infection, notably by pneumococci, which may be related to low levels of immunoglobulin and be manifest as peritonitis or pneumonia.

Serum calcium levels are low partly because the serum albumin is decreased. In addition, in many patients there is impaired conversion of hydroxycholecalciferol to 1,25-dihydroxycholecalciferol, presumably due to impaired function of the proximal convoluted tubules, and increased

---

Some causes of the nephrotic syndrome
Intrinsic glomerulonephrtis (GN)
Minimal lesion nephropathy:
  idiopathic
  secondary to Hodgkin's disease or drugs
Membranous GN:
  idiopathic
  secondary to tumours or drugs
Proliferative GN
Mesangiocapillary GN (subgroups)
Focal sclerosing GN
Systemic disease
Diabetes mellitus
Systemic lupus erythematosus
Henoch–Schönlein purpura
Amyloidosis
IgG/IgM cryoglobulinaemia
Shunt nephritis
Raised renal venous pressure
Renal vein thrombosis
Severe right heart failure
Constrictive pericarditis

---

loss of protein-bound 1,25-dihydroxycholecalciferol in the urine. Dysfunction of the proximal tubules may rarely cause aminoaciduria or glycosuria.

The clinical features depend on the cause of the nephrotic syndrome and show considerable variability in severity, which relates only roughly to the magnitude of the proteinuria and the degree of hypoalbuminaemia. The patient is classically pale and puffy, with gross oedema causing swelling of legs, scrotum, labia, hands and face. There may be ascites and pleural effusions. The oedema has a postural distribution, and periorbital facial oedema which is worse on waking may be severe enough to close the palpebral fissures.

In children the most likely cause of the nephrotic syndrome is idiopathic minimal lesion glomerulonephritis, but most forms of glomerulonephritis (intrinsic and secondary), many metabolic diseases (including diabetes and amyloidosis), drug-induced hypersensitivity, some infections, and grossly increased renal venous pressure, as in constrictive pericarditis, can cause the nephrotic syndrome.

Laboratory features

Laboratory findings include those relating to any underlying disease (see Ch. 9). The serum may be turbid. There is hypoalbuminaemia and a variable decrease in serum concentrations of other globulins and proteins. Some factors, e.g. fibrinogen, are increased. Serum sodium is normal or low (sometimes 'spurious' from hyperlipidaemia) and serum potassium is often low with elevated bicarbonate levels reflecting secondary hyperaldosteronism. Serum cholesterol, triglyceride and phospholipids are usually elevated.

The urine

The urine may froth when passed or if shaken. Dipstick testing shows proteinuria but this must always be measured in 24-hour collections. The protein in the urine is predominantly albumin but the relative proportion of higher molecular weight proteins relates roughly to the type of histological lesion and inversely to the likelihood of therapeutic response to steroid administration. Various indices of selectivity of proteinuria have been proposed to predict the response to therapy and the likely pathological lesion.

Microscopic examination of urine usually shows hyaline casts, oval fat bodies and fatty casts. Haematuria is present in some types of glomerulonephritis — both intrinsic and secondary. It is more likely to be present in membranous than in minimal lesion idiopathic nephrotic syndrome. Granular and other casts may be present, depending on the underlying renal lesion. During the acute phase the urinary sodium will often be very low, i.e. less than 10 mmol/l, reflecting the avid tubular reabsorption of sodium.

Table 6.1 compares the features associated with the nephritic and nephrotic syndromes.

ASYMPTOMATIC URINARY ABNORMALITY

Various combinations of haematuria, proteinuria, bacteriuria and excess excretion of white cells in the urine may be found in otherwise apparently normal asymptomatic patients. Although fever and

Table 6.1 Comparison of clinical features of the nephritic and nephrotic syndromes

	Nephritic syndrome	Nephrotic syndrome
Urine	Blood ++	Blood 0–+
	Protein +	Protein ++++
Plasma	Urea ↑	Urea normal or ↑
	Creatinine ↑	Creatinine normal or ↑
	Albumin normal	Albumin ↓
	Cholesterol normal	Cholesterol ↑
Total body sodium	↑	↑
Blood volume	↑	Normal or ↓
Blood pressure	↑	Normal or ↑
Oedema	+	++++

heavy exercise may cause proteinuria or haematuria, the discovery of blood or protein in the urine in patients with no apparent renal symptoms should always be confirmed and extended as discussed in Chapter 4. The finding of coincident hypertension, or a combination of haematuria and proteinuria makes renal disease more likely, as does the presence of granular, cellular or haem casts in the urinary sediment. In a number of forms of chronic renal disease, including some forms of glomerulonephritis, urinary abnormalities may vary widely from time to time.

In all cases, but particularly in asymptomatic haematuria, the most probable diagnosis relates to the age and gender of the patient, e.g. microscopic haematuria in a young male is more likely to be due to glomerulonephritis but in an older male is

---

Some causes of asymptomatic urinary abnormality
Glomerulonephritis:
  primary
  secondary
Thin basement membrane nephropathy
Orthostatic proteinuria
Pregnancy hypertension
Interstitial nephritis
Drugs
Exercise, fever
Urological tumour
Renal calculi
Renal cyst (rare)
Polycystic disease

more likely to be due to a tumour of the transitional endothelium of the urinary tract.

Asymtomatic patients with proteinuria, haematuria or bacteriuria are commonly identified when the urine is tested as part of a routine examination for insurance or employment. In these patients further investigation is necessary but may identify no significant disease. It is important not to arouse excessive inappropriate anxiety in individuals who have no overt ill health, particularly as further procedures may not identify any condition whose natural history will be modified by treatment.

URINARY TRACT INFECTION

Infection in the urinary tract may be asymptomatic or cause a variety of symptoms and signs. Frequency of micturition, urgency, and burning or scalding pain on passing urine may indicate active infection but can also occur in the absence of identifiable infection. Some patients note an unpleasant offensive odour of the urine. Strangury or a painful urge to void with an empty bladder is a particularly unpleasant symptom. Visible haematuria may occur, particularly in acute cystitis, but haematuria and proteinuria are not classic diagnostic features. Pyelonephritis with renal parenchymal involvement may cause pain and tenderness in the renal angle but this is not invariable. Systemic signs and symptoms of infection — rigors, headache, nausea, aching — may accompany urinary tract infection, and septicaemia may arise in susceptible individuals, particularly with coincident obstruction or following instrumentation.

Laboratory findings

Active infection will often cause a polymorphonuclear leucocytosis and rarely, unless there is coincident disease such as chronic renal failure or obstruction and infection, a rise in serum creatinine.

The urine

The diagnostic findings are discussed in Chapters 4 and 16. Significant pyuria in fresh urine should always suggest urinary infection, but it may occur in sterile urine in analgesic nephropathy, renal stones, treated or incompletely resolved infection, or tuberculosis.

ACUTE RENAL FAILURE

Acute renal failure occurs when the kidneys are unable to excrete metabolic products which then accumulate. It may be due to intrinsic renal disease or be the result of impaired perfusion or urinary obstruction.

The wide variety of clinical causes includes those which cause cardiovascular insufficiency or shock, particularly with coincident septicaemia (see Ch. 20). It can also be caused by toxins and nephrotoxic drugs, acute tubulointerstitial disease, several forms of glomerulonephritis, systemic vasculitis and intravascular coagulation which can also present as acute renal failure. Often the condition is insidious and is diagnosed because the underlying clinical state of the patient causes the condition to be sought, e.g. following complex

---

Some causes of acute renal failure

Tubulointerstitial disease
Trauma, shock, sepsis
Drug-induced
Hypercalcaemia
Urate nephropathy
Oxalate nephropathy
Drugs and toxins
Papillary necrosis and obstruction
Myeloma protein
Rapidly progressive glomerulonephritis (GN) —
   usually crescentic
Anti-GBM GN
Idiopathic GN
Post-streptococcal GN, etc.
Systemic vasculitis
Polyarteritis
Wegener's granulomatosis
Intravascular coagulation
Haemolytic–uraemic syndrome
Cortical necrosis
Acute transplant rejection
Renal artery occlusion
Post-partum renal failure

surgery with sepsis, in prolonged cardiogenic shock, etc.

Rapidly progressive forms of glomerulonephritis must be identified and distinguished from acute tubular necrosis.

Oliguria is usual but not invariable, and blood concentrations of urea, creatinine and uric acid are raised, the rate of increase being determined by the metabolic status of the patient and the degree of renal failure. While the cause and onset may be obvious, as in crush injury or mismatched blood transfusion, acute renal failure has many causes (see Ch. 20) which may be overlooked in patients with multiple problems including surgery, infection or trauma.

Biochemical abnormalities

Biochemical abnormalities in the blood include elevated urea, creatinine and uric acid, acidosis, hyperkalaemia, hypocalcaemia, hyperphosphataemia and hyponatraemia from accumulation of ingested water and water of metabolism.

The urine

The urine often contains red blood cells and numerous casts (including haem, cellular and granular casts) but the sediment may be relatively benign. Myoglobin can be identified in conditions associated with muscle destruction. In established acute renal failure due to acute tubular necrosis the osmolality of urine approaches that of plasma, urinary creatinine and urea are less than 10 times the serum concentrations, and the urinary sodium is relatively elevated, exceeding 20 mmol/l and usually greater than 40 mmol/l. These abnormalities reflect the impaired renal tubular function and disturbed glomerulotubular balance which is usually present. Rarely, and usually in milder forms of acute renal failure, there is polyuria and a 'normal' output of dilute urine. If acute renal failure is suspected it is essential to save all urine for chemical analysis before administering diuretics.

Acute renal failure has a multitude of causes, many of them reversible, and these are described in Chapter 20.

CHRONIC RENAL FAILURE

This term includes a very wide range of metabolic disturbances ranging from asymptomatic reduction of glomerular filtration rate in apparently normal patients to terminal uraemia. Seldin suggested a useful classification into four stages.

1. Diminished renal reserve
2. Renal insufficiency (creatinine clearance less than 35 ml/min) — patients somewhat precariously balanced and susceptible to rapid decompensation and clinical deterioration
3. Renal failure — patients with anaemia, severe azotaemia, acidosis, hyperphosphataemia
4. Uraemia — patients with preterminal manifestations of renal failure.

A very early symptom may be nocturia reflecting impaired renal concentrating capacity, but patients with slowly developing chronic renal failure characteristically evolve a number of compensatory physiological mechanisms. In contrast to patients with acute renal failure, hyperkalaemia is rare except when complications occur and the metabolic acidosis is usually 'compensated'. Patients may be identified by the finding of asymptomatic urinary abnormalities such as proteinuria, or they may present with hypertension, recurrent urinary infection (e.g. analgesic nephropathy, reflux nephropathy), vague ill health, anaemia and its sequelae, poor intellectual concentration, nausea, anorexia, twitching, restless legs, cramps, peripheral neuropathy, increasing pigmentation, gastrointestinal disturbances, bone pains, crystalline arthropathy or a tendency to easy bruising and bleeding.

Clinically, chronic renal failure may not be obvious but there is a characteristic combination of pallor of the mucosae and palms, and yellowish brown skin pigmentation in more advanced chronic renal failure. The fingernails may be abnormal, with pallor of the proximal portion and a thin rim of distal pigmentation (Lindsay's nails), and calcium phosphate deposition in the conjunctivae on both sides of the pupil may help to suggest the diagnosis.

The common causes of chronic renal failure include glomerulonephritis, the various forms of interstitial nephritis, including analgesic nephropathy and reflex nephropathy, and adult polycystic kidney disease. They may be identified from the history. Episodes of infection, obstruction or dehydration and administration of tetracyclines may precipitate acute renal failure with rapid deterioration into acute severe uraemia.

Laboratory findings

The diagnosis is confirmed by measurement of sustained elevated blood urea and creatinine concentrations. There is hyperphosphataemia, a tendency to hypocalcaemia and, later, compensated metabolic acidosis. Except in polycystic disease and bilateral hydronephrosis the kidneys are usually small. The numerous other biochemical and metabolic anomalies are described in Chapter 22.

Anaemia is often present and may be normocytic or microcytic. The fully developed syndrome of preterminal uraemia should now be seen only in patients for whom maintenance dialysis is inappropriate. The patient is pigmented, and there is massive spontaneous bruising, twitching, anorexia, vomiting, often with severe central chest pain from pericarditis, and mental obtundation leading to convulsions and coma.

URINARY TRACT OBSTRUCTION

Because the muscular urinary tract generates pressure to allow the onward and outward passage of urine, obstruction will lead to back pressure and ultimately to impaired renal function as well as susceptibility to urinary infection. The combination of obstruction and infection is particularly destructive and may lead to pyonephrosis with extensive damage to renal parenchyma. Sloughing of papillae as in analgesic nephropathy may lead to renal colic and episodes of obstruction. Calcification occurs in necrotic infarcted medullary tissue.

Obstruction may be complete (as by an impacted stone) or, more often, incomplete or intermittent.

Some causes of urinary tract obstruction
Congenital
Bladder neck obstruction, pelviureteric obstruction
Urethral valves
Vesicoureteric reflux
Ectopia vesicae
Spina bifida
Ectopic ureters
Ectopic or fused kidneys
Acquired
Renal stones
Papillary necrosis
Retroperitoneal fibrosis
Urethral stricture
Radiation strictures
Urinary tuberculosis
Neoplasms
Benign prostatic hyperplasia
Carcinoma of the prostate
Papillary tumours (bladder, ureter, pelvis)
Carcinoma of the bladder
Gynaecological malignancy
Retroperitoneal tumour

In young patients obstruction in the urethra may be valvular and in older men prostatic hypertrophy is an important cause. Grade 3 vesicoureteric reflux is also a form of functional obstructive uropathy. In a variety of conditions, including inherited anomalies such as spina bifida, paraplegia or diabetes, neurogenic bladder dysfunction may lead to obstruction with overflow. Such patients may present with recurrent infections, constant dribbling and wetting or progressive uraemia. Early recognition is important because surgical relief will often reverse renal failure. Bladder neck obstruction or dysfunction may be recognized by palpation of a full bladder after attempted voiding.

Investigation

Lesser degrees of urinary stasis and retention may be revealed by a variety of techniques, including careful post-micturition catheterization, post-voiding films during pyelography and voiding cystometrograms.

Laboratory findings

Obviously, complete obstruction will cause anuria and the biochemical features of acute renal failure leading to uraemia. Intermittent or partial obstruction will produce the biochemical changes of chronic renal failure as a result of renal parenchymal damage. In both cases superimposed infection will cause an exacerbation of renal failure and is particularly likely to lead to septicaemia. The laboratory features are described under 'Urinary tract infection' above.

TUBULOINTERSTITIAL SYNDROMES

These are best divided into:

a. Diseases causing progressive tubulointerstitial destruction and fibrosis. These often cause progressive chronic renal failure with small scarred kidneys, e.g. analgesic nephropathy. This condition used to be called chronic pyelonephritis — a term which must be discontinued.

b. A variety of other conditions — see box — some of which also lead to progressive renal tubular destruction.

The variety of disorders includes cystic diseases, interstitial nephritis (see Ch. 18), functional tubular abnormalities, renal tubular acidosis, Fanconi syndrome, cystinuria, pseudohypoparathyroidism and nephrogenic diabetes insipidus. In the first two groups there is ultimately a significant reduction in glomerular filtration rate but earlier manifestations, particularly of interstitial nephritis (e.g. analgesic nephropathy) and medullary cystic disease, include disproportionate polyuria and failure to concentrate the urine. In the earlier stages proteinuria is absent or minimal but this may increase significantly, especially when chronic renal failure intervenes. A particularly important condition is adult polycystic disease. Its protean clinical manifestations, occurring usually in adult life, include haematuria, renal pain, palpable renal masses, hypertension, chronic renal failure, renal colic, cystic changes in other organs and subarachnoid haemorrhage from aneurysms.

Chronic interstitial nephritis is more likely to cause disproportionate sodium loss than primary glomerulonephritis. Nevertheless, hypertension may occur and ultimately renal failure.

There is a wide variety of metabolic renal tubular defects. They may occur as inherited disorders or as a result of certain toxins or other conditions, e.g. Bence Jones protein, sarcoidosis. Major groups include the various forms of renal tubular acidosis which cause hyperchloraemic acidosis, nephrocalcinosis and recurrent renal calculi. Disorders of the proximal tubule can cause aminoaciduria, sometimes selective as in cystinuria or non-selective as in cystinosis. Other proximal tubular defects include impaired reabsorption of phosphate, glucose and urate and bicarbonate. These are manifest as glycosuria with normal blood glucose concentrations, hypophosphataemia and hypouricaemia respectively. Other inherited tubular disorders include sodium wasting, potassium wasting and magnesium loss. There may also be specific tubular resistance to the effect of hormones, as in nephrogenic diabetes insipidus and pseudohypoparathyroidism. All of these con-

---

Tubulointerstitial syndromes

1. Cystic diseases (see Ch. 18)
   Polycystic kidneys (adult)
   Polycystic kidneys (infantile)
   Medullary cystic disease
   Medullary sponge kidneys
   Single or multiple cysts
2. Interstitial nephritis
   Analgesic nephropathy
   Reflux nephropathy
   Gouty nephropathy
   Sickle cell disease
   Drug-induced
   Lead nephropathy
   Infection
   Balkan nephropathy
3. Functional tubular abnormalities
4. Renal tubular acidosis
5. Fanconi syndrome
6. Cystinuria
7. Pseudohypoparathyroidism
8. Nephrogenic diabetes insipidus
   Familial rickets
   Bartter's syndrome
   Liddle syndrome
   Gordon syndrome

ditions may be identified by the occurrence of metabolic abnormalities, e.g. unexplained acidosis, hypokalaemia, bone disease, polyuria, renal calculi, or, in children, failure to thrive.

RENAL CALCULI

Renal stones should always be seen as evidence of identifiable metabolic abnormalities, particularly if recurrent or multiple, as emphasized by Coe (1981). Stones may be asymptomatic, or they may present as classic renal colic radiating from loin to labia or testis, or they may be recognized by the passage of solid material in the urine. In the differential diagnosis of abdominal pain and swelling it is important to recognize that renal colic may cause a degree of ileus and distension.

Whether the stone is identified by X-ray or ultrasound or recognized in the urine, macroscopic or microscopic non-dysmorphic haematuria is supportive diagnostic evidence. Persistent dilatation of the urinary tract may also be identified after passage of the stone. Urate calculi are generally not radiopaque and should be suspected not only in patients with gout but also in those with active myeloproliferative disease or in climates where dehydration is likely. In cystinuria, examination of the urinary sediment may identify the characteristic hexagonal crystals.

Calcified stones are due to metabolic disturbances causing hypercalciuria with or without hypercalcaemia, renal tubular acidosis or hyperoxaluria. They can also occur as a consequence of papillary necrosis in analgesic nephropathy, in medullary sponge kidney or as the result of persistent urinary infection, particularly with coexistent urinary stasis. Large staghorn calculi do not cause renal colic but may present with pain or urinary infection.

The laboratory findings are described in Chapter 19.

UROLOGICAL TUMOURS

Benign and malignant tumours can occur in the kidneys or in the urinary collecting system.

Renal tumours in children (usually a nephroblastoma) and adults (usually a Grawitz carcinoma) may present with systemic features including fever, weight loss, leucocytosis and anaemia; thrombophlebitis; non-metastatic complications such as hypercalcaemia or polycythaemia; or as the result of secondary deposits in lung or bones. The classic triad of macroscopic haematuria, weight loss and a palpable renal mass is a presenting feature in some patients. An important complication of analgesic nephropathy is transitional cell carcinoma of the renal pelvis. It should be suspected when patients deteriorate or develop macroscopic haematuria.

More common tumours, particularly in older patients, are papillary neoplasms in the bladder, ureters or renal pelves. They usually present as frank blood in the urine and should be suspected in all patients with this symptom. Persistent microscopic haematuria may also occur as an incidental finding in early cases.

The urine

Examination of the urine shows haematuria or casts without significant proteinuria. The red cells are non-dysmorphic. In specialized cytological laboratories malignant cells may be identified in fresh urine.

The diagnosis is confirmed by endoscopic examination and biopsy, usually following pyelography.

HYPERTENSION

Many forms of renal disease, including nephritis, interstitial nephritis, polycystic disease and reflux nephropathy, cause hypertension. Although essential hypertension is common and occurs in up to 20% of the community, the finding of hypertension should always lead to consideration of possible underlying renal disease, the commonest cause of secondary hypertension. This may be manifest by proteinuria, haematuria, a history of recurrent urinary infection, or evidence of disease such as polyarteritis, but is often inapparent.

Some patients with hypertension caused by renal artery stenosis can be cured by surgery or dilatation of the narrowed segment. This is more likely if the patient is young and the onset recent. Particularly in younger patients a bruit over the aorta in the epigastrium and radiating to one side suggests this diagnosis. Confirmation of the diagnosis depends on visualization of the renal artery and assessment of the functional significance if a stenosis is identified (see Ch. 27).

HAEMATURIA/LOIN PAIN SYNDROME

Inevitably there are a number of other presentations which include overlapping features of the 'classic' syndromes outlined in this chapter. One of the more difficult is the haematuria/loin pain syndrome characterized by microscopic or macroscopic haematuria and severe loin pain occurring in intermittent attacks. Many patients are young women taking the oral contraceptive pill. This syndrome is particularly likely in acute focal glomerulonephritis, but other histological and vascular abnormalities have been described which are not consistently present or precisely characterized.

REFERENCES AND RECOMMENDED READING

Black D A K 1972 Diagnosis in renal disease. In: Black D A K (ed) Renal disease, 3rd edn. Blackwell, Oxford, pp 827–840

Cassidy M J D, Kerr D N S 1992 The assessment of the patient with chronic renal insufficiency. In: Cameron S, Davison A M, Grunfeld J-P, Kerr D, Ritz E (eds) Oxford Textbook of clinical nephrology. Oxford Unviersity Press, New York, vol 2, pp 1149–1173

Coe F L 1981 Clinical and laboratory assessment of the patient with renal disease. In: Brenner B M, Rector Jr F C (eds) The kidney, 2nd edn. Saunders, Philadelphia, ch 23, p. 1135

Coe F L 1989 Renal colic and flank pain. In: Massry S G, Glassock R J (eds) Textbook of nephrology. Williams & Wilkins, Baltimore, pp 501–505

Eliahau H E 1989 Oliguria and anuria. In: Massry S G, Glassock R J (eds) Textbook of nephrology. Williams & Wilkins, Baltimore, pp 475–478

Firland M 1989 Dysuria and frequency. In: Massry S G, Glassock R J (eds) Textbook of nephrology. Williams & Wilkins, Baltimore, pp 487–490

Glassock R J 1989 Hematuria and pigmenturia. In: Massry S G, Glassock R J (eds) Textbook of nephrology. Williams & Wilkins, Baltimore, pp 491–500

Glassock R J 1989 Proteinuria. In: Massry S G, Glassock R J (eds) Textbook of nephrology. Williams & Wilkins, Baltimore, pp 530–534

Mallick N P, Short C D 1992 The clinical approach to haematuria and proteinuria. In: Cameron S, Davison A M, Grunfeld J-P, Kerr D, Ritz E (eds) Oxford Textbook of clinical nephrology. Oxford University Press, New York, vol 1, pp 227–240

Ooi B S, Jao W, First M R, Mancilla R, Pollak V E 1975 Acute interstitial nephritis: a clinical and pathologic study based on renal biopsies. American Journal of Medicine 59: 614

Rainford D J, Stevens P E 1992 The investigative approach to the patient with acute renal failure. In: Cameron S, Davison A M, Grunfeld J-P, Kerr D, Ritz E (eds) Oxford Textbook of clinical nephrology. Oxford University Press, New York, vol 2, pp 969–982

Schreiner G E 1989 Uremia. In: Massry S G, Glassock R J (eds) Textbook of nephrology. Williams & Wilkins, Baltimore, pp 540–550

Sinniah R, Pwee J S, Lim C H 1976 Glomerular lesions in symptomatic macroscopic hematuria discovered on routine medical examination. Clinical Nephrology 5: 216

7. Diagnostic pathways in renal disease

J. R. Lawrence   J. A. Whitworth

The basic renal investigative techniques are described in Chapters 4 and 5 and some of the basic clinical syndromes in Chapter 6. In the diagnosis of renal disease, particularly glomerulonephritis, it is helpful to characterize the triad of:

1. clinical features (pathophysiology and pathobiochemistry);
2. histological features (pathology, light and electron microscopy and immunopathology); and
3. pathogenesis and aetiology.

In this chapter, beginning with common presenting features of syndromes, a brief basic and practical sequence of important investigations is defined. It should be recognized that a comprehensive list of appropriate patterns of renal investigation would be inordinately long and contain an almost infinite number of variations.

Investigations are aimed primarily at establishing the aetiology and pathological diagnosis. They are also essential to identify reversible and life-threatening metabolic disturbances such as acidosis, hyperkalaemia or acute uraemia.

Although protocols are useful they only provide guidelines. Investigation and management of patients must always be individual. Thus, before each step the clinician must pose a question to be answered. The answer will have further investigative or therapeutic consequences. In this chapter we have developed skeletons of investigative pathways trying to identify the questions to be answered to avoid the risk of promulgating mindless and expensive 'cook book' approaches to the investigation and management of the nominated clinical problem.

HAEMATURIA

Haematuria must be distinguished from various other causes of reddish-brown discoloration of the urine, including methmyoglobin, methaemoglobin and free haemoglobin. Systemic bleeding disorders must be considered. There are many causes of visible haematuria but it is most likely to be due to urological tumours, stones or trauma. It can arise from any level in the renal tract. Although urological causes are most common, particularly in the older patient, frank haematuria can be caused by nephritis, notably IgA nephropathy, thin basement membrane nephropathy, or crescentic forms of glomerulonephritis, and also by cystitis. It is necessary to exclude a diagnosis of nephritis before embarking on the search for a urological lesion. Careful microscopic examination of fresh urinary sediment is essential and can distinguish between glomerular and non-glomerular bleeding. In IgA nephropathy mixed red cell morphology is often found. Coincident proteinuria strongly favours nephritis.

Diagnostic pathways in haematuria, macroscopic or microscopic		
Q:	*Site of origin?*	
Test:	Dipstick, blood, protein, microscopic examination and culture of urine, red cell morphology, casts, bacteria	

A:	Glomerular bleeding (± protein)		A:	Non-glomerular bleeding
Q:	*Acute or chronic disease?*		Q:	*Site of origin and cause? (renal function)*
Test:	Ultrasound, KUB or CT scan		Test:	Ultrasound, CT/KUB, cystography,
A:	Normal to large kidneys			endoscopy, cytology
			A:	Stone, tumour, cystitis, etc.
Q:	*Glomerulonephritis?*			
Test:	? Biopsy (renal function)			
A:	Small kidneys			
Q:	*Chronic glomerulonephritis or interstitial nephritis?*		Q:	*Renal trauma?*
			Test:	Arteriography
Q:	*Renal function?*			

THE NEPHRITIC SYNDROME

In this condition renal biopsy is commonly indicated. Exceptions include obvious post-streptococcal glomerulonephritis in children in whom biopsy is indicated only if expected recovery does not occur, or if anomalous clinical features suggest unusual lesions or severe renal failure or oliguria suggests crescentic nephritis. When only one kidney is present it may be preferable to consider open biopsy. To obtain maximal diagnostic information from biopsy it is necessary to include immunological and electron microscopic studies. The diagnostic triad should lead to appropriate therapy and is often important in establishing prognosis. In IgA nephropathy, for example, a confirmed diagnosis will often save the patient from repeated endoscopic investigation of attacks of renal pain and haematuria.

Diagnostic pathway in the nephritic syndrome

Q: *Acute or chronic?*
Test: a. Renal function
          Blood — creatinine, urea, pH, electrolytes, calcium, phosphate, haemoglobin
       b. Renal size
          Ultrasound, KUB, CT scan

Q: *Aetiology, prognosis?*
Test: Immunological function tests (see Ch. 9)
       Tests for systemic diseases

Test: Renal biopsy

PROTEINURIA

Persistent proteinuria usually indicates renal disease. Glomerular proteinuria is predominantly albumin and usually exceeds 500 mg per 24 hours. True orthostatic proteinuria has an excellent prognosis even though some patients have minor histological glomerular abnormalities. Proteinuria occasionally indicates tubulointerstitial disease — in this case the protein is not predominantly albumin and rarely exceeds 1 g in 24 hours. However, in the later stages of interstitial nephritis, notably in analgesic nephropathy and reflux nephropathy, focal glomerular lesions of hyalinosis/sclerosis can be associated with persistent significant proteinuria, usually less than 3 g/24 hours.

THE NEPHROTIC SYNDROME

In patients with the nephrotic syndrome it is usually desirable to identify the glomerular pathology by renal biopsy, including electron microscopy and immunopathology. Children with uncomplicated nephrosis are an exception, as the presence of minimal lesion nephropathy is often assumed. Failure of therapeutic response to steroids is then an indication for biopsy. Some consider that a similar approach is justifiable in adults with 'idiopathic' nephrotic syndrome but we advocate early biopsy so that therapy and prognosis can be based on knowledge of the glomerular lesion. It is essential to search carefully for underlying systemic or other disease in all nephrotic patients. However, nephritis may coexist with another underlying lesion, e.g. diabetic nephropathy. Membranous nephropathy in adults may be due to occult malignancy.

Diagnostic pathway in proteinuria including the nephrotic syndrome

Q: *Pathological?*

Test: Repeated dipstick testing of urine for blood, protein, glucose

Microurine — blood, red cell morphology, casts

A: 1. Blood, casts, etc. — probable nephritis (investigate as under *Nephritic syndrome*)

2. Orthostatic proteinuria — observe; review after 6 months

3. Persistent or heavy proteinuria

Q: *Quantity of proteinuria?*

Test: 24-hour urinary protein

A: **A. Proteinuria exceeding 0.5 g/24 hours**

Q: *Nephrotic syndrome (particularly if protein > 3 g/24 h)?*

Test: Blood — albumin, cholesterol

Q: *Renal function? (see under* Nephritic syndrome*)*

Q: *Renal size?*

Test: X-ray, IVP, ultrasound

A: 1. Small scarred kidneys — probable interstitial nephritis and focal hyalinosis/sclerosis

2. Normal or large kidneys — probable primary or secondary glomerulonephritis or other systemic disease

Q: *Systemic disease?*

Test: Immunological and other tests for systemic lupus erythematosus, diabetes mellitus, amyloidosis, etc.

Q: *Aetiology, appropriate therapy, prognosis?*

Test: Renal biopsy (histology, immunofluorescence, electron microscopy)

A: **B. Proteinuria less than 0.5 g/24 hours**

Q: *Glomerular or tubular proteinuria?*

Tests: Determination of urine protein type

X-ray, etc., to determine renal morphology and size

Q: *Early diabetes or a form of interstitial renal disease?*

Tests: As appropriate. Renal biopsy

ACUTE RENAL FAILURE (See Ch. 20)

Many of the numerous causes of this syndrome are obvious from the history but acute renal failure can also occur insidiously in the course of other diseases, e.g. cardiogenic shock or septicaemia. Investigation is directed towards identification of urinary obstruction or 'pre-renal' causes of poor renal perfusion and confirmation of established acute renal failure by biochemical analysis of urinary and blood sodium, creatinine and osmolality. Renal calculi and shed papillae are not always radio-opaque and evidence of obstruction may be obtained atraumatically by ultrasound examination. Oliguric crescentic rapidly progressive glomerulonephritis (RPGN) may not present with gross haematuria or proteinuria. Both RPGN and acute interstitial nephritis can be confirmed by urgent renal biopsy.

The other essential aspect of diagnosis in acute renal failure is identification of life-threatening metabolic disturbances such as acidosis, hyperkalaemia, acute progressive uraemia or septicaemia.

Diagnostic pathway in acute renal failure

Q: *Metabolic consequences?*
Test: Blood: urea, creatinine, potassium, pH, calcium, phosphate, P_aO_2, ECG, culture

Q: *Established, pre-renal or obstructive?*
Tests: Urine volume, osmolality
        Urine and plasma: sodium, creatinine, urea
A: Oliguria

Q: *Pre-renal, poor renal perfusion?*
Tests: Postural blood pressure, central venous pressure, cardiac output: ?radionuclide scan

Q: *Not pre-renal? Obstructive?*
Tests: Rectal examination, bladder volume, catheter
        Renal size, calculi, ureteric obstruction
        Ultrasound, X-ray, CT (scan)
        IVP, antegrade or retrograde pyelography, endoscopy, aortography
A: Established renal failure

Q: *Aetiology?*
Tests: Urine: dipstick microscopy
        Blood: film, coagulation studies
        Blood/urine: culture, serology, etc.
        Blood: Sodium, urate, protein-paraprotein
        Kidney size (as above)
A: Normal or large kidneys, no obvious cause

Q: *Glomerulonephritis or acute interstitial nephritis?*
Test: Renal biopsy
A: Small kidneys

Q: *Acute on chronic?*
Tests: Blood — haemoglobin, etc.
        Infection — urine and blood

CHRONIC RENAL FAILURE

Investigation of chronic renal failure may identify its cause and, although this is not always helpful in immediate management, it may be useful subsequently, e.g. after transplantation. In analgesic nephropathy, some forms of nephritis and in obstructive uropathy accurate diagnosis may lead to effective therapy. Investigation follows two other important paths:

1. The severity of the metabolic consequences of chronic renal failure is established to guide therapy and assess subsequent progress.

2. In all cases, but particularly when there has been recent acute deterioration, it is essential to seek and reverse infection, urinary obstruction, uncontrolled severe hypertension, acute metabolic overload or cardiac failure.

Diagnostic pathways in acute deterioration in chronic renal failure

Q: *Metabolic status?*
Test: Blood: creatinine, urea, bicarbonate, pH, K

Q: *Are reversible factors present?*
        (e.g. infection, obstruction, dehydration, overload, uncontrolled hypertension, cardiac failure)
Tests: Urine and blood cultures, bladder catheter, ultrasound, X-ray of abdomen, pyelography, cystoscopy/
        retrograde (to identify any obstruction)

Diagnostic pathways in chronic renal failure

Q: *Degree of renal functional loss?*
Tests: Blood: creatinine, urea, phosphate, bicarbonate, pH, creatinine clearance, glomerular filtration rate

Q: *Renal size, morphology?*
Tests: Ultrasound, X-ray of abdomen, IVP, CT, radionuclide scan

Q: *Obstruction?*
Tests: Ultrasound, pyelography, endoscopy, CT

Q: *Metabolic effects of renal failure?*
Tests: Blood: pH, electrolytes, haemoglobin, platelets, Ca, PO_4, alkaline phosphatase, parathormone and
        vitamin D. Bone X-rays, bone biopsy (renal osteodystrophy). Nerve conduction times (neuropathy).
        X-ray of chest, ECG (hypertensive vascular disease)

Q: *Urinary infection?*
Test: Urine microscopic examination and culture

Q: *Aetiology of renal failure?*
Tests: Renal anatomy and histology
        Exclude systemic disease

DYSURIA AND FREQUENCY

This presentation is more common in females, but particularly in children and males the possibility of underlying correctable pathology must be considered. An underlying structural lesion is more likely if infection involves the upper tract or is not 'cured' by one-dose therapy.

Males and children should always be investigated, but in women further investigation may not be necessary in uncomplicated cases.

Diagnostic pathways in dysuria and frequency in non-pregnant women

Q: *Is infection present?*

Test: Microscopic examination and culture of fresh urine, dipstick

A: Infection

Test: 3-day treatment followed by repeat culture at one week

A: Persistent infection

Q: *Underlying structural/functional cause?*

Tests: Renal function studies, pyelography, voiding cystography, cystoscopy

---

HYPERTENSION

If there is a clinical suspicion of renal artery stenosis and likely clinical benefit from its correction the condition should be identified. This has been a controversial area but is being simplified by new methods of screening and therapy.

Diagnostic pathways in hypertension

Q: *Renal cause of hypertension?*

Tests: Urine: dipstick testing for protein and blood; microscopy, culture, creatinine clearance, pyelography, radionuclide scan (morphology/perfusion)

A: Acute or chronic renal disease

Q: *Renal artery stenosis?*

Tests: Pyelography, radionuclide scan, digital subtraction angiography

A: Probable renal artery stenosis

Test: Confirmatory arteriography

ACUTE AND CHRONIC INTERSTITIAL NEPHRITIS

These conditions have a variety of presentations and causes. The investigative protocols are suggested for patients in whom the condition is suspected on other clinical grounds.

Diagnostic pathways in suspected acute interstitial nephritis

Q: *Interstitial nephritis, glomerulonephritis or acute renal failure?*

Tests: Renal function — urine output
Blood: eosinophils. Urine: dipstick testing; microscopy; eosinophils; culture.
Ultrasound, pyelography and possibly CT to determine renal anatomy.
Evidence of drug sensitivity

A: Normal size kidneys, polyuric renal failure

Tests: (Gallium scan); renal biopsy

Diagnostic pathways in suspected chronic interstitial nephritis

Q: *Cause of chronic renal failure?*

Tests: Renal function studies
Ultrasound, pyelography and possibly CT to determine renal anatomy

A: Small/scarred kidneys

Tests: Bladder function/anatomy
Voiding cystogram, urethrogram
Cystometrography
Endoscopy (retrograde pyelography)

Glomerulonephritis

8. Pathogenesis of glomerulonephritis

S. R. Holdsworth   R. C. Atkins

INTRODUCTION

Most cases of human glomerulonephritis are believed to result from immunologically induced, inflammatory injury in the glomerulus. The presence of immune reactants can be demonstrated in the majority of patients with glomerulonephritis. The predominant immune reactants demonstrated are immunoglobulin and complement. However, it must be acknowledged that in some forms of glomerulonephritis there is little evidence of the direct participation of immune reactants in the glomerular lesion (e.g. minimal lesion glomerulonephritis and 'pauci immune' crescentic glomerulonephritis).

Our understanding of the pathogenesis of glomerulonephritis comes primarily from two sources. In human glomerulonephritis, studies of renal biopsies allow the detection of components of the immune system that are believed to initiate glomerular injury, i.e. immunoglobulin and T cells, as well as the involvement of inflammatory mediator components including complement and coagulation factors. Our current classification of glomerulonephritis is largely based on the patterns of histological injury detected at both light and electron microscopic levels, together with the patterns of immunoglobulin (and its subfractions) and complement deposition demonstrated by immunofluorescence or peroxidase (Table 8.1).

The second source of our knowledge on the immunopathogenesis of glomerulonephritis is derived from studies in animals. The mechanisms by which glomerulonephritis can be induced and

Table 8.1 Immunopathological features in idiopathic glomerulonephritis

	Immunohistology	Electron microscopy	Serological features	HLA DR	Mechanisms of injury
Minimal lesion	Nil	Podocyte foot process fusion	Nil	B8, 12 DR7	?T cell products
Membranous GN	Granular IgG C3	Subepithelial deposits	Nil	B8, 18, DR3	ICGN ? antigp330
Focal glomerulosclerosis	Segmental IgM C3	Segmental sclerosis	Nil		Unknown
IgA Mesangial GN	Mesangial IgA C3	Mesangial deposits	$\uparrow$ IgA (50%)	Bw35, DR4	ICGN
Mesangiocapillary GN					
Type I	Granular IgG C3	Subendothelial and intramembranous deposits	$\pm \downarrow$ C3	—	ICGN
Type II	Granular C3 deposits	Intramembranous	$\downarrow$C3, C3 NeF	—	Unknown
Anti-GBM GN	Linear IgG	Crescentic GN	Circulatory anti-GBM antibody	DR2	anti-GBM autoimmunity

Key: ICGN — immune complex glomerulonephritis;
C — complement;
C3 NeF — C3 nephritic factor;
± — occasionally present.

Table 8.2 Initiation of glomerulonephritis

A. *Autoimmune responses to glomerular antigens*
   1. Antiglomerular (and tubular) basement membrane
      (GBM)
   2. Anti-epithelial cell (gp330) and thymocyte
      responses — shown only experimentally
B. *Immune responses to extrarenal antigens*
   1. Exogenous — microbial products, drugs, foreign
      serum
   2. Endogenous — autoimmune disease, tumour antigens

the means by which the mediation of injury can be manipulated have provided us with most of our understanding of the events occurring in the pathogenesis of glomerulonephritis.

INITIATING EVENTS IN GLOMERULONEPHRITIS (Table 8.2)

The primary event initiating immune glomerular injury in most circumstances is the deposition of immunoglobulin or accumulation of sensitized T lymphocytes within glomeruli. Immunoglobulin deposition is found in the glomeruli of most patients and has been most intensively studied. Recent investigations show that T lymphocytes also participate in a minority of cases (typically the most aggressive). Immunoglobulin deposition can

be a result of a number of different mechanisms (Fig. 8.1). Host immune response to antigen results in specific immunoglobulin and sensitized T cells as the primary components of the effector arm of the immune response. Antigens to which host immune responses resulting in glomerulonephritis develop can be exogenous (e.g. microbial antigens) or endogenous (renal or extra-renal) (Table 8.2). Immune responses to endogenous antigens are typically part of an autoimmune disease process (often with extra-renal manifestations). The major autoimmune diseases associated with glomerulonephritis are systemic lupus erythematosus, the various connective tissue diseases and the vasculitides.

True autoimmunity to structural components of the glomerulus is uncommon. The best characterized example is anti-GBM disease (< 5% of all cases of glomerulonephritis). Because of the uniformly dense distribution of the target antigens in the GBM, antibody deposition gives a linear appearance when biopsies are stained for antibody by immunofluorescence or immunoperoxidase immunohistology, Figure 8.2a. In most situations antibody deposits in the glomerular filter originate from circulating immune complexes comprising antibody complexed to endogenous or exogenous

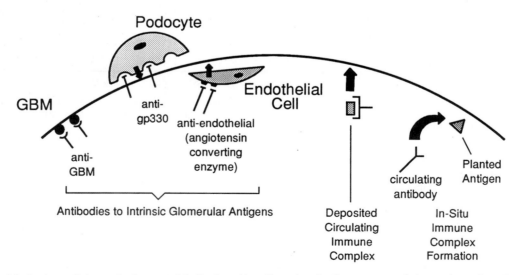

Fig. 8.1 Mechanisms of glomerular immunoglobulin deposition. Several antibodies to structural glomerular antigens have been demonstrated. Only anti-GBM antibodies give linear deposition in the glomerulus. Granular deposits can result from antibody to epithelial or endothelial antigens, deposition of circulating immune complexes or from the reaction of circulatory antibody with deposited antigen — 'in-situ' immune complex formation

soluble antigens. The irregular deposition of these immune complexes gives a granular appearance of immunoglobulin in the glomerular capillary wall with immunohistological staining techniques, Figure 8.2b. Experimental models of glomerulonephritis have shown that autoantibodies to sparsely distributed glomerular antigens can also give granular distribution of immunoglobulin deposition in the glomerulus (Fig. 8.1).

It is now known that some circulating soluble antigens, because of their particular physicochemical properties (principally cationic charge and lectin-like characteristics), may have a high affinity for the glomerular capillary wall and consequently may become 'planted' there. In a sensitized host local deposition of specific antibody can result in an 'in-situ' formed immune complex (Fig. 8.1). These also produce a granular pattern by immunohistological staining.

Immune responses associated with development of glomerulonephritis (Table 8.3)

Identification of the antigens initiating immune responses leading to glomerular antibody deposition is only possible in a small minority of patients. However, recognition of specific antibody–antigen responses can be important in diagnosis.

Exogenous antigens associated with immune complex glomerulonephritis

An immune response to exogenous antigens is appropriate when part of host defence against an

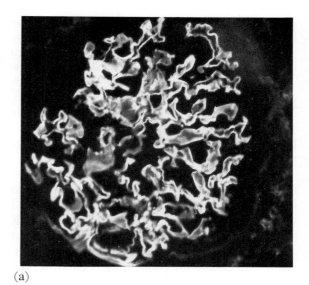

(a)

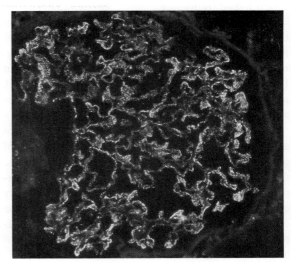

(b)

Fig. 8.2 Renal immunofluorescence with fluorescence-conjugated anti-IgG showing: (**a**) linear deposition of antibody in a patient with anti-GBM antibody-associated glomerulonephritis; (**b**) granular deposition of antibody in a patient with immune complex-associated glomerulonephritis

Table 8.3 Specific antigen–antibody responses diagnostic in glomerulonephritis

---

Antibodies to:
  GBM — Goodpasture's syndrome
  Neutrophil cytoplasmic antigens (ANCA) — vasculitis with glomerulonephritis
  Streptococcal products (e.g. ASOT) — post-streptococcal GN
  IgG (cryoglobulins) — cryoglobulinaemia
  DNA — SLE

Detectable glomerulonephritis-associated antigens
  Hepatitis B
  Malaria
  Drugs (penicillamine, gold)

---

invading microorganism but under certain conditions it may lead to circulatory immune complexes that can be deposited in the glomerulus. Factors that determine this outcome relate to both antigen and the host immune response. Antigens that have the greatest potential to lead to immune complex glomerulonephritis are those that persist particularly in the circulation, e.g. on infected cardiac valves as in bacterial endocarditis or on foreign intravascular material such as infected A-V shunts. These conditions are frequently associated with glomerulonephritis. Similarly, chronic persistence of antigen, e.g. hepatitis B virus, or chronic re-presentation of antigens, e.g. malaria, can also be associated with immune complex glomerulonephritis.

The particular characteristics of certain antigens may also render them more likely to be associated with the type of host immune response associated with immune complex glomerulonephritis. This has been best demonstrated with streptococcal antigens in post-streptococcal glomerulonephritis. Many other acute infections have been associated with acute transient glomerulonephritis, but with a much lower frequency.

The mode of presentation of antigens can determine the nature of the host immune response. Antigens presented at mucosal surfaces, e.g. respiratory pathogens or food allergens, lead to an IgA-associated response. Such situations are likely to occur in IgA-associated forms of glomerulonephritis.

Clearly, immune complex formation is not always associated with the development of glomerulonephritis. A number of factors influence the formation and clearance of immune complexes. Some of the important influences that may determine their glomerular deposition are the charge of the antigen (cationic being more nephritogenic), the size of the complex (those formed at antibody–antigen equivalence being more nephritogenic), antibody class and affinity, the capacity of the body's mononuclear cell phagocytic system to clear immune complexes, and local glomerular haemodynamic factors.

The best studied model of immune complex glomerulonephritis in animals is serum sickness, induced typically with foreign serum proteins. These antigens are associated with glomerulonephritis because if given in high enough doses they have the following characteristics: they are highly immunogenic (reliably lead to a strong antibody response) and persist in the circulation for sufficient time and in sufficient quantity to allow establishment of host antibody production with the associated immune complex formation and deposition. Serum sickness occasionally occurs in man with an associated transient form of glomerulonephritis.

Many exogenous antigens have been associated with glomerulonephritis in man. Most of these are products of invading microorganisms. However, use of some drugs (e.g. gold and penicillamine) has been associated with presumed immune complex glomerulonephritis in man. Although recognition of a particular exogenous antigen–antibody response in patients with glomerulonephritis in uncommon, it should always be considered as eliminating these antigens can result in the remission of the associated glomerulonephritis.

Endogenous extraglomerular antigens

Host immune response to endogenous antigens is typically associated with autoimmunity. A number of specific antigens commonly found in patients with immune complex diseases are important in diagnosis. The best examples are the nuclear antigens used to diagnose and classify SLE and the related connective tissue disesae. Autoantibodies to immunoglobulins themselves (e.g. in cryoglobulinaemia) can induce glomerulonephritis. Other antibodies to immunoglobulins (rheumatoid factor) or anti-idiotype antibodies may secondarily bind to the antibody component of deposited immune complexes which in these situations act as planted antigens.

Recently, a strong association between those forms of vasculitis commonly associated with glomerulonephritis and the presence of anti-neutrophil cytoplasmic antibodies (ANCA) has been established. Interestingly, these forms of glomerulonephritis typically have little evidence of glomerular deposition of immune reactants ('pauci' immune glomerulonephritis). These autoantibodies may be an epiphenomenon or they may be capable of interacting with neutrophils in a manner that augments or induces glomerular injury. The exact role of these antibodies in glomerulonephritis remains to be defined.

Some forms of glomerulonephritis can occasionally be associated with tumours (minimal lesion with Hodgkin's disease and membranous with solid tumours). Host immune responses to these tumours are likely to be involved in the initiation of the associated glomerulonephritis. Removal of the tumour or chemotherapy can lead to remission of these forms of glomerulonephritis.

Endogenous glomerular antigens

Glomerular basement membrane. Spontaneous development of antibody (and probably sensitized T cells) to GBM occurs uncommonly in man. The specific target antigen, a component of the non-collagenous domain of type IV collagen, has recently been cloned. These antibodies cross-react with lung basement membrane and frequently also cause pulmonary haemorrhage. Initiation of the disease has been associated with viral infections and hydrocarbon exposure but case-controlled studies do not lend support to these agents as specific initiators of this type of antoimmune glomerulonephritis. In susceptible rats mercuric chloride induces autoreactive T cells which induce transient anti-GBM antibodies as part of a polyclonal B cell response. In man, anti-GBM autoantibodies are not usually associated with other autoantibodies. The pathogenicity of human anti-GBM antibodies has been demonstrated by observing the disease in primates injected with antibody eluted from diseased human kidneys.

The association of anti-GBM antibodies, ANCA or the presence of granular IgG deposition in some patients with crescentic glomerulonephritis has allowed for an aetological classification of crescentic forms of glomerulonephritis (Table 8.4).

Epithelial cell antigens. Rats injected with homologous renal tubular preparations develop glomerulonephritis with features very similar to human membranous glomerulonephritis. This appears to be due to the induction of an autoantibody to an antigen present on tubular cells but also expressed on the coated pits of the glomerular epithelial cell surface. One of the major targets is a 330 kd glycoprotein (gp330). Immune complexes are formed in-situ which covert the antigen to an insoluble form bound to the cytoskeleton. The

Table 8.4 Immunopathological features of crescentic glomerulonephritis

Type	Immuno-histology	Serology	Associated disease	Mechanism
I	Linear IgG	anti-GBM	Pulmonary involvement	Auto reactive T cells + antibody to GBM
II	Granular Ig	ANA, HepB	IC diseases (e.g. SLE, SBE)	ICGN
III	Pauci immune	ANCA	Vasculitis	Uncertain

Key: ANA — antinuclear antibody;
SLE — systemic lupus erythematosus;
SBE — bacterial endocarditis;
Pauci immune — sparse glomerular immune reactants.

immune complexes are subsequently deposited on the subepithelial side of the GBM. While there is little evidence for the presence of equivalent anti-epithelial cell antibodies in human glomerulonephritis, similar mechanisms may potentially be operative.

Mesangial antigens. Antibodies have been shown to react with material taken up by the mesangium in rats. Thymocytes in the rat have a surface antigen that cross-reacts with mesangial cells. Injection of anti-thymocyte sera causes profound complement-dependent mesangial cell lysis. This model has allowed factors regulating subsequent mesangial matrix proliferation in the recovery phase to be studied. Antibodies functionally and specifically blocking transforming growth factor beta (TGF-β) prevented this mesangial proliferation, thus suggesting that TGF-β may be an important regulator of mesangial cell proliferation in disease, e.g. human mesangial proliferative glomerulonephritis.

Endothelial antigens. Antibodies to angiotensin-converting enzyme (ACE) present on endothelial cells can bind to the glomerular endothelia when injected into experimental animals. Subsequently immune deposits develop in the GBM along the filtration slits, suggesting that these in-situ reactants are processed by the endothelium. These experiments provide another potential mechanism of immune complex formation in glomerulonephritis. In humans antiendothelial cell antibodies (AECA) can be detected in the serum in some patients with glomerulonephritis (particularly in lupus nephritis and mesangial proliferative glomerulonephritis). Whether these are playing an injurious role or are an epiphenomenon remains to be defined.

Other glomerular antigens. A variety of monoclonal antibodies, some of which can induce proteinuria, have been developed that react with a number of characterized (e.g. podocytes, mesangial matrix components, GBM) and undefined antigens. Hopefully, these will provide tools to better define specific structural components and characterize their functional role.

Host factors in nephritogenic immune responses

Experimental models of glomerulonephritis have shown clear genetic differences in the capacity of various animal strains to be sensitive to the initiation of glomerulonephritis. In man there has been considerable study to identify genes within the major histocompatibility complex which confer susceptibility to glomerulonephritis. The strongest established association is observed with DR2 in anti-GBM antibody associated glomerulonephritis. A number of other associations with different types of idiopathic glomerulonephritis have been observed and are listed in Table 8.1.

Defined antigen–antibody interactions of diagnostic use in glomerulonephritis (Table 8.3)

In the clinical situation detection of antibodies to a number of characterized endogenous and exogenous antigens is very useful in the diagnosis of specific types of glomerulonephritis. These include antibodies to GBM (Goodpasture's syndrome), cryoglobulins (cryoglobulinaemia), DNA (lupus nephritis), ANCA (vasculitis-associated glomerulonephritis), and streptococcal antigen (post-streptococcal glomerulonephritis).

Detection of several specific antigens known to be associated with glomerulonephritis, or the exposure of antigens known to induce immune responses associated with glomerulonephritis,

should also be considered in newly presenting cases to allow precise diagnosis (Table 8.3).

MECHANISMS OF IMMUNE GLOMERULAR INJURY (Fig. 8.3)

Deposition of antibody usually does little direct injury, however, antibody initiates the activation of a number of inflammatory mediator molecules which may ultimately induce injury (Table 8.5). Efforts at therapeutic intervention in glomerulonephritis include preventing exposure to potentially nephritogenic antigens preventing glomerular deposition of antibody, and, since most patients unfortunately present with established injury, use of anti-inflammatory agents to modulate glomerular injury. An understanding of the mechanisms of glomerular injury allows a more rational means of devising therapeutic strategies.

Antibody. Antigen-bound immunoglobulin can activate a number of humoral and cellular mediators through receptors on the Fc piece. These include receptors for complement components and inflammatory cells, including monocytes and

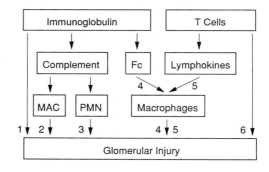

Fig. 8.3 Mediation systems of immune glomerular injury. The action of B cells (immunoglobulin) or T cells can induce glomerular injury by a number of recognized pathways: (1) antibody can directly induce injury; (2) antibody-activated complement via the membrane attack complex (MAC) can directly induce injury, or (3) chemoattractant complement fragments can recruit injurious polymorphonuclear leucocytes (PMN), (4) macrophages can be recruited and activated to induce glomerular injury by immune adherence receptors on the Fc piece of deposited immunoglobulin, or (5) by lymphokines produced by sensitized T cells in a manner akin to delayed type hypersensitivity (DTH); (6) T cells may directly induce glomerular injury

Table 8.5   Mediators of injury in glomerulonephritis

Humoral
1. Deposited antibody
2. Complement fragments
3. Complement MAC
4. Coagulation factors
5. Eicosanoids
6. Cytokines

Cellular
1. Neutrophils
2. Platelets
3. Monocytes/macrophages
4. T cells

neutrophils. In very high quantities anti-GBM antibodies can directly induce proteinuria without the involvement of either complement or inflammatory cells. It is not known if these concentrations of glomerular antibody are achieved in human glomerulonephritis.

Complement. Complement is the humoral inflammatory mediator most widely observed in human and experimental glomerulonephritis. The patterns of distribution and prominence of particular components as well as the alteration of serum levels are important in the diagnosis and classification of glomerulonephritis (Table 8.1). Depression of complement levels in the serum may indicate primary deficiencies in complement components (rare conditions but associated with increased incidence of glomerulonephritis) or consumption of complement in active inflammation. Several types of glomerulonephritis are characterized by hypocomplementaemia. Transient depression occurs in post-streptococcal glomerulonephritis and may occur in bacterial endocarditis. Persistent depression is seen in active lupus and mesangiocapillary glomerulonephritis (once called hypocomplementaemic glomerulonephritis).

Binding of antibody with antigen activates the complement cascade. Many cleavage products with profound pro-inflammatory functions are released including vasoactive chemotactic and leucocyte-activating factors. The complete activation of all components of the cascade forms the membranolytic membrane attack complex (MAC). Both classic (initiated by Clq) and

alternate (initiated by C3) complement pathways are involved in glomerulonephritis.

The best described complement-mediated mechanism of injury in glomerulonephritis is recruitment of neutrophils. However, complement-mediated neutrophil-independent forms of experimental glomerulonephritis have recently been described. The failure of animals congenitally deficient in C6 to fully develop these forms of injury and the beneficial effects of experimental depletion of late components provide evidence that the MAC is involved in inducing injury. Such models include Heyman's nephritis and some anti-GBM and immune complex-induced models of glomerulonephritis.

Continuous activation of the alternate complement pathway and possibly its glomerular deposition can be induced by an antibody to the C3 convertase (protecting it from degradation) termed C3 nephritic factor. This factor is most closely associated with mesangiocapillary glomerulonephritis.

Coagulation factors. Fibrin is an important mediator of crescent formation and renal failure in both anti-GBM and immune complex-induced glomerulonephritis. This has been shown by observing the benefit of anticoagulation or fibrinolytic agents, e.g. tissue-type plasminogen activator (tPA) or Ancrod, in these experimental models. Fibrin deposition is prominent in crescentic human glomerulonephritis but the benefits of anticoagulation are less clear cut. Recent evidence links inflammation and coagulation through receptors on mononuclear cells and their elaboration of cytokines. The major molecules involved are tissue factor (which activates factor VII, i.e. the intrinsic coagulation cascade) expressed by activated macrophages infiltrating nephritic glomeruli, and the enhanced production of plasminogen activator inhibitor (PAI) by glomerular endothelial cells under the stimulatory influence of pro-inflammatory cytokines synthesized by macrophages.

Eicosanoids. Arachidonic acid is metabolized by cyclo-oxygenase to the prostaglandin family or through lipo-oxygenase to the leukotrienes. These products play a role in haemodynamics and immune processes. Intrinsic glomerular cells as well as infiltrating inflammatory cells can synthesize these molecules. Variations in the levels of a number of these products are observed in glomerulonephritis. It is likely that they play a role in the altered haemodynamics and the fall in GFR observed in glomerulonephritis. Manipulation of the levels of various components by infusion or inhibition or by essential fatty acid depletion has variable effects but in general modulates the intensity of glomerular inflammation.

Neutrophils. Neutrophil participation is prominent in proliferative forms of glomerulonephritis. These cells are recruited by antibody-initiated chemoattractant complement fragments. Recent data suggest that monocyte and endothelial derived cytokines (such as IL-8) may also recuit these cells. In most situations of inflammation neutrophils induce injury by their release of reactive oxygen species including hydrogen peroxide, hydroxyl and superoxide ions as well as by their production of lysosomal proteolytic enzymes (including myeloperoxidase and cathepsin-G).

Macrophages. Monocytes are potentially potent mediators of inflammatory injury and are also prominent participants in proliferative forms of glomerulonephritis. They are recruited and activated within glomeruli by interaction with cell adherence receptors on the Fc fragment of glomerular immunoglobulin and by lymphokines such as migration inhibition factor (MIF) and procoagulant-inducing factor (MPIF) secreted by sensitized T cells. Macrophages can orchestrate a variety of outcomes in glomerulonephritis. They can produce a vast array of biologically active molecules capable of inducing proteinuria (e.g. reactive oxygen species, lysosomal enzyme) inducing coagulation (procoagulant activity, plasminogen activator and its inhibitor), and influencing the function of intrinsic glomerular cells by their release of cytokines and growth factors. They have an important role in inducing proteinuria and fibrin deposition, and they have the potential to be involved in repair or sclerosis but their specific involvement in these processes remains to be defined.

Cytokines and growth factors. A number of pro-inflammatory cytokines have been shown to be present in glomerulonephritis. Tumor necrosis factor (TNF) and interleukin 1 (IL-1) subserve a number of roles in augmenting inflammation. They activate inflammatory cells as well as targeting intrinsic glomerular cells. Interleukin 6 (IL-6) can stimulate mesangial cell proliferation, and the levels of this cytokine are increased in the urine of patients with mesangial proliferative IgA glomerulonephritis. Infiltrating monocytes are a major source of cytokines in nephritic glomeruli but intrinsic glomerular cells, particularly mesangial cells, are also capable of their production. Cytokines can stimulate cell proliferation, as can a number of specific growth factors. A role for TGF-β in facilitating mesangial matrix proliferation in anti-thymocyte serum-induced glomerular injury has been confirmed.

Intrinsic glomerular cells. Evidence is now accumulating to suggest that intrinsic glomerular cells may be active participants in the processes of glomerular injury induced by antibody or T cells. Proliferation of intrinsic cells is a major feature of many types of glomerulonephritis.

Mesangial cells. These cells proliferate in response to a number of immune inflammatory signals present in glomerulonephritis including cytokines, growth factors, complement components, immune complexes and endotoxin. In addition, mesangial cells can produce IL-1 and 6, TNF, TGF-β, prostaglandins, and platelet activating factor.

Endothelial cells. These cells subserve a number of important roles including the maintenance of an anticoagulant state, permeability and extracellular matrix production. Immune stimulation by cytokines enhances the expression of procoagulant molecules, downregulates anticoagulant function, increases permeability and upregulates the expression of leucocyte adhesion molecules and HLA molecules.

Epithelial cells. These cells also produce coagulant molecules, including plasminogen activator inhibitor, and proliferate in response to cytokines and growth factors. Their proliferation, together with monocyte accumulation in Bowman's space, forms crescents in situations of intense glomerular inflammation and injury in glomerulonephritis (Fig. 8.4) and is associated with development of renal failure.

Cell-mediated immunity in glomerulonephritis

Recent observations highlight the potential role for glomerular T cells to induce injury in glomerulonephritis. Glomerular T cell accumulation has now been confirmed in human and experimental proliferative/crescentic glomerulonephritis. These cells are activated (evidenced by their expression of interleukin 2 receptors and production of cytokines including MIF, interleukin 4 and γ-interferon) and are thus specifically sensitized. Their capacity to induce injury has been confirmed by depletion and adoptive transfer studies in experiment glomerulonephritis. T cells are known to be important in forms of chronic inflammation such as delayed type hypersensitivity reactions (DTH). In the skin DTH is manifest by sensitized T cell induced monocyte recruitment and activation to induce fibrin deposition causing skin induration in response to re-presentation of antigen to a sensitized host. Evidence in crescentic glomerulonephritis in man and animals suggests similar mechanisms may contribute to crescent formation. T cells macrophages expressing enhanced procoagulant activity, together with fibrin deposition, are simultaneously observed in crescentic glomerulonephritis (Fig. 8.4).

As well as local glomerular T cell involvement in glomerulonephritis, evidence suggests that cell-mediated immunity acting systemically may be involved in minimal change glomerulonephritis. There is evidence that these patients may have a clone of T cells inducing proteinuria by the production of vasoactive lymphokines.

Involvement of the interstitium in the evolution of glomerulonephritis

Progression of renal injury is associated with interstitial inflammatory cell infiltration, tubular damage and sclerosis. The intensity of these changes correlates with the severity of the glomerular lesion and is related to loss of GFR. However,

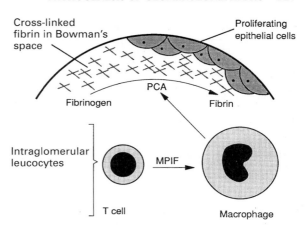

Fig. 8.4   Sensitized glomerular T cells recruit and activate macrophages by the production of lymphokines including macrophage procoagulant-inducing factor (MPIF). Activated macrophages express enhanced procoagulant activity (PCA) that induces fibrin deposition leading to crescent formation. Crescents are composed of fibrin, accumulating mononuclear leucocytes and proliferating epithelial cells

these changes are also observed in non-immune renal injury so their relationship to glomerular events and immune glomerular signals is unclear. Whether they contribute to progressive glomerular injury or represent a consequence of it remains to be resolved.

Sclerosis and repair

The balance of cytokines and growth factors is likely to play an important role in chronic injury. The complex interaction of these molecules with infiltrating and intrinsic glomerular cells together with the persistence of immune stimulating glomerular antigens will eventually determine proliferation, sclerosis or resolution. Several non-immune factors are also important in the progression of glomerular injury in glomerulonephritis. These include hypertension, glomerular hyperfiltration and the involvement of elevated levels of lipoproteins.

Principles of therapy (Table 8.6)

Preventing nephritogenic immune response to exogenous antigens. Over the last century the

Table 8.6 Principles of therapy in glomerulonephritis

1. Eliminate environment antigens associated with GN — public health
2. Eliminate GN-associated antigens in individuals — treat infections, e.g. endocarditis, cease associated drugs
3. Reduce immune response — steroids, immunosuppressives
4. Reduce glomerular inflammation
   — steroids
   — plasmapheresis (remove circulating immune reactants)
5. Reduce perpetuating factors
   — hypertension
   — hyperlipoproteinaemia

incidence of glomerulonephritis in Western countries has fallen appreciably. This reflects the reduction in current and persistent bacterial infections and thus infection-related glomerulonephritis. Public health measures and antibiotics have eliminated many of the antigenic stimuli causing immune responses leading to glomerulonephritis. Unfortunately, in 'Third-World' countries and in Australia in the aboriginal community a higher incidence of infection and glomerulonephritis is still observed. In individual cases, although uncommon, a removable initiating antigen may be identified, e.g. in bacterial endocarditis. It was hoped that the identification of common antigens associated with glomerulonephritis would lead to effective therapy but this has not occurred.

Endogenous antigens. As these responses are observed in the autoimmune diseases, modification of these reactions will await development of the capacity to manipulate specific tolerance.

Treatment of established immune glomerular injury. In most patients with established glomerulonephritis the principles of treatment are directed at reducing the immune response — usually with steroids or immunosuppressive drugs, such as cyclophosphamide or azathioprine to reduce antibody and T cell accumulation in glomeruli — or by intervening in the mechanisms of inflammation within nephritic glomeruli. Steroids are potent inhibitors of many aspects of inflammation and anticoagulants may reduce fibrin deposition. Plasmapheresis has the theoretical benefit of removing antibody and inflammatory reactants, e.g. fibrinogen and complement, from the circulation.

Therapeutic intervention is clearly of benefit in minimal change glomerulonephritis, anti-GBM disease and in many cases of glomerulonephritis associated with lupus and vasculitis. Benefit may be observed in other forms of glomerulonephritis although results are not as uniform or easily achieved.

A number of non-immune factors are also of importance in determining the outcome of glomerulonephritis. These include hypertension and hyperfiltration as well as elevated levels of lipoproteins. Lowering systemic blood pressure normalizing glomerular capillary hydraulic pressure, reducing lipoprotein levels and, perhaps, protein restriction reduce progressive renal injury in glomerulonephritis.

REFERENCES

Atkins R C 1991 Pathogenesis of glomerulonephritis. Proceedings of the XIth International Congress of Nephrology. Springer-Verlag, Berlin, pp 3–18
Druet P, Glotz D 1992 Immune mechanisms of glomerular damage. In: Cameron S, Davison A M, Grunfeld J P, Kerr D, Ritz E (eds). Oxford Textbook of clinical nephrology. Oxford Medical Publications, Oxford, pp 240–262

Glassock R 1992. Treatment of immunologically mediated glomerular disease. Kidney International 42: S121–126
Holdsworth S R, Tipping P G 1991 Cell mediated immunity in glomerulonephritis. pp 97–122. In: Pusey C D (ed) Immunology of renal disease. Kluwer Academic Publishers, Dordrecht
Wilson C B 1991 The renal response to immunologic injury. In: Brenner B M, Rector F C (eds) The kidney. W B Saunders, Philadelphia pp 1062–1181

9. Classification, pathology and clinical features of glomerulonephritis

N. M. Thomson   J. Charlesworth

PRIMARY GLOMERULONEPHRITIS

INTRODUCTION

Although glomerulonephritis was first described by Richard Bright in 1827, it is only in the last three decades that there have been major developments in our understanding of the disease. This has largely resulted from the widespread use of renal biopsy for investigating suspected glomerulonephritis and evaluation of the biopsy by a combination of light microscopy, electron microscopy and immunohistological techniques, as well as from the study of experimental glomerulonephritis in animals and developments in our understanding of immunological processes underlying the disease. Over 20 histological categories and subcategories of glomerulonephritis are now recognized and the natural history of most categories has largely been determined. However, little recent progress has been made in the prevention and treatment of glomerulonephritis and this disease remains the commonest cause of progressive irreversible renal failure in Australia.

INCIDENCE

While glomerulonephritis is an uncommon disease in general practice, it is the commonest cause of chronic renal failure requiring dialysis and transplantation. Over the last few decades there has been a remarkable reduction in developed countries in the prevalence of post-infectious glomerulonephritis, largely as a result of better hygiene and nutrition, and the widespread use of antibiotics whenever streptococcal infection is suspected. This is reflected in the statistics for the incidence of death from glomerulonephritis in the United Kingdom.

In 1848, 615 per million population died from glomerulonephritis, compared to 41 per million in 1941. However, post-infectious glomerulonephritis remains a major problem in communities with poor hygiene and nutrition, both in developed countries (e.g. Australian Aboriginals) and in developing countries. In South Africa 2% of all black patients admitted to hospital have acute post-infectious glomerulonephritis which has been induced by streptococcal superinfection of scabies. In Nigeria in 1973 nephrotic syndrome induced by malaria accounted for 2.4% of all admissions to hospital. However, with the control of malaria in that country the incidence of malarial nephropathy has been reduced by 90%. Despite the eradication in the Western world of the common infections associated with glomerulonephritis, the disease still has an incidence of between 30 and 100 cases per million population per year. The aetiological agents are largely unknown and, until they are known, it is unlikely that the incidence of glomerulonephritis will fall further.

PATHOPHYSIOLOGY

The function of the glomerulus is to produce glomerular filtrate while at the same time retaining serum proteins and the formed elements of the blood. This process depends on blood flow through the glomerulus and on the structural

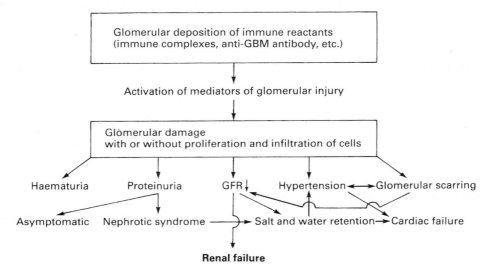

Fig. 9.1 Flow chart depicting the consequences of glomerulonephritis. GFR — glomerular filtration rate

integrity of the filtration barrier (see Ch. 1). In glomerulonephritis this integrity may be impaired by damage to the glomerular basement membrane (GBM), proliferation of endogenous glomerular cells, infiltration by circulating leucocytes, release of inflammatory mediators or glomerular scarring (either singly or in combination) resulting in one or more of the following: proteinuria, haematuria, impairment of glomerular filtration, salt and water retention and hypertension (Fig. 9.1).

Proteinuria

The mechanisms of proteinuria have been discussed in Chapter 1. The factors inducing proteinuria are complex but include: deposition of immunoreactive substances (immunoglobulin, complement) in and around the GBM; release of vasoactive substances and catheptic enzymes from infiltrating leucocytes; possible release of vascular permeability factors from circulating lymphocytes; and haemodynamic changes within the glomerulus. Along with haematuria, proteinuria is probably the most sensitive indicator of glomerular disease. However, the degree of proteinuria does not reflect the severity of the glomerulonephritis.

Haematuria

The source of red cells in the urine in glomerulonephritis remains an enigma. Although it is conceivable that they could be lost through large holes in the GBM, on histological examination red cells are seen only occasionally in Bowman's space, and on electron microscopy holes in the GBM are rare except in severe proliferative glomerulonephritis. Again, the degree of haematuria bears little relation to the severity of the disease except perhaps in mesangial IgA glomerulonephritis, where episodes of macroscopic haematuria may be associated with crescent formation.

Renal failure

Renal failure in glomerulonephritis has multiple causes:

1. Acute impairment in glomerular filtration may be related to proliferation and physical changes of glomerular cells and infiltrating leucocytes, producing a physical impedance to filtration as well as to haemodynamic consequences induced by the many humoral factors released by this inflammatory event. If proliferative

glomerulonephritis is accompanied by crescent formation, constriction of the glomerular tuft by the cellular crescent and proteinaceous exudate may rapidly produce severe renal failure.

2. In slowly progressive renal impairment, reduced glomerular filtration is due to glomerular scarring with ultimate glomerular deletion, reflecting a continuing immune insult.

3. The concomitant development of chronic hypertension in glomerulonephritis will produce glomerular ischaemia and scarring and thus worsening of renal function.

4. Occasionally, in the severe nephrotic syndrome, acute renal failure may develop due to hypovolaemia as a consequence of severe hypoproteinaemia.

Salt and water retention

Salt and water retention is common in many phases of glomerulonephritis and has a number of causes.

1. In the nephrotic syndrome salt retention may be related to secondary hyperaldosteronism due to hypovolaemia induced by hypoproteinaemia.

2. In severe chronic renal failure (CRF) salt retention is related principally to reduced glomerular filtration rate (GFR).

3. Concomitant hypertensive cardiac failure is also an important cause of salt retention in CRF.

4. In the acute nephritic syndrome associated with acute proliferative glomerulonephritis, salt retention is often disproportionately greater than any fall in GFR, and this may be due to a fall in peritubular venous capillary hydrostatic pressure.

Hypertension

Hypertension in glomerulonephritis is probably multifactorial in origin and it is often quite difficult to determine which of the following factors is most important:
1. Salt and water retention
2. Glomerular capillary and arteriolar scarring associated with advanced glomerulonephritis
3. Increased responsiveness of normal pressor mechanisms

4. Activation of the renin–angiotensin system
5. Possible failure of a chronically diseased kidney to produce a vasodilator.

Hypertension in glomerulonephritis is very common, particularly in chronic progressive disease. If uncontrolled it has deleterious effects on the glomeruli, resulting in glomerular ischaemia and obsolescence. Thus in chronic glomerulonephritis hypertensive changes may dominate those of the primary glomerular disease.

CLINICAL FEATURES

Glomerulonephritis may present with any of the following clinical features: haematuria, proteinuria, nephrotic syndrome, renal failure or hypertension. Although it may seem convenient to assign an individual patient to one of these presentations, classification of glomerulonephritis on such a basis is quite inappropriate. The clinical presentation should be used only as a guide to the most likely type of glomerular pathology or as part of the subclassification of various histological types of glomerulonephritis. Thus, although the prime indicators of glomerulonephritis are an abnormal urinary sediment and proteinuria, the ultimate diagnosis of the presence and type of glomerulonephritis should rest upon renal biopsy.

Asymptomatic haematuria and proteinuria

With the widespread use of routine urinalysis, asymptomatic haematuria and/or proteinuria are now the commonest presentations of glomerulonephritis. Haematuria and mild proteinuria may of course be seen in any urinary tract disease (e.g. glomerulonephritis, infection, tumour, calculi, trauma), but the concomitant finding of an abnormal urinary sediment containing red cell or granular casts, or red cells of morphology indicating origin from the kidney (dysmorphic red cells), makes the diagnosis of glomerulonephritis highly likely.

Anyone with asymptomatic haematuria or proteinuria should be thoroughly investigated for renal disease. Proteinuria should always be accurately quantitated on a 24-hour urine collection (significant proteinuria is defined as greater than

---

Presenting features of glomerulonephritis
Haematuria
    Macroscopic
    Microscopic (asymptomatic)
Proteinuria
    Asymptomatic
    Nephrotic syndrome
Nephritic syndrome
Renal failure
    Acute oliguric
    Chronic
Hypertension

100–200 mg/24 h). The detection of orthostatic proteinuria (proteinuria in urine formed in the upright but not in the recumbent position), with an increase in the 24-hour urinary excretion of protein of less than 2 g, is probably insignificant although in some patients orthostatic proteinuria is associated with a mild glomerular lesion. Asymptomatic haematuria and proteinuria may be presenting feature(s) of any type of glomerulonephritis. However, in the absence of renal impairment this presentation is likely to indicate a more slowly progressive type of glomerulonephritis.

Nephrotic syndrome

The essential feature of the nephrotic syndrome is a urinary protein excretion exceeding 3 g/24 h.

The other features of the nephrotic state (hypoproteinaemia, oedema and hyperlipidaemia) are a consequence of the urinary protein leak (Fig. 9.2). Clinically, the patient does not usually present until oedema becomes evident. It is likely that the oedema of the nephrotic syndrome is a function of hypoproteinaemia. The degree of hypoproteinaemia correlates moderately well with the degree of proteinuria. Other factors determining the severity of the hypoproteinaemia include the patient's initial general nutrition and the capacity of the liver to increase protein synthesis. The liver's capacity to increase protein synthesis may be impaired in the nephrotic syndrome because of the protein-deficient state itself, consequent upon a combination of urinary loss, bowel oedema reducing absorption and reduced appetite. It has been postulated that protein leak from the intravascular space may occur in sites other than the glomerulus as part of an overall increase in capillary permeability. There is little evidence for this in the nephrotic syndrome except perhaps in minimal change (minimal lesion) glomerulonephritis. In fact, the protein concentration of interstitial, ascitic and pleural fluid collecting in the nephrotic syndrome is usually very low.

The development of oedema in the nephrotic syndrome has been thought to be related to the renal response to hypoproteinaemia. With the fall in plasma oncotic pressure, fluid would leak into

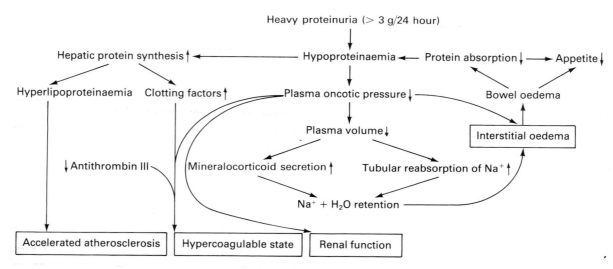

Fig. 9.2   Flow chart depicting the pathophysiology of the nephrotic syndrome

the interstitial space, resulting in a reduction in circulating blood volume. The resultant reduction in renal blood flow would lead to activation of the renin–angiotensin system and thus an increase in aldosterone secretion. At the same time there would be a reduction in GFR leading to increased tubular sodium and water reabsorption. The circulating blood volume would thus be sustained, but at the expense of increasing interstitial collection of salt and water. However most recent evidence suggests that the kidney may be retaining salt by mechanisms not dependent on the renin–angiotensin system and that blood volume may actually be increased in some nephrotic patients. Thus most people with the nephrotic syndrome are able to maintain a normal blood volume although about 20% show a fall in volume. The more severe the degree of hypoproteinaemia the more difficult it is for the kidney to maintain blood volume. Marked falls in blood volume occasionally occur (especially as a result of injudicious use of diuretics), leading to acute renal failure and unexplained abdominal pain. In most patients oedema develops when the serum albumin concentration falls below 16 g/l. Although there is a good correlation between serum albumin concentration and the severity of oedema, some patients can present with gross anasarca with serum albumin concentrations of 25 g/l while others occasionally show no oedema with serum albumin concentrations of less than 15 g/l. This difference is probably due to variations in renal sodium conservation, dietary sodium and the use of diuretics.

Not all serum proteins are lost to the same degree in nephrotic syndrome, largely because of differences in molecular size, but also because of charge. Thus in some patients albumin and the smaller molecular weight globulins show reduced serum concentrations while the larger molecular weight α_2-globulins and β-globulins and fibrinogen may be normal or increased in concentration. The observed variations in renal clearance are to some degree related to the type of glomerulonephritis. In minimal change glomerulonephritis smaller molecular weight proteins are lost while larger molecules are retained by the glomerulus (selective proteinuria). In contrast, in proliferative glomerulonephritis proteins of all sizes and charge are lost (non-selective proteinuria). These differences in the selectivity of proteinuria have in the past been correlated with the histological type of glomerulonephritis with the aim of detecting steroid-responsive minimal change disease. However, there is considerable overlap of selectivity between these groups and this, coupled with the almost universal use of renal biopsy in the investigation of the nephrotic syndrome, has led to the abandonment of this investigation by most physicians.

The consequences of the nephrotic state may be considerable.

1. Nutrition is commonly impaired, leading to worse nephrosis.

2. Anorexia and abdominal pains and diarrhoea (in children) may result from oedema of the bowel wall.

3. Impairment of renal function may develop because of reduced blood volume.

4. Hyperlipidaemia is very common in the nephrotic syndrome and is largely related to the increase of liver synthesis of lipoproteins. Other factors in hyperlipidaemia include a fall in lipoprotein removal and diminished activity of lipoprotein lipase. Both cholesterol and triglycerides are affected. Although hyperlipidaemia is probably of little importance in short-lived nephrotic states (e.g. steroid-responsive minimal change disease) it undoubtedly leads to accelerated atherosclerosis when the nephrotic syndrome is long-lasting (e.g. in membranous glomerulonephritis).

5. An increase in the incidence of thrombotic episodes is seen in the nephrotic syndrome. This is related to venous stasis in the legs, a reduction in blood volume and alterations in the concentration of several blood clotting factors (an increase in fibrinogen and factor VIII, a fall in antithrombin III and an increase in fibrinolytic inhibitors).

6. Impaired immunological capacity leads to susceptibility to infection.

The nephrotic syndrome may occur in any type of primary or secondary glomerulonephritis. In children 75–85% of cases of the nephrotic syndrome are due to minimal change disease. In adults

---

Causes of the nephrotic syndrome

1. Primary glomerulonephritis (GN)
   Common presentation
   Minimal change disease
   Membranous nephropathy
   Focal glomerulosclerosis
   Membranoproliferative GN
   Diffuse endocapillary or mesangial proliferative GN
   Uncommon presentation
   Focal and segmental proliferative GN
   Diffuse exudative endocapillary proliferative GN
   Diffuse proliferative GN with crescents
2. GN of systemic immunological disorders
   Systemic lupus erytematosus
   Vasculitis (polyarteritis nodosa, microscopic, polyarteritis, Wegener's granulomatosis)
3. Glomerulopathy of metabolic disorders
   Diabetes mellitus
   Amyloidosis
4. Toxic glomerulopathy
   Drug-induced (penicillamine, gold, mercurials)
   Venoms
5. Nephropathy of pre-eclampsia and eclampsia
6. Vascular
   Renal vein thrombosis
   Raised venous pressure (constrictive pericarditis, thrombosis, chronic cardiac failure)
7. Nephropathy of malignancy
   Lymphoproliferative malignancy — minimal change lesion
   Carcinoma — membranous nephropathy

---

this dominance of minimal change disease is lost. The commonest causes (accounting for 90% of cases) of the nephrotic syndrome in adults are minimal change disease, membranous glomerulopathy, focal glomerulosclerosis, mesangial proliferative glomerulonephritis, membranoproliferative glomerulonephritis and diabetes. Again, renal biopsy is essential for the accurate identification of the type of glomerulonephritis in a nephrotic patient.

Nephritic syndrome

The nephritic syndrome as commonly seen in acute post-infectious glomerulonephritis is charac-terized by the following four features: oliguria, haematuria (macroscopic or microscopic), hypertension, and oedema, particularly facial oedema. It is now recognized that the nephritic syndrome may occur in any type of proliferative glomerulonephritis, mesangial proliferative glomerulonephritis (with or without mesangial IgA deposition), rapidly progressive proliferative glomerulonephritis with crescents, and in systemic diseases such as systemic lupus erythematosus (SLE), Henoch–Schönlein purpura and polyarteritis. More commonly one or more of the features of the nephritic syndrome are absent in patients presenting with proliferative glomerulonephritis.

Macroscopic haematuria

Glomerulonephritis presenting as macroscopic haematuria is nearly always proliferative in type, and especially mesangial proliferative glomerulonephritis with mesangial IgA deposition. Again, the presence of proteinuria and an active urinary sediment and morphology of the red cells help in the differentiation of glomerulonephritis from other causes of macroscopic haematuria such as urinary tract malignancy and calculi. However, in IgA nephropathy the morphology of the red cells is often 'mixed'.

Acute oliguric renal failure

Glomerulonephritis presenting as acute renal failure (ARF) is a feature of proliferative disease, particularly if glomerular crescents are present. Previously, post-infectious glomerulonephritis was the predominant type of glomerulonephritis presenting with ARF although nowadays the commonest causes are diffuse proliferative glomerulonephritis with crescents (rapidly progressive crescentic glomerulonephritis), proliferative glomerulonephritis of SLE, systemic vasculitis and Henoch–Schönlein purpura.

Chronic renal failure

Unfortunately, because of the asymptomatic nature of many cases of slowly progressive glomerulonephritis, chronic renal failure (CRF) remains a major presentation of glomerulonephritis. However, this presentation may decline in frequency with the wider use of routine urinalysis and blood pressure measurement.

Hypertension

Hypertension is very common in any type of chronic renal disease. Thus the finding of asymptomatic hypertension on routine screening is not an unusual way for glomerulonephritis to be detected.

CLASSIFICATION OF GLOMERULONEPHRITIS

The classification of glomerulonephritis has for decades been a confusing mixture of histological and clinical facets of the disease, reflecting our poor understanding of the disease and the lack of use of renal biopsy. The ideal classification would take into account aetiology, pathogenesis and, possibly, clinical features. However, as discussed in Chapter 8, we can only rarely determine the aetiological agents in glomerulonephritis. Classification is further complicated by the fact that the same aetiology and pathogenesis can produce quite different histological entities in different patients. This phenomenon is due largely to differences in the individual's immune response to the aetiological agent and thus differences in the resultant degree of activation of the mediators of glomerular injury. For example, in rabbits with chronic immune complex glomerulonephritis induced by foreign serum protein, a wide variety of histological lesions occurs, varying from mild proliferative glomerulonephritis to severe proliferative disease with multiple glomerular crescents. Similarly, the same histological lesion can be induced by different pathogeneses and aetiologies; for example, diffuse proliferative glomerulonephritis with crescents may be induced by glomerular deposition of anti-GBM antibody, deposition of circulating immune complexes or by other mechanisms.

The classification of glomerulonephritis according to clinical presentation alone is even more misleading and unhelpful since the same presenta-

---

Elements of the ideal classification of glomerulonephritis

1. Aetiology, e.g.
   Infection
   Drugs
   Toxins
   Tumour antigens
2. Pathogenesis
   Circulating immune complexes
   Circulating antibody to glomerular antigens
   Delayed hypersensitivity
3. Histology of the glomerular injury
4. Clinical features

---

tion may be induced by a variety of types of glomerulonephritis which may have quite different natural histories and responses to therapy. The modern classification of glomerulonephritis is therefore based primarily on histological changes but incorporates where possible various facets of aetiology, pathogenesis and clinical presentation, e.g. 'diffuse endocapillary proliferative exudative glomerulonephritis due to glomerular deposition of immune complexes subsequent to streptococcal skin infection and presenting as an acute nephritic syndrome'.

There are limited number of ways in which a glomerulus may be altered in glomerulonephritis. The endogenous glomerular cells (endothelial, epithelial, mesangial) may proliferate; exogenous circulating leucocytes (polymorphonuclear leucocytes, macrophages, lymphocytes) and platelets may accumulate in the glomerulus; mesangial matrix may increase; the basement membrane may undergo a variety of changes; and hyalinosis and sclerosis may develop. Thus the pathological classification of glomerulonephritis is based on these possible alterations to the glomerulus. Before considering the classification it is important to define several terms.

Proliferative — proliferation of endogenous glomerular cells
Exudative — infiltration by polymorphonuclear leucocytes
Diffuse — involving all glomeruli
Global — involving the whole glomerular tuft

Focal — involving some glomeruli only

Segmental — involving only a part or segment of the glomerular tuft.

Although the term 'proliferative' has traditionally been used to indicate proliferation of the endogenous glomerular cells (see above) there is now considerable evidence to suggest that at least some of the cells producing the proliferative appearances are infiltrating leucocytes such as macrophages. It is often quite difficult on light or electron microscopy to identify accurately the origin of a cell in the glomerulus. However, new techniques of glomerular culture, histochemistry and examination by monoclonal antibodies which have been raised against each cell type allow more accurate determination of which cells (endogenous or circulating or both) are involved in the proliferative change.

The modern classification of glomerulonephritis no longer rests solely on the light microscopic appearance of the kidney. The concomitant evaluation of the biopsy by immunohistology (fluorescent-antibody microscopy or immunohistochemistry) to detect glomerular deposition of immunoglobulins and complement components, is essential for characterization of all renal biopsy specimens. For example, in early membranous glomerulonephritis the glomerulus may appear normal on light microscopy whereas on immunohistology it can be seen to contain extensive regular immune deposits. Similarly, electron microscopy is a valuable aid in determining the type of glomerulonephritis and in some situations is essential for correct diagnosis. Diagnosis by light microscopy has been aided by the use of very thin sections prepared from plastic-embedded tissue. The evaluation of a renal biopsy requires considerable experience on the part of the pathologist and the renal physician.

The current classification of glomerulonephritis (GN) was developed by a worldwide group of renal pathologists under the auspices of the World Health Organization. This classification is based on histological changes but also incorporates to some degree the immunopathogenesis of glomerulonephritis. Although this classification refers only to primary glomerulonephritis it is

---

Histological classification of primary glomerulonephritis (GN)

Minimal or no glomerular lesion on light microscopy
Minimal change disease (minimal lesion GN; lipoid nephrosis)
Minimal lesion GN with immune deposits (especially mesangial IgA)
Thin basement membrane disease
Diffuse glomerular lesions
Non-proliferative
   Membranous nephropathy (membranous GN; epimembranous nephropathy)
Proliferative
   Diffuse exudative endocapillary proliferative GN (post-infectious GN; post-streptococcal GN)
   Diffuse endocapillary proliferative GN (without polymorph exudation)
   Diffuse mesangial proliferative GN
   (a) with mesangial IgA
   (b) without mesangial IgA
   Diffuse proliferative GN with crescents
   (a) with anti-GBM antibody
   (b) with immune complex deposition
   (c) pauci-immune
   Membranoproliferative GN (mesangiocapillary GN; lobular GN)
   (a) type I — subendothelial deposits
   (b) type II — dense intramembranous deposits (dense deposit disease)
Focal glomerular lesions
Non-proliferative
   Focal and segmental glomerulosclerosis and hyalinosis
Proliferative
   Focal and segmental proliferative GN
   (a) with mesangial IgA
   (b) without mesangial IgA

---

important to note that many systemic diseases also produce glomerulonephritis. The glomerular changes in systemic diseases may have distinctive characteristics to indicate the disease. However, frequently the glomerular changes in systemic disease are very similar or identical to those of primary glomerulonephritis. For example, a diagnosis on renal biopsy of membranoproliferative or membranous glomerulonephritis should always raise the possibility of systemic lupus erythematosus.

Histologically glomerulonephritis can be divided into three main groups: (1) minimal or no glomerular lesion on light microscopy; (2) diffuse glomerular lesion; and (3) focal glomerular lesions. Detailed discussion of the pathology of each type of glomerulonephritis is available in several texts.

Minimal or no glomerular lesion

The definition of a normal glomerulus on light microscopy is often quite difficult. Thus concomitant evaluation of the biopsy by immunohistology and electron microscopy is essential when classifying a renal biopsy in which the light microscopy appears normal or near-normal.

Minimal change disease (minimal lesion glomerulonephritis)

This term is generally used to describe the histological appearance of the kidney in patients presenting with the nephrotic syndrome if the glomeruli appear normal on light microscopy (Figs 9.3, 9.4), lack any significant immunoglobulin or complement deposition on immunohistology, and reveal extensive spreading of podocyte foot processes on EM (Figs 9.5, 9.6). Some areas may show gaps in the podocytic layer, leaving segments of externally bare glomerular basement membrane (Fig. 9.7); such areas may be sites of leakage of plasma protein from the glomerular capillaries to the urinary space. This disease, which is characteristically responsive to corticosteroid therapy, has an excellent prognosis in that progressive renal failure is extremely rare. It must be distinguished from other diseases in which light microscopy reveals minimal abnormalities:

1. Focal and segmental glomerulosclerosis and hyalinosis (FSGS) in which the early segmental hyalinotic lesion may be missed on light microscopy, particularly if the biopsy does not include juxtamedullary glomeruli. This disease also presents as the nephrotic syndrome. Whether minimal lesion glomerulonephritis may progress to FSGS is still a matter of some controversy (see below).

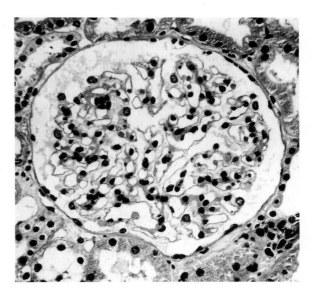

Fig. 9.3   Minimal change disease. Light micrograph of glomerulus showing apparently normal appearance. (HE × 250)

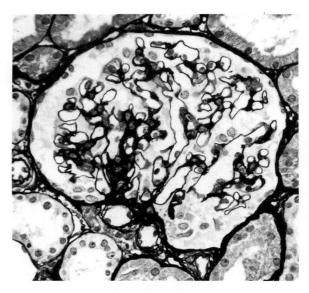

Fig. 9.4   Minimal change disease. Light micrograph of glomerulus, stained with silver, showing normal appearance. (PAS–silver × 250)

2. Mesangial IgA disease in which there are minimal changes on microscopy. However, prominent IgA is seen on immunohistology and

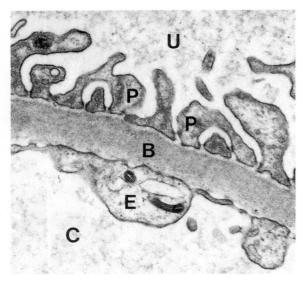

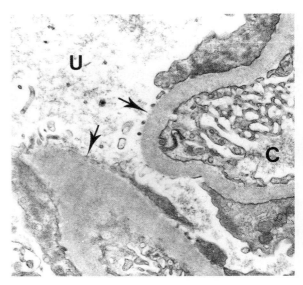

Fig. 9.5 Normal human kidney. Electron micrograph of glomerular capillary wall showing normal epithelial foot processes (P) applied to outside of basement membrane (B). C — capillary lumen; E — endothelium; U — urinary space. (× 25 000)

Fig. 9.7 Minimal change disease. Electron micrograph of portion of glomerulus showing gaps (arrows) in the epithelial covering on the outside of the basement membrane. C — capillary lumen; U — urinary space. (× 15 000)

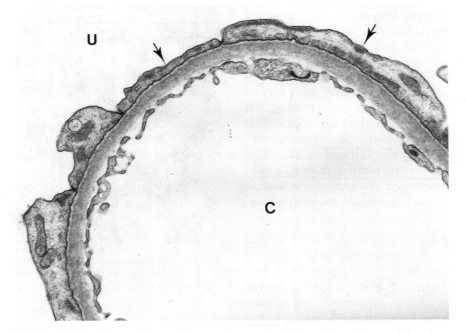

Fig. 9.6 Minimal change disease. Electron micrograph of glomerular capillary wall showing extensive epithelial spreading (arrows). C — capillary lumen; U — urinary space. (× 15 000)

mesangial deposits are seen on electron microscopy.

3. Early membranous glomerulonephritis in which the extramembranous deposits and GBM thickening are not yet evident on light microscopy but regular immune deposits along the GBM are apparent on fluorescence and electron microscopy.

4. Minor or doubtful cellular proliferation or increase in mesangial matrix on light microscopy (with minimal or no immune deposits on immunohistology or electron microscopy) occurring with presentations other than the nephrotic syndrome. Such minor glomerular abnormalities typically present as mild asymptomatic haematuria or proteinuria and many of these patients have what is now termed thin basement membrane disease (see below). Occasionally these findings represent a healed or healing phase of post-infectious glomerulonephritis (months or years later).

Minimal change disease by definition presents as the nephrotic syndrome, with a peak incidence in children aged 1–6 years, where it accounts for 75–85% of cases of the nephrotic syndrome. It does, however, occur in all age groups, even the elderly, although after childhood it accounts for only 20–30% of cases of the nephrotic syndrome. Hypertension is seen in 20% of children with minimal change disease even in the presence of a reduced intravascular volume. Urine microscopy is usually unremarkable (microscopic haematuria is seen in only 20%) and red cell casts are rare. Renal impairment is unusual except in the presence of intravascular volume depletion or sepsis.

Renal biopsy is required for diagnosis. However, in children where the nephrotic syndrome (in the absence of heavy microscopic haematuria) has an 80% chance of being due to minimal change disease, biopsy is usually only performed in those children not responding to steroid medication. Prednisolone is commenced at a dose of 2 mg/kg/day for children (50–60 mg per day in adults) and continued at that dose for 1–2 weeks after remission of the disease. Thereafter the dose is slowly reduced to zero over a period of 1–2 months. Whilst awaiting response to steroids care needs to be paid to the detection of volume depletion which may require intravenous albumin. Although over 90% of patients will undergo a remission 7–28 days after commencing corticosteroid therapy, about 60–70% subsequently have one or more relapses of the disease and 25–30% become steroid-dependent. Relapses are treated as for the initial episode although after remission tapering of the dose is prolonged. The length of the remission in patients with frequently relapsing steroid-dependent disease can be markedly prolonged by a course of oral cyclophosphamide of 2–3 mg/kg/day for 8–10 weeks. This regimen is unlikely to result in sterility. Complications of the disease are those of the nephrotic state and steroid medication and an increased incidence of infection unrelated to therapy. Before the development of antibiotics the 1-year survival was only 50%, death being due to infection. Nowadays 1-year survival is virtually 100%. As remission is usually evident within 2–4 weeks, hyperlipidaemia does not require therapy.

Thin basement membrane disease

Thin basement membrane disease (benign recurrent haematuria or benign familial haematuria) is a benign entity characterized pathologically by extensive and severe thinning of the glomerular basement membrane (on electron microscopy) and clinically by persistent microscopic haematuria and very often a strong family history of haematuria. Little or no abnormalities are found on light microscopy of the glomeruli and immune deposits are absent. Thin basement membrane disease is found in 20–40% of children and adults who present with isolated microscopic haematuria. Recurrent macroscopic haematuria is seen in some cases. The urinary red cells are usually dysmorphic. Proteinuria is usually absent but occasionally moderate to heavy. Renal function is almost always normal and remains so although cases of progressive renal failure have been reported. Hypertension is unusual.

Morphometric studies of the GBM show a GBM thickness of less than 300 nm in adults with thin basement membrane disease compared to a normal GBM thickness of 350±50 nm. As the normal thickness of the GBM increases throughout childhood, the disease is thought to represent a failure of development of the GBM rather than a destruction of the GBM. The changes in the GBM are quite different from Alport's syndrome, which may also present initially as isolated haematuria.

Diffuse glomerular lesions

Membranous nephropathy (membranous glomerulonephritis; epimembranous nephropathy)

Membranous nephropathy is characterized by the progressive deposition on the outside of the GBM on immune deposits, with subsequent thickening of the GBM (Figs. 9.8–9.10) and ultimate glomerulosclerosis. The glomerular involvement is diffuse and associated with little, if any, cellular proliferation although mesangial matrix may be increased. The development of the disease occurs in four stages (Fig. 9.11). In stage I the GBM may be of normal thickness, yet on immunohistology (Fig. 9.12) and electron microscopy (Fig. 9.13) immune deposits are easily recognized on the outer (extramembranous) aspect of the GBM. In stage II spikes of basement membrane material grow out between the immune deposits, ultimately enclosing them so that they become intramembranous and

the GBM considerably thickened (stage III). The sites of intramembranous deposits may later become electron-lucent as though the deposits have been absorbed. Ultimately the GBM becomes very

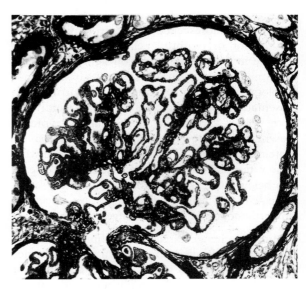

Fig. 9.9 Membranous glomerulonephritis. Light micrograph of glomerulus, stained with silver, showing extensive spike formation. (Silver methenamine × 250)

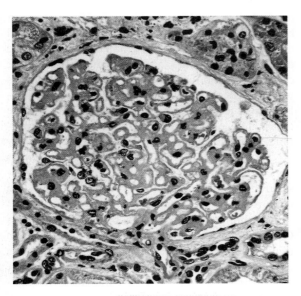

Fig. 9.8 Membranous glomerulonephritis. Light micrograph of glomerulus showing thickening of capillary walls. (HE × 250)

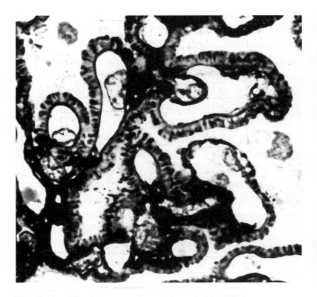

Fig. 9.10 Membranous glomerulonephritis. High power light micrograph of glomerulus, stained with silver, showing detailed view of spikes projecting from the outside of the basement membrane. (Silver methenamine × 1000)

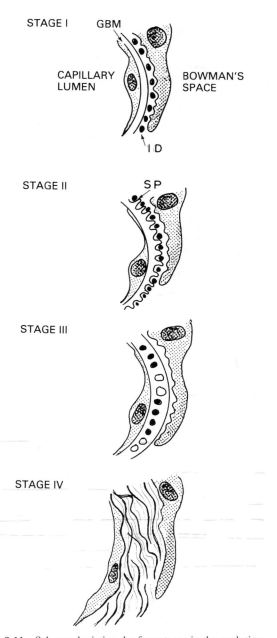

STAGE I

GBM

CAPILLARY
LUMEN

BOWMAN'S
SPACE

I D

STAGE II

S P

STAGE III

STAGE IV

Fig. 9.11 Scheme depicting the four stages in the evolution of membranous glomerulonephritis. Stage I: immune deposits (ID) on the outer aspect of glomerular basement membrane (GBM) beneath foot processes of epithelial podocytes. Stage II: projections of GBM appearing as spikes (SP) between the immune deposits. Stage III: incorporation of immune deposits (some now electron-lucent) within a thickened GBM. Stage IV: sclerosis with marked thickening of the capillary wall.

irregular, thickened and sclerotic (stage IV). The early stage (stage I) may not be detected on light microscopy, thus requiring immunohistology and electron microscopy for diagnosis. In stage II PAS stains reveal a thickened basement membrane and silver stains clearly demonstrate the spikes of silver-positive GBM extending between the deposits (see Fig. 9.10). The regular granular immune deposits on the extramembranous aspect of the GBM contain IgG (see Fig. 9.12) in virtually every patient, C3 in 80–90% of patients and other immunoglobulins in 30–60% of patients.

70–80% of cases of membranous nephropathy are idiopathic whilst the remainder are due to systemic immune diseases such as SLE, drugs (especially non-steroidal anti-inflammatory agents, penicillamine, gold and ACE inhibitors), infections (especially hepatitis B) and occasionally solid tumours or lymphoproliferative disease. The pathogenesis of idiopathic membranous nephropathy is poorly understood. There is quite a strong genetic association with the MHC antigens HLA B8 and DR3. Experimentally the disease can be produced in rats by immunization with a glycoprotein, gp330, which is found in the luminal brush border of the renal tubular cells as well as in the pits on the glomerular epithelial cell membrane. The terminal

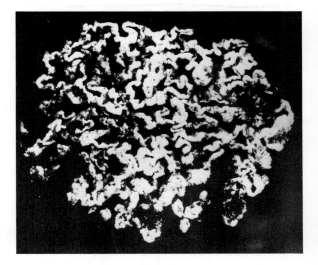

Fig. 9.12 Membranous glomerulonephritis. Immunofluorescence of glomerulus showing intense granular staining for IgG in capillary wall. (× 300)

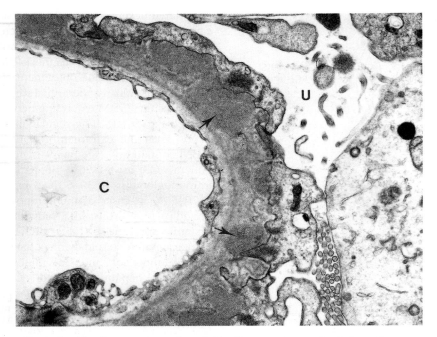

Fig. 9.13 Membranous glomerulonephritis. Electron micrograph of glomerular capillary wall showing multiple subepithelial deposits (arrows). C — capillary lumen; U — urinary space. (× 12 600)

attack complex C5b–9 of the complement system seems to be very important in the induction of proteinuria in membranous nephropathy.

Most patients with membranous nephropathy present with proteinuria and usually with the nephrotic syndrome. Microscopic haematuria is very frequent (50–70% of patients) but presentation with macroscopic haematuria is very unusual (less than 5%). Many patients already have significant impairment of renal function at presentation. The mean age at presentation is 50 years and the disease is quite rare in childhood.

Membranous nephropathy usually progresses only slowly to end-stage renal failure over a mean period of 15–20 years. Patients presenting with asymptomatic proteinuria rather than the nephrotic syndrome appear to have a better prognosis but this may simply reflect earlier presentation. The prognosis for children with membranous nephropathy is considerably better than for adults. Spontaneous clinical and histological resolution of the disease has been reported, although uncommonly. However, the nephrotic syndrome spon-

taneously remits in 25–35% of patients, either permanently or temporarily. This latter event makes the evaluation of therapy difficult without a clinical trial. Treatments which have been used in membranous nephropathy include corticosteroids, cyclophosphamide and chlorambucil, but there is little evidence that these therapies are of overall benefit, see Chapter 10. Some patients deteriorate much more rapidly.

Diffuse exudative endocapillary proliferative glomerulonephritis (acute diffuse exudative PGN; post-infectious GN)

Diffuse exudative PGN is characterized by proliferation of endocapillary cells (endothelial and mesangial) within all glomeruli and accumulation of polymorphonuclear leucocytes (Fig. 9.14). The capillary basement membrane is usually well preserved. In severe cases crescent formation may also occur. Immunofluorescent microscopy reveals immune deposits around the capillary loops consisting of C3 (Fig. 9.15) in 100% of patients, IgG in 50%, and IgA and IgM in 10–20% of patients. On electron microscopy (and on thin section light microscopy) these deposits are manifested as large electron-dense humps (Fig. 9.16) on the outer aspect of the GBM beneath the epithelial podocytes (subepithelial humps). Humps and immunoglobulin deposition are transient, disappearing within 6–8 weeks of the development of the disease, although C3 deposition may persist for longer.

This disease used to be called 'acute post-streptococcal glomerulonephritis', as the commonest presentation was a nephritic illness following within 7–14 days of a β-haemolytic streptococcal infection. The concomitant development of hypocomplementaemia and recovery after 2–3 weeks suggested an acute immune complex genesis for the disease. It is not clear whether the immune complexes circulate and then deposit in the glomerulus or whether they are actually formed in situ in the glomerulus following the glomerular deposition of the 'nephritogenic' antigen of the streptococcus. It is now recognized that this histological and clinical entity may follow other than streptococcal infections, and that some patients have no preceding clinical infection. Conversely, the whole disease may be subclinical, microscopic haematuria being detected by routine urinalysis and diffuse exudative PGN by renal biopsy. Very rarely this disease presents as the nephrotic syndrome. As mentioned above, the incidence of post-infectious GN has declined dramatically in the developed world because of better nutrition, hygiene and use of antibiotics. Most nephrological referral centres now see only two or three cases a year. Although the disease is commonest in childhood it may occur throughout adult life.

Almost all children (99%) and adults (95%) recover from the acute nephritic illness, with histological resolution and normalization of serum complement concentration. Those who do not recover usually have extensive crescent formation and die from acute renal failure and its associated complications. Recovery depends on the provision of temporary therapy for salt and water retention and for hypertension (and dialysis for the occasional patient who develops reversible acute renal failure). Asymptomatic haematuria and protein-

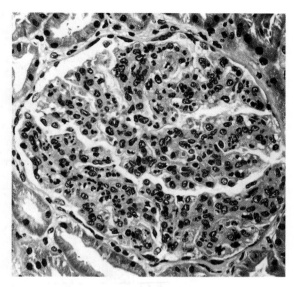

Fig. 9.14   Diffuse exudative endocapillary proliferative glomerulonephritis. Light micrograph of glomerulus showing extensive endocapillary proliferation associated with the accumulation of polymorphonuclear leucocytes. (HE × 200)

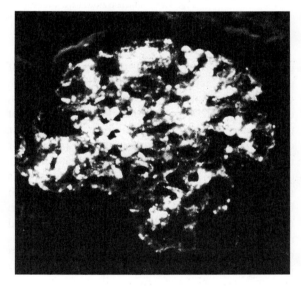

Fig. 9.15   Diffuse exudative endocapillary proliferative glomerulonephritis. Immunofluorescence of glomerulus showing extensive staining for C3. (× 200)

uria may persist for several months and an increase in mesangial matrix may be obvious on follow-up renal biopsy for one or two years.

Although the short-term natural history is well defined, argument continues about long-term

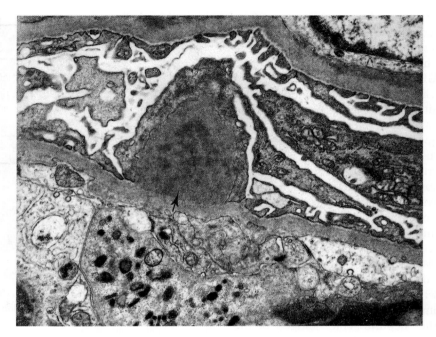

Fig. 9.16　Diffuse exudative endocapillary proliferative glomerulonephritis. Electron micrograph of glomerular capillary wall showing large subepithelial hump (arrow). (× 18 000)

prognosis. It is suggested that up to 10% of patients with acute diffuse exudative PGN will, within 20 years of recovery from the acute illness, develop chronic renal failure. Others claim that progressive chronic renal failure virtually never occurs. It is true to say that proteinuria persists for more than 5 years after the acute disease in 25% of adults and 5–10% of children. The consensus is that chronic renal failure is very rare (1–2%) following childhood disease and uncommon (around 5%) in adults. More accurate data would require renal biopsy with comprehensive assessment (immunohistology and electron microscopy) in all patients with clinical acute disease and identification of subclinical disease.

Diffuse endocapillary proliferative glomerulonephritis (without polymorph exudation)

This disease is histologically similar to diffuse exudative PGN without polymorph accumulation. However, immune reactants identified by immunofluorescence or as humps on electron microscopy are less frequently detected. Unlike most cases of diffuse exudation PGN, the proliferative changes may persist for years. Whether the disease is a separate entity or reflects resolution of exudation is not easy to determine. Patients rarely show hypocomplementaemia at presentation or a changing antistreptolysin titre. This form of glomerulonephritis is most likely to present as asymptomatic proteinuria or haematuria, rarely as an acute nephritic illness and occasionally as the nephrotic syndrome. The true long-term prognosis is unknown although progression to chronic renal failure has been documented in some patients.

Diffuse mesangial proliferative glomerulonephritis

In this disease proliferation of the mesangial cells (Fig. 9.17) is associated with an increase in the mesangium of the glomerular tuft due to an increase in the mesangial matrix and/or an accumulation of immune deposits. Varying degrees of mesangial sclerosis are also seen. The capillary wall is relatively uninvolved, unlike endocapillary PGN (with and without exudation) in which immune deposits and some mesangial expansion are seen in the capillary loops. Occasionally crescents may develop. Although the lesion is diffuse some glomeruli may be more severely affected than others. The few patients who show no immune deposits within the mesangium may include those with resolving post-infectious glomerulonephritis. Most patients, however, show extensive mesangial immune deposits readily identified by immuno-histology (Fig. 9.18) and electron microscopy (Fig. 9.19).

In about 50% of patients the dominant immu-noglobulin is IgA (Fig. 9.18), usually accompanied by C3 and not infrequently by other immuno-globulins. This is one of the three main histological patterns in which the so-called 'mesangial IgA' disease may be manifested and reflects the diffi-culty of equating pathogenetic with histological classifications of glomerulonephritis. Histologically mesangial IgA disease may be: (1) diffuse me-sangial proliferative GN; (2) focal and segmental proliferative GN; or (3) minimal or no glomerular lesion on light microscopy. Mesangial IgA deposi-tion is also seen in the glomerulonephritis associated with Henoch–Schönlein purpura.

Diffuse mesangial proliferative GN may present in a number of ways:

1. Recurrent episodes of macroscopic haem-aturia, frequently precipitated by (and occur-ring within one or two days of) an upper respiratory tract infection. This presentation is particulary associated with mesangial IgA depo-sition (70%).

2. Asymptomatic haematuria and proteinuria. This group includes some patients with previous post-infectious GN as well as those with mesangial IgA deposition.

3. Nephrotic syndrome (uncommon).

4. Nephritic syndrome (uncommon but especially associated with mesangial IgA depo-sition).

5. Acute renal failure (less than 5% of patients).

A small group of patients presenting with chronic renal failure have diffuse proliferative GN

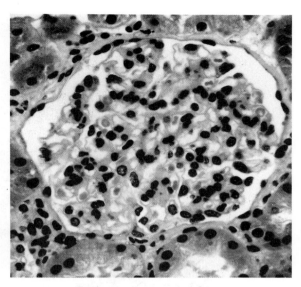

Fig. 9.17 Diffuse mesangial proliferative glomerulonephritis. Light micrograph of glomerulus showing mesangial hypercellularity. (HE × 325)

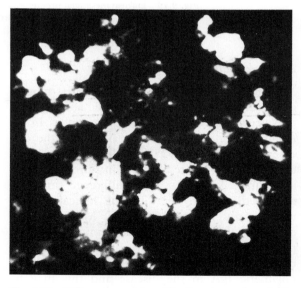

Fig. 9.18 Diffuse mesangial proliferative glomerulonephritis. Immunofluorescence of glomerulus showing intense staining for IgA in mesangial areas. (× 400)

with mesangial IgA deposition but by this stage extensive glomerulosclerosis has occured and the original histological type of glomerulonephritis is not obvious.

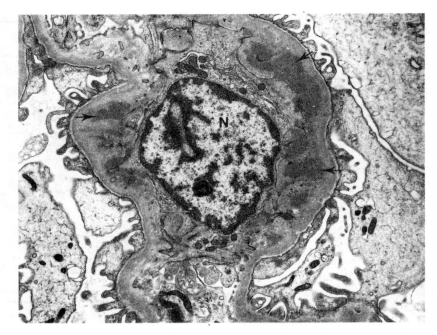

Fig. 9.19 Diffuse mesangial proliferative glomerulonephritis. Electron micrograph showing glomerular mesangial deposits (arrows). N — mesangial cell nucleus. (×9100)

IgA nephropathy

Mesangial IgA disease is the commonest type of glomerulonephritis in the world although its prevalence varies from country to country. In the Asian–Pacific area (including Australia) the disease comprises about 25% of all cases of glomerulonephritis compared to 10% in Europe and 5% in North America. This difference may be explained in part by different indications for renal biopsy in these countries. Mesangial IgA disease is thought to have an immune complex pathogenesis, but the nature of the antigen(s) is unknown. There is an increased production of polymeric IgA in the disease and this may be related to abnormalities of IgA synthesis. There is a high incidence in patients with chronic alcoholic liver disease.

The natural history of diffuse mesangial proliferative GN (with or without deposition) is in general excellent. Progression to renal failure is very uncommon in children, and in adults presenting simply with recurrent episodes of macroscopic or microscopic haematuria but normal renal function. Overall about 10–20% of patients show progression to renal failure, especially if they present in late adulthood or have associated hypertension. Progression is more likely if renal biopsy shows glomerulosclerosis, crescent formation, or interstitial scarring and in patients with heavy proteinuria.

Diffuse proliferative glomerulonephritis with crescents

Accumulation of cells in Bowman's space to form crescents (Figs 9.20, 9.21) may occur in any type of diffuse or focal proliferative glomerulonephritis, whether primary or associated with systemic disease (e.g. polyarteritis, Wegener's granulomatosis, SLE, Henoch–Schönlein purpura). Crescent formation has even been reported in membranous nephropathy. However, in some patients the development of crescents dominates the endocapillary cell proliferation. The severity of the lesion is commonly graded according to the proportion of glomeruli in which crescents are

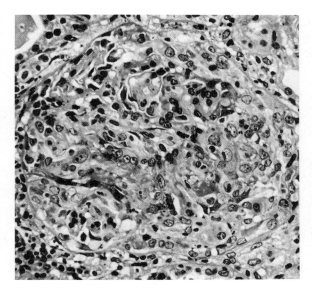

Fig. 9.20 Diffuse proliferative glomerulonephritis with crescents. Light micrograph of glomerulus showing extensive crescent formation in a patient with Goodpasture's syndrome. (HE × 250)

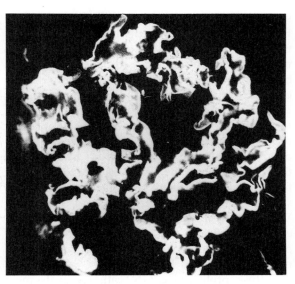

Fig. 9.22 Diffuse proliferative glomerulonephritis with crescents. Immunofluorescence of glomerulus from patient with Goodpasture's syndrome showing intense linear staining for IgG in capillary walls. (× 300)

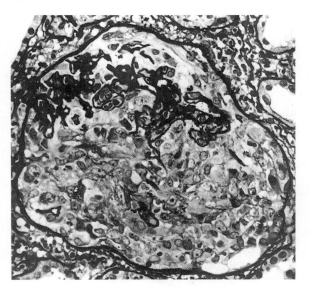

Fig. 9.21 Diffuse proliferative glomerulonephritis with crescents. Light micrograph of same glomerulus as in Fig. 9.20, stained with silver, showing remnants of glomerular basement membrane (stained black) and crescent cells filling Bowman's capsular space. (PAS–silver × 250)

found, e.g. (1) more than 80% crescents; (2) 50–80% crescents; (3) less than 50% crescents. Such a grading has prognostic value. When crescents involve more than 60% of glomeruli the term 'rapidly progressive crescentic glomerulonephritis' is used. Crescent formation is commonly associated with segmental necrosis of capillary loops.

Proliferative glomerulonephritis with crescents may result from a variety of immunological insults:

1. Anti-GBM antibody, as indicated by linear deposition of immunoglobulin along the GBM (Fig. 9.22) and by circulating anti-GBM antibody. This pathogenetic mechanism may be associated with concomitant pulmonary haemorrhage (Goodpasture's syndrome).

2. Glomerular immune complex deposition, as evidenced by granular deposition of immune reactants along the capillary loops.

3. Pauci-immune. In some patients no immune reactants are found within the glomerulus. This type of crescentic glomerulonephritis is thought to be a form of vasculitis limited to the kidney, and in 80% of these patients anti-neutrophil cytoplasmic antibodies (ANCA) are detected in the serum.

Whatever the pathogenesis of proliferative glomerulonephritis with crescents, there is exten-

sive deposition of fibrin within the crescent and
Bowman's space and often within the glomerular
tuft. The development of crescents seems to be
related to extensive damage to the GBM induced
by the immunological insult and leading to leakage
of proteinaceous fluid (including fibrinogen) into
Bowman's space where the fibrinogen is converted
to fibrin (Fig. 9.23). Macrophages accumulate in
the glomerular tuft and, in response to fibrin
deposition, migrate into Bowman's space where
they phagocytose the fibrin and become transformed into epithelioid cells; these cells form a
substantial part of the cellular crescent (Fig. 9.24).
Whether the crescent is also composed of proliferating epithelial cells is uncertain. In some
patients the glomerular tufts show typical focal
necrotizing lesions.

Diffuse proliferative GN with crescents most
commonly presents as acute renal failure with
oliguria or anuria. A non-specific prodromal illness
(malaise, lethargy, fever) is sometimes seen but

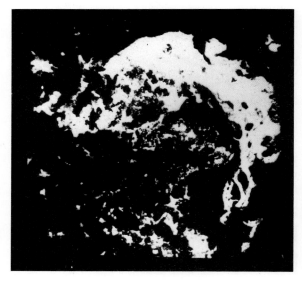

Fig. 9.23   Diffuse proliferative glomerulonephritis with
crescents. Immunofluorescence of glomerulus from patient
with Goodpasture's syndrome showing intense staining for
fibrin in crescent. (× 250)

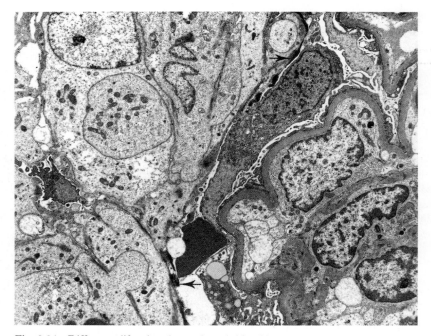

Fig. 9.24   Diffuse proliferative glomerulonephritis with crescents. Electron
micrograph showing large, pale, epithelioid crescent cells adjacent to glomerular tuft in
patient with Goodpasture's syndrome. Note fibrin (arrows). (× 4200)

such a history should always alert the clinician to the possibility of a systemic illness such as polyarteritis. Less commonly the patient presents with macroscopic or microscopic haematuria, or with the nephritic syndrome. Hypertension is not common, in contrast to diffuse exudative endocapillary PGN. The disease in uncommon compared to other types of glomerulonephritis and quite rare in children.

The prognosis of crescentic glomerulonephritis is predominantly related to the severity of crescent formation. About 50% of patients with crescents involving more than 50% of glomeruli will have stable useful renal function 6 months after diagnosis. If crescents involve more than 80% of glomeruli only 30% recover, and if all glomeruli are affected (100% crescents) less than 10% of patients show spontaneous recovery. If the patient is oliguric at presentation the likelihood of recovery is further reduced, and if anuria is present recovery is very rare. There is now increasing though uncontrolled evidence that therapy with immunosuppressive drugs, steroids (intravenous methylprednisolone followed by oral prednisolone), anticoagulants and plasma exchange may markedly improve the short-term prognosis. However this benefit is not seen in patients who are anuric at presentation. Even if a patient shows stability or recovery of renal function in the short term, long-term survival is poor in that, for patients with more than 80% crescents, less than 20% have useful renal function at 2 years. Whether long-term survival can also be improved by therapy remains to be determined. Progressive later renal damage may not necessarily be due to continued glomerular inflammation but may result from a vicious cycle induced by glomerular scarring and hypertensive vascular damage.

Membranoproliferative glomerulonephritis (mesangiocapillary GN; lobular GN)

In membranoproliferative glomerulonephritis (MPGN) there is diffuse thickening of capillary walls associated with proliferation of mesangial cells and an increase in mesangial matrix. The thickening is due to expansion of mesangium into the capillary wall, between the GBM and the endothelial cell (hence the term mesangiocapillary GN) and deposition of a second layer of basement membrane-like material. The mesangial interposition and expansion may be so extensive as to give a lobular appearance to the glomerulus (hence the old term lobular GN).

Crescent formation is not uncommon and may be extensive. Two major types of MPGN are now recognized:

Type I MPGN or MPGN with subendothelial deposits (Figs 9.25–9.29). This is the commonest type of MPGN (70–80%) and is characterized on electron microscopy and immunohistology by immune deposits (IgG, IgM, C3, C4 and, in 30%, IgA) along the subendothelial aspect of the GBM, particulary near the mesangial areas of the capillary loops and the mesangial stalk. Such deposits further increase the capillary wall thickness and, by separating the GBM from the interposed mesangium, produce a 'double contour' of the capillary wall, best appreciated on PAS or silver stain.

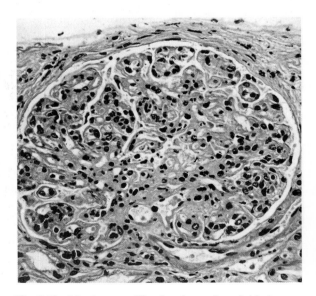

Fig. 9.25 Membranoproliferative glomerulonephritis (type I). Light micrograph of glomerulus showing thickening of capillary walls and mesangium associated with prominent hypercellularity. (HE × 175)

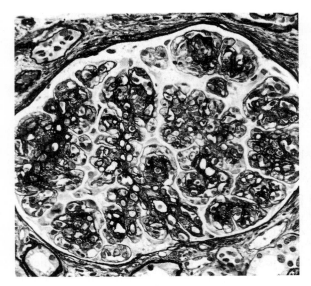

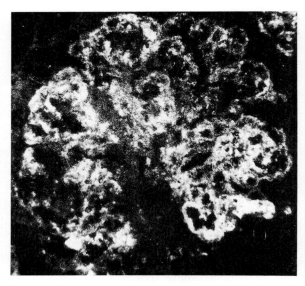

Fig. 9.26 Membranoproliferative glomerulonephritis (type I). Light micrograph of same glomerulus as in Fig. 9.25, stained with silver, showing extensive 'double contour' appearance. (Silver methenamine × 175)

Fig. 9.28 Membranoproliferative glomerulonephritis (type I). Immunofluorescence of glomerulus showing extensive staining for IgG. (× 200)

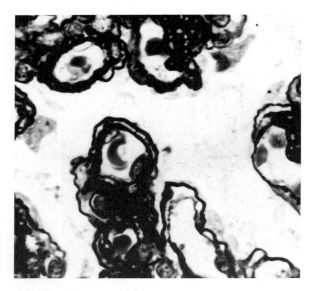

Fig. 9.27 Membranoproliferative glomerulonephritis (type I). High power light micrograph of glomerulus, stained with silver, showing detailed view of 'double contours' around capillary loops. (Silver methenamine × 1000)

Type II MPGN or dense deposit disease (Figs 9.30–9.34). This is characterized by a relatively continuous, intramembranous deposit

creating a ribbon-like layer of electron-dense material within the basement membrane not only of the glomerulus but also of Bowman's capsule and the tubules. It is unknown whether this 'deposit' is an immune deposit or a transformation of GBM constituents. The dense deposit may also be seen on light microscopy using thin sections. Immunofluorescence reveals continuous but irregular deposits of C3 along the capillary loop and more discrete deposits within the mesangium. However, unlike in type I MPGN, immunoglobulin is only rarely found in the glomerulus. A type III MPGN is also described in which there are both subendothelial and epimembranous deposits.

MPGN most commonly presents as the nephritic syndrome or nephrotic syndrome and less commonly as macroscopic or microscopic haematuria. The disease is rare in children under 5 years of age but thereafter occurs in all decades of life. There is an association between dense deposit disease and partial lipodystrophy. The most outstanding feature of MPGN is the frequent presence (in 70–80%) of hypocomplementaemia which seems to be persistent and unrelated to activity of disease. In type I MPGN

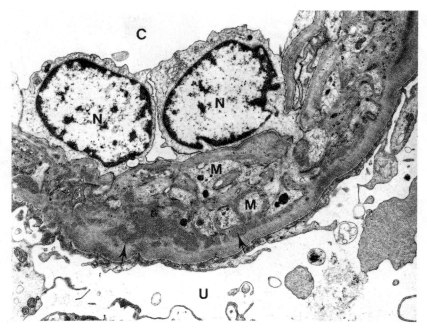

Fig. 9.29 Membranoproliferative glomerulonephritis (type I). Electron micrograph of glomerular capillary wall showing subendothelial deposits (arrows) and interposition of mesangial cell processes (M). C — capillary lumen; N — endothelial cell nuclei; U — urinary space. (× 5600)

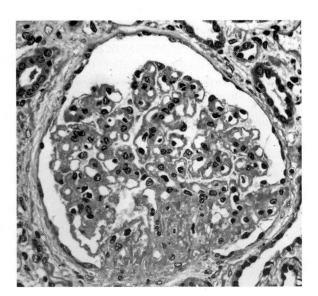

Fig. 9.30 Membranoproliferative glomerulonephritis (type II, dense deposit disease). Light micrograph of glomerulus showing thickening of capillary walls and mesangium associated with some hypercellularity. (HE × 200)

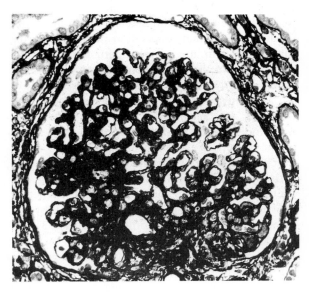

Fig. 9.31 Membranoproliferative glomerulonephritis (type II, dense deposit disease). Light micrograph of same glomerulus as in Fig. 9.30, stained with silver, showing some 'double contours'. (Silver methenamine × 200)

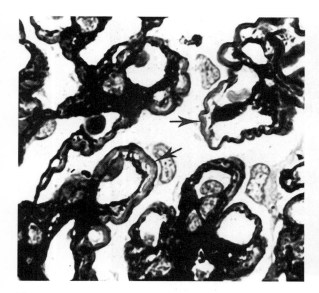

Fig. 9.32 Membranoproliferative glomerulonephritis (type II, dense deposit disease). High power light micrograph of glomerulus, stained with silver, showing detailed view of 'double contours' and partial replacement of basement membrane with 'dense deposit' material (arrows). (Silver methenemine × 1000)

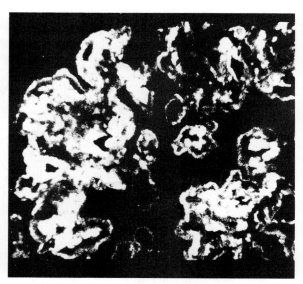

Fig. 9.33 Membranoproliferative glomerulonephritis (type II, dense deposit disease). Electron micrograph of glomerulus showing staining for C3 around capillary loops and in clumps within the mesangium. (× 300)

the profile of serum complement components suggests activation of the complement cascade by the classic pathway (i.e. low C3, C4, C1q). This profile in the serum, coupled with immunoglobulin and complement deposition in the glomeruli, suggests an immune complex pathogenesis.

By contrast, the serum complement component profile in dense deposit disease indicates activity of the alternative pathway of complement activation (low C3, but normal C4 and C1q). In dense deposit disease C3 nephritic factor (NeF) is found in the serum of 70–80% of patients. C3 NeF, which is an autoantibody, stabilizes the alternative-pathway C3 convertase (C3bBb), allowing uncontrolled activation of complement. Whether dense deposit disease is directly caused by intravascular activation of complement by C3 NeF is unknown.

The natural history of MPGN is progressive, with a gradual decline of renal function so that 50% of patients reach end-stage renal failure in 10–11 years. The progression is more rapid in dense deposit disease than in the subendothelial deposit variety. Bad prognostic signs are persist-

ent nephrotic syndrome and crescents on renal biopsy. There is little if any evidence that steroids or immunosuppression or anticoagulation are of benefit in MPGN although promising results have been reported with the use of anti-platelet drugs.

Not all patients with MPGN fit into one of the two main categories (type I or II). There seems to be a small group in whom features of both types are seen. Moreover, it is important to remember that the histological features of MPGN may also be seen in the proliferative GN of SLE and in the glomerulonephritis occurring in infected ventriculo-atrial shunts (shunt nephritis) and bacterial endocarditis.

Focal glomerular lesions

Focal and segmental glomerulosclerosis and hyalinosis (FSGS)

In FSGS the glomeruli characteristically show segmental hyalinosis and sclerosis (Fig. 9.35), the former predominantly at the periphery of the glomerular tuft, often with adhesion to Bowman's capsule, while sclerosis may be more mesangial in

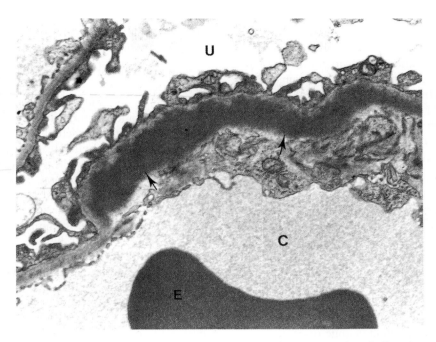

Fig. 9.34 Membranoproliferative glomerulonephritis (type II, dense deposit disease). Electron micrograph of glomerular capillary wall showing 'dense deposit' material (arrows) replacing extensive segments of basement membrane. C — capillary lumen; E — erythrocyte; U — urinary space. (× 7000)

distribution. Hyaline consists of protein, lipid and mucopolysaccharide and is seen as an acellular homogenous mass staining with PAS and eosin but not with silver stains. Sclerosis is a mixture of mesangial matrix and basement membrane-like material and appears as solid areas of silver and PAS-positive material. Hyalinosis is probably the primary pathological change, with sclerosis occurring subsequently. Ultimately the process of hyalinosis and sclerosis will involve the whole glomerulus, leading to extensive interstitial fibrosis. However, even in very advanced disease the segmental and focal nature of the lesion is often still in evidence. Not uncommonly hyalinosis is also seen within the subendothelial areas of arterioles. Interstitial foam cells are frequently found. In the early stage of the disease the segmental hyalinotic lesions may be confined to the juxtamedullary glomeruli and thus may be missed on superficial renal biopsy. Electron microscopy confirms the hyalinotic and sclerotic lesion but also characteristically shows spreading

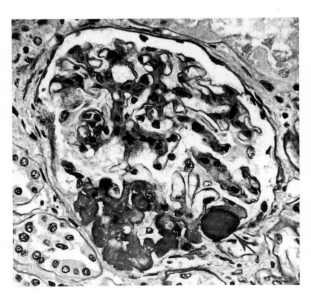

Fig. 9.35 Focal glomerulosclerosis. Light micrograph of glomerulus showing segmental sclerosis and a rounded mass of PAS-positive hyaline material (arrow). (PAS × 300)

of the podocyte foot processes (Fig. 9.36) similar to that seen in minimal change disease. Podocytic degeneration is common, leaving segments of externally bare glomerular basement membrane — possibly sites of leakage of plasma proteins into the urinary space. Immunohistology reveals segmental deposits of IgM and C3 which probably represent proteins which have leaked into the area of hyalinosis rather than immunoreactants initiating the disease.

FGS may be confused with a number of other diseases:

1. The healing phase of focal and segmental proliferative GN.

2. Focal and global sclerosis. The latter does not show the segmental nature of the FSGS lesions and has an entirely different pathogenesis and natural history. Focal and global sclerosis may result from the normal ageing process, renal ischaemia or possibly prolonged nephrotic syndrome due to minimal change disease.

3. Focal and segmental sclerosis may occur in chronic renal interstitial disease such as reflux nephropathy and analgesic nephropathy.

The commonest presentation of FSGS is the nephrotic syndrome with microscopic haematuria. However, some patients present with microscopic haematuria and asymptomatic proteinuria. The disease occurs in both children and young adults and accounts for about 10% of patients with the nephrotic syndrome. FGS is characteristically insensitive to corticosteroids although some reports claim that up to 25% of patients will undergo complete remission with steroid therapy. The relation of this disease to minimal change disease is also controversial. It has been suggested that some patients with minimal change disease may progress to FGS and that this may be related to glomerular damage induced by persistent proteinuria. The existing controversy may in part be due to misdiagnosis of FSGS if the first biopsy misses the early segmental hyalinotic lesion, par-

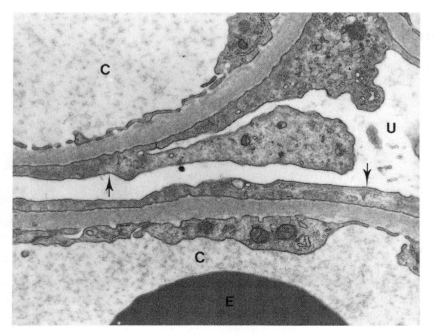

Fig. 9.36 Focal glomerulosclerosis. Electron micrograph of portion of glomerulus showing extensive epithelial spreading (arrows). C — capillary lumen; E — erythrocyte; U — urinary space. (× 16 000)

ticularly if the biopsy is too superficial to sample the juxtamedullary glomeruli.

FSGS is usually progressive, resulting in end-stage renal failure after approximately 6–8 years. Some patients presenting with gross nephrotic syndrome may run a rapidly progressive course to renal failure over 2–3 years. Presentation with asymptomatic proteinuria/haematuria is usually associated with a slower progression of disease. Spontaneous remission of the nephrotic syndrome is rare but when it occurs progress of the hyalinotic/sclerotic lesions appears to halt. There is a very high rate (30–50%) of recurrence of FSGS in renal allografts, and heavy proteinuria may be in evidence within days of transplantation.

Focal and segmental proliferative glomerulonephritis

Focal and segmental proliferation (Fig. 9.37) is common is glomerulonephritis associated with systemic diseases such as Henoch–Schönlein purpura, bacterial endocarditis and Goodpasture's syndrome. As a primary entity it is a particularly associated with mesangial deposition of IgA. However, in some patients there is capillary loop deposition of IgG, C3 and other immunoglobulins while in others there are no glomerular immune deposits. Healing focal and segmental proliferative GN may be difficult to differentiate from focal glomerulosclerosis, as discussed above.

Patients with this type of glomerulonephritis present either with asymptomatic proteinuria, microscopic haematuria, recurrent episodes of macroscopic haematuria or nephrotic syndrome. The natural history of this lesion has been poorly studied but is thought to be good, with less than 20% of patients progressing to end-stage renal failure over 10–15 years.

CORRELATION OF CLINICAL AND LABORATORY FEATURES OF GLOMERULONEPHRITIS WITH HISTOLOGICAL DIAGNOSIS

The diagnosis of glomerulonephritis can often be made from a thorough history, physical examination and urinalysis and microscopy, especially if

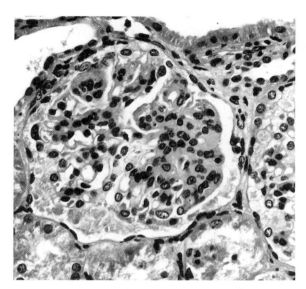

Fig. 9.37 Focal and segmental proliferative glomerulonephritis. Light micrograph of glomerulus showing prominent segmental proliferative lesions, with other segments being apparently normal (from a patient showing IgA deposition in glomerular mesangial regions). (HE × 300)

the patient presents with the nephritic or nephrotic syndrome. However, for the diagnosis of the type of glomerulonephritis, clinical and laboratory features on their own are notoriously unreliable. For example, the nephrotic syndrome may occur with any histological type of glomerulonephritis, and nephritic syndrome with any type of proliferative GN. Although a certain profile of clinical and laboratory features may be strongly suggestive of a particular histological diagnosis (Table 9.1) it may be sufficiently inaccurate to make such an approach dangerous unless combined with the ultimate diagnostic tool, renal biopsy. Renal biopsy allows accurate diagnosis and an assessment of severity of the glomerular lesion, both of which are essential for therapy and prognosis. It must be stressed, however, that the patient's presenting features and laboratory findings may greatly aid the interpretation of the renal biopsy and are essential in the detection of systemic disease.

Thus renal biopsy should be performed in most patients with suspected glomerulonephritis provided there are no contraindications (see Ch. 4). However, renal biopsy is not performed initially in

Table 9.1 Correlation of clinical and laboratory features of glomerulonephritis with histological diagnosis

Histology	Clinical features — Proteinuria — Asymptomatic	Nephrotic	Macro-haematuria	Micro-haematuria	Nephritic syndrome	ARF	CRF	Anti-GBM antibody	Laboratory findings — Hypo-complementaemia	Rising ASOT	High serum IgA
Minimal change disease	0	++++	0	+	0	0	0	−	−	−	−
Minimal lesion with IgA	+++	+	+	++++	0	0	0	−	−	−	+++
Membranous nephropathy	+++	+++	+	+++	0	0	+	−	−	−	−
Diffuse exudative endocapillary PGN	+	+	+	++++	++++	+	0	−	C3↓ C4↓ C1q↓ (early)	+++	−
Diffuse endocapillary PGN	+++	++	+	+++	0	0	+	−	−	+	++
Diffuse mesangial PGN	+++	++	+++	++++	+	+	+	−	−	−	++
Diffuse PGN with crescents	0	+	+	++++	++	+++	+	++	−	+	−
Membranoproliferative GN	+	+++	+	++++	++	0	+	−	C3↓ Factor B↓ (C4, C1q) (normal)	−	−
Focal and segmental glomerulosclerosis	+++	++++	0	++++	0	0	+	−	−	−	−
Focal and segmental PGN	+++	+	+++	+++	+	+	+	+	−	−	−

Key: ARF — acute renal failure; CRF — chronic renal failure; ASOT — anti-streptolysin O titre; PGN — proliferative glomerulonephritis

0	Never or rarely (< 2–3%)
+	Occasionally (< 10%)
++	Not uncommonly (10–30%)
+++	Commonly (30–80%)
++++	Very commonly or always (80–100%)

children presenting with the nephrotic syndrome, if there is minimal activity of the urinary sediment (no granular or red cell casts or microscopic haematuria), as they have a greater than 90% chance of minimal change disease. Only those in whom the nephrotic syndrome does not respond to steroid therapy are biopsied. Patients with mild or moderate microscopic haematuria (dysmorphic red cells) but no proteinuria and who have normal renal function are often not biopsied as they are likely to have benign conditions such as thin membrane disease or mild IgA nephropathy.

Laboratory investigations in glomerulonephritis

The most important indications of glomerulonephritis are the clinical presentation, findings on urinalysis and urine microscopy, and the presence of a normal upper and lower urinary tract on intravenous pyelography or ultrasound without gross renal scarring. Further investigations give clues to the likely type of glomerulonephritis but do not negate the need for renal biopsy.

Microscopy and urinary sediment (see Ch. 4)

Granular and red cell casts indicate a diagnosis of glomerulonephritis in over 90% of cases, distortion and fragmentation of red cells (dysmorphic red cells) in the urine strongly suggest glomerulonephritis.

Serum complement profile

Activation of the complement cascade occurs in several types of glomerulonephritis, giving two predominant profiles of complement components. In diseases with circulating immune complexes the cascade is activated through the classic pathway, resulting in low total complement, C3, C4 and C1q. Such a profile is frequently seen in the glomerulonephritis of SLE, bacterial endocarditis and serum sickness. Post-infectious glomerulonephritis may show a similar profile early in the disease, although later the alternative pathway seems to be dominant since C3 is low while C4 and C1q may be normal in concentration. In

membranoproliferative glomerulonephritis, and especially in the dense deposit disease variety, complement is activated through the alternative pathway because of the presence of C3 nephritic factor in the serum (see above). Thus the profile of complement components in this disease is low total complement and C3, with normal concentrations of C4 and C1q. Whereas serum complement concentrations reflect disease activity in the first group there is no correlation with activity of MPGN.

Anti-GBM antibody

Anti-GBM antibody in the serum can be readily detected by a number of techniques, including haemagglutination tests and indirect immunofluorescence. However, the most sensitive technique (giving the least number of false negative and false positive results) is a radioimmunoassay in which

---

Laboratory investigations of glomerulonephritis (GN)

To indicate a likely diagnosis of GN
Clinical presentation
Urinalysis (haematuria, proteinuria)
Microscopy of urinary sediment (granular and red cell casts, dysmorphic red cell morphology)
Intravenous pyelogram or renal ultrasound (smooth renal outline, normal pelvicalyceal system and lower urinary tract)

To indicate the likely type of GN
Serum complement profile
Evidence of recent infection with β-haemolytic streptococcus (throat or skin swab, rising ASOT)
Circulating anti-GBM antibody
Circulating immune complexes (limited value)
Investigations to detect systemic disease (e.g. anti-DNA antibody, skin biopsy)
Serum IgA concentrations
Urine protein selectivity
Renal biopsy (light, immunofluorescent and electron microscopy)

To assess the consequences of GN
24-hour urinary protein excretion
Serum protein concentrations (if nephrotic syndrome)
Serum lipids (if nephrotic syndrome)
Renal function
Severity of lesion on renal biopsy

radiolabelled GBM-soluble antigens are used as the target.

Circulating immune complexes in the serum

While circulating immune complexes may be detected in the serum of patients with a variety of types of glomerulonephritis (particularly if due to a systemic disease such as SLE, bacterial endocarditis, polyarteritis), they have no discriminant value in identifying types of glomerulonephritis. Nor does their detection separate glomerulonephritis from other diseases with an immune complex pathogenesis.

Other circulating antibodies — see Chapters 4 and 11.

PART 2
SECONDARY GLOMERULONEPHRITIS

Several diseases cause glomerular inflammation as part of a more generalized process. The renal component may be the dominant lesion or represent an incidental or unexpected finding. In either case its precise definition may become an important determinant of both diagnosis and treatment. This part of Chapter 9 will review those generalized diseases where glomerulonephritis may be a significant component. Other forms of glomerular involvement in systemic disease will be discussed in Chapter 11.

GLOMERULONEPHRITIS IN MULTISYSTEM DISEASES

Systemic lupus erythematosus

Systemic lupus erythematosus (SLE) constitutes a small but significant percentage of patients with glomerulonephritis. The frequency of detection will depend on the patient population, criteria for diagnosis and, to some extent, the interests of the department involved. The majority of patients do not develop severe renal failure; among the Australian community, approximately 5% of patients with glomerulonephritis on dialysis have SLE as their primary diagnosis. The geographical distribution of the disease is highly variable with severe cases observed particularly in Asian and black communities.

Lupus constitutes a complex profile of clinical and laboratory abnormalities and it is tempting to consider that these reflect an exaggerated response to a common environmental agent by a genetically susceptible host. Dietary and endocrine factors have also been implicated in pathogenesis. The evidence for genetic predisposition is convincing: there is high concordance of disease in monozygotic twins compared to their dizygotic counterparts, and considerable data document familial aggregation and specific ethnic susceptibility. Studies of HLA support the concept of a lupus haplotype and spontaneous lupus syndromes have been described in C5-deficient mice. Furthermore, there are many reports of an increased incidence of SLE among patients with inherited deficiency of complement proteins, particularly components of the classic pathway. C2 deficiency is the most important of these abnormalities. About one third of such patients have a lupus-like illness while the frequency of C2-deficient homozygotes in Caucasoid populations is 1 in 10 000.

Pathology and pathogenesis

The World Health Organization (WHO) recognizes five types of lupus glomerulonephritis and these are shown in Table 9.2. A further category (type VI) encompasses advanced sclerosing lesions. Each category may have additional active or chronic features and these are also shown in the Table. The majority of changes are not pathognomonic of lupus and occur in various forms of glomerular disease. However, two lesions have a high degree of specificity: firstly, wire loop changes which result from segmental (eosinophilic) thickening of capillary walls by subendothelial immune deposits and, secondly, the haematoxylin body — the tissue equivalent of the LE cell — which results

Table 9.2 Histological classification of lupus glomerulonephritis

| Type | Light microscopy | Deposit on EM and on IF (IgG and C3) | | |
		Mesangial	Subendothelial	Subepithelial
Type I	Normal	+	–	–
Type II Mesangial proliferation	Diffuse mesangial hypercellularity	++	±	–
Type III Focal and segmental proliferation	Segmental proliferation and necrosis; occasional hyaline thrombi	+++ (often IgA+M)	+	–
Type IV Diffuse proliferation	Diffuse hypercellularity; membranoproliferative change. Necrosis, crescents, wire loops	+++	+++	++++
Type V Diffuse membranous	Capillary wall expansion; subepithelial deposits; usually some mesangial hypercellularity	++ (often IgM)	+	+++
Type VI Advanced sclerosing	Segmental, mesangial or global sclerosis	–	–	–

EM — electron microscopy; IF — immunofluorescence

from interaction between altered nuclear material and autoantibodies. It is important to emphasize that features of disease activity or chronicity may occur with several of the major histological categories, especially types III, IV and V. Tubulointerstitial lesions are common, particularly in more severe cases. There may be mononuclear cell infiltration, tubular atrophy and interstitial fibrosis. Immune deposits may be demonstrated along the tubular basement menbrane. Vascular lesions are less prominent and true arteritis is relatively uncommon.

Immunofluorescence microscopy emphasizes the polyclonal B-cell activation that is characteristic of lupus. The glomerular deposits are granular and usually involve more than one immunoglobulin as well as classic pathway complement components. Typically, the distribution of immunoreactive proteins is diffuse with involvement of both capillary walls and the mesangium. Where crescent formation occurs, there will be fibrin deposition. Similar granular deposits may be observed along the tubular basement membrane. Not all tubulointerstitial lesions will show deposits comparable to those in glomeruli which suggests the possibility of additional immunological mechanisms. Indeed, it is recognized that this component of the disease may progress independently to lupus glomerulitis.

Electron microscopy confirms the presence of dense deposits which may be distributed throughout the capillary wall and within the mesangium. They are usually homogenous or finely granular but occasionally become organized in a whorl-like pattern that is often referred to as 'finger printing'. Electron microscopy may also show virus-like particles in the cytoplasm of endothelial cells; their significance is uncertain.

While the immunoregulatory factors that lead to this hyperglobulinaemic state remain to be clarified, the primary effector system appears to involve antigen–antibody interaction. Indeed, lupus glomerulonephritis represents one of the few forms of inflammatory glomerular injury where circulating immune complexes seem likely to be a major contributor. However, their antigenic content remains uncertain. This matter has been reviewed recently and substantial data support a role for DNA–anti-DNA complexes in the pathogenesis of lupus glomerulonephritis. However, the site of immune complex formation remains uncertain; it seems possible that both circulating and in-situ systems are involved.

The association of lupus with complement deficiency is well documented. However, the mechanisms by which this promotes immunological damage are far less certain. Two major proposals have been made: firstly, that the physiological processes of complement are modified such that the metabolism of immune complexes is altered in favour of extra-ordinary deposition and secondly, that the complement defect simply marks a genetic site that renders patients susceptible to the disease.

An important advance in the understanding of lupus syndromes is the realization that serum

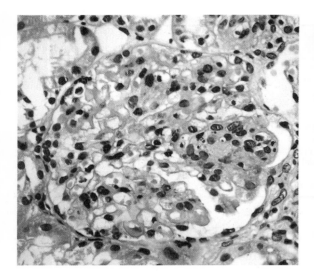

Fig. 9.38   Lupus nephritis. Light micrograph of glomerulus showing focal and segmental proliferative lesion. (HE × 300)

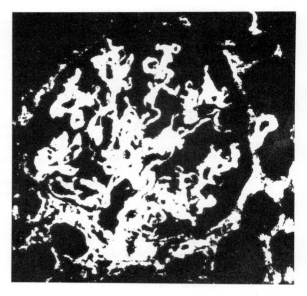

Fig. 9.39   Lupus nephritis. Immunofluorescence of glomerulus (same patient as shown in Fig. 9.38) with intense staining for IgG. Note also the presence of some intertubular staining. (× 350)

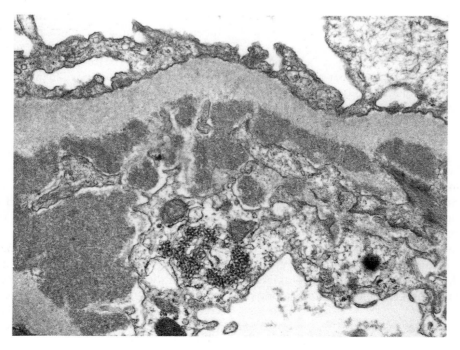

Fig. 9.40   Lupus nephritis. Electron micrograph of glomerular capillary wall (same patient as shown in Fig. 9.38) showing extensive subendothelial deposits and prominent endothelial tubulovesical inclusion bodies. (× 17 500)

antibodies to anionic phospholipids may be associated with specific clinical features such as recurrent thrombosis and miscarriage. While these antibodies have been recognized for many years (and paradoxically known as the lupus anticoagulant) it is only more recently that their impact has been recognized. Such patients are frequently thrombocytopenic but the link between this abnormality and the features of lupus glomerulonephritis is not clear. However, altered intraglomerular coagulation may play a role in lupus glomerulonephritis and it will be of interest to observe the place (if any) of these phospholipid antibodies.

Clinical manifestations

The frequency of renal involvement in SLE at the time of clinical presentation varies from 50–90%, and it is often stated that all patients will develop this component during their lifetime. The patient may exhibit a variety of features of renal disease. These range from asymptomatic minor urinary abnormalities to rapidly progressive renal failure. Glomerulonephritis is the dominant lesion in most patients but the coexistence of tubular and vascular abnormalities adds to the diversity of clinical manifestations.

There is reasonable correlation between the microscopic lesion and clinical features. For example, focal proliferative (type III) glomerulonephritis is associated typically with haematuria and non-nephrotic proteinuria while the type V membranous lesion produces significant proteinuria (often within the nephrotic range) and a similar clinical pattern to that observed with the idiopathic form of membranous nephropathy. The type IV mesangiocapillary (or membranoproliferative) form shows a wide range of clinical abnormalities and is responsible for the majority of severe cases. Many of these patients are hypertensive and it is quite probable that the susceptibility of certain ethnic communities to this complication contributes to the severity of their lupus glomerulonephritis.

A minority of patients will show clinical evidence of tubular abnormalities such as aminoaciduria or, more commonly, impairment of urinary acidification (i.e. renal tubular acidosis). These changes reflect the simultaneous involvement of the tubulointerstitial areas of the renal cortex in the same pathogenetic process that affects the glomerulus. Indeed, a significant percentage of patients will show tubulointerstitial inflammation even though the clinical features indicate predominant glomerular disease.

Some patients will show glomerular lesions on renal biopsy despite the lack of serum and urinary abnormalities. While the majority of such cases will show mild glomerular changes, it is well recognized that certain patients may have a serious lesion despite the absence of positive laboratory findings. This observation has contributed to the debate on whether all patients with SLE should undergo renal biopsy, irrespective of laboratory findings.

Diagnosis

The diagnostic process commences with the clinician's awareness that the manifestations of renal disease may reflect a more generalized disorder. Many clinical and laboratory features may support the diagnosis of SLE. However, in certain cases the renal manifestations will be the only presenting feature. SLE must be considered as an explanation for any glomerular lesion, particularly in the young female. Screening tests are mandatory in such cases. The full range of diagnostic criteria, established by the American Rheumatism Association (ARA), is shown in Table 9.3. Patients with four or more criteria may be classified as having SLE. Tests for anti-nuclear antibodies (ANA) and, more specifically, antibodies to double-stranded DNA assist in the confirmation of diagnosis. Measurement of complement proteins and immune complexes provides supportive evidence for diagnosis and disease activity. Typically, the latter produces activation of the classic complement pathway with reduction in serum concentration of early components such as $C1q$, $C4$ and $C3$. (The level of serum $C4$ may be influenced by the coexistence of one or more null alleles at the two $C4$ genetic loci.) It should be emphasized that elevation of immune complexes occurs in many

Table 9.3　Criteria for diagnosis of SLE

1.　Malar rash
2.　Discoid rash
3.　Photosensitivity
4.　Oral ulcers
5.　Arthritis
6.　Serositis
7.　Renal disease (proteinuria > 500 mg/day or cellular casts)
8.　Neurological disorder (seizures or psychosis)
9.　Haematological disorder (haemolytic anaemia, lymphocytopenia, leucopenia or thrombocytopenia)
10.　Immunological disorder (positive LE cell test, anti-DNA antibody, anti-Sm antibody)
11.　Positive antinuclear antibody

diseases — not all immune — and offers only limited assessment in terms of both diagnosis and disease activity.

Treatment

Renal involvement is the commonest serious manifestation of SLE and warrants consideration for aggressive therapy. Selection of treatment will be determined by three major criteria:

(i)　clinical and laboratory assessment of renal function
(ii)　renal histology
(iii)　lupus serology

All the manifestations of glomerular disease may be present in a single patient. However, the degree of proteinuria and renal failure will provide the best guidelines for selection of therapy. The type IV (diffuse proliferative) lesion is commonly associated with changes in both of these parameters. It should be emphasized that symptomatic therapy and, in particular, the control of hypertension will be a simultaneous requirement.

There have been some recent changes in the approach to specific therapy of lupus glomerulonephritis. In general, it is considered that significant renal involvement will warrant the use of combined steroid/cytotoxic therapy and that only patients with relatively minor involvement or who demonstrate a rapid response to treatment should be treated with steroids alone. Several regimens of steroid therapy have been tried in such patients: high dose oral therapy (prednisolone, 1 mg/kg/day) or intermittent pulse therapy given as intravenous methylprednisolone 500–1000 mg

per day for 3–5 days. There is no statistical evidence that this latter regimen has any advantage over the former.

Most physicians consider that cyclophosphamide is the cytotoxic drug of choice. Again, this may be given orally in a dose of 2–3 mg/kg/day or as intermittent intravenous therapy ($0.5–1$ g/m^2 body surface area, given monthly for approximately six months). There is often difficulty in the choice of a regimen for the maintenance of remission. Many approaches have been used including the continuation of intermittent intravenous cyclophosphamide (perhaps every 3–4 months), a change to oral azathioprine or cyclosporin A or the use of low dose steroids alone. Individual patient requirements vary considerably in this regard and the final choice will be determined substantially by patient progress. A major trial in North America suggests that intermittent i.v. cyclophosphamide provides a favourable means of maintaining control of the disease.

Two other major forms of aggressive therapy require consideration. Firstly, plasma exchange has been used extensively in the treatment of the severe, acute lupus lesion. However, its value has not been proven conclusively by controlled trials. In general, such treatment should be considered when combined steroid/cytotoxic therapy fails to control the renal abnormality. The major indication is progressive renal failure. The use of cyclosporin in autoimmune diseases continues to increase as it is realized that disease control is often accomplished with a minimum of side effects. The introduction of this agent is best reserved until the lesion is under control, at which time it can be introduced at a relatively low dose in order to titrate beneficial effects more precisely.

The symptomatic therapy of major renal syndromes that result from lupus nephritis is discussed in other chapters. Specifically, the approach to the nephrotic patient with SLE does not differ markedly from that used in other patients. Similarly, the renal impairment that may result requires treatment in its own right.

Pregnancy and SLE

The patient with lupus nephritis faces additional complications and risks during pregnancy. Fertility may be impaired, both by the primary disorder and subsequent management (i.e. with alkylating agents), and the coexistence of anti-phospholipid antibodies may increase the predisposition to miscarriage. However, renal involvement need not preclude a successful pregnancy. The determinants of outcome will be similar to those observed in other patients with renal disease where pre-existing renal failure and/or hypertension will lead to increased maternal and fetal risk. Such risks do not occur in the patient with nephrotic syndrome, although it is well recognized that fetal size may be reduced.

The reports of variation in disease activity during pregnancy are highly variable. It appears that the likelihood of exacerbation of lupus is declining, possibly as a result of more effective treatment.

It is important to emphasize the potential risks of certain therapeutic agents that are commonly used in lupus and are potentially toxic to the fetus. Specifically, patients should not become pregnant while on cyclophosphamide, calcium channel blockers or angiotensin converting enzyme inhibitors. It is important that the clinician makes the patient aware of the risks of pregnancy if such medications are to be used.

Renal vasculitis

The early descriptions of systemic vasculitis documented the involvement of middle-sized blood vessels and clinical syndromes that reflected organ ischaemia. More recent series emphasize features that result from inflammation of small-calibre vessels, such as the glomerular capillary. The classification of systemic vasculitis has been revised on numerous occasions as clinical features become better defined and pathogenetic factors are characterized. Of the various forms that are now recognized, the two disorders that affect the kidney most significantly are microscopic polyarteritis nodosa (PAN) and Wegener's granulomatosis (WG). The Hammersmith group has proposed the following definitions of these two entities:

(i) Microscopic PAN is vasculitis that affects small vessels (i.e. small arteries and arterioles) without macroscopic aneurysms and without particular involvement of the respiratory tract.

(ii) WG is vasculitis that affects predominantly small vessels with early and major disease of the respiratory tract, excluding asthma. Granulomata are a characteristic (but not essential) feature.

Pathology and pathogenesis

In most cases, the renal histology of PAN and WG cannot be distinguished. The major sites of injury are the glomerulus and small- or medium-calibre blood vessels. However, tubulointerstitial inflammation is commonly observed as part of the disease process. The glomerular lesion may resemble that of endocarditis with both necrosis and a tendency to crescent formation. Renal granulomata are not seen in the majority of patients with WG. The number of glomeruli involved is highly variable and the lesion tends to be segmental rather than diffuse. The vascular abnormality typically involves the intima and/or media with fibrinoid necrosis and a mixed cellular infiltrate; in the acute phase, the main element is the polymorph. In the microscopic form of either disease, the interlobular arteries and veins are the primary site of involvement.

The immunofluorescence findings in both diseases are disconcertingly variable. Immunoglobulins and complement proteins are found in some cases but there is no dominant protein nor typical pattern. Electron microscopy shows immune deposits that are small and scanty compared to other immune glomerular lesions. In contrast, there is significant fibrin deposition and platelet aggregation at sites of fibrinoid necrosis.

The pathogenesis of both conditions remains uncertain. Immunopathological evidence does not support a direct role for the traditional mediators of glomerular inflammation, namely specific antibody and immune complexes. It has long been suspected that the mononuclear phagocyte plays an important part because of the finding of (extra-renal) granulomata, particularly in WG. A more recent finding is the detection of antibodies to the neutrophil cytoplasm (ANCA). These were first demonstrated by immunofluorescence microscopy in patients with necrotizing glomerulonephritis and have been observed subsequently in both microscopic PAN and WG. Two major patterns have been observed: diffuse cytoplasmic staining (the classic cANCA) and perinuclear staining (pANCA). It is now recognized that the latter phenomenon is caused by interaction between antibodies and cytoplasmic antigens that undergo redistribution during fixation in vitro. cANCA appears to have a high degree of specificity for PAN and WG, while pANCA is observed with other immunological disorders, including SLE. Target antigens have been identified for both reactions: cANCA is reactive with a 29 kd protein that is homologous to neutrophil proteinase 3 (NP 3) while pANCA reacts with myeloperoxidase and elastase. Longitudinal studies show that the identification of ANCA has value for both diagnosis and monitoring of disease activity. However, it remains uncertain whether they play a role in the pathogenesis of microvascular lesions. It should be mentioned that the perinuclear pattern may be positive in various other immunological and infectious diseases (see Table 9.4).

Clinical features

The diagnosis of renal involvement of PAN or WG cannot be made on clinical grounds alone. The features may range from asymptomatic urinary abnormalities to rapidly progressive renal failure. In the majority of cases, damage predominantly affects the glomerulus. Haematuria and/or

Table 9.4 Disorders associated with ANCA

1. Wegener's granulomatosis
2. Microscopic polyarteritis nodosa
3. Segmental necrotizing glomerulonephritis
4. SLE, rheumatoid disease, anti-GBM disease
5. Kawasaki disease, Churg–Strauss syndrome
6. Atrial myxoma
7. HIV infection

Key: GBM — glomerular basement membrane; HIV — human immunodeficiency virus; 1, 2 and 3 — frequently detected; 4, 5, 6 and 7 — occasionally detected.

proteinuria are common findings, although the latter rarely reaches nephrotic proportions. Hypertension is a frequent accompaniment and may be the dominant finding when larger-calibre vessels are involved.

The extra-renal distribution of disease is critical to both diagnosis and management. Both disorders share several non-specific constitutional features which include fever, weight loss, fatigue and arthralgia/myalgia. Patients with PAN may also show one or more of the following: localized neurological abnormalities — such as mononeurittis — muscle tenderness, cutaneous vasculitis and symptoms and signs that reflect organ ischaemia (such as angina). Many of these features, including constitutional symptoms, are commonly less severe in WG. However, there is a predominance of upper respiratory symptoms including sinusitis, epistaxis, pharyngeal lesions and otitis media or externa.

While many patients will present with a pattern of disease that is typical of either PAN or WG, other patients may have features that are initially confined to the urinary tract. Indeed, the final diagnosis may not be evident until additional features occur or specific serology is undertaken, such as the detection of ANCA.

Diagnosis

Until recently, the diagnoses rested with two major components: (i) the realization that the patient had multisystemic involvement, and (ii) the histological demonstration that this involvement reflected a leucocytoclastic vasculitis. It is now recognized that the demonstration of ANCA constitutes an important third component. In many cases, several additional possibilities require consideration and may have important implications for therapy: SLE, endocarditis-associated nephritis, Henoch–Schönlein purpura and essential cryoglobulinaemia. The diagnostic separation of microscopic PAN and WG may have therapeutic implications. Two major practical considerations are the acknowledged resistance of the latter to steroid therapy alone and the frequent role of infection in this disorder. The clinical distinction of the two entities is easiest when there is involvement of the upper respiratory air passages. While the involvement of the nasopharynx is widely appreciated, a significant percentage of patients will also have abnormalities of the external ear. The constitutional effects of both diseases are comparable; however changes in the white cell count and, in particular, eosinophilia point to the Churg–Strauss variant of polyarteritis.

As with SLE, a controversy exists as to whether all patients with PAN or WG warrant renal biopsy, i.e. should patients without manifestations of renal disease undergo such a procedure? There is no consensus on this issue. However, it seems unlikely that biopsy data would change the clinical management of such a case.

Treatment

The renal manifestations of PAN and WG may be the major indication for treatment. The majority of such patients will have undergone both clinical and laboratory assessment, including a renal biopsy. All of these parameters will require consideration in the formulation of appropriate therapy. For example, the patient with minor urinary abnormalities, normal renal function and insignificant histological involvement may warrant observation rather than specific treatment (i.e. from a nephrological point of view). However, extra-renal manifestations may indicate the need for therapy in such a case.

In contrast, the patient with an active urine sediment, impaired renal function and significant changes on biopsy will require specific, aggressive therapy. The drugs of choice are steroids and cyclophosphamide. However, their mode of administration remains somewhat unresolved. Certain major questions require consideration: does intravenous administration of one or both drugs provide better results than oral treatment?; must both drugs be used in all patients? Unfortunately, there are no controlled trials to demonstrate superiority of one regimen over another. For example, it is uncertain whether pulse therapy with methylprednisolone is superior to high dose oral prednisolone (e.g. 1 mg/kg/day). Similarly, success with the use of intermittent intravenous cyclophosphamide in patients with lupus has not been reproduced in patients with PAN or WG; in fact, there is evidence that this approach produces more side effects than oral therapy. While some groups advocate the use of steroids alone in patients with PAN, this approach seems less successful with WG where it may be associated with incomplete control of disease activity and subsequent resistance to therapy. In the case of polyarteritis, the clinician must be prepared to add cyclophosphamide if the early response to steroid therapy is unsatisfactory.

The role of plasma exchange in the treatment of severe renal vasculitis remains uncertain. Again, there have been no controlled trials of this therapy, although many anecdotal observations suggest that it may be of assistance in the control of disease activity. It should be reserved for those cases where orthodox steroid/cytotoxic therapy has proved unsatisfactory.

The selection of a regimen for the maintenance of remission is also difficult. Continued high doses of prednisolone raise the prospect of side effects. What alternatives are available? Recent reports of small numbers of patients suggest that cyclosporin A may provide a suitable alternative when patients are at risk of toxicity from steroid and cytotoxic therapy. The value of other cytotoxic agents — such as azathioprine — has been disappointing in this group of diseases. Review of renal histology (i.e. by repeat renal biopsy) may be valuable and the clinician should consider supervised periods without immunosuppressive therapy in the patient who is convincingly in remission.

HENOCH–SCHÖNLEIN PURPURA (HSP)

The familiar combination of glomerulonephritis and specific extra-renal features makes the diagnosis of Henoch–Schönlein purpura (HSP) relatively easy in most circumstances. The propensity for mucosal surfaces is striking and may involve both the upper and lower digestive tracts, the bronchi and the eyes. The majority of patients are between the ages of 5 and 15 years with a slight preponderance of males. In this group, the usual outcome is a full recovery. The disorder is less predictable in adults where a higher percentage of patients develop progressive renal failure. However, HSP is comparatively rare in this age group.

There are striking immunopathological similarities between HSP and primary mesangial IgA nephropathy. These are discussed elsewhere. As with that disorder, there is a frequent association with a non-specific respiratory or gastrointestinal infection. Many different antigens have been implicated (including drugs and allergens) but no direct association with preceding streptococcal infection has been demonstrated. In this regard, it should be emphasized that children in the susceptible age group show a high frequency of positive streptococcal serology, irrespective of renal involvement.

The incidence of glomerular disease in HSP varies widely among different reports and has been suggested to be as high as 90%. However, the criteria for diagnosis of renal disease will influence this incidence and many reports suggest an occurrence of 10–30%. There are occasional cases where more than one member of a family has been affected or, alternatively, one or more other members have had IgA nephropathy.

Pathology and pathogenesis

The morphology of the glomerulus in HSP is very similar to that in IgA nephropathy, although the changes in the former tend to be more severe. In particular, necrosis and crescent formation are both more common in HSP. Both conditions show an increase in mesangial cells and matrix. The considerable range of severity of morphological changes in the systemic form of the disorder has led to a suggested classification based on the distribution of mesangial changes, the degree of crescent formation and the occasional development of a mesangiocapillary glomerulonephritis. This classification is summarized in Table 9.5. Electron microscopy shows deposits in both the mesangial matrix and mesangial cells and is similar in the two conditions. Widely distributed capillary wall deposits occur in the mesangiocapillary variant.

The pathogenesis of HSP and IgA nephropathy remains uncertain. The two disorders share immunological abnormalities, both within the glomerulus and the circulation. Central to these findings is the deposition of IgA within the mesangium; this is usually accompanied by C3, IgG and, to a lesser extent, IgM. Other components of the alternative complement pathway (such as properdin) may also be detected; in a minority of patients, classic pathway proteins such as C1q and C4 may also be found. There is now consensus that IgA1 is predominant over IgA2 and that secretory component is not present. However, J chain may be demonstrated in most cases. As with IgA nephropathy, about 50% of patients show a high serum concentration of IgA and elevated levels of immune complexes which tend to vary according to clinical disease activity. It is unresolved whether the polymeric IgA found in the plasma of such patients reflects an antigen–antibody complex or true IgA polymers. Several studies have reported increased IgA production in cell culture although the technical details of these reports vary considerably.

It is recognized that both IgA nephropathy and HSP may recur after transplantation, although the incidence varies among different populations and the severity is generally less than in the original disorder. Of interest are the results of transplantation of kidneys with IgA deposits into recipients without evidence of IgA disease: subsequent

Table 9.5 Histological classification of Henoch–Schönlein glomerulonephritis

Type I — minimal abnormalities
Type II — mesangial proliferation
Type III — focal or diffuse mesangial proliferation with
         crescent formation
Type IV — membranoproliferative lesion

biopsy showed disappearance of IgA deposits. Such an observation raises the question of the efficiency of immune complex solubilization in such patients. Two reports demonstrate impaired (complement-dependent) dissolution of IgA deposits, in vitro, by serum from such patients.

Clinical features

The commonest manifestation of renal damage is either macroscopic or microscopic haematuria. Of greater prognostic significance is the occurrence of heavy proteinuria or the nephrotic syndrome, hypertension or renal failure. The duration of these latter features will influence long-term prognosis for renal function and it appears that this is more important in the adult patient.

The correlation between extra-renal features and nephropathy in HSP is poor. Involvement of other organs reflects a leucocytoclastic vasculitis of small-calibre blood vessels. These clinical manifestations will not be reviewed in further detail.

Diagnosis

There is no specific laboratory test for HSP. The diagnosis lies with the clinical findings and the changes on renal biopsy. Perhaps the most striking of the extra-renal manifestations is the presence of a purpuric rash on the buttocks and lower limbs. Typically, these lesions do not blanch and may subsequently extend to other areas. The coexistence of arthralgia and, occasionally, frank arthritis as well as various abdominal symptoms (including melaena) adds support to the clinical suspicion of HSP. In the absence of a rash, the renal manifestations may be of particular diagnostic importance and immunofluorescent abnormalities will be critical to the diagnosis. Without these data, the clinical features may resemble other forms of systemic vasculitis including PAN/WG, SLE or essential cryoglobulinaemia.

Treatment and prognosis

In general, HSP is a self-limiting disorder. However, a minority of patients (variably reported between 5 and 20%) will show persistent urinary abnormalities and even renal failure 5 years after the initial episode. There is wide consensus that specific forms of treatment are not warranted in most cases.

The worst outlook is seen in patients with severe disease at the time of presentation. These will include patients with acute crescentic disease, persistent nephrotic syndrome and significantly impaired glomerular filtration rate. While such patients have been subjected to various protocols of treatment (including steroids, cytotoxics and plasma exchange) there have been no random trials to confirm whether such therapy is effective. Recurrence of disease in the transplanted kidney has been reported in a few cases.

Other multisystem diseases

It is not surprising that many other forms of multisystem disease show glomerular inflammation, given their overlap in terms of both pathogenesis and clinical manifestations; however, in most cases the glomerular lesion is not a major component of renal injury. These diseases include rheumatoid arthritis and Sjögren's syndrome, mixed connective tissue disease and sarcoidosis. In many, the light microscopy and immunofluorescent changes resemble those of primary membranous nephropathy. There are occasional reports of more severe glomerular involvement. It is rare for the glomerular abnormality to contribute significantly to impairment of renal function in such patients, although other forms of renal damage (e.g. those associated with therapy) may be more serious. Indeed, in patients with rheumatoid arthritis, a membranous lesion will occur most commonly as a result of treatment with gold or penicillamine.

THE KIDNEY AND BACTERIAL ENDOCARDITIS

The association between heart valve infection and renal abnormalities has been appreciated for over 100 years. However, during that time there have been major changes in the understanding of pathogenesis and the efficacy of treatment. Prior to the introduction of antibiotics, the majority of patients developed renal disease as a consequence of subacute valvular infection. The incidence of clinical renal involvement dropped significantly with the introduction of effective treatment so that most reports suggested that less than 30% of patients were affected. However, it must be emphasized that no entirely satisfactory study has been performed. Post-mortem reports tend to over-emphasize the severity of renal involvement while papers based on renal biopsy material exaggerate the incidence of severe disease. Similarly, assessment based on urine sediment can be very deceptive because of the coincidence of renal infarction, abscess formation or treatment-induced damage.

In recent years, the increased incidence of endocarditis in intravenous drug users has changed the profile of this disease. Specifically, the percentage of patients with acute endocarditis from *Staphylococcus aureus* has increased and this, in turn, has led to a higher frequency of diffuse glomerular disease. Indeed, the relative frequency of types of cases will be determined by the social and medical background of individual patients — i.e. in countries where rheumatic fever is still common, the lesion will be different to those where drug-related infection dominates.

Pathology and pathogenesis

Early reports suggested that the renal lesion of endocarditis involved embolization and/or infarction. However, subsequent data suggest an immunological basis for most lesions. This is supported by the detection of immune deposits within glomeruli (by both immunofluorescence and electron microscopy), the involvement of the complement system during active disease and the occasional isolation of bacterial-specific antibodies (and antigens) from intraglomerular lesions.

Typically, endocarditis causes glomerulonephritis. There are two major categories of lesion. The focal/segmental abnormality occurs classically with subacute infection. Necrosis may be a feature and there is deposition of eosinophilic material at these sites. There may be neutrophil infiltration and involvement of the overlying Bowman's capsule. In contrast, a high percentage of patients with acute bacterial endocarditis will have diffuse glomerular lesions that, in most respects, resemble post-streptococcal glomerulonephritis. There is diffuse endocapillary and mesangial proliferation and neutrophil infiltration may be prominent. In severe cases, crescent formation may be a major feature.

The immunological basis for most of these lesions is emphasized by the deposition of one or more immunoglobulins (predominantly IgG) in a granular fashion, either globally or at sites of focal lesions. Electron microscopy confirms the frequent occurrence of subepithelial deposits in acute cases while subacute disease tends to be associated with subendothelial lesions.

Clinical features

The assessment of renal involvement in endocarditis may be difficult, with only minor and transient changes in urine sediment. This applies particularly to focal and segmental lesions, where creatinine clearance is often normal. It is widely accepted that the correlation between urinary abnormalities and histological changes is very poor. One group studied the renal histology of 8 patients at a time when there was no evidence of clinical renal disease: all had evidence of focal glomerular lesions. In contrast, diffuse glomerulonephritis is associated frequently with renal impairment and significant abnormalities of urine sediment. Some of these patients will progress to severe renal failure and require dialysis. This complication becomes a major contributor to morbidity and mortality. Both histological types usually manifest as acute glomerulonephritis rather than as nephrotic syndrome.

It is important to emphasize again that not all the renal abnormalities observed during the course of endocarditis reflect glomerular inflammation. The clinician must also recognize the role of impaired cardiac output and, later in the disease, the potential risk of antibiotic nephrotoxicity. The assessment of renal function at the time of presentation assists the clarification of these issues, in that the majority of patients will not have received treatment.

Diagnosis

Subsequent to the diagnosis of endocarditis, nephrological assessment lies initially with examination of the urine sediment and biochemical quantitation of renal function. This includes measurement of proteinuria, serum creatinine and, if necessary, creatinine clearance. Such parameters may be important in monitoring disease activity and efficacy of treatment. Endocarditis-associated glomerulonephritis may be associated with changes in the serum concentration of complement components and the detection of circulating immune complexes. Complement proteins remain normal or elevated in the uncomplicated case of endocarditis but a high percentage of patients will show transient reduction in serum level when there is renal involvement. It is thought that this results from immune complex-mediated activation of the classic pathway. The complement changes return to normal with effective treatment. Immune complexes have been reported in up to 95% of cases, irrespective of renal disease, and these, to some extent, reflect progress with treatment. It should also be emphasized that a significant percentage of patients with subacute disease will develop antinuclear antibodies and rheumatoid factors.

Definitive assessment of renal involvement requires renal histology. However, a renal biopsy is not undertaken in all cases because the diagnosis of endocarditis implies that the renal abnormalities result from this disorder and that effective treatment demands the use of antibiotics. Difficulties may arise when renal function deteriorates despite apparently effective treatment. In such circumstances, biopsy may become mandatory.

Treatment

Treatment of the renal lesion will involve effective elimination of heart valve infection. A minority of patients will also require specific treatment of renal abnormalities, such as severe renal failure (i.e. by dialysis). It is rare to resort to immunosuppressive treatment for control of the immune glomerular lesion. Such measures would only be undertaken with extreme caution and under carefully supervised antibiotic cover.

As with many disorders in modern medicine, renal failure will not be the final determinant of outcome. This will depend on the nature of the cardiac lesion, the severity of ensuing sepsis and the involvement of other vital organs such as the central nervous system.

GLOMERULAR LESIONS IN OTHER INFECTIONS

Many forms of infection may be complicated by glomerulonephritis although only a minority of patients will be involved. A detailed description of each condition is not possible in this text. The most classic lesion, i.e. that which follows streptococcal infection, is described in Chapter 9 Part 1. This section describes three other infections where significant glomerular inflammation may occur.

Hepatitis B

The association between glomerulonephritis, vasculitis and hepatitis B has been recognized for over twenty years. The incidence varies widely among different ethnic populations and socio-economic groups. Many of the cases of glomerulonephritis associated with hepatitis B occur in children and may result from transfusion or materno–fetal transfer. The lesions may occur independently of active liver disease. Hence, young patients with glomerular disease should be screened for hepatitis B antigens and antibodies as part of the investigative process. Several reports also document an association between hepatitis B and the microscopic form of PAN. Analysis of glomerular deposits has, occasionally, yielded both hepatitis B antigens as well as traditional immunoreactive proteins such as IgG and C3.

Interpretation of immunological abnormalities may be difficult in patients with significant liver cell injury. For example, many such cases will have detectable immune complexes irrespective of the immunological nature of the disease. Similarly, complement levels may be lowered by impaired synthesis since the majority of complement proteins are produced predominantly by hepatocytes. The association between cirrhosis and mesangial IgA nephropathy is well recognized and is discussed in the chapter on primary glomerular disease.

Shunt nephritis

Mesangioproliferative and mesangiocapillary lesions may follow infection of ventriculo-atrial shunts. The typical organism is a coagulase-negative staphylococcus. Only a minority of patients with infected shunts suffer this complication which, in most respects, resembles an immune complex-mediated disease. There are granular deposits of immunoglobulins and complement, serum complement levels are often reduced. The majority of patients recover with adequate treatment although diagnosis may be delayed and recovery may take months or years after the apparent eradication of infection.

Similar glomerular lesions may occur following severe systemic infection, such as septicaemia and/or abscess formation.

Malaria

Infection by *Plasmodium malariae* is an important cause of glomerular damage in certain countries. The typical clinical presentation is nephrotic syndrome (particularly of the child) and various glomerular changes have been reported on biopsy. The most characteristic is that of mesangiocapillary nephritis, with duplication of the basement membrane and typical IgG/C3 deposits. However, other lesions — both diffuse and focal — have been described. The logical treatment is the effective eradication of the parasite but this does not assure healing of the lesion which may be established for some time before treatment is commenced (see Chapter 12).

NEOPLASIA

The association between malignancy and glomerular lesions is well established although comparatively rare. Many forms of carcinoma have been implicated, the most common of which originate from the lung and lower gastrointestinal tract. Typically, renal histology shows a membranous lesion although various other types of glomerulonephritis have been described. Most patients present over the age of 40 years, and the renal abnormality precedes the diagnosis of tumour in a significant number of cases.

Several forms of lymphoma have also been associated with glomerular lesions. The link between Hodgkin's disease and minimal change nephrotic syndrome is well documented and this association is instructive in understanding the pathogenesis of the glomerular abnormality.

The finding of membranous glomerulonephritis in the older nephrotic patient should prompt the clinician to consider a possible diagnosis of underlying neoplasia. In patients over 60 years of age it has been estimated that such an association exists in 25% of patients. Reduction in proteinuria has been reported following the excision or effective treatment of various tumours and recurrence has been observed with the development of metastases. However, the decision to investigate older patients for underlying malignancy remains controversial. It would appear appropriate to apply clinical and non-invasive diagnostic techniques to such cases but it must be emphasized that the diagnostic yield is low.

ESSENTIAL MIXED CRYOGLOBULINAEMIA

A wide range of disorders is associated with the formation of cryoglobulins. These are summarized in Table 9.6. The cold-precipitable proteins that result are usually divided into three classes, the latter two of which are called mixed cryoglobulins because there is interaction between IgG and a second (monoclonal or polyclonal) immunoglobulin. While most patients exhibit clinical features of another disease, about 25–30% of cases with mixed cryoglobulinaemia will have features that relate to the cryoglobulin itself. This group is termed essential mixed cryoglobulinaemia. These cases represent an unusual form of systemic vasculitis and their recognition is important because of the therapeutic implications.

Table 9.6   Classification of cryoglobulins and their associated diseases

Type I	Monoclonal (IgG, M or A or BJP)	Myeloma, macroglobulinaemia, CLL, essential cryoglobulinaemia
Type II	Mixed polyclonal/monoclonal (e.g. IgG–IgM)	Essential mixed cryoglobulinaemia, rheumatoid arthritis, Sjögren's syndrome
Type III	Mixed polyclonal (e.g. IgG–IgM; IgG–IgM–IgA)	a. Infections e.g. cytomegalovirus, hepatitis B, endocarditis, malaria b. Autoimmune disease e.g. SLE, rheumatoid, PAN, HSP, biliary cirrhosis c. Lymphoid diseases e.g. lymphoma d. Essential mixed cryoglobulinaemia

Key: BJP — Bence Jones protein;
         CLL — chronic lymphatic leukaemia.

Pathology and pathogenesis

The renal manifestations of essential cryoglobulinaemia tend to occur quite late in the disorder and typically involve the glomerulus. The majority of lesions show diffuse proliferation and, in some cases, the changes of mesangiocapillary glomerulonephritis. Specific staining or electron microscopy confirms the presence of substantial eosinophilic deposits, either intraluminally or at subendothelial sites. Immunofluorescence shows distinctive multi-immunoglobulin deposition that coincides closely with the content of the cryoglobulin. C3 deposition occurs in the majority of cases.

The pathogenesis of essential cryoglobulinaemia remains uncertain although there is a general view that the reaction resembles that observed with (other) rheumatoid factors. Similar hypotheses have been put forward as to the stimulus for such reactivity.

Clinical features

A substantial range of extra-renal manifestations have been described. These include arthralgia, palpable purpura and abnormalities of liver function. The renal features most commonly involve an acute nephritic picture (in about one quarter of patients) or a syndrome based on heavy proteinuria.

Diagnosis

The condition may be confused with other causes of systemic vasculitis. The diagnostic process will involve the exclusion of such conditions as well as elucidation of specific features of essential cryoglobulinaemia. Specifically, patients will show typical light and immunofluorescent microscopic changes, distinctive complement abnormalities (i.e. classic pathway activation in the absence of ANA) and large quantities of cryoglobulin. These proteins can be further characterized by several techniques including isoelectric focussing. The identification of a protein with a single isoelectric point will distinguish the type II (monoclonal) form from the type III (polyclonal) abnormality.

Treatment

The basic requirement of therapy is to lower the plasma level of cryoglobulin. This can rarely be achieved with steroid therapy alone. Similarly, the use of plasma exchange may enchance cryoglobulin production. Hence the most logical therapy is a combination of steroids, cytotoxics and, where indicated (i.e. by severe tissue injury), plasma exchange. The regular measurement of cryoglobulin offers an accessible method of monitoring disease activity, although it is generally thought that the level of cryoprotein correlates poorly with disease activity. Monitoring of complement levels may also be valuable.

Aggressive treatment may lead to improvement and stabilization of the glomerular lesion. However, such patients warrant long-term supervision, as there may be recurrence of active disease.

Other gammopathies

Several other plasma cell disorders cause renal damage. Both multiple myeloma and Waldenström's macroglobulinaemia may be associated with membranous glomerular lesions although, in the former, this is much less important than other features such as light chain nephropathy, amyloidosis and the effects of hypercalcaemia (Ch. 11).

PROGRESSIVE SYSTEMIC SCLEROSIS (PSS)

This condition is characterized by increased fibrosis of the skin and, in many cases, of internal organs. Its pathogenesis is uncertain. It has been suggested that the fibrotic process is triggered by vascular injury, immunological mechanisms and/or stimuli to collagen synthesis. There is considerable support for each of these theories and they may not be mutually exclusive. As with most other multisystem disorders, humoral immunological abnormalities have been demonstrated, including a high incidence of antinuclear antibodies (of variable pattern) and, more recently, the demonstration of antibodies to sites within the centromere. Various other specificities have also been reported. Whether any of these antibody systems plays a role in pathogenesis remains to be clarified.

Clinically, PSS may follow a relatively benign course or lead to relatively rapid involvement of vital organs and early death. The former group often show quite distinctive features including calcinosis, Raynaud's phenomenon, oesophageal hypomotility, sclerodactyly and telangiectasia; this group of features is commonly referred to as the CREST syndrome.

Clinical features

The frequency of involvement of the kidneys in scleroderma syndromes (whether benign or progressive) has been reported to be between 50 and 100%. This incidence will depend on selection criteria and the relative frequency of benign and malignant forms of the disorder. Pathologically, several structures may be involved. The predominant lesion involves blood vessels, particularly of the calibre of the interlobular arteries and arterioles. Changes may be acute or chronic and their distribution may be variable. Affected vessels show luminal narrowing and intimal areas may be arranged in a concentric pattern that is often described as an onion-skin appearance. Glomeruli may show intracapillary fibrin deposition with endothelial cell swelling and mesangiolysis. Rarely, there are more definite changes to suggest glomerular inflammation, including mesangial hypercellularity and crescent formation. Neither blood vessels nor glomeruli show any consistent pattern on immunofluorescence microscopy.

The two most prominent clinical features in PSS are hypertension and impaired renal function. The rate of progress of these two features varies considerably and only a small percentage will present with accelerated hypertension. Most patients will have mild proteinuria but this rarely reaches nephrotic proportions. No specific treatment has been shown to be effective and, for the renal lesion, control of blood pressure will be a major issue. Recent work suggests that the use of angiotensin-converting enzyme inhibitors is of particular value.

RECOMMENDED READING

Atkins R C, Thomson N M 1992 Rapidly progressive glomerulonephritis. In: Schrier R W, Gotschalk C W (eds) Diseases of the kidney. Little, Brown and Co., Boston, pp 1689–1713

Austin H A III, Balow J E 1983 Henoch-Schönlein nephritis: Prognostic features and the challenge of therapy. American Journal of Kidney Disease 2: 512–520

Baldwin D S 1982 Chronic glomerulonephritis: Non-immunologic mechanisms of progressive glomerular damage. Kidney International 21: 109–120

Balow J E 1987 Lupus nephritis (NIH Conference). Annals of Internal Medicine 106: 79–94

Boulton-Jones J M, Sissons J G Evans D J, Peters D K 1974 Renal lesions of subacute infective endocarditis. British Medical Journal 2: 11–14

Broyer M, Meyrier A, Niaudet P, Habib R 1992 Minimal changes and focal segmental glomerular sclerosis. In: Cameron S, Davison A M, Grunfeld J-P, Kerr D, Ritz E (eds) Oxford Textbook of clinical nephrology. Oxford University Press, Oxford, pp 298–339

Clarkson A R, Woodroffe A J, Bannister J D, Lomax-Smith J D, Aarons I 1984 The syndrome of IgA nephropathy. Clinical Nephrology 21: 7–14

Coovadia H M, Adhikari M 1989 Outcome of childhood minimal change disease. Lancet i: 1199–1200

Couser W G 1988 Rapidly progressive glomerulonephritis. Classification, pathogenic mechanisms and therapy. American Journal of Kidney Diseases 11: 449–464

Couser W G, Norass C P 1988 Pathogenesis of membranous nephropathy. Annual Revue Medicine 39: 517–530

D'Amico G, Colasanti G, Farrario F, Sinico A R, Bucci A, Fornasier A 1988 Renal involvement in essential mixed cryoglobulinemia: A peculiar type of immune complex mediated disease. Advances in Nephrology 17: 219–239

Emancipator S N, Lamm M E 1989 IgA nephropathy. Pathogenesis of the most common form of glomerulonephritis. Laboratory Investigation 60: 168–183

Falk R J 1990 ANCA-associated renal disease (Nephrology Forum). Kidney International 39: 998–1010

Fauci A S, Haynes B F, Katz P, Wolff S M 1983 Wegener's granulomatosis: Prospective clinical and therapeutic experience with 85 patients for 21 years. Annals of Internal Medicine 98: 76–85

Fogo A, Hawkins E P, Berry P L et al 1990 Glomerular hypertrophy in minimal change disease predicts subsequent progression to focal glomerular sclerosis. Kidney International 38: 115–123

Glassock R J, Cameron J S 1988 The nephrotic syndrome. Marcel Dekker, New York

Heptinstall R H 1992 Thin basement membrane disease. In: Heptinstall R H (ed) Pathology of the kidney, 4th edn. Little, Brown and Co., Boston, pp 285–289

Kincaid-Smith P 1975 The kidney. A clinico-pathological study. Blackwell, Oxford

Lai K N, Lai F M, Chan K K W, Chow C B, Tong K L, Vallance-Owen J 1987 The clinicopathologic features of hepatitis B virus-associated glomerulonephritis. Quarterly Journal of Medicine 63: 323–333

Meadows R 1978 Renal histopathology. A light, electron and immunofluorescent microscopy study of renal disease. Oxford University Press, Oxford

Pinching A J, Lockwood C M, Pussell B A et al 1983 Wegener's granulomatosis: Observations on 18 patients with severe renal disease. Quarterly Journal of Medicine 208: 435–460

Rodriguez-Iturbe B 1984 Epidermic poststreptococcal glomerulonephritis. Kidney International 25: 129–136

Savage C O S, Winearls C G, Evans D J, Rees A J, Lockwood C M 1985 Microscopic polyarteritis: Presentation, pathology and prognosis. Quarterly Journal of Medicine 56: 467–483

Tiebosch A T M G, Frederik P M, van Breda Vriesman P J C 1989 Thin-basement membrane nephropathy in adults with persistent haematuria. New England Journal of Medicine 320: 14–18

10. Therapy of glomerulonephritis

T. H. Mathew

INTRODUCTION

Primary glomerulonephritis (GN) accounts for about 35% of patients requiring dialysis in Australia. This makes it three times more frequent than any other single cause of renal failure. However, in absolute terms only 2 new patients/100 000 of population present each year, making it by most criteria an uncommon condition.

This low prevalence underlies the difficulty in developing therapy for GN. A multicentre approach has been required to gather sufficient numbers for a controlled trial. The paucity of numbers has been one of the factors leading to the abundance of uncontrolled and often anecdotal studies in the literature. Other difficulties in assessing the therapy of GN include the great variety of causes of primary GN even with a similar histopathological appearance. In membranous nephropathy for instance it is recognized that there may be many aetiologies and that it is probably not a single disease despite apparently similar immunopathogeneses. The altered immune status of the individual susceptible to GN varies both in character and severity and may have a genetic basis. This may mean not only that a heterogeneous response occurs within an ethnic group but, as one crosses racial groups and indeed continents, considerable variation in the clinical course and the response to treatment could be expected. Further difficulty ensues with the recognition that our understanding of the pathogenesis is still rudimentary. The tailoring of specific therapy to particular pathogenetic mechanisms has not yet occurred. It is hoped that the next decade will see the application of molecular biological advances to the therapy of GN (Table 10.1).

Reviewing therapy of GN at the present time is thus somewhat disappointing. Most recent reports involve therapy (e.g. steroids, cyclophosphamide) introduced twenty or more years ago which is clearly imperfect both in efficacy and side effect profile. The advances in therapeutic knowledge that have occurred have been mainly through the conduct of large multicentre controlled trials. However in most types of GN there is enough anecdotal evidence (in addition to the controlled data) to give the therapeutic optimist some encouragement.

Table 10.1 Theoretical approaches to treatment*

Immune event	Treatment
1. Elimination of provoking antigens	Genetics engineering Public health measures Antibiotics, surgery
2. Interference with immune response	Monoclonal antibodies Corticosteroids Cyclosporin (other cytotoxics) Soluble particles
3. Interference with formation of immune aggregates	Plasma exchange Antigen excess 'Primed' columns
4. Interference with inflammatory reaction	Corticosteroids Oxygen scavengers Anticoagulants Specific inhibitors (Antiplatelet, antikinin)
5. Interference with fibrogenesis	Corticosteroids inhibit IL-1 and growth factors

* Modified from Cameron J S 1990 Nephrology Dialysis Transplantation (suppl 1) 16–22

175

Many reviews of GN therapy have stressed the caveat *primum non nocere*. This is a pertinent reminder that most GN therapies have been broad in immunological effect and have carried the risk of important side effects such as bone marrow depression, sterility and increased oncogenesis. The focus of treatment has necessarily been on GN known to have a tendency to progress into renal failure. Subsequent transplantation would then usually involve the same type of immunosuppressive therapies and the same risks. The equation of risk versus benefit can now be drawn with more confidence than twenty years ago, yet the decision to actively intervene in the individual patient remains difficult and the subject of controversy amongst renal physicians.

GENERAL MEASURES IN THE TREATMENT OF GN (Table 10.2)

1. Follow-up

Patients diagnosed to have a persistent GN in practice should be offered regular renal follow-up. This facilitates the application of general measures. One important benefit that accrues with this policy is that the opportunity exists to educate patients about the chronic renal failure programme, should the need for that develop. This avoids the highly undesirable situation of having a patient, identified as having a persistent renal problem, being lost to follow-up and then precipitated into the chronic programme with no warning and much disruption to patient and family.

2. Hypertension

For many years it has been observed that hypertension often develops coincident with progression in renal failure. The obvious suggestion has been that the two are linked as cause and effect although

proving this link is difficult. When hypertension accelerates, as evidenced by diastolic pressures consistently above 120 mmHg and fundal changes of haemorrhages and exudates, there is little doubt as to its contribution to deterioration of renal function. From these observations has arisen the belief and, hence, the practice that hypertension in all patients with persistent renal disease, particularly those with GN, should be treated aggressively. In practice this means the introduction of antihypertensive agents when the blood pressure readings are consistently above 145/95 mmHg. This advice seems especially pertinent in patients with IgA nephropathy, a condition in which the development of severe hypertension is common even when the basic GN process is not severe.

3. Fluid control

The development of oedema in patients with GN is usually due either to a nephrotic state or to difficulty handling the normal load of salt and water at a time of renal function deterioration. In either instance the use of diuretics is indicated once oedema is creating discomfort or the fluid overload is in danger of causing left heart failure. Diuretics are preferred to restriction in salt and water intake, for compliance with the latter regime tends to be short-lived. The combination of restriction in input and loop-acting diuretics should be avoided because in most patients it is too severe and will lead to the possibility of dehydration and a pre-renal component to renal failure.

4. Dietary management

Considerable effort has recently been devoted to delineating the role of protein restriction in slowing down the progression of renal disease (not only in patients with GN). A reasonable approach at this time is to modestly reduce protein intake (to 0.8–1.0 g/kg/day) to minimize nephron workload whilst avoiding protein malnutrition, see Chapter 22. The special care for dietary protein treatment in the nephrotic state is dealt with below.

Table 10.2   General measures in treatment of GN

1. Follow-up
2. Meticulous control of hypertension
3. Fluid control
4. Early institution of protein restriction
5. Measures to reduce proteinuria

5. Measures to reduce proteinuria

Recently considerable attention has been paid to the potential benefit of reducing the quantity of urine protein excreted. There are some patients with nephrotic range proteinuria in whom a modest reduction in proteinuria will remove the risk of a full-blown nephrotic syndrome developing. Some have argued that the reduction in proteinuria itself may be beneficial in allowing the kidney to heal.

Non-steroidal anti-inflammatory agents have been known for many years to reduce the glomerular filtration rate and it has not been possible to divorce this action from the reduction in proteinuria which occurs with their use. ACE inhibitors likewise have been credited with the same characteristics but after careful studies there is now agreement that these two actions are not always linked. Accordingly, there is now a vogue for the use of ACE inhibition for this indication. It remains to be seen from longer-term studies whether there is benefit from their use in this fashion.

In the absence of specific treatment these general measures are helpful in minimizing morbidity and hopefully in slowing down the progress of persistent disease.

Table 10.3 Specific treatment of GN

Type of GN	Treatment	Effectiveness
Minimal change	Corticosteroids	+++
	Cyclophosphamide	+++
	Chlorambucil (etc)	++
	Cyclosporin	++
Membranous	Corticosteroids	+ (?)
	Cyclophosphamide	++
	Chlorambucil	++
	IgG (i.v.)	+
	Cyclosporin	+
Mesangial IgA (nephrotic)	Corticosteroids	++
Mesangiocapillary (Type I)	Corticosteroids	+ (?)
	Cytotoxics	+/−
Rapidly progressive	Plasma exchange	++
1. ANCA-associated	Corticosteroids	
2. Immune complex	Cyclophosphamide	
3. Anti-GBM Ab-induced		
Focal necrotizing	Corticosteroids	+++
	Cytotoxics	+++

SPECIFIC TREATMENT OF GLOMERULONEPHRITIS (Table 10.3)

Minimal change glomerulonephritis

The efficacy of corticosteroids in inducing a remission in this condition is well established although understanding of the pathogenesis of minimal change nephrotic syndrome has progressed little in recent years. An abnormality of T cell function leading to changes in the charge of the membranes, particularly in the glomerular capillaries with consequent alteration in membrane permeability, remains the main and yet unproven hypothesis. Response to steroids or alkylating agents has been used by some as a means of proving the presence of this condition.

The case for treatment rests on the reduction of morbidity and mortality which occurs with a shortened period of nephrotic state. The pattern of response to a course of high dose prednisolone in children has been determined by controlled trials although several questions remain. In untreated adults, complete or partial remission can be expected in about 65% of patients over 3 years, and these figures are probably similar in children.

About 95% of children will initially respond to the first course of steroids within 8 weeks of commencement, whereas in adults the percentage responding is less (80%) and the response is slower, taking up to 16 weeks. The ideal initial dose of steroid is still being defined although in adults most physicians would use oral prednisolone in a single daily dose of about 1 mg/kg and in children a somewhat higher dosage on a weight basis. Alternate day oral therapy is considered less efficacious in inducing remission though it is preferred by some physicians as a first course because of reduced side effects. Intravenous 'pulse' methylprednisolone (e.g. 1 g methylprednisolone daily for 3 days) followed by low dose oral steroids has been shown recently to shorten time to remission, reduce side effects and to induce remission in some patients resistant to oral prednisolone. Remission can also be achieved with cyclophosphamide, chlorambucil, azathioprine, cyclosporin and other agents.

After remission is induced about 20% of patients will have no further problem. Around 50% of patients will have multiple relapses, mostly in the first year after presentation, with the remainder having an occasional relapse over the next few years. Those patients who have multiple relapses can be divided into those who become free of proteinuria with treatment but remain in remission for only short periods off steroids and those who relapse whilst still on reducing doses of steroid. In the latter group continuing use of steroid becomes necessary to maintain the patient in the non-nephrotic state, and steroid side effects become a major issue in management.

The use of alkylating agents (mainly cyclophosphamide or chlorambucil) has been shown to induce a longer-lasting remission in those patients subject to frequent relapses but a considerable portion still relapse within a few years. It is now clear that those with steroid dependence tend to be resistant to the usually recommended course of an alkylating agent (e.g. 8 weeks of low dose [2–3 mg/kg] cyclophosphamide). In this group an improved response may occur with a higher dosage and longer course of cyclophosphamide (e.g. 12 weeks at a dose of 2 mg/kg). In this situation the equation of risks versus benefit needs to be individualized, for bone marrow depression and sterility become real concerns. Azathioprine given in continuing dosage for some years has been claimed to be effective in remitting the steroid-dependent and cyclophosphamide non-responsive group. Adults tend to have a more stable response to treatment and relapses are relatively rare over the age of 60 years.

Renal biopsy is not indicated in the child who presents with a straightforward picture of minimal change GN. Adults should be biopsied in view of the much increased likelihood of alternative diagnoses. Some of the biopsies in the steroid-dependent group of children will show changes of focal glomerulosclerosis. The relationship between minimal change disease and focal glomerulosclerosis has been debated, with many now believing that the two conditions are at different ends of the same spectrum and are joined by a small number of cases who may first present with the picture of steroid-sensitive or steroid-dependent nephrotic syndrome. At the far end of the spectrum are those who at first presentation demonstrate steroid and cyclophosphamide non-responsiveness. This group is destined for continuation of the nephrotic state and the risk of progression into renal failure at a variable rate.

The role of cyclosporin in treating minimal change disease remains unclear. In most trials cyclosporin on its own appears equally successful to steroids in inducing a remission but durable remissions are comparatively rare. Cyclosporin dependency has been described in some cases. In both adults and children cyclosporin used in combination with steroids markedly reduces the threshold of steroid sensitivity and thereby allows a substantial reduction in corticosteroid dosage. In one trial 50% of cases resistant to steroids and alkylating agents remitted completely, suggesting that the mode of action of cyclosporin is different and that it may have a role in the treatment of this condition.

Recent work has thus considerably clarified treatment in this condition and increased therapeutic options. Several questions remain including the optimum dose, route and length of the steroid course used to induce the first remission and what agent to use in multiple relapsers or those with steroid dependence. Pulse therapy seems likely to become the established induction therapy, with low dose cyclophosphamide for no more than 8 weeks remaining the preferred agent for those needing additional therapy.

MEMBRANOUS NEPHROPATHY

The issue of treatment in membranous nephropathy has been contentious for many years. The last decade has seen more publications in the treatment of this condition than in any other type of GN, indicating both the frequency which the condition is seen and the continuing uncertainties in choice and timing of therapy.

Recent evidence has helped to resolve some of the questions. There is now substantial controlled trial evidence showing a response to therapy, at least as measured by reduction in proteinuria and in some trials by the maintenance of or improvement in renal function. The question is no longer 'Should membranous nephropathy be treated?' but 'Which patients?' and 'With which agent?'.

Two major schools of thought have developed. The first believes that all patients with idiopathic membranous nephropathy and a fully developed nephrotic syndrome should be treated at diagnosis whereas the second believes that a waiting period is in order before proceeding to treatment to select the patients who are destined to progress into renal failure. Central to this issue is an assessment of just how many fully nephrotic patients with membranous nephropathy are destined to go into renal failure and whether there are any risk factors that can be determined at presentation. Some recently published studies suggest that between 20 and 50% of these patients, if untreated, will go into renal failure within 10 years and that the number is less in children and young adults. This information can be used either way in the debate about treatment. Within this group, can risk factors be defined? Here again there is no clear agreement but most series would show an increased risk with age, female sex, impaired initial renal function and marked tubulointerstitial change on the renal biopsy. Opinion varies on the role of staging glomerular basement membrane change as a predictor of progression.

It is important to stress that initial efforts should be directed at detecting an underlying aetiology. Around 20% of recent adult series have been shown to have an associated or underlying condition such as malignancy, drug use or infections. Treatment of these conditions or removal of the causal antigen will usually result in stabilization or improvement of the membranous nephropathy, and steroid or immunosuppressive treatment is not warranted.

The patients with non-nephrotic range proteinuria and normal renal function will in general do well with a conservative approach and certainly do better as a group than those with heavy proteinuria. The consensus in this group would be to watch and wait. Those destined to progress will become fully nephrotic in time and treatment can then be considered.

Real debate continues about the majority of patients in most series who present with persistent proteinuria in excess of 3.5 g/24 hours. Therapeutic enthusiasts rest their case on evidence showing that there is treatment responsiveness early in the course of membranous nephropathy which is lost if initiation of therapy is delayed. Those in favour of making a delayed decision point to the spontaneous remission rate, the toxicity of all the proven therapies and some evidence that a satisfactory response is still seen if treatment does not start until renal function has shown definite signs of deterioration. Further trials are needed to resolve this matter.

Once a decision in favour of treatment is made, further debate surrounds the choice of agents. Five controlled trials have been published in the last 15 years addressing the question of whether prednisolone, alone or with an alkylating agent, alters the short or medium-term outcome. It is difficult to summarize this experience for two of the trials using identical regimes (alternate day prednisolone only) came to opposite conclusions, another using daily oral steroids concluded in the negative, and two Italian trials comparing methylprednisolone/prednisolone with prednisolone alternating monthly with chlorambucil gave impressive positive results. Other recent uncontrolled data have shown methylprednisolone to be successful in rescuing patients who had shown progressive decline in renal function. Many physicians have expressed concern about the dose and course of chlorambucil and have found its therapeutic index too narrow to use without significant difficulty. In most reports the observation is made that the longer and stronger the course of immunosuppression the greater the response rate. It is particularly important to note that the response to alkylating agents is often delayed beyond the course of administration and may be seen some months later.

Other reports have examined the role of cyclosporin, and although a definitive conclusion is not yet possible there is encouragement that it may prove to be effective. Some of the apparent improvement in proteinuria may be due to the effect of cyclosporin on GFR, and along with other non-specific drug-induced remissions in proteinuria there is a significant relapse rate. High dose intravenous IgG has also been reported to be effective in this condition although there is current concern about side effects including an adverse effect on renal function.

What can one conclude and recommend to the individual patient? Firstly every effort should be made to identify the cause and to treat it effectively. In those adult patients presenting with non-nephrotic range proteinuria observation is appropriate. When a patient has at presentation, or develops under observation, the full nephrotic syndrome or shows a trend towards deterioration of renal function, a recommended approach (despite the conflicting evidence) is a trial of steroids (i.v. methylprednisolone followed by oral prednisolone 125 mg on alternate days for 8 weeks). If that course does not result in improvement, cyclophosphamide 1.5–2 mg/kg/day for no more than 6 months is tried. In those not responding, measures to reduce proteinuria (see above) and to control hyperlipidaemia are in order.

MESANGIAL IgA NEPHROPATHY

The overall conclusion in considering therapy for patients with mesangial IgA nephropathy is that no agent has been established to affect outcome favourably. A major difficulty in assessing therapy in this condition is the paucity of adequately controlled trials. This relates to the fact that progression is uncommon and, even when it can be predicted (by the presence of hypertension, proteinuria, impaired renal function and tubulointerstitial change on biopsy), the course is slow. This means that any trial must follow a special cohort of patients for some years to have any chance of demonstrating a conclusion.

Phenytoin, fish-oil, cyclosporin, danazol and non-steroidal anti-inflammatory agents have been sufficiently well investigated to establish that they are ineffective in most patients with mesangial IgA nephropathy. Cyclophosphamide, warfarin and dipyridamole, in combination, have been shown to reduce proteinuria significantly but show no consistent ability to prevent renal function deterioration.

Recent interest has focused on the identification of a subgroup of patients with heavy proteinuria. In a high proportion of these, steroids have been successful in inducing a complete remission in proteinuria. Whether this subgroup represents a distinct entity or merely the coincidence of two reasonably common conditions (minimal change GN and IgA nephropathy) remains unclear. For patients with heavy proteinuria a trial of steroids (as in minimal change GN) is justified. Beyond this, an aggressive approach to the group with poor prognostic factors is favoured by some nephrologists, with plasma exchange and cytotoxic agents being used. The majority of nephrologists however await clearer evidence of efficacy and currently would not offer any active therapy in the vast majority of patients with IgA nephropathy.

Henoch–Schönlein purpura (HSP)

The majority of patients with HSP are children and have a mild nephritis. These children do well in the short term with no specific therapy. However, a recent report looking at long-term outcome of a hospital-acquired series of 78 patients has stressed the need for long-term follow-up and special monitoring, particularly during pregnancy. In this series over one third of pregnancies developed complications. Of those patients with a severe initial presentation almost half developed hypertension or impaired renal function later in life.

Patients presenting with more severe episodes of HSP have marked crescent formation on renal biopsy and qualify for inclusion in the group labelled 'rapidly progressive GN' (RPGN). The treatment for these cases should be the same as for those with RPGN (see below).

The presentation in the adult tends to be more severe than in children; there may be some crescents on biopsy, heavy persisting proteinuria and a tendency to deterioration in renal function. In this situation a trial of steroids or immunosuppression is warranted and may be effective in slowing down or remitting the process. Anticoagulants and antiplatelet agents, whilst attractive considering the prominence of a coagulation system disturbance in HSP, have not been shown to affect the outcome.

MESANGIOCAPILLARY GN (TYPE 1)

This important type of GN has attracted much therapeutic interest. The outcome for about 50% of untreated patients is to survive free of renal failure at 10 years. This survival seems to have improved in recent years but the apparent improvement may relate in part to different indications for biopsy and hence incomparable starting points in assessment. It also appears that this condition is not being seen as frequently as in the past, at least in developed countries, and this makes it even more difficult to aggregate enough patients for a clinical trial.

A recent critical review has concluded that no treatment for children or adults with idiopathic MCGN has been proved effective. This review stresses the paucity of prospective, randomly controlled trials, the need for long-term follow-up and the need carefully to define end-points.

Treatments assessed and claimed to be ineffective included steroids alone, cyclophosphamide, warfarin, dipyridamole, non-steroidal anti-inflammatory agents and prednisolone in various combinations, and platelet inhibitor therapy on its own.

The Cincinatti group have for many years reported an advantage to their children with MCGN of using alternate day steroids. Their most recent report of a 56% 20-year renal survival with few side effects from steroids is impressive. However, a concerted attempt to replicate these results in an international controlled trial failed in part because of a high withdrawal rate due to steroid-associated hypertension.

Despite the negative controlled trial evidence many physicians still advocate a trial of alternate day steroids in children with severe disease evidenced by a persisting nephrotic syndrome or impaired renal function where the untreated course is predictably poor. In the adult presenting with severe disease similar arguments apply and some would be influenced by anecdotal evidence favouring a trial of i.v. pulse methylprednisolone followed by oral steroids or cytotoxic agents. If the initial presentation is acute and the renal biopsy is dominated by crescents, treatment as for RPGN is indicated.

MESANGIOCAPILLARY GN (TYPE 2)

Although patients with MCGN Type 2 have been included in the uncontrolled reports of alternate day steroid therapy from Cincinatti which indicate a favourable effect, there is a dearth of other favourable reports. Much anecdotal evidence supports the conclusion that this condition is not responsive to therapy.

RAPIDLY PROGRESSIVE GLOMERULONEPHRITIS

1. Anti-neutrophil cytoplasmic antibody (ANCA) associated GN. This condition was previously called pauci-immune or idiopathic and when confined to the kidney was considered to be a form of renal polyarteritis. The recognition that ANCA was a reliable marker and perhaps part of the pathogenesis of this condition has allowed this group to be more clearly identified and treatment to be planned with more certainty.

The presentation may be slow and grumbling with mild impairment of renal function and an active urine sediment. Biopsy at this time will reveal a focal and segmental necrotizing proliferative GN with little crescent formation. Treatment at this stage with steroids or cytotoxic therapy will stabilize the condition or allow improvement.

If the presentation and treatment are delayed, progression will occur and eventually acute renal failure will ensue. Biopsy at this time is characterized by cellular crescents affecting up to 100% of glomeruli. Treatment at this stage is a medical emergency for any delay allows more fibrotic scarring to occur.

2. Immune complex-associated RPGN. In this type of RPGN, which accounts for about 30–40% of cases, there is evidence of immune complex deposition (IgG and C3 deposition on capillary walls in a granular pattern) in the clinical context of post-infectious states, SLE or cryoglobulinaemia.

3. Antiglomerular basement membrane antibody-induced RPGN. This condition is called Goodpasture's syndrome when the acute nephritic episode is accompanied by lung haemorrhage. Approximately 20–40% of cases of RPGN are accounted for by this condition.

The appropriate treatment for these three conditions, which whilst similar in clinical expression have diverse pathogenesis, remains contentious. With the exception of post-infectious states, where supportive measures alone are usually successful, an aggressive therapeutic approach is favoured since untreated, persistent renal failure is the outcome in 90% of cases within days or weeks.

All reports stress the emergency nature of these conditions, with a favourable outcome being dependent on early diagnosis and the institution of treatment without delay; this means renal biopsy being performed on that day that the diagnosis is suspected and appropriate treatment commencing later that same day.

Treatment with immunosuppressives, steroids and anticoagulants was shown in the 1970s to probably improve the outcome in all forms of RPGN. Plasma exchange was introduced in the late 70s and followed soon after by pulse therapy with i.v. methylprednisolone. The precise indications for these therapies are still being established, with the literature marked by a paucity of controlled experience. In ANCA-associated and in immune complex-induced RPGN a trial of i.v. methylprednisolone pulses (10–30 mg/kg/day) for 3 or more doses followed by high dose oral steroids is warranted with resort to plasma exchange and cytotoxic drugs if this is not successful. If the diagnosis of Wegener's granulomatosis is suspected cyclophosphamide should be added from the beginning.

ANCA-associated RPGN often responds to an aggressive regime even if treatment is not started until renal failure has supervened. This contrasts with experience in anti-GBM antibody-induced RPGN where it has been shown that there is little reward if treatment is delayed till oliguria has occurred. In ANCA-associated RPGN long-term treatment is indicated since relapses are frequent. The length of active treatment for the other types of RPGN remains contentious.

It is hoped that better understanding of the pathogenesis of RPGN will lead to more specific therapies in the near future.

MANAGEMENT OF NEPHROTIC SYNDROME

When the nephrotic state is likely to be persistent, important aspects of management arise. These include non-specific measures to reduce the proteinuria (see above), control of hyperlipidaemia and oedema, dietary aspects and monitoring for the development of vitamin D and iron deficiency.

Dietary management

Increasing the oral intake of protein in order to increase the serum albumin is not successful in practice. Likewise the intravenous administration of albumin to correct the serum albumin level is of temporary benefit only, for the administered albumin is largely lost into the urine within a few hours. In keeping with advice in all forms of persistent renal disease it is considered advisable to avoid excesses of dietary protein (particularly animal in origin). Thus in the persistent nephrotic state dietary protein intake should be at normal levels (e.g. 1–1.25 g/kg/day).

Control of hyperlipidaemia

The characteristic increase in serum cholesterol and the high ratio of low density lipoprotein to high-density lipoprotein seen in the persistent nephrotic state is assumed to be associated with accelerated atherosclerosis. Dietary measures to restrict cholesterol intake are not effective and most of the drugs available until recently were poorly tolerated, ineffective and had an increased rate of side effects when used in the nephrotic state. The role of simvastatin and lovastatin in managing the hyperlipidaemia of the nephrotic state is still being defined. The efficacy of these agents has been established but the risk, particularly of myositis and myopathy, has not. When hypercholesterolaemia is severe it seems reasonable to use these agents with careful monitoring of side effects. The muscle side effects are reversible when detected early.

Vitamin D and iron deficiency

The urinary loss of vitamin D and transferrin in the persistent nephrotic syndrome can result in vitamin D and iron deficiency respectively. Should this be suspected, appropriate replacement therapy is usually successful.

Hypercoagulable state

Various markers of hypercoagulability are found in the nephrotic state and are believed to contribute to the occurrence of renal vein thrombosis which is sometimes seen in this condition and has indeed been suspected to be a cause rather than a complication. Oral anticoagulation is not indicated in the nephrotic state unless thrombotic events have occurred.

FURTHER READING

Cameron J S 1990 How can we treat glomerulonephritis? Nephrology Dialysis Transplantation (suppl 1):16–22
Cameron J S 1992 Membranous nephropathy and its treatment. Nephrology Dialysis Transplantation (in press)
Donadio J V Jr 1990 Treatment of glomerulonephritis in the elderly. American Journal Kidney Disease 16: 307–311
El Nahas A M 1989 Glomerulosclerosis: Insights into pathogenesis and treatment. Nephrology Dialysis Transplantation 4: 843–853

Falk R J, Charles Jennete J 1991 The third international workshop on antineutrophil cytoplasmic autoantibodies. American Journal Kidney Disease 28: 145–147
Haycock G B 1988 The treatment of glomerulonephritis in children. Pediatric Nephrology 2: 247–255
Ponticelli C, Fogazzi G B 1989 Methylprednisolone pulse therapy for primary glomerulonephritis. American Journal of Nephrology 9 (suppl 1): 41–46

11. Miscellaneous glomerular diseases

A. R. Clarkson   A. J. Woodroffe   A. C. Thomas

DIABETES MELLITUS

In recent years diabetic nephropathy has become an increasingly important cause of end-stage renal failure. Retinopathy, neuropathy and vascular disease usually accompany the renal lesion and complicate management. Small vessel disease (microangiopathy), which is the basis of pathological changes, develops in the majority of long-term diabetes but the clinical expression varies in individual patients. Renal failure causes death in up to 40% of diabetics, being 17 times more common than in non-diabetics. The incidence of diabetes mellitus varies from 5–30% in the community, higher incidence frequently being found in ethnic groups emerging from a primitive background and embracing western lifestyles. The vast potential pool of patients with diabetic nephropathy thus is a challenge to the planners of end-stage renal failure programmes and a stimulus to researchers charged with developing better understanding and treatment of the basic disease. Over the past 20 years the natural history of diabetic nephropathy has been clarified, and experience with life extension programmes (dialysis and transplantation) has demonstrated that effective rehabilitation can be achieved. It is clear now that the development of uraemia in a diabetic subject does not signal inevitable death and current outlooks are far more positive than 20 years ago.

Diabetic glomerulosclerosis

Insulin-dependent (type I) diabetics develop progressive thickening of glomerular capillary basement membrane (Fig. 11.1b), widening of mesangium by PAS-positive material (Fig. 11.2), narrowing of glomerular capillaries and focal and global sclerotic lesions (Fig. 11.2). Severity of change, in general, is dependent upon length of time since onset of diabetes. This is not necessarily the case in non-insulin-dependent diabetes mellitus (type II) where advanced pathological changes may be found at the time of diagnosis. In both, however, distinctive changes, fibrin caps, capsular drops and gross hyalinization of arterioles, together with the non-specific but characteristic linear immunofluorescence along glomerular capillary walls for IgG and albumin (Fig. 11.3), serve to facilitate diagnosis. Interstitial scarring, tubular dropout and infiltration in the interstitium of mononuclear cells accompany glomerulosclerosis and reflect progressive renal damage more accurately.

Studies early in the course of diabetes mellitus, both in man and in streptozotocin-induced diabetes in animals, demonstrate increased kidney size, glomerular diameter, tubular size and filtration surface area. As glomerulosclerosis progresses, the kidneys contract. These pathological changes reflect alteration in function throughout the course of the disease.

Functional changes

Proteinuria after exercise is seen early in diabetic patients but usually disappears when good blood glucose control is achieved. Continuous or persistent proteinuria is not usually found until 10–15 years later but may be preceded by several years of microalbuminuria, increased excretion of β_2-microglobulin and elevated glomerular filtration

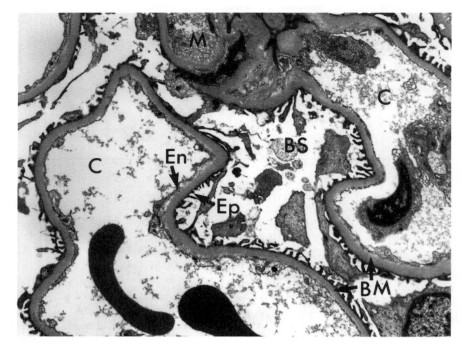

Fig. 11.1a

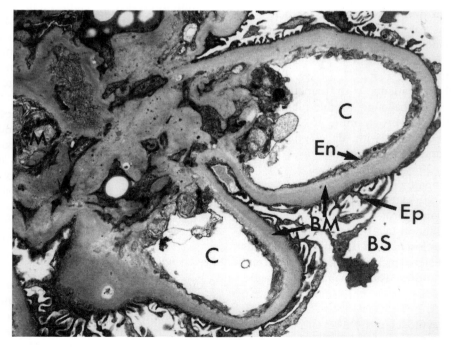

Fig. 11.1b

Fig. 11.1a–b   Electron micrographs of glomerular basement membranes demonstrating alterations of membrane thickness: (**a**) normal; (**b**) diabetic.

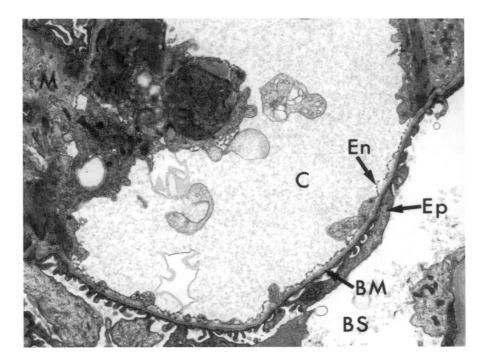

Fig. 11.1c Thin membrane nephropathy. The normal basement membrane thickness is in the order of 350–430 nm. The diabetic glomerulus illustrated has a basement membrane thickness of around 1000 nm whilst in the thin membrane nephropathy illustrated it is around 220 nm. BM — basement membrane, C — capillary lumen, Ep — visceral epithelium, En — endothelium, M — mesangium, BS — Bowman's space. (× 4900)

rate. Various factors have been proposed to account for these changes including hyperfiltration, systemic and glomerular hypertension, hyperlipidaemia, abnormal hypercoagulability and metabolic changes in the basement membrane. It is likely that each plays a part and contributes variably to the development and progression of diabetic glomerulosclerosis. Once proteinuria is established prognosis is poor as hypertension, nephrotic syndrome and renal impairment ensue at a rate variable from one diabetic to another but constant in individuals.

Natural history and complications

The typical development of diabetic nephropathy, as shown in Table 11.1, may be punctuated, altered or complicated by urinary tract infections, neuropathic changes in the bladder causing ob-struction and incomplete emptying, papillary ne-crosis, degenerative arterial changes leading to renal artery stenosis resulting in accelerated hyper-tension or atheroembolic renal disease, and increased susceptibility to toxins such as radio-paque contrast materials, antibiotics and diuretics.

The ill-defined nature and older age at onset of type II diabetes make predictability of natural history more difficult.

Treatment (Table 11.1)

The ideal treatment of diabetic nephropathy begins at the onset of diabetes with education, cessation of smoking, optimal control of blood glucose by insulin or diet and coordination of speciality consultants such as diabetologist, neph-rologist, ophthalmologist, podiatrist, vascular surgeon and dietician. Such multidisciplinary

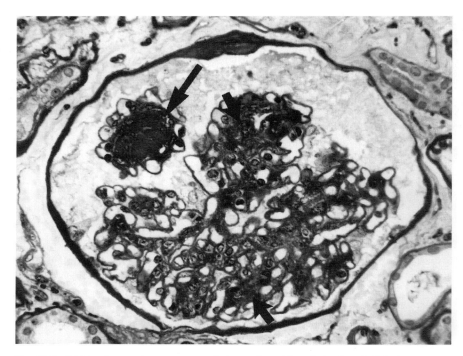

Fig. 11.2 Light microscopic appearance of glomerulus with well-developed diabetic glomerulosclerosis. There is both diffuse glomerulosclerosis (small arrows) and nodular glomerulosclerosis or Kimmelstiel–Wilson lesion (large arrow) with PAS-positive material expanding the mesangia and forming discrete segmental nodules. Note also narrowing of some of the glomerular capillary lumina and thickening of capillary loop walls, Bowman's capsule and adjacent tubular basement membranes. (PAS × 350)

Table 11.1 Natural history and therapy of diabetic nephropathy

Stage	GFR	Treatments
Early (silent)	Normal	Euglycaemia (insulin, diet). Stop smoking.
Microalbuminuria	Increased	Control hypertension (Ace inhibition).
Fixed proteinuria (albuminuria)	Increased to normal	Control hypertension, hyperlipidaemia. (Ace inhibition) Treat retinopathy. ? Pancreatic transplantation.
Nephrotic syndrome	Normal to low	Control oedema, salt restriction.
Renal failure	Low	Protein restriction. Dialysis access.
End-stage renal failure	Zero	CAPD. Haemodialysis. Transplantation: renal, pancreatic

management should be continued life-long, with emphasis in management shifting from one specialist to another as complications develop. Treatment of diabetic nephropathy should ideally be introduced when microalbuminuria develops and glomerular filtration rate is elevated. Angiotensin-converting enzyme inhibitors reverse these features as well as controlling hypertension. In addition these drugs reduce proteinuria once established and potentially retard the progression of diabetic nephropathy. Control of hypertension may require further agents such as calcium channel blocking drugs. Dietary protein restriction and low fat diets should be introduced judiciously and consideration given to using HMGCoA reductase inhibitors and other lipid lowering agents. As renal failure worsens, the range of options in end-stage renal failure treatment should

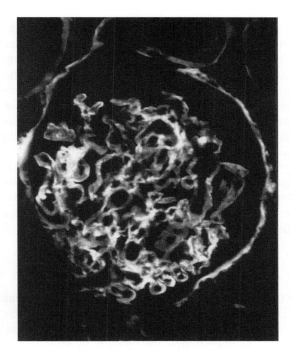

Fig. 11.3 Immunofluorescence of diabetic glomerulus demonstrating non-specific linear staining for anti-human IgG along glomerular capillary walls, Bowman's capsule and adjacent tubular basement membranes. Similar staining may also be seen with antibodies against albumin. (Anti-human IgG × 280)

be discussed fully with the patient while every effort is made to avoid and treat complications such as infections, retinopathy, and coronary, cerebral and peripheral vascular disease.

Renal transplantation alone does not preclude the continuing need for insulin therapy. For this reason combined renal and pancreatic transplantation has recently been introduced. Early results are sufficiently encouraging to suggest continued support of this strategy and further development of islet-cell transplantation even though reversal of retinopathy, neuropathy and vascular disease is not yet observed.

Maintenance of good eyesight is of paramount importance as visual impairment compounds the difficulties of dialysis treatment.

Management of end-stage renal failure

In general, renal replacement therapy in diabetics should be introduced at an earlier stage of renal impairment than in non-diabetics to avoid serious visual, cardiac and neuropathic complications detracting from the efficacy of treatment. Of the dialysis modalities available CAPD has proved popular with diabetics because of the continuous nature of the treatment, better blood glucose control with insulin given intraperitoneally at the time of dialysate infusion, and maintenance of a higher level of haemoglobin. On the other hand, haemodialysis is effective provided that vascular access is satisfactory, ocular haemorrhage is avoided (dialysis anticoagulation must be controlled rigorously) and cardiac function is sufficient to withstand the extracorporeal circulation. Infection complicates both forms of dialysis more frequently in diabetics than in others and must be treated vigorously.

Renal transplantation is a viable form of treatment for end-stage renal failure in diabetics and is capable of restoring normal renal function. Patient and graft survivals are shorter than in those with other renal disease, the increased incidence of infection, progressive vascular disease and development of diabetic nephropathy in the graft accounting for the poorer results.

HEREDITARY GLOMERULAR DISEASES

Thin membrane nephropathy (benign familial haematuria)

This condition is extremely common in the Australian community, being found in 15–20% of renal biopsies from patients with primary glomerular disease. Haematuria is usually microscopic but occasional patients develop macroscopic blood loss in association with an upper respiratory infection. As its name implies, the condition is benign, the haematuria persists life-long without evidence of renal impairment, and it is familial — the inheritance being autosomal dominant. Important facets of investigation include microscopy of the urine, which reveals dysmorphic red cells (their finding precludes the need for expensive and unnecessary urological investigations), and the taking of a full family history. Renal biopsy, which is required in only one member of a kindred, demonstrates characteristic electron microscopic appearances of glomerular basement membrane thinning (Fig. 11.1c). Blood leaks probably occur through small breaks in the basement membrane. Immunofluorescence is negative, but light microscopy reveals subtle increases in the size of mesangial and juxtaglomerular regions.

Thin membrane nephropathy is an important diagnosis to confirm as life insurance, superannuation and other benefits may not be offered without it. Moreover other more sinister causes of persistent microscopic haematuria such as IgA nephropathy, Alport syndrome and uroepithelial malignancy require exclusion.

Alport syndrome

The classic features include neurosensory deafness and nephritis. Clinically and pathologically similar hereditary nephritis is often found in kindreds with no extra-renal manifestations while others may have ocular defects such as anterior lenticonus (bulging of the anterior surface of the lens), macular lesions and cataracts in addition to deafness, or a platelet defect characterized by macrothrombocytopathic thrombocytopenia. It is considered appropriate to link all forms under the embracing term Alport syndrome. The inheritance is dominant with variable penetrance. In some kindreds there is clear evidence of X-linkage while differing ages of onset of clinical features and variable occurrence of extra-renal pathology in others suggest that inheritance may not be through a single gene.

Pathology

Characteristic ultrastructural changes in the glomerular basement membrane occur in all cases (Fig. 11.4a). Even in juveniles presenting with microscopic haematuria and with a normal appearance of glomeruli under the light microscope, lamellation, splitting, thinning and inclusion 'granules' may be seen in the basement membrane under the electron microscope. This so-called 'basket-weave' appearance becomes more prominent as the disease progresses, as do light microscopic abnormalities.

Diffuse mesangial enlargement, focal and segmental glomerular sclerosis, periglomerular fibrosis, crescent formation, tubular atrophy, interstitial fibrosis, vascular changes and the presence of interstitial foam cells denote advancing disease. Immunofluorescence studies are negative or demonstrate non-specific accumulation of IgM, C3 and other proteins in sclerotic lesions.

Abnormalities similar to those occurring in the glomerular basement membrane are found in the basement membrane of the stria vascularis of the cochlea and the basement membrane that forms the anterior lens capsule.

Clinical features

Haematuria is the cardinal feature, being present from birth in most cases. Usually detected only by dip-stix urinalysis or microscopy, it may become gross or macroscopic in relation to intercurrent illnesses such as sore throats or childhood exanthemata. Dysmorphic red cells and casts are seen in the urinary sediment.

Proteinuria is minimal in early cases but increases as the disease advances and may reach nephrotic ranges. Heavy proteinuria is indicative of a poor prognosis. Renal impairment may be absent for years but once apparent progresses to end-stage renal failure within a few years. It seems that renal failure is inevitable in males (often in the second and third decades of life), but in females it occurs variably and at a much later age.

Treatment

No specific treatment affects the underlying pathological process. Hypertension control and protein restriction are the cornerstones of therapy for advancing renal failure. Dialysis is usually uncomplicated but occasional patients have developed antiglomerular basement membrane (GBM) glomerulonephritis in their renal transplant due to the development of antibodies against GBM antigens not present in their native kidneys.

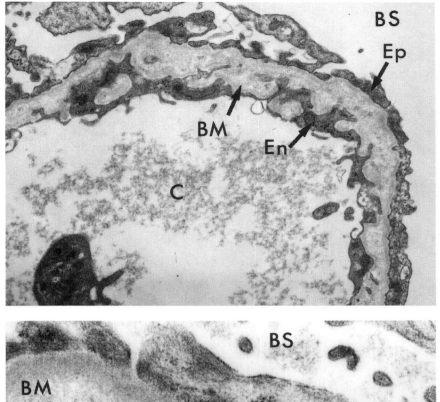

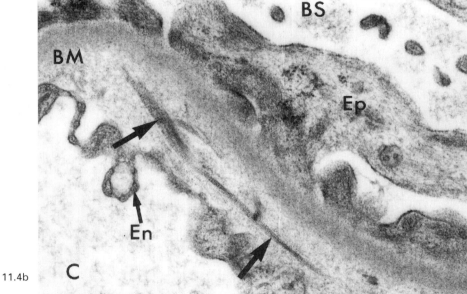

Fig. 11.4a, b Electron micrographs of glomerular basement membranes demonstrating alterations in ultrastructural appearance. **(a)** Alport syndrome. There is marked irregularity of the basement membrane thickness with splitting into multiple interweaving lamellae enclosing electron-lucent areas ('basket-weave' appearance). Electron-dense granules approximately 500 Å may also be seen within the basement membrane. ($\times 6500$). **(b)** Nail–patella syndrome. There is thickening of the basement membrane with electron-lucent areas. Fibrils with the periodicity of collagen (arrows) may be seen within the lucent areas, subendothelial space and mesangium. In some cases, similar fibrils may also be seen in the interstitial space adjacent to tubular basement membranes. ($\times 35\,000$). BM — basement membrane, Ep — visceral epithelium, En — endothelium, C — capillary lumen, BS — Bowman's space.

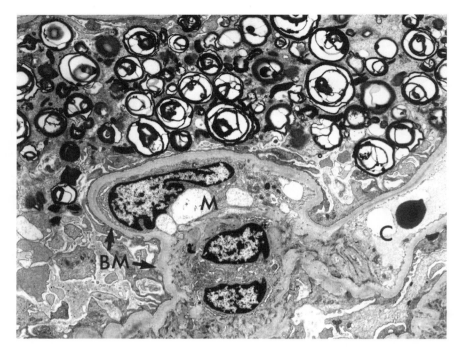

Fig. 11.5 Electron micrograph demonstrating ovoid or round bodies of concentric osmophilic lamellae ('myelin bodies') within a glomerular visceral epithelial cell in Fabry's disease. In some cases, similar bodies may also be found in glomerular endothelial cells, mesangial cells, tubular epithelium and endothelial and smooth muscle cells of small arteries. C — capillary lumen, M — mesangium, BM — basement membrane. (× 4000).

Fabry's disease

This uncommon condition, angiokeratoma corporis diffusum universale, results from deficiency of the enzyme α-galactosidase. This defect leads to tissue accumulation of the neutral glycosphingolipids cerebroside dihexoside and cerebroside trihexoside. The inheritance is X-linked so that hemizygous males are severely affected while heterozygous females are often asymptomatic, sometimes have a mild form of the disease and rarely are severely afflicted.

Clinical manifestations are due to progressive accumulation of glycophospholipids in all tissues. Particularly prominent are mucous membrane and skin lesions (angiokeratomas) which consist of red papules in the mouth, lower abdomen, buttocks and pubic region, renal and cardiac involvement. Periodic episodes of severe pain due to involvement of dorsal root ganglia, fever and excessive sweating may also be observed.

Renal involvement causes slowly progressive renal impairment, but this is usually preceded by proteinuria, haematuria and hypertension. Renal biopsy is diagnostic. Lipid-laden glomerular visceral epithelial cells are seen on light microscopy and electron microscopy reveals dense osmophilic concentric laminated 'myelin bodies'. Similar abnormalities are found in tubular epithelial cells and endothelial cells of arterioles (Fig. 11.5). Fabry's disease usually causes death from renal failure or cardiac involvement in the fourth or fifth decades.

Screening of family members for α-galactosidase deficiency in serum, peripheral leucocytes, hair follicles and biopsy specimens is advised and genetic counselling recommended. Detection of the carrier state by identification of two distinct clones of cells, one with normal, the other with deficient α-galactosidase activity, is usually performed by hair bulb analysis and is important in predicting the possibility of disease transmission.

Treatment is supportive. Dialysis is not contra-indicated and renal transplantation provides excellent relief of uraemic symptoms, although it does not replace the missing enzyme.

Nail–patella syndrome

This syndrome, hereditary onycho-osteodys-plasia, consists of dysplasia of the nails, multiple osseous abnormalities, particularly hypoplastic displaced patellae, metacarpal anomalies, de-formed elbows, iliac horns, scoliosis, scapular thickening and renal involvement. Nail–patella syndrome is an autosomal dominant trait and renal involvement results from a generalized disturbance in the synthesis of collagen. About 40% of patients develop proteinuria or haem-aturia but nephrotic syndrome and chronic renal failure are uncommon.

Light microscopic changes are non-specific, but ultrastructural changes are characteristic and occur within the glomerular basement membrane which is irregularly thickened. The membrane contains numerous lucent areas within which are electron-dense fibrils with the periodicity of collagen (Fig. 11.4b). Immunofluorescence is negative. Treat-ment is supportive and renal replacement therapy is not contraindicated.

DYSPROTEINAEMIAS (Table 11.2)

These are conditions in which there are abnormali-ties of immunoglobulin production with the appearance of 'paraproteins' in blood, urine or both, and frequently deposition of these proteins in the kidney. Clinical manifestations of renal involvement in these diseases include acute renal failure, proteinuria, nephrotic syndrome and end-stage renal failure from more chronic disease. A primary renal presentation is quite common, requiring that these conditions be considered in the above clinical settings and screened for by protein electrophoresis/immunofixation of blood and urine. Renal biopsy (with special stains) corrobo-rates the individual diagnosis and treatment is tailored accordingly.

Table 11.2 Dysproteinaemias

Multiple myeloma
Light-chain nephropathy
Waldenström's macroglobulinaemia
Cryoglobulinaemia
Amyloidosis
Fibrillary glomerulonephritis

Multiple myeloma

This is a disease characterized by proliferation of bone marrow plasma cells which results in a clone of B cells secreting a paraprotein. Such para-proteins, whether heavy or light chain immuno-globulins, are monoclonal and are identified by electrophoresis (this includes the detection of light chains in urine — previously by thermal solubility tests as 'Bence Jones protein'). IgG myeloma is more common than IgA (as is kappa than lambda) and IgD is rare, but probably often missed.

Renal involvement is multifactorial (Table 11.3).

Myeloma kidney

This histological designation refers to the extensive presence of large lamellated, eosino-philic tubular casts with interstitial inflammation (with or without giant cell reaction) and fibrosis (Fig. 11.6). The casts are composed of para-protein, Tamm–Horsfall protein and albumin. Clinical features are usually those of acute renal failure.

Light-chain nephropathy

Here there are dominant glomerular lesions, notably nodular glomerular sclerosis (Fig. 11.7), with linear glomerular capillary wall deposition of light chains (Fig. 11.8) and electron-dense depos-

Table 11.3 Renal involvement in multiple myeloma

'Myeloma kidney'
Light-chain nephropathy
Renal amyloidosis
Hypercalcaemia
Hyperuricaemia

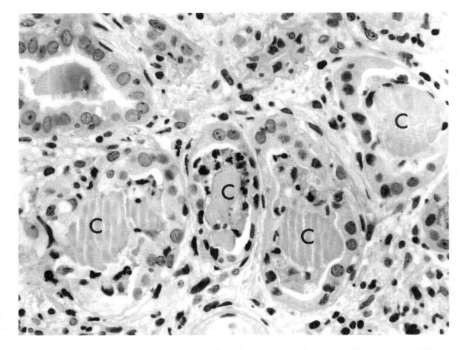

Fig. 11.6 Light microscopic appearance of myeloma cast nephropathy. Dense eosinophilic lamellated or fractured casts (C) can be seen surrounded by macrophagic cells and cellular debris within damaged and partially ruptured tubules. The interstitium shows a patchy inflammatory infiltrate and early fibrosis. (HE × 450)

its in the lamina rara interna of the glomerular basement membrane (Fig. 11.9). There are superficial similarities to diabetic nephropathy and to dense deposit disease but, when light immunofluorescence and electron microscopy are taken together, the lesions are specific. Clinical features are proteinuria, nephrotic syndrome and progressive renal failure.

Renal amyloid

This is less common in multiple myeloma than the above and will be discussed separately.

Hypercalcaemia

This is a very important factor in acute renal failure from multiple myeloma and one which usually can be controlled by hydration and the administration of corticosteroid drugs.

Hyperuricaemia

This complication frequently occurs soon after the introduction of chemotherapy and may hasten renal failure. Hydration, systemic alkalinization and allopurinol therapy are important preventative measures.

In the event of progression to end-stage renal failure, the issues of dialysis and transplantation will obviously be influenced by the presence of extra-renal disease (e.g. bone, bone marrow). With modern chemotherapy, and in the absence of significant extra-renal disease, such strategies should not necessarily be withheld.

Light-chain nephropathy

Only one third of these patients have overt myeloma. Clinical presentations are proteinuria, nephrotic syndrome and chronic renal failure. The light, immunofluorescence and electron micro-

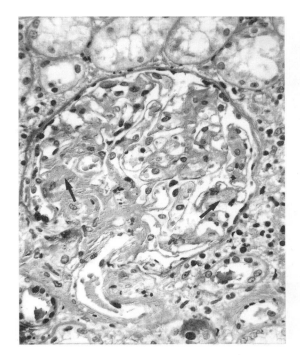

Fig. 11.7 Light microscopic appearance of glomerulus in a case of kappa light-chain nephropathy. The glomerulus is enlarged, with mesangial expansion by PAS-positive material leading to nodular glomeruloscerosis (arrows) which may be confused morphologically with diabetic glomerulosclerosis. Frequently, however, there are additional foci of mesangial interposition (see Fig. 11.9) which may superficially resemble a mesangiocapillary glomerulonephritis. (PAS × 280)

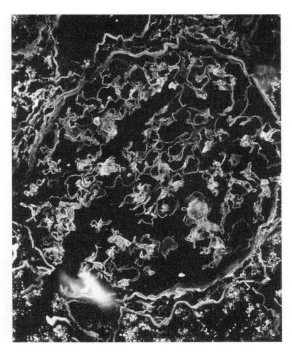

Fig. 11.8 Immunofluorescence of a glomerulus in kappa light-chain nephropathy demonstrating homogeneous staining of mesangial nodules and linear deposition of light chains along glomerular basement membranes. Focal staining of Bowman's capsule and adjacent tubular basement membranes is also present. (Anti-human kappa × 280)

scopic appearances have already been mentioned and illustrated (see Multiple myeloma). Importantly, the diagnosis will be missed unless anti-light-chain immunofluorescent reagents are used on all renal biopsies that show PAS-negative and Congo red-negative glomerular deposits. Clinical features are also subtle, often with no bone pathology or haematological abnormality to suggest myeloma. Results of plasma exchange and chemotherapy are inconclusive but these should not necessarily preclude supportive therapy, including chronic dialysis and transplantation.

Waldenström's macroglobulinaemia

This is caused by the production by large plasmacytoid cells of a monoclonal IgM which is responsible for hyperviscosity of the blood, hepatosplenomegaly, lymphadenopathy and frequently renal involvement. The latter is most often glomerular in nature, either with a mesangiocapillary lesion associated with large intracapillary deposits of IgM or with amyloidosis. Proteinuria and nephrotic syndrome occur but acute and progressive chronic renal failure are much less common than in multiple myeloma.

Cryoglobulinaemia (Table 11.4)

Cryoglobulins are immunoglobulins that precipitate in the cold. They are found in association with lymphoproliferative diseases, connective tissue diseases and liver disease, but in one third are 'essential', ('essential mixed cryoglobulinaemia'). Clinical manifestations are purpura, arthralgias, Raynaud's phenomenon, palpable vasculitis, proteinuria and nephrotic syndrome. The diagnosis is

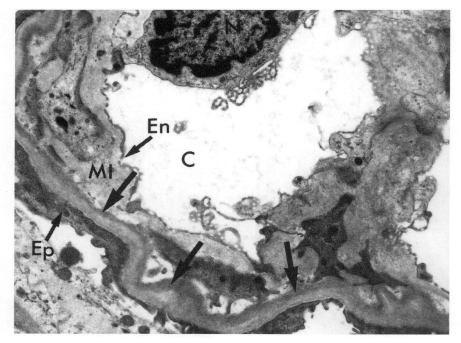

Fig. 11.9 Electron micrograph of glomerular capillary loop in kappa light-chain nephropathy. There is a band of electron-dense material representing kappa light chains within the lamina rara interna of the basement membrane (arrows). Similar material can be seen within the mesangium which is interposing itself between the fenestrated endothelial cytoplasm and basement membrane. C — capillary lumen, En — endothelium, N — endothelial cell nucleus, MI — mesangial interposition, Ep — visceral epithelium. (× 9000)

made by screening for and characterizing blood cryoglobulins. IgM rheumatoid factor is often positive and serum complement concentrations low. Some patients will be hepatitis B or C positive. Renal biopsy most frequently shows a mesangiocapillary pattern, often with huge deposits (IgM, IgG and C3 on immunofluorescence) which by electron microscopy appear 'crystalloid'.

Treatment strategies include immunosuppression and plasma exchange but the results are

Table 11.4 Cryoglobulinaemia

Type I Monoclonal	—	mainly myeloma proteins and macroglobulins
Type II Mixed	—	e.g. monoclonal IgM anti-IgG
Type III two or more polyclonal	—	e.g. polyclonal IgM anti-IgG

inconclusive. Prognosis is guarded; the condition tends to undergo remissions and exacerbations but decline may occur due to infection, renal involvement and the underlying disorder.

Amyloidosis

Two major clinicopathological groups of amyloidosis exist — the deposited fibrils in one group consist mostly of light chains (AL) and in the other mostly of 'protein A' (AA) (Table 11.5). Renal involvement occurs with both, usually as nephrotic syndrome with or without renal impairment. Postural hypotension and other features of autonomic neuropathy often are clues in the differential diagnosis. Renal biopsy findings are of PAS-negative, Congo red-positive mesangial deposits (Fig. 11.10). Similar deposits occur in and around blood vessels. In advanced cases amyloid

Table 11.5 Amyloidosis

Primary	AL
Multiple myeloma	AL
Secondary:	
(rheumatoid arthritis, chronic infection)	AA

deposits may obliterate the whole glomerulus. Little cellular proliferation occurs. Electron microscopy (Fig. 11.11) shows fibrils in a random distribution and arrangement, approximately 80–100 Å in diameter with a 50 Å periodicity. The fibrils spread from the mesangium to the subendothelium and through the glomerular basement membrane. The ultimate renal prognosis in primary amyloidosis is poor despite treatments such as melphalan and corticosteroids. However, dialysis and transplantation might still be clinically appropriate.

Fibrillary glomerulonephritis (immunotactoid nephropathy)

Mentioned in the context of the above conditions, this glomerular lesion is newly identified and caused by fibrillary deposits (230–400 Å in diameter) as seen by electron microscopy. These deposits are Congo red-negative. IgG deposits are present in the absence of paraproteins, cryoglobulins or systemic lupus erythematosus.

RHEUMATOID ARTHRITIS

Renal involvement in patients with rheumatoid arthritis can be due to many factors. Analgesic nephropathy and the adverse affects on the kidney of non-steroidal anti-inflammatory drugs are usually the immediate concern, but membranous nephropathy caused by treatment with gold salts or d-penicillamine may give rise to proteinuria and nephrotic syndrome. Amyloidosis and vasculitis also occur. Proteinuria in such patients requires that renal biopsy be performed to delineate the diagnosis as therapy varies according to the cause. Drug-induced membranous nephropathy usually resolves with cessation of the offending drug treatment. Amyloidosis secondary to rheumatoid arthritis

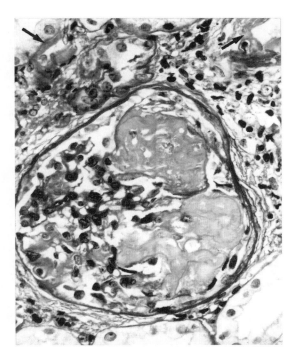

Fig. 11.10 Light microscopic appearance of a glomerulus in renal amyloidosis. Homogeneous, eosinophilic, PAS-negative and Congo red-positive deposits of amyloid have expanded the mesangium and led to nodule formation obliterating approximately half the glomerulus. Similar deposition may be seen in adjacent small blood vessels (arrows). (PAS × 400)

frequently has a much longer natural history than primary amyloidosis.

HEROIN NEPHROPATHY

A fairly specific pattern of glomerular lesions has been described in intravenous heroin users during the last decade. Nephrotic syndrome occurs often with advancing renal failure and hypertension, and this clinical presentation is associated with the finding of focal glomerulosclerotic lesions on renal biopsy. Immunofluorescence is positive for IgM and C3 and occurs independently from glomerular lesions associated with hepatitis B and HIV infections, which frequently complicate the heroin addiction. In addition, infective endocarditis and acute renal failure from rhabdomyolysis must also be considered when renal disease occurs in intravenous drug users.

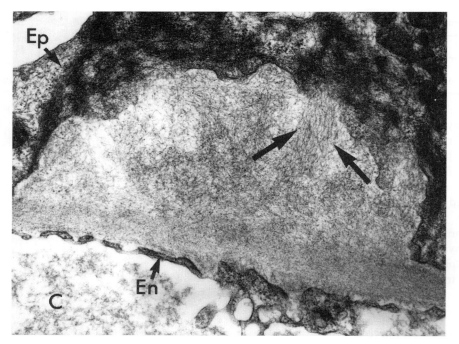

Fig. 11.11 Electron micrograph of glomerular basement membrane with characteristic amyloid fibrils diffusely permeating it and giving rise to a subepithelial deposit. Just beneath the epithelial cell cytoplasm, the amyloid fibrils tend to be orientated in a parallel arrangement (arrows) compared with the more random arrangement elsewhere. C — capillary lumen, Ep — visceral epithelium, En — endothelium. (× 24 000)

RENAL DISEASE IN HIV INFECTION

Initial clinical experience of renal disease in patients with AIDS was related to cryoglobulinaemia and the nephritis associated with hepatitis B infection and heroin abuse. However renal function was noted to deteriorate far more quickly in those patients with AIDS compared with non-AIDS patients with similar renal diseases. Experience is now larger and includes patients who were not drug abusers. In these a variety of immune complex-mediated glomerular changes have been identified. Mesangial, mesangiocapillary and diffuse proliferative glomerulonephritis with positive immunofluorescence for IgM and C3 and electron-dense deposits in mesangia and along capillary walls have been described. In addition, tubular ne-crosis, interstitial lesions and opportunistic infections of the kidney (e.g. cryptococcal abscesses) may be found. The need for multiple and potentially nephrotoxic antibiotics may contribute to the interstitial changes. Finally haemolytic uraemic syndrome has been described in AIDS patients with Kaposi's sarcoma.

Evidence for renal disease is found in approximately 50% of patients with AIDS. Proteinuria, nephrotic syndrome and varying degrees of renal failure are the commonest presentations. Supportive therapy is all that can be offered and dialysis may extend useful life. Initial transplant experience is poor as the added immunosuppression seemingly renders the already compromised patients more liable to develop infections and malignancies.

RECOMMENDED READING

Aarons I, Smith P S, Davies R A, Woodroffe A J, Clarkson
  A R 1989 Thin membrane nephropathy: a clinico-
  pathological study. Clinical Nephrology 32: 151
Cunningham E E, Brentjens J R, Zielezny M A 1980 Heroin
  nephropathy: a clinicopathologic and epidemologic study.
  American Journal of Medicine 68: 47
Gardenswartz M H, Lerner C W, Seligson G R 1984 Renal
  disease in patients with AIDS: a clinicopathological study.
  Clinical Nephrology 21: 197
Grunfeld J-P 1985 The clinical spectrum of hereditary
  nephritis. Kidney International 27: 83

Mogensen C E, Mauer S M, Kjellstrand C M 1988 Diabetic
  nephropathy. In: Schrier R W, Gottschalk C W (eds)
  Diseases of the kidney, 4th edn, Vol 3. Little Brown,
  Boston, Ch. 79, p. 2395
Vaamonde C A, Pardo V 1988 Multiple myeloma and
  amyloidosis. In: Schrier R W, Gottschalk C W (eds)
  Diseases of the kidney, 4th edn, Vol 3. Little Brown,
  Boston, Ch. 80, p. 2439

12. Tropical renal diseases

V. Sitprija

Nephropathies in the tropics are largely determined by the tropical environment. The hot climate, poor nutrition, shortage of health care in certain areas, cultural and social background and genetic variations are important predisposing factors. Tropical renal diseases therefore cover renal diseases exclusively seen in the tropics with unique characteristics as well as renal diseases seen worldwide but common in the tropical area. In the latter category the diseases may have a different natural history and presentation. The topic is thus broad and includes (Table 12.1):

1. Renal diseases caused by tropical infections
2. Renal diseases caused by toxins
3. Renal diseases due to metabolic and nutritional disorders
4. Renal disease caused by antimicrobial and chemical agents.

In this chapter emphasis will be placed on renal diseases caused by infections and toxins.

GENERAL PRINCIPLE

Clinical renal manifestations

Urinary sediment changes and proteinuria

A few erythrocytes and leucocytes in the urine are commonly seen in febrile diseases and mild proteinuria of less than 1 g per 24 hours is frequent. The proteinuria and abnormal urinary sediment disappear quickly when infection is under control. However, in occasional cases nephrotic range proteinuria can occur, but resolves when infection is treated.

Persistent glomerulonephritis and proteinuria have been noted in the diseases that run a chronic course, such as quartan malaria, viral hepatitis, leprosy, schistosomiasis and filariasis. Autoimmune mechanisms may play a contributing role and treatment of infection does not resolve the glomerulonephritis.

Haematuria

Gross haematuria or significant microscopic haematuria is seen commonly in viper snake bite. This is attributed to bleeding diathesis. Russell's viper venom activates factors X and V, while the venoms of green pit viper and malayan pit viper have thrombin-like action.

Haemoglobinuria

Intravascular haemolysis is common in tropical diseases. Viper venom can cause intravascular haemolysis through the activity of phospholipase A and the direct lytic factor. Bacterial haemolysin can induce haemolysis. The high incidence of glucose-6-phosphate dehydrogenase deficiency in the tropics makes erythrocytes susceptible to haemolysis during infection and certain drug therapy. Certain chemical agents such as naphthalene and copper sulphate and plant toxins can also cause haemolysis. Haemoglobinuria is common in the tropics and can contribute to the development of acute renal failure.

Myoglobinuria

Rhabdomyolysis is often noted in sea-snake bite and wasp, hornet and bee stings. Certain infectious

Table 12.1   Spectrum of tropical renal diseases

Tropical infections causing renal diseases
Bacterial infections
Leptospirosis
Melioidosis
Salmonellosis
Shigellosis
Cholera
Scrub typhus
Leprosy
Diphtheria
Clostridial infection
Parasitic infections
Malaria
Trichinosis
Filariasis
Toxoplasmosis
Schistosomiasis
Opisthorchiasis
Leishmaniasis
Ecchinococcosis
Viral infections
Viral hepatitis
Dengue haemorrhagic fever

Toxins causing renal diseases
Animal toxins
Snake bite
Insect stings
Centipede bite
Scorpion sting
Spider bite
Carp raw bile
Jelly fish sting
Plant toxins
Pithecolobium lobatum
Amanita phalloides
Galerina venenata
Vicis favus
Semecarpus anacardium
Callilepis laureola
Securicada longipedunculata
Euphorbia matabelensis
Crotalaria laburnifolia

Metabolic and nutritional disorders causing renal diseases
Renal stone disease
Renal tubular acidosis
Hypokalaemic periodic paralysis

Antimicrobial and chemical agents causing renal diseases
Aminoglycosides
Cephalosporin
Sulpha drugs
Paraquat
Non-steroidal anti-inflammatory drugs
Copper sulphate
Naphthalene
Carbon tetrachloride

diseases affecting muscles such as trichinosis and leptospirosis can cause rhabdomyolysis, and any condition that induces ischaemia of the muscles can also cause rhabdomyolysis and myoglobinuria. Therefore, myoglobinuria may be observed in infectious diseases which compromise microcirculation resulting in muscular ischaemia. Hypokalaemia, hypophosphataemia, alcohol, heroin addiction and viral diseases are uncommon causes of rhabdomyolysis.

Electrolyte changes

Hyponatraemia is observed in 67% of patients with febrile illness. Both delayed and brisk responses to water load have been observed in febrile diseases.

Hypernatraemia due to water deficit may be observed in the patient with loss of consciousness. Diabetes insipidus is rare.

Hypokalaemia is not uncommon in febrile illness, and this is attributed to respiratory alkalosis. Interestingly, kaliuresis can be of significant degree in the icteric type of leptospirosis and in obstructive jaundice and could account for hypokalaemia despite renal failure. Hypokalaemia may also be observed in severe diarrhoea, especially in cholera.

Hyperkalaemia is seen in association with intravascular haemolysis, rhabdomyolysis and renal failure. It may be severe enough to need treatment.

Hypocalcaemia and hypophosphataemia may be observed in severe sepsis and malaria with heavy parasitaemia. The causes of hypocalcaemia are multiple. Respiratory alkalosis could be responsible for hypophosphataemia.

Acute renal failure

Tropical acute renal failure is usually characterized by hypercatabolism with rapid rises in blood urea and serum creatinine. Hyperuricaemia and hyperphosphataemia may be noted. The blood urea and serum creatinine ratio often rises except in the patients with rhabdomyolysis in whom the ratio may be lower. Jaundice is frequently present. It is cholestatic in type with only mild elevation of liver enzymes but with high levels of serum alkaline phosphatase. Intravascular coagulation and intravascular haemolysis may be present in severe infection or in animal toxin poisoning. The duration of renal failure averages 2 weeks, but may be from a few days to several weeks. Non-oliguric renal failure is not uncommon. Renal failure is reversible except for those with cortical necrosis.

Treatment

Treatment of the basic tropical disease should be instituted. Persistent glomerulonephritis may require corticosteroid and perhaps immunosuppressive therapy, but the results vary.

For management of renal failure the scheme of treatment does not differ from that given for renal failure due to the other causes. Hypercatabolism dialysis, when indicated, should be performed frequently. Haemodialysis is preferred to peritoneal dialysis, but, in the developing countries with a poor socioeconomy, peritoneal dialysis is still used because of convenience. Fortunately, control of infection improves solute transport.

Exchange blood transfusion is useful in the patient with falciparum malaria with heavy parasitaemia. Severe jaundice with total serum bilirubin over 425 μmol/l can compromise renal function and should be handled by either exchange blood transfusion or plasmapheresis. Decrease in jaundice has been reported to improve renal function. Exchange blood transfusion has also been used in renal failure due to heat stroke and severe poisoning due to toxins or venoms.

Renal pathology

Pathological changes are seen in every structure of the kidney.

Vascular changes

Hyaline deposition in the glomerular afferent arteriole may be observed in tropical infection. By immunofluorescence there is C3 deposition in the afferent arterioles; the clinical significance is not understood.

Arteritis and thrombophlebitis of the interlobular artery and vein may be seen in viper bite. C3 deposition without immunoglobulin is demonstrated in the vascular wall. Arteritis indicates severe envenomation, and when associated with tubular necrosis can cause severe and prolonged renal failure.

Peritubular capillaries are engorged with erythrocytes and mononuclear cells. This finding is present in severe infection, especially in falciparum malaria and septicaemia, and could be important in the pathogenesis of renal failure

Glomerular changes

Various types of glomerular lesions are seen. Mesangial proliferative glomerulonephritis is common in acute tropical diseases. Granular deposition of IgM and C3 is usually observed in the mesangial area and the glomerular capillary wall. Except for occasional cases of nephritic and nephrotic syndrome, in most cases glomerulonephritis is mild and transient.

In snake bite mesangiolysis and membranolysis suggestive of direct nephrotoxicity have been observed. Diffuse proliferative glomerulonephritis without deposition of immunoglobulins and complement presenting with nephritic syndrome has been described in green pit viper bite. Extracapillary proliferative glomerulonephritis has been reported in Russell's viper bite.

Membranous glomerulonephritis and membranoproliferative glomerulonephritis have been found in chronic infections such as viral hepatitis, leprosy and schistosomiasis.

Tubulointerstitial changes

Tubular necrosis is present in the majority of patients with acute renal failure. Interstitial changes characterized by oedema and mononuclear cell infiltration are common, especially in severe tubular necrosis. Tubular necrosis with marked interstitial changes may present with renal failure of prolonged clinical course. However, interstitial changes alone can be seen in leptospirosis without tubular necrosis and with normal renal function. Interstitial nephritis has been described in scrub typhus, leprosy, viral infections and snake bite.

Cortical necrosis

Cortical necrosis can be observed in association with disseminated intravascular coagulation in infectious diseases and toxin poisoning. Shigellosis is a common infectious cause, and may present with the haemolytic uraemic syndrome. In the toxin group viper bite can cause cortical necrosis. Russell's viper envenomation is a well-known cause of cortical necrosis in India. Certain plant toxins, such as the sap of the marking nut tree (*Semecarpus anacardium*), have been reported to cause renal failure and cortical necrosis.

Other pathological changes

Other renal changes include papillary necrosis, abscess and amyloidosis. Papillary necrosis is usually associated with obstructive uropathy with severe infection or diabetes mellitus. Renal abscess is common in the septicaemic form of melioidosis. Amyloidosis is seen in leprosy and schistosomiasis.

Pathogenesis of renal changes

Three mechanisms are involved in the pathogenesis of renal lesions: immunological reactions, non-specific effects of inflammation and direct nephrotoxicity (Table 12.2).

Table 12.2 Pathogenesis of renal lesions in tropical diseases

1. Immunological mechanisms
    Immune complex-mediated
    Cell-mediated
2. Non-specific inflammatory effects
    Mediators and cytokines
    Free oxygen radicals
    Complement activation
    Hypovolaemia
    Hypotension
    Haemorrheological changes
    Pigmenturia
    Intravascular coagulation
    Cardiac dysfunction
    Jaundice
    Hyperthermia
3. Direct nephrotoxicity
    Bacterial invasion
    Parasitic migration
    Toxins
    Chemical agents

1. Immunological reactions

Evidence of immune mechanism is reflected by the presence of circulating immune complexes in the plasma, the decrease in serum compliment and the deposition of immune complexes in the renal tissue, in various infectious diseases. Mesangial proliferation glomerulonephritis in infection is an example of immune complex glomerulonephritis. Corresponding antigens are demonstrable in the glomeruli. In some models this is evidence of implanted antigen or immune complex in situ.

As in the other forms of glomerulonephritis cell-mediated immune responses are important in the pathogenesis of glomerular lesions in tropical disease, and particularly in interstitial nephritis. The granulomatous lesion of the lower urinary tract in *S. haematobium* infection is also cell-mediated. In addition, alteration in T cell function may perpetuate infection. In severe malaria, defect in natural killer cells through decreased interleukin 2 could impair eradication of malarial parasites and favour secondary infection leading to renal dysfunction.

The immediate type of hypersensitivity reaction plays an important role in the pathogenesis of lesions due to parasitic migration such as visceral larva migrans and filarial infection.

2. Non-specific inflammatory effects

Several factors in the inflammatory process can interfere with microcirculation of the kidney and cause renal injury. Various chemical mediators are released during inflammation: these substances include prostaglandins, thromboxane A_2, kinins, leukotrienes, angiotensin, endorphin, endothelin, endothelium-derived relaxing factor (EDRF), serotonin, histamine, adenosine, catecholamines, atrial natriuretic peptides (ANP) and platelet-activating factor (PAF). It is obvious that these mediators have two opposing effects — vasoconstriction and vasodilatation. Yet the net effect on renal haemodynamics is usually renal vasoconstriction with ischaemia. In addition, cytokines released can have further adverse effects on renal haemodynamics. Tumour necrosis factor (TNF), interleukins (IL), myocardium depressant factor and various growth factors are among those under extensive study. TNF, platelet-derived growth factor (PDGF) and IL are involved in several inflammatory diseases. TNF injection can result in the clinical picture resembling endotoxin shock. Oxygen radical generation in the inflammatory process and the reflow is an additional insult to the renal injury.

At the clinical level there are several risk factors that contribute to the development of renal injury.

2.1 Hypovolaemia. Hypovolaemia is common in severe tropical diseases. It can result from decreased fluid intake or increased fluid loss through skin, urine, respiratory and gastrointestinal tracts, or a combination of both. In viper bite bleeding can contribute significantly to hypovolaemia. Increased vascular permeability due to mediators with fluid shift from intravascular to interstitial space occurs. Dengue haemorrhagic fever, anthrax, falciparum malaria and leptospirosis are among the known diseases that cause hypovolaemia.

2.2 Hypotension. Hypotension can be the result of hypovolaemia or vasodilatation. Systemic vasodilatation with renal vasoconstriction can occur in sepsis and snake envenomation. Wasp, hornet and bee stings and snake bite often cause hypotension which may be sufficient to induce renal failure.

2.3 Haemorrheological change. In acute infections there is an increase in acute phase proteins in the plasma. Plasma fibrinogen can rise significantly and erythrocyte viscosity is also increased in intraerythrocytic parasitic infection such as malaria and babesiosis. The rise in blood viscosity and rouleaux formation can interfere with the renal microcirculation. Cytoadherence between parasitized erythrocytes and the vascular endothelium in malaria can also compromise the microcirculation. Cytoadherence of leucocytes to the vascular endothelium also occurs in inflammation through the effects of cytokines, further decreasing the renal blood flow.

2.4 Pigmenturia. Intravascular haemolysis and rhabdomyolysis are common in tropical disease, and haemoglobinuria or myoglobinuria can cause renal failure by decreasing renal blood flow, direct tubulotoxicity and tubular obstruction.

2.5 Intravascular coagulation. Intravascular coagulation can be induced by sepsis and animal toxins but in most infectious diseases it is of low grade and local.

2.6 Cardiac dysfunction. Decreased cardiac function may be observed in certain infectious diseases which involve myocardium, such as typhoid fever, leptospirosis and diphtheria, and in severe sepsis. Renal blood flow can thus be compromised.

2.7 Jaundice. Severe jaundice is one of the risk factors for the development of acute renal failure, especially when the total serum bilirubin exceeds 425 μm/l.

2.8 Hyperthermia. It would require a very high temperature, at the level of 42°C, to cause direct renal injury through complement activation and oxygen radical release. Although fevers of 42°C are not common it is possible that a combination of high fever and other non-specific factors may induce renal injury.

These factors are non-specific and can be shared by several inflammatory diseases. In most cases of renal injury the causes are multiple. Therefore, severe infection of any aetiology can cause acute renal failure.

3. Direct nephrotoxicity

Direct toxicity to the kidney has been shown in several models, including bacteria, parasites and toxins. In bacterial infection leptospirosis is a good example. Leptospires penetrate the skin and gain access via the circulation to various organs. In the kidney they produce mild glomerulonephritis within a few hours. Bacterial penetration through the peritubular capillaries causes interstitial nephritis. This occurs before invasion to the renal tubules to cause tubular necrosis. Renal changes therefore consist of glomerulonephritis, interstitial nephritis and tubular necrosis.

In the parasitic model parasites can migrate to the kidney and cause renal lesions through cellular reactions. These reactions include cellular proliferation, infiltration and cystic and granulomatous changes around the parasites. The model is exemplified in ecchinococcosis, with ecchinococcal cysts of the kidney, and in filariasis.

In the toxin model viper venoms, especially Russell's viper venom and green pit viper venom, are vasculotoxic and capable of causing vasculitis and glomerulonephritis. Russell's viper venom is also tubulotoxic. A number of plants are toxic to the kidney; many exert nephrotoxicity indirectly through the non-specific inflammatory effects but a few are directly nephrotoxic. Direct toxicity has been reported in the ingestion of djenkol bean (*Pithecolobium lobatum*).

COMMON TROPICAL RENAL DISEASES

Nephropathy in falciparum malaria

Renal changes in falciparum malaria vary from mild glomerulonephritis to tubular necrosis.

Glomerulonephritis

Glomerular changes are usually mild and consist of hypertrophy or proliferation of mesangial cells. Pigment carrying mononuclear cells may be seen in the mesangial area. There is granular deposition of IgM and C3 in the mesangial area and along the luminal side of glomerular capillaries. Granular deposition of malarial antigen is demonstrable in the mesangial region and the capillary wall. The findings are consistent with immune complex glomerulonephritis. Fibrin deposition may be seen occasionally in the paramesangial areas. Electron microscopy shows paramesangial and subendothelial deposits. These changes are transient and disappear within a few weeks. They are responsible for mild proteinuria and abnormal urinary sediment. In occasional cases nephrotic range proteinuria may be present but resolves completely when malaria is treated. Reversible nephritic syndrome has also been described.

Tubular necrosis

Tubular necrosis with or without tubulorrhexis is present in the patient with renal failure. Severe lesions appear in distal and collecting tubules. Necrotic tubules usually contain granular and amorphous casts containing haemoglobin. There is dilatation of the proximal tubules and interstitial oedema and mononuclear cell infiltration. Dilated peritubular capillaries congested with erythrocytes, malarial pigment-laden macrophages and mononuclear cells are found early in the disease.

Non-specific inflammatory effects previously mentioned are involved in the pathogenesis of tubular necrosis in malaria. These factors include hypovolaemia, blood hyperviscosity, catecholamine effects, intravascular haemolysis, intravascular coagulation and jaundice. Adherence of the knobs of infected erythrocytes to the vascular endothelium receptor protein thrombospondin and interadherence among erythrocytes interfere with renal microcirculation. There is also adherence of leucocytes to the vascular endothelium and TNF is believed to play an important role in the symptomatology of malaria and endotoxaemia.

Falciparum malaria is a common cause of acute renal failure in the tropics. The patient usually has high fever and heavy parasitaemia or intravascular haemolysis. There may be alteration of consciousness. Renal failure is often associated with cholestatic jaundice with marked elevation of serum alkaline phosphatase but mild elevation of liver enzymes. Intravascular haemolysis may be present in the patient with glucose-6-phosphate dehydrogenase deficiency. Blackwater fever is probably related to this enzyme deficiency. Myoglobinuria may be observed. Renal failure is hypercatabolic with rapid rises of blood urea and creatinine. Hyperuricaemia occurs, and hyperkalaemia may be alarming when associated with intravascular haemolysis. Non-oliguric renal failure is not uncommon. The duration of renal failure averages 2 weeks, with a range from a few days to several weeks. The prognosis is grave when associated with multiple organ involvement, especially when there is acute respiratory distress syndrome.

Treatment is focussed on malaria. Quinine is the drug of choice. The dose need not be altered except in severe renal failure. Due to hypercatabolism dialysis, when indicated, should be performed frequently. Haemodialysis is preferred to peritoneal dialysis since solute transport through the peritoneal membrane is compromised by impaired microcirculation in malaria but because of the ease of the procedure peritoneal dialysis is often used and solute transport is improved when malaria is treated. Exchange blood transfusion is useful in decreasing parasites when there is heavy parasitaemia or severe hyperbilirubinaemia. In less severe forms of renal failure with serum creatinine lower then 0.5 mmol/l a combination of frusemide and dopamine has been shown to attenuate the progression of renal failure.

More important is the prevention of renal failure in the patient with heavy parasitaemia or intravascular haemolysis. Hydration must be kept at an adequate level because the malarial patient may have high secretion of antidiuretic hormone. Fluid must be given cautiously. With delayed response to fluid load a small dose of frusemide may be needed. With good urine flow the urine volume must be replaced with proper electrolyte solution to avoid volume depletion. Urine should be made alkaline when there is intravascular haemolysis.

Nephropathy in quartan malaria

Quartan malaria is caused by *Plasmodium malariae*. The disease is common in Africa, and can be associated with both a transient form of glomerulonephritis and persistent glomerulonephritis.

Glomerular changes are the common lesion in quartan malaria. In persistent glomerulonephritis membranous glomerulonephritis is often observed in children, while membranoproliferative glomerulonephritis is frequent in adults. Crescentic glomerulonephritis may occur. Immunofluorescence study shows deposition of IgG, IgM and C3 along the glomerular capillary wall. *P. malariae* antigens are detectable in 25% of cases. IgG_3 deposition is usually associated with a coarse granular deposit, while IgG_2 deposition is seen with a fine and diffuse deposit. The basement membrane is irregularly thickened with electron-dense material. Glomerulonephritis in quartan malaria runs a chronic course leading to glomerular sclerosis, interstitial cell infiltration and tubular atrophy.

The reason for the persistent glomerular renal lesion in contrast to the mild and reversible lesion in falciparum malaria is not apparent.

Clinically, the patient may present with the nephrotic syndrome or persistent proteinuria which is usually poorly selective. Urinary sediment is non-specific with few leucocytes and granular casts. Hypertension may occur as the disease progresses. There may be associated infection. The disease runs a chronic course leading to renal failure within 3–5 years.

In contrast to falciparum malaria in which renal lesions resolve following antimalarial therapy, in quartan malarial nephropathy antimalarial treatment usually fails to cause remission. Prednisolone is not effective in most cases, although some patients with highly selective proteinuria may respond favourably. Cyclophosphamide should be used in steroid-resistant cases.

Nephropathy in schistosomiasis

Renal changes in man are observed in infections caused by *Schistosoma mansoni*, and *S. haematobium*. The changes are predominantly in the glomeruli. Membranous glomerulonephritis, membranoproliferative glomerulonephritis, crescentic glomerulonephritis and focal glomerulonephritis have been described. Amyloidosis of the kidney may occur. Immunofluorescent microscopy reveals granular deposits of IgM, IgG, IgA, IgE, C3 and fibrin in the mesangium and the capillary wall. The glomerular lesions are immune complex-mediated. The intestinal lining and tegument of the adult worm are important antigens. There is also evidence of in-situ immune complex formation. In *S. haematobium* infection, besides the glomerular changes, there are also tubulointerstitial changes secondary to obstructive uropathy.

Proteinuria and abnormal urinary sediments are noted in 25–33% of hepatosplenic schistosomiasis. Nephrotic syndrome is observed in 9%. Proteinuria is of poor selectivity. Hypertension is seen in 3%. The nephrotic syndrome and hypertension are bad prognostic signs. Treatment by corticosteroids and immunosuppressive agents is ineffective. In *S. haematobium* infection there is obstructive uropathy in 77% of affected patients. Natriuresis and urine concentration defect are noted even in the early stage of hydronephrosis.

Nephropathy in leptospirosis

Renal involvement invariably occurs in leptospirosis even without clinical renal manifestations. Interstitial nephritis is the basic renal lesion, and can be seen in the patient with normal blood creatinine. Tubular necrosis occurs in patients with renal failure. Glomerular changes are mild. There is mesangial hyperplasia with increased mesangial matrix and deposition of IgM and C3 in some cases. Renal failure and cholestatic jaundice are usually associated with severe infection and this combination is known as Weil's syndrome. Non-oliguric renal failure is not uncommon. Anicteric renal failure represents a milder form of infection. Haemolytic uraemic syndrome may be observed, but is rare. Although renal failure is hypercatabolic accompanied by hyperuricaemia, hyperphosphataemia and hyperkalaemia, hypokalaemia due to kaliuresis may also occur in some cases with severe jaundice.

Renal lesions in leptospirosis are attributed mainly to bacterial invasion and non-specific inflammatory effects. Renal failure is therefore due to both non-specific inflammatory factors and bacterial invasion. Humoral immune response plays a minor role in the pathogenesis of glomerular changes.

Nephropathy in gastrointestinal infections

Transient glomerulonephritis with mild urinary sediment changes is a common finding in infectious diseases affecting the gastrointestinal tract. Mesangial proliferative glomerulonephritis with IgM and C3 depostition is usually observed. Occasionally, IgA deposition has been detected in typhoid fever and intestinal tuberculosis.

Persistent glomerulonephritis has been observed in hepatitis B infection. Membranous glomerulonephritis is often reported, although mesangial proliferative glomerulonephritis, diffuse proliferative glomerulonephritis and focal glomerulosclerosis can occur. There is electron-dense deposition in the glomerular basement membrane, subendothelial, mesangial and subepithelial areas and granular deposition of IgG, IgM, C3, HBcAg and HBsAg in the mesangium and along the capillary wall. Tubular atrophy and interstitial mononuclear cell infiltration have been described. The findings are consistent with immune complex glomerulonephritis. The development of the persistent lesion requires a continuous supply of antigen with limited antibody response. Early and rapid immune response would result in mesangial proliferative glomerulonephritis with rapid resolution. Those patients who have no antibody response show no evidence of renal disease.

Patients with hepatitis B infection may present with nephrotic syndrome, asymptomatic proteinuria and microscopic haematuria. Serum C3 is decreased in 30% of cases. The clinical picture of cryoglobulinaemia with purpura, arthralgia and splenomegaly has been reported. Nephritic syndrome and oliguria associated with progressive glomerular injury can also be seen. Response to corticosteroids and immunosuppressive agents is variable. Leucocyte interferon has been used in membranous glomerulonephritis with good result. Spontaneous remission within 6 months may be seen.

Tubular necrosis with acute renal failure may occur in many diarrhoeal diseases, of which cholera, shigellosis and salmonellosis are good examples. Haemolytic uraemic syndrome has been described in shigellosis and diarrhoeal diseases, especially in children. Acute renal failure may also occur in hepatitis A infection. Opisthorchiasis with cholangiocarcinoma and severe obstructive jaundice may present with acute renal failure, hyponatraemia and hypokalaemia due to natriuresis and kaliuresis. Improvement of renal function follows the decrease in degree of jaundice by biliary decompression.

Nephropathy in leprosy

Renal involvement is most frequent among lepromatous patients although it can also be seen in the other types of leprosy.

Diffuse proliferative glomerulonephritis and mesangial proliferative glomerulonephritis are common but focal proliferative glomerulonephritis and glomerulosclerosis have been reported. Immunofluorescence study shows granular deposition of IgM, IgG, IgA and C3 in the mesangial areas and along the glomerular capillary walls. There is electron-dense deposition in the mesangial, subendothelial, intramembranous and subepithelial areas. The findings are compatible with immune complex glomerulonephritis. Secondary amyloidosis is noted in up to 10%, predominantly in lepromatous and borderline lepromatous leprosy.

The clinical spectrum covers nephrotic syndrome, nephritic syndrome, asymptomatic proteinuria, haematuria and even renal failure. Circulating immune complexes and cryoglobulinaemia are detectable in the majority of patients. Serum complement may be low. Cell-mediated immune response is depressed in the lepromatous type. Nephrotic syndrome is common in the patient with amyloidosis, and may be observed in the patient with membranous and diffuse proliferative glomerulonephritis. Concentration and acidification defects have been described. Chronic renal failure from amyloidosis is common.

Treatment should concentrate on leprosy. Management of renal involvement is usually supportive. Corticosteroid therapy is not effective.

Nephropathy in filariasis

Mesangial proliferative glomerulonephritis and membranous glomerulonephritis can occur in filariasis. Eosinophilic infiltration in the glomeruli has been shown. Microfilariae may be seen in the glomeruli with glomerular deposition of C3 and IgM. Amyloidosis has been reported in the animal model.

Clinically, the patient usually has a history of lymphatic obstruction, presenting with chyluria before the onset of glomerular symptoms. Nephrotic syndrome and nephritic syndrome may be seen. Mild impairment of renal function and hypertension may be observed. While nephritic patients may respond to the antifilarial treatment, nephrotic patients may not.

Nephropathy in snake bite

Renal involvement is common in snake bite. Proteinuria with urinary sediment changes is noted in 4% and gross haematuria occurs in 35%, mostly in viper bite. Renal failure is life-threatening and is observed in 5.5% of cases. Snakes known to cause renal failure include sea snake, Russell's viper, green pit viper, Puff adder, saw scale viper, *Bothrop jararaca*, crotalid snake, *Cryptophis nigrescens*, boomslang, *Agkistrodon hypnale*, tiger snake, dugite and gwardar. Systemic manifestations include intravascular haemolysis, disseminated intravascular coagulation, rhabdomyolysis and hypotension. Reversible heavy proteinuria has been described in Russell's viper bite in Burma.

Glomerular changes in snake bite are usually mild. Mesangial proliferative glomerulonephritis with or without immune complex deposition is common. Mesangiolysis is occasionally seen in viper bite. Diffuse proliferative glomerulonephritis and extracapillary proliferative glomerulonephritis may also be observed in viper bite without immune complex deposition. Tubular necrosis is a common renal pathological change and is responsible for the majority of cases of acute renal failure in snake bite.

Renal changes in snake bite are due to non-specific inflammatory effects, immunological reactions and direct nephrotoxicity. Viper venoms are vasculotoxic. Direct tubulotoxicity of Russell's viper venom has been shown.

Nephropathy in insect stings

Bee stings may be associated with glomerular lesions; minimal change nephropathy, mesangial proliferative glomerulonephritis, membranous glomerulonephritis and glomerulosclerosis have been decribed.

The patient may present with nephrotic syndrome 2–14 days after the sting. Serum complement and renal function are usually normal and corticosteroid therapy yields a favourable response in 50% of the cases.

Multiple wasp or hornet stings may result in acute renal failure. Myoglobinuria and haemoglobinuria have been observed.

Nephropathy due to carp raw bile

Ingestion of the raw bile of fresh water grass carp (*Ctenopharyngodon idellus*) or Jullien's golden price carp in the Chinese traditional belief that it will improve visual acuity and rheumatic symptoms can cause abdominal pain, diarrhoea, jaundice and acute renal failure. Renal failure is due to non-specific inflammatory factors.

Nephropathy due to plant toxins

Nephrotoxicity has been reported following ingestion of several kinds of plants (Table 12.1), yet the renal injury induced by most plant toxins is through non-specific effects such as diarrhoea, volume depletion, haemolysis and hepatic failure. Direct nephrotoxicity has been described in djenkol bean toxicity and ingestion of *Callilepis laureola*. Djenkol beans are usually consumed by people in southern Thailand and Indonesia. Renal failure, abdominal pain and haematuria can result from ingestion of the raw beans in large amounts with low fluid intake. Djenkolic acid, which is an active ingredient of djenkol bean, can cause irritation of renal tubules due to crystallization at acid pH and low urine flow. Tubular obstruction can occur.

Callilepis laureola is a herb with tuberous rootstock in Africa. An infusion of the tubers is used as a traditional medicine in the treatment of various diseases. *Callilepsis laureola* ingestion can cause renal failure and jaundice, perhaps through direct nephrotoxicity and hepatotoxicity. It is one of the causes of nephropathy due to plant toxins in Africa. Atracytyloside, an alkaloid ingredient, is believed to be nephrotoxic.

The sap of the marking nut tree (*Semecarpus anacardium*) has an irritant effect. Skin exposure to the sap can cause marked skin reactions accompanied by fever, dysuria and haematuria. Renal failure with cortical necrosis has been reported.

Renal stone disease

While uric acid stones are seen in Western countries, calcium stones are still common among the people of poor socioeconomy in the tropics and may present as bladder stones. The cause is not clear. Low urine citrate may be the cause in some in north-eastern Thailand. Hypercalciuria is not common. Distal renal tubular acidosis is responsible in some. Renal stone disease, distal renal tubular acidosis and hypokalaemic paralysis are fascinating syndromes commonly seen in north-eastern Thailand, representing metabolic problems of environmental origin. Sudden unexplained nocturnal death among these people could be attributed to cardiac arrhythmia induced by inhibition of Na,K-ATPase and potassium depletion. A minority of renal stones seen in Indonesia, Burma and southern Thailand are caused by djenkolic acid resulting from djenkol bean ingestion. Alkalinization of urine and forced fluid intake help in dissolving the stone in this clinical setting.

Nephropathy due to chemical agents

Paraquat, a bipyridylium compound, is a widely used herbicide. Acute poisoning occurs by ingestion, inhalation and exposure of abraded skin. Toxicity includes acute renal failure, hepatocellular injury and respiratory failure. Plasma levels greater than 2 mg/l at 24 h or 1 mg/l at 48 h are bad prognostic indices. Treatment should concentrate on preventing paraquat absorption by administration of bentonite or Fuller's earth, cathartics or gastric lavage. Haemodialysis, charcoal haemoperfusion and forced diuresis should be performed.

Copper sulphate, commonly used in India in the leather industry, can cause haemoglobinuria, haematuria and renal failure associated with gastrointestinal symptoms. Renal failure is attributed to intravascular haemolysis and hypovolaemia.

RECOMMENDED READING

Andrade Z A, Rocha H 1979 Schistosomal glomerulopathy. Kidney International 16: 23–29

Chugh K 1989 Nephrology forum: snake bite induced acute renal failure in India. Kidney International 35: 891–907

Chugh K S, Sakhuga V 1990 Glomerular disease in the tropics. American Journal of Nephrology 10: 437–450

Gold C H 1980 Acute renal failure from herbal and patent remedies in Blacks. Clinical Nephrology 14: 128–134

Sitprija V 1984a The kidney in acute tropical disease. In: Kibukamusoke J W (ed) Tropical nephrology. Citforge, Canberra, pp 148–169

Sitprija V 1984b Acute renal failure in the tropics. In: Husain I (ed) Tropical urology and renal disease. Churchill Livingstone, London, pp 49–58

Sitprija V 1988 Nephrology forum: nephropathy in falciparum malaria. Kidney International 34: 867–877

Sitprija V, Boonpucknavig V 1986 Tropical diseases and glomerulonephritis. Proceedings of the 3rd Asian Pacific Congress of Nephrology, Singapore, pp 262–271

Sitprija V, Boonpucknavig V 1989 Renal involvement in parasitic diseases. In: Tisher C C, Brenner B M (eds) Renal pathology. JB Lipppincott, Philadelphia, pp 575–604

Sitprija V, Tungsanga K, Eiam-Ong S, Tosukhowong P, Leelhaphunt N, Sriboonlue P, Prasongwatana P 1991 Metabolic syndromes caused by decreased activity of ATPase. Seminars in Nephrology 11: 249–252

Interstitial and tubular disease

13. Interstitial nephritis — acute and chronic

K. L. Lynn   R. A. Robson

ACUTE INTERSTITIAL NEPHRITIS

Interstitial nephritis is a pathological term describing inflammation of the tubules and interstitium. Acute interstitial nephritis (AIN) is a common renal syndrome that may be associated with a variety of infections and drug therapies, or may develop without an identified cause. AIN is the cause of up to 15% of cases of acute renal failure. Histologically there is interstitial oedema with a mononuclear cell infiltrate, usually in the cortical interstitium. The glomeruli and vessels are usually spared. The inflammatory cells are a mixture of lymphocytes, macrophages and occasional plasma cells. Most lymphocytes are T cells. Eosinophils, neutrophils and basophils can be present depending on the aetiology. Virtually any form of acute interstitial nephritis can become chronic if the pathological disturbance is unrelenting. Chronic forms of AIN may present with acute renal failure, e.g. multiple myeloma (see Ch.11).

Recent observations have re-emphasized the significance of the interstitial cellular infiltrate in the acute and progressive phases of glomerulonephritis.

Aetiology

There are three main causes of AIN, namely drug-induced, infection-related, and idiopathic immune-mediated diseases, such as systemic lupus erythematosus and Sjögren's syndrome, which may also cause AIN, are discussed in Chapter 11.

Infection-related AIN may result from direct invasion of the renal interstitium by the offending organism or be associated with a systemic infection without direct renal involvement. In the first form a neutrophilic inflammatory infiltrate is seen which is often focal. In renal infections such as acute pyelonephritis the medulla is primarily involved. Acute renal failure is rare with this form of AIN. Infectious agents causing AIN include bacteria, mycoplasma, rickettsia, spirochetes and viruses (Table 13.1). The pathogenesis is unknown although an immunologically mediated mechanism is suspected.

Idiopathic AIN is distinguished by exclusion of infection, drugs or underlying immune disease.

Table 13.1 Infectious causes of acute interstitial nephritis

Bacteria
  Streptococcus
  Diphtheria
  Brucellosis
  Legionella
  Pneumococcus
  Tuberculosis
  Mycoplasma
  Leprosy

Spirochetes
  Syphilis
  Leptospirosis

Viruses
  Epstein–Barr virus
  Measles
  BK virus
  Cytomegalovirus
  Hanta virus

Protozoa
  Toxoplasmosis

Rickettsia
  Rocky Mountain spotted fever

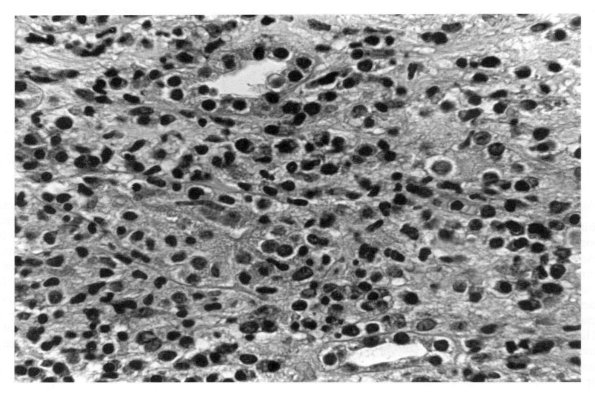

Fig. 13.1   Acute interstitial nephritis. The patient received diflunisal and developed acute renal failure, eosinophilia and a skin rash. The renal cortex shows a heavy mixed interstitial inflammatory cell infiltrate consisting of lymphocytes, plasma cells, eosinophils and neutrophils. Several intact tubules seen here are infiltrated by inflammatory cells (HE × 360). (Photomicrograph kindly supplied by Dr J. Gardner.)

Pathology

The kidneys are of normal size or enlarged. There are two principal histological lesions — interstitial oedema and inflammatory infiltrates (Fig. 13.1). The pathological appearances in tubules may vary from normal to necrosis. The glomeruli and vessels remain normal. It is assumed that an immune mechanism causes most forms of AIN. Cell-mediated immune mechanisms are more important than humorally mediated mechanisms in the pathogenesis of AIN. Occasionally there is evidence of a humoral mechanism with the deposition of anti-tubular basement membrane antibodies or immune complexes. The inflammatory cells are predominantly lymphocytes and plasma cells. Phenotypic analysis of the renal interstitial infiltrates in non-drug AIN has revealed a preponderance of T lymphocytes (both CD4+ and CD8+ cells) and monocyte macrophages. Immunofluorescence studies reveal linear or glomerular immune deposits in the tubular basement membrane in a minority of cases. Electron microscopy is consistent with the immunofluorescence findings.

Clinical presentation

The different mechanisms underlying AIN result in a variety of clinical presentations. Depending on the drug or infectious agent involved and the individual response the presentation of AIN can range from a hypersensitivity syndrome — fever, rash, eosinophilia and acute renal failure — to an asymptomatic increase in plasma creatinine or abnormal urinary sediment without evidence of renal insufficiency.

The idiopathic interstitial nephritis–uveitis syndrome has been recognized recently. Diagnosis requires the exclusion of other causes of interstitial nephritis and uveitis. The condition usually affects girls in the pubertal age group. Presentation is with non-specific constitutional symptoms and uveitis which is usually anterior and may be recurrent. Most patients make a full recovery.

Diagnosis

Renal biopsy is the only definitive diagnostic test for AIN. It is important to take a full drug history. Fever, rash, eosinophilia, haemolytic anaemia, proteinuria (usually < 1 g/24 h), pyuria and haematuria may be present. The urine should be examined specifically for eosinophils using Wright's stain. The differential diagnoses include renal vasculitis, acute tubular necrosis, rapidly progressive glomerulonephritis and atheromatous embolic renal disease.

Treatment

In most patients full recovery of renal function occurs but occasionally renal impairment will persist. Any drugs with a potential for causing AIN should be withdrawn. The treatment of acute interstitial nephritis with steroids remains unproven and controversial. There is some evidence that steroids may shorten the course of an illness and prevent permanent renal damage.

Drug-induced acute interstitial nephritis

Antibiotics are the most commonly implicated drugs in acute interstitial nephritis. Methicillin is the most frequently reported but penicillin, ampicillin, rifampicin, phenindione, sulphonamides, co-trimoxazole, thiazides and phenytoin are frequently implicated and are more important clinically. Drugs that are less often associated with acute interstitial nephritis include other antibiotics, non-steroidal anti-inflammatory drugs, diuretics, analgesics, and H_2 antagonists.

The interval between exposure to a drug and the onset of symptoms varies from hours to months.

Clinical presentation is variable and includes an allergic phenomenon, skin rash (50%), fever (75%) and eosinophilia. Bilateral or unilateral loin pain has been described. Urinalysis demonstrates mild to moderate proteinuria and haematuria.

Microscopy shows only moderate amounts of red and white cells, white cell casts and eosinophils. The absence of eosinophils does not exclude the diagnosis. Biopsy shows a mixed inflammatory cell infiltrate — including neutrophils, eosinophils, lymphocytes and plasma cells — indistinguishable from other forms of AIN. The cellular infiltrate tends to be diffuse in the cortex and heavier and more focal in the medulla. The glomeruli are usually normal or show only minor secondary changes.

CHRONIC INTERSTITIAL NEPHRITIS

There are many conditions that may cause a chronic interstitial nephritis (Table 13.2). Some of these conditions are considered in other chapters,

Table 13.2   Causes of chronic interstitial nephritis

Chronic phase of acute interstitial nephritis
Glomerulonephritis
Drugs
Analgesic nephropathy*
Lithium
Heavy metals
Cadmium toxicity
Lead toxicity*
Mercury
Reflux nephropathy*
Medullary cystic disease*
Sickle cell disease
Neoplastic
Myeloma*
Lymphoma/leukaemia
Sjögren's syndrome*
Sarcoidosis
Metabolic
Gout
Hyperoxaluria
Hypercalcaemia*
Obstructive uropathy*
Renal ischaemia
Balkan nephropathy
Radiation nephritis
Infections*
Leprosy
Syphilis
Tuberculosis

* In other chapters

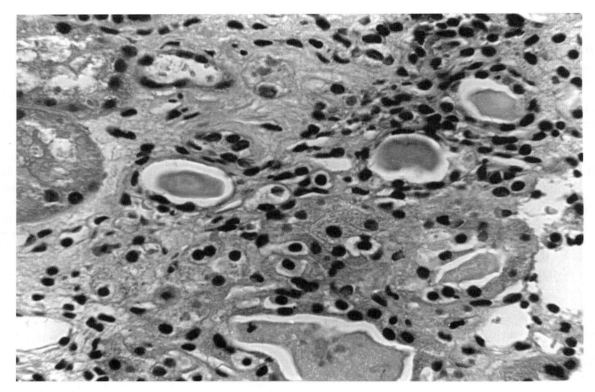

Fig. 13.2   Chronic interstitial nephritis. This patient had been treated with lithium for many years and presented with mild chronic renal failure. The renal cortex shows tubular atrophy with cast formation, interstitial fibrosis and patchy chronic inflammatory cell infiltration (HE × 360). (Photomicrograph kindly supplied by Dr J. Gardner.)

and only those not covered elsewhere are described here in brief.

Chronic interstitial nephritis produces a nonspecific histological picture characterized by an increase in interstitial fibrosis and chronic inflammatory cells, and associated tubular atrophy (Fig. 13.2).

Radiation nephropathy (nephritis)

Radiation nephritis occurs as a result of inadvertent renal irradiation, usually during radiotherapy for malignant disease. Antineoplastic agents administered concomitantly may enhance the potential for the development of radiation nephritis. Radiation nephritis may develop acutely (6–12 months after irradiation) or not for 18 months or several years. The acute presentation is with hypertension, often accelerated, oedema, protein-

uria and signs and symptoms of chronic renal failure. The chronic presentation is insidious. The kidneys are small with widespread glomerular sclerosis, tubular atrophy and arteriolar fibrinoid necrosis.

Balkan nephropathy

Balkan endemic nephropathy is a chronic interstitial nephritis of unknown cause occurring in geographically discrete areas of Romania, Bulgaria and the former Yugoslavia. Typically, there is a history of having lived in an endemic village for over 20 years before the insidious onset of chronic renal failure during the fifth and sixth decades of life. Males and females are affected equally. Proteinuria is usually less than 1 g per day and mostly of low molecular weight species. Blood pressure is frequently normal. Associated transitional cell neoplasms are common. The pathological and clinical features closely resemble those of analgesic nephropathy.

Gouty nephropathy

The pathogenesis of gouty nephropathy remains controversial with debate about the relative importance of intratubular uric acid crystal deposition with tubular blockage and subsequent tubular atrophy and interstitial scarring or the interstitial deposition of sodium urate crystals as a cause of interstitial inflammation. The only distinctive histological feature of gouty nephropathy is the presence of urate crystals within the parenchyma of the renal pyramid. This does not imply a pathogenetic role for crystal deposition in the accompanying inflammation as medullary urate deposits were found in 8% of unselected autopsies by Linnane et al (1981). Hyperuricaemia per se does not appear to cause progressive renal failure.

Sickle cell nephropathy

Patients with sickle cell disease may develop papillary necrosis as the result of the ischaemic effects of sickling and eventual occlusion of the vasa recta. Renal failure is a common cause of death in older patients with sickle cell anaemia.

Lithium-induced interstitial nephritis

The effects of lithium on the renal tubule are well established. More controversial is the association or otherwise of lithium with chronic interstitial nephritis and chronic renal failure. There is experimental animal evidence that lithium therapy is associated with chronic interstitial nephritis. Similarly, in man there are reports of a characteristic histological lesion consisting of tubular dilatation, microcyst formation and interstitial fibrosis. Prospective histological studies in man, however, have failed to confirm that well-monitored lithium therapy is associated with progressive histological damage. Similarly, longitudinal clinical studies have failed to confirm progressive renal impairment.

On balance, it is probable that individual case reports of chronic interstitial nephritis associated with lithium therapy are due either to episodes of toxicity or alternatively represent an idiosyncratic adverse drug reaction.

REFERENCES AND FURTHER READING

Linnane J W, Burry A F, Emmerson B T 1981 Urate deposits in the renal medulla. Prevalence and associations. Nephron 29: 216–222

Luxton R W 1961 Radiation nephritis: a long term study of 54 patients. Lancet 2: 1221–1224

Neilson E G 1989 Pathogenesis and therapy of interstitial nephritis. Kidney International 35: 1257–1270

Ten R M, Torres V E, Milliner D S, Schwab T R, Holley K E, Gleich G J 1988 Acute interstitial nephritis: immunologic and clinical aspects. Mayo Clinic Proceedings 63: 921–930

Toto R D 1990 Review: acute tubulointerstitial nephritis. American Journal of Medical Sciences 229: 392–410

Walker R G, Kincaid-Smith P 1992 The patient with chronic interstitial disease – lithium. In: Cameron S, Davison A M, Grünfeld J-P, Kerr D, Ritz E (eds) Oxford textbook of nephrology. Oxford University Press, Oxford, p. 853–857

14. Analgesic nephropathy

R. S. Nanra

Analgesic nephropathy is a form of chronic renal disease usually associated with excessive long-term use of common proprietary analgesic mixtures. It is characterized by renal papillary necrosis (RPN) and chronic interstitial nephritis, and may lead to a distinct clinical syndrome including chronic renal failure and hypertension. Similar renal disease also results from prolonged misuse of non-steroidal anti-inflammatory drugs (NSAIDs).

HISTORY AND EPIDEMIOLOGY

The association between analgesic consumption and renal disease with papillary necrosis and chronic interstitial nephritis was first recognized by Spuhler and Zollinger in Switzerland in 1953. Initial reports of analgesic-associated renal disease appeared in the English literature in the early 1960s. Although analgesic nephropathy is particularly prevalent in the developed Western countries, the disease is now recognized in most parts of the world.

Analgesic nephropathy is a disease of the twentieth century. In Australia the excessive use of 'headache powders' was recognized as a social habit, particularly in women, as early as 1907. Surveys of different segments of communities throughout the world indicate that 2–40% regularly use analgesics. In the Scandinavian countries the consumption of phenacetin-containing analgesic mixtures reached epidemic proportions during 1950–1960. The number of deaths from uraemia, RPN and chronic interstitial nephritis rose in parallel. In several countries, an increase in the prevalence of RPN at autopsy has been noted since the early 1950s. In Sydney,

Australia, the autopsy incidence of RPN rose from 3.7% in 1962 to 21.4% in 1977. Analgesic nephropathy was also found to contribute significantly to the numbers of patients requiring dialysis and transplantation. The reported figures varied from 2–2.5% in North America to 4.8–16.7% in the United Kingdom and Europe, and up to 21.5% in Australia. The introduction in 1961 of legislation to restrict the sales of analgesics in the Scandinavian countries was followed by a decline in consumption of phenacetin-containing mixtures and a slow decrease in mortality from these causes. In Sweden there was also a gradual decline in the number of patients with analgesic nephropathy and end-stage renal disease who required replacement therapy by renal dialysis and transplantation. In contrast, in Switzerland, where no restrictions had been placed on analgesic sales, analgesic nephropathy was responsible for approximately 20% of the renal replacement programme in 1979. In Australia the introduction of analgesic legislation in 1979, which restricted the sale and advertisement of analgesic mixtures, has also led to a decrease in total analgesic usage, and there has been a progressive decline to 11% in 1991 in the number of patients with analgesic nephropathy and renal failure who are accepted for dialysis and transplantation.

Gault et al (1968) in Canada noted that the per capita consumption of phenacetin-containing analgesic mixtures in a number of developed Western countries appeared to correlate with the prevalence of analgesic nephropathy in those countries. A government study in Australia found that the high per capita sales of analgesic mixtures in two states corresponded to a high incidence of analgesic-associated renal disease and renal failure. The association between regular analgesic consumption and renal disease was confirmed by a prospective longitudinal epidemiological study in Switzerland which demonstrated a significant increase in renal impairment and mortality in the population at risk compared to the control group.

PATHOLOGY

The basic pathological lesions in analgesic nephropathy are:

1. RPN
2. Chronic interstitial nephritis
3. Capillary sclerosis
4. Transitional cell carcinoma of the urothelium.

The primary lesion in analgesic nephropathy is RPN resulting from medullary cytotoxicity and an ischaemic infarct. The pathological changes of chronic interstitial nephritis in the overlying cortex are largely secondary to obstruction to tubules in the necrotic medulla. However, there is some experimental and clinical evidence that chronic interstitial nephritis may also occur in the absence of RPN. This has been attributed to direct aspirin-related cytotoxicity in the renal cortex. In recent years the presence of a characteristic vascular lesion, affecting small arterioles and venules in the renal medulla and in the submucosa of the renal pelvis and the urinary tract, has been emphasized in analgesic nephropathy. There is homogeneous thickening and sclerosis of the vessel walls, which stain strongly with periodic acid-Schiff (PAS) reagent. This change is independent of age, hypertension and diabetes mellitus, and its identification in a histological specimen should raise the serious possibility of an analgesic aetiology. Tumours of the transitional cell urothelium develop in approximately 8% of patients with analgesic nephropathy.

Macroscopic appearance

Typically the kidney in chronic analgesic nephropathy is reduced in size. The capsule tends to be thickened and adherent, with prominent scars and multiple small cysts on its cortical surface. The pale tumour-like nodular tissue between the scars represents hypertrophy of the viable nephrons in the columns of Bertin. The distinctive features on the cut surface of the kidney are the brownish-black necrotic papillae, atrophy of the overlying cortex and hypertrophy of the intervening columns of Bertin (Fig. 14.1). The necrotic papillae are sclerotic and reduced in size in contradistinction to the pale swollen papillae of diabetic papillitis necroticans.

Microscopic appearance

Renal papillary necrosis

Histologically, RPN may be divided into three grades.

Grade I: necrobiosis. There is loss of nuclei from loops of Henle and vasae rectae. The basement membrane of the 'ghost' structures appears thickened and stains heavily with periodic acid-Schiff (PAS) stain. There is also loss of interstitial cells. These changes are most prominent towards the tip of the papilla.

Grade II: partial RPN. All elements of the medulla undergo necrosis but there is selective sparing of the collecting tubules.

Grade III: total RPN. All structures in the papilla are involved: the loops of Henle, the vasae rectae, the collecting ducts and the interstitium, including the interstitial cells. There is a clear line of demarcation between viable and necrotic tissue. The appearances are those of a coagulative necrosis in which outlines of 'ghost' medullary structures may be identified. The interstitium may appear glassy (hyaline) and there is a striking absence of an inflammatory infiltrate. Calcification involving tubular casts, tubular walls and the interstitium is common. Bone formation may occur. These features are highly suggestive of ischaemic infarction. Separation and loss of a necrotic papilla results in the formation of a medullary cavity which becomes lined with fibrous tissue. Tubules of remaining viable nephrons open into the pelvicalyceal system through this cavity.

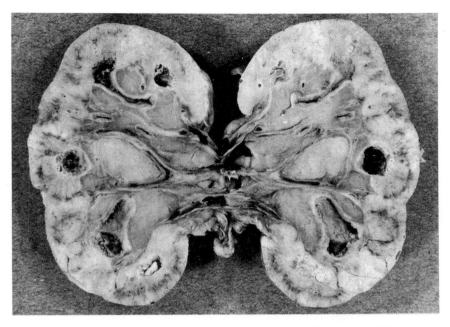

Fig. 14.1 Macroscopic appearance of renal papillary necrosis. Cut surface of kidney showing black necrotic papillae with atrophy of overlying cortex. (Reproduced with permission from Nanra 1983)

Chronic interstitial nephritis

The cortex overlying the necrotic medulla shows the histological features of chronic interstitial nephritis. The major microscopic findings are tubular atrophy, interstitial fibrosis and a variable round cell infiltrate (Fig. 14.2). Careful microscopic examination usually reveals a golden-brown lipofuchsin-like pigment in the interstitium and tubules, indicating an analgesic aetiology for the interstitial disease. The glomeruli are relatively unaffected. However, definite glomerular changes do occur and include global glomerular sclerosis, focal and segmental sclerosis and hyalinosis, glomerular hypertrophy, and periglomerular fibrosis. It has been suggested that the glomerular changes may be due to hyperfiltration affecting a reduced nephron population. Other glomerular lesions such as membranous nephropathy and mesangial IgA glomerulonephritis have been described, but no association with analgesic nephropathy has been established. The arteries often show changes of benign nephrosclerosis, with thickening of the arterial wall, reduplication of elastica, intimal fibrosis, and hyaline sclerosis, especially of small arterioles. Arterial lesions of malignant hypertension and atheroma may also be seen.

During episodes of acute analgesic RPN, the overlying cortex may become oedematous and the tubules may contain renal tubular epithelial casts.

Transitional cell carcinoma of urothelium

The commonest analgesic-associated tumour is transitional cell carcinoma of the urothelium; however, hypernephroma, sarcoma and chorionepithelioma have also been reported. Analgesic-associated tumours have a reversed distribution in the urinary tract. The ratio of bladder to renal pelvis tumours in analgesic nephropathy is 1:11 whereas tumours unrelated to analgesic abuse occur in a ratio of 15:1. Ureteric tumours also occur. Morphologically, the tumours may be solitary pedunculated papillomatous tumours or,

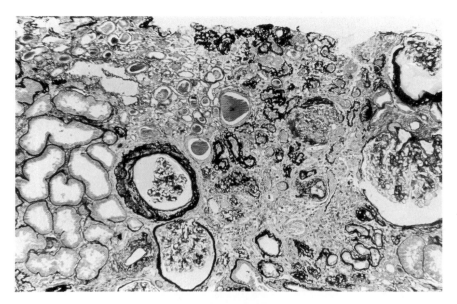

Fig. 14.2 Chronic interstitial nephritis. Photomicrograph showing marked tubular atrophy, interstitial fibrosis and a non-specific round cell infiltrate. The glomerular tufts appear normal. Note periglomerular fibrosis, and arteriolar thickening and sclerosis

more commonly, broad-based solid infiltrating tumours which may extend over large areas of the surface of the renal pelvis. Surrounding epithelial hyperplasia and dysplasia are common and may extend into the upper ureter. Analgesic tumours may be multifocal and tend to be poorly differentiated and more malignant.

AETIOLOGY AND PATHOGENESIS

Renal papillary necrosis and chronic interstitial nephritis

There is now overwhelming evidence — epidemiological, clinicopathological and experimental — to incriminate analgesics in renal disease.

Epidemiological evidence

The epidemiological evidence, summarized above, clearly demonstrates a significant association between analgesic sales and consumption, and renal disease, prevalence of terminal renal failure and mortality.

Clinical and pathological evidence

The clinical syndrome of analgesic nephropathy and the pathological features of RPN are distinctive. More than 3500 cases of analgesic nephropathy have been described in the literature, and in two states of Australia and some parts of Europe analgesic nephropathy is responsible for 20–25% of all patients requiring renal dialysis or transplantation. Continued consumption of analgesics is associated with progressive decline in renal function, and analgesic withdrawal usually results in stabilization or improvement in the renal disease.

Experimental evidence

Experimental RPN with chronic interstitial nephritis can be induced with most analgesic mixtures and NSAIDs. The pathological features are identical to those seen in patients with analgesic nephropathy. In animal studies, aspirin appears to be more nephrotoxic than phenacetin and its major metabolite, paracetamol. Analgesic mixtures containing aspirin and phenacetin or aspirin and paracetamol appear to have greater nephrotoxicity than the individual drugs and there is sound biochemical evidence to suggest that their combined toxicity is additive and synergistic.

Clinical analgesic nephropathy is almost exclusively related to long-term abuse of proprietary analgesic mixtures obtainable 'over the counter'. In the English-speaking countries, the analgesic mixtures originally contained aspirin and phenacetin with either caffeine or codeine. In some mixtures, phenacetin was later replaced by paracetamol or salicylamide. In Europe, the most widely used and popular analgesic mixtures contain antipyrine, phenacetin and caffeine. In some, antipyrine has been replaced by amidopyrine or aspirin. The absence of aspirin from these mixtures partly explains the almost complete absence of peptic ulcer from the analgesic syndrome in Europe.

Although a definite link has been established between RPN and long-term use of individual analgesic agents, the overall number of reported cases is small. The major culprit is aspirin but paracetamol, indomethacin, phenylbutazone, fenoprofen, ibuprofen, naproxen and alcofenac alone have also been incriminated.

Clinical and experimental studies suggest that aspirin has significant acute and chronic nephrotoxicity: haematuria, tubular epithelial celluria, aminoaciduria, enzymuria, impaired concentrating ability with reduced free water clearance, transient renal tubular acidosis, transient reduction in glomerular filtration rate (GFR) and urinary PSP (phenolsulfonphthalein) excretion, RPN, chronic interstitial nephritis and acute tubular necrosis with acute renal failure have all been described. Some of the acute effects are related to suppression of intrarenal prostaglandin (PG) synthesis, and their relevance to the chronic lesions of RPN and chronic interstitial nephritis is questionable.

Patients with rheumatoid arthritis often take aspirin over many years and therefore afford an apportunity to evaluate the clinical nephrotoxicity of aspirin. At autopsy up to one fifth of rheumatoid patients have RPN and chronic interstitial nephritis. The renal disease, however, is much milder than that seen in patients who abuse analgesic mixtures, and patients with rheumatoid arthritis rarely develop terminal renal failure. This difference is due to the fact that analgesic nephropathy patients consume much larger quantities of analgesics and that the nephrotoxicity of the analgesic mixture is greater than that of aspirin alone.

The documented effects of phenacetin and its major metabolite paracetamol are fewer and milder, and include haematuria, tubular epithelial celluria, transient impairment of concentrating ability, and mild and patchy RPN. The nephrotoxicity of phenacetin is probably related to its metabolite paracetamol, and it is paracetamol and not phenacetin that concentrates in the renal medulla.

The pathogenesis of analgesic nephropathy has been best studied in animal experiments in relation to the nephrotoxicity of aspirin, phenacetin and paracetamol. In hydropaenic animals, aspirin and paracetamol concentrate in the renal medullary cells and interstitium. Their concentrations in the medulla after a large therapeutic dose are equivalent to those in the liver and renal cortex following an overdose. Unlike paracetamol, aspirin also appears to accumulate in the renal cortex. Overall, the concentrations achieved by aspirin are higher than those of paracetamol and this may partly explain the greater experimental nephrotoxicity of aspirin. Phenacetin, on the other hand, does not accumulate in the medulla or cortex. It is therefore very likely that the nephrotoxicity of phenacetin is related to paracetamol.

At a cellular level, both aspirin and paracetamol undergo activation by a microsomal cytochrome P-450-dependent mono-oxygenase, leading to the formation of reactive alkylating metabolites which are cytotoxic. The metabolites bind covalently to cellular proteins, resulting in intracellular glutathione depletion, probably via the hexose–monophosphate shunt. The combined cytotoxicity of aspirin and paracetamol is therefore synergistic. In addition, aspirin also inhibits prostaglandin synthetase, reduces red blood cell 2,3-diphosphoglyceride, uncouples renal cortical oxidative phosphorylation, and inhibits amino acid incorporation into cellular proteins (Table 14.1). The net effects of these intracellular metabolic derangements are cytotoxicity and cell death, tissue ischaemia, and hypoxia. The renal concentrating

Table 14.1　Intracellular effects of aspirin and paracetamol

Intracellular effect	Aspirin	Paracetamol
Formation of P-450 dependent reactive metabolite	+	+
Covalent protein binding	+ (inhibitis PG synthesis)	+
Glutathione depletion	+	+
Uncoupling of oxidative phosphorylation	+	
Inhibition of amino acid incorporation	+	
Reduction of RBC 2,3-diphosphoglyceride	+	

PG — prostaglandin

mechanism plays a crucial role in the development of RPN and the effect of dehydration in clinical and experimental RPN has been abundantly documented. Dehydration leads to toxic concentrations of aspirin and paracetamol in the medulla, particularly at the tips of the loops of Henle and in the vasae rectae and papillary interstitium. It also contributes to the development of medullary ischaemia, which plays an important role in the pathogenesis of RPN. Conversely, a constant water diuresis effectively protects the renal medulla in experimental RPN. The various stages in the development of RPN and chronic interstitial nephritis are summarized in Figure 14.3.

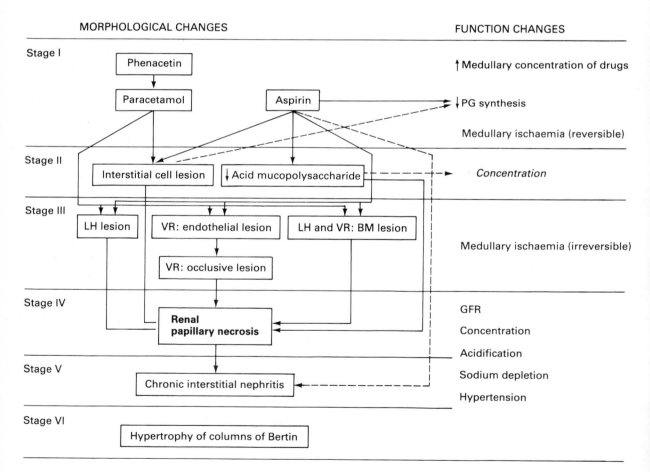

Fig. 14.3　Stages in the development of analgesic nephropathy – renal papillary necrosis and chronic interstitial nephritis.
PG — prostaglandin; LH — loop of Henle; VR — vasae rectae; GFR — glomerular filtration rate; BM — basement membrane

Stage I. Aspirin and paracetamol, the major metabolite of phenacetin, are concentrated in the medulla by the countercurrent mechanism. The covalent acetylation of cellular proteins in the medulla by aspirin leads to suppression of vasodilator prostaglandin synthesis and reversible medullary ischaemia.

Stage II. The earliest detectable histological lesion in experimental RPN is interstitial cell injury and loss of acid mucopolysaccharide in the medullary interstitium.

Stage III. The cytotoxic effects of the reactive metabolites of aspirin and paracetamol lead to glutathione depletion and necrobiosis in the loops of Henle, endothelial lesions in vasae rectae, and the characteristic basement membrane change of capillary sclerosis. Occlusive lesions develop in the vasae rectae and lead to irreversible medullary ischaemia.

Stage IV. The combination of irreversible medullary ischaemia, cytotoxic cell necrosis and interstitial damage results in RPN with the histological features of ischaemic infarction.

Stage V. Obstruction to tubules in the necrotic medulla causes atrophy of the overlying cortex with the histological features of chronic interstitial nephritis. The direct cortical cytotoxicity of aspirin and the altered distribution of cortical renal blood flow by suppression of prostaglandin synthesis may contribute to chronic interstitial nephritis.

Stage VI. Nephrons in the column of Bertin which are unaffected by obstructive atrophy undergo compensatory hypertrophy and form the tumour-like nodules seen in chronic analgesic nephropathy.

The development of analgesic nephropathy may be more complex than direct duration- and dose-related nephrotoxicity of analgesics. For example, there are some patients who have no evidence of any detectable renal disease, despite a significant history of analgesic abuse, suggesting that other factors may be important in the pathogenesis of RPN. These may include fluid intake, climatic factors, sex, and a genetic predisposition. An increased frequency of HLA A3 and B12 has been described in analgesic nephropathy. Although

the female to male ratio of analgesic abuse in the Australian community is 2:1, analgesic nephropathy affects females 7:1.

Transitional cell carcinoma of urothelium

More than 400 cases of urothelial tumours associated with analgesics have been reported in the literature. The distinctive features of analgesic-associated urothelial tumours are summarized below.

1. A high incidence in countries such as Sweden, Switzerland and Australia where analgesic nephropathy is common.

2. Female predominance in contradistinction to the male preponderance in non-analgesic patients.

3. A mean total phenacetin consumption of 9.1 kg in the form of analgesic mixtures.

4. Frequent accompaniment of RPN and renal insufficiency (in 92% of patients).

5. Reversed distribution of tumour in the urinary tract.

6. Increased malignancy.

7. Analgesic abuse is associated with a relative risk of 5.7 to 13 for renal pelvic carcinoma, and of 2.6 for bladder carcinoma. 8% of analgesic abusers may develop urothelial tumours.

Most investigations have linked phenacetin to the development of analgesic-associated urothelial tumours, and attention has focussed on the 2-hydroxy and N-hydroxy metabolites of phenacetin. However, definitive proof of the carcinogenicity of phenacetin is still lacking. The role of other factors, including cigarette consumption, caffeine, artificial sweeteners, urinary infections, calculi and unknown factors, such as in Balkan nephropathy which has a strikingly high incidence of carcinoma, cannot be ignored.

AGE AND SEX DISTRIBUTION

Analgesic nephropathy is predominantly a female disease, with a female-to-male ratio of 6–7:1. The only exception to this was noted in the Swedish town of Huskvarna, where analgesic abuse was prevalent among male factory workers. The male-to-female ratio of 3.6:1 in this town provided further causative evidence incriminating analgesics in renal disease.

Analgesic nephropathy occurs predominantly between the ages of 40 and 60 years. It is uncommon under the age of 30 years and an alternative diagnosis should be considered in these patients. Analgesic nephropathy may have a familial tendency.

CLINICAL MANIFESTATIONS

Analgesic nephropathy is part of a much wider clinical syndrome — the analgesic syndrome — in which there are multi-organ manifestations including gastric ulcer, anaemia, neuropsychiatric manifestations, cardiovascular disturbances, pregnancy and gonadal manifestations, generalized pigmentation and premature ageing.

Analgesic nephropathy may be asymptomatic and renal disease may only become apparent when

Table 14.2 Analgesic nephropathy: manifestations and complications

Manifestions and complications	Mechanism
Functional	
Changes in GFR:	
Normal GFR	Partial RPN or necrobiosis in papillae without significant chronic interstitial nephritis
Chronic renal failure	Nephron loss
	Nephrosclerosis
Acute renal failure	Acute intravascular volume depletion (dehydration, gastric ulcer haemorrhage)
	Acute RPN
	Ureteric obstruction
	Septicaemia
	Malignant hypertension
	Acute myocardial infarction
	Renal artery thrombosis
	Bilateral renal artery stenosis and ACE inhibition
Impaired concentrating capacity	Necrobiosis and necrosis of loops of Henle
	Loss of acid mucopolysaccharide from medullary matrix
Partial and complete RTA	Distal nephron damage with disturbed acidifying mechanism
Salt-losing state	Loss of sodium-conserving juxtamedullary nephrons
Hypertension	Nephron loss
	Loss of vasodilator medullary prostaglandins and activation of renin–angiotensin system
	Renal artery stenosis and thrombosis
Secondary gout	Hyperuricaemia due to reduced GFR, sodium depletion and diuretics
UTIs	Loss of mucopolysaccharides from medullary matrix
Proteinuria	Glomerular lesions causing glomerular proteinuria
	Tubular proteinuria from chronic interstitial nephritis
Microscopic or macroscopic haematuria	Cystitis
	Renal calculi/nephrocalcinosis
	Analgesic abuse
	Acute RPN
	Malignant hypertension
	Transitional cell tumour
Morphological	
Renal calculi/nephrocalcinosis	Calcification of necrotic papilla
RTA	UTI with urea-splitting organism
Hydronephrosis/pyonephrosis	Ureteric obstruction due to necrotic papilla, calculus, transitional cell tumour, or post-inflammatory stricture
Renal artery stenosis/thrombosis	Atheroma
Glomerular lesions	Hyperfiltration
	Immunological

Key: GFR — glomerular filtration rate; RPN — renal papillary necrosis; RTA — renal tubular acidosis; UTI — urinary tract infection.

abnormal laboratory findings are detected on routine medical examination. The clinical manifestations of analgesic nephropathy are summarized in Table 14.2. At the time of presentation approximately 80% of patients have a reduced GFR; 10–15% of these have terminal renal failure with GFR values below 10 ml/min per 1.73 m^2 body surface area. The clinical manifestations of renal insufficiency have a tubulointerstitial pattern characterized by a concentrating defect (all patients), prominent sodium-losing state, disproportionate systemic acidosis related to secondary renal tubular acidosis (30% of patients), and intermittent renal tubular epithelial celluria with cellular casts. Enzymuria consistent with tubular dysfunction may be present. These functional defects are commonly associated with nocturia and nocturnal cramps which are most prominent in summer months. In patients with chronic renal failure, renal osteodystrophy tends to be common and severe. These functional changes reflect damage to and loss of the juxtamedullary nephrons with their long loops of Henle, which extend deeply into the renal medulla. This leads to a failure to generate a concentration gradient in the renal medulla and thus to impairment of concentrating capacity and sodium conservation, and an acidifying defect.

Episodes of acute-on-chronic renal failure are usually precipitated by severe dehydration with intravascular volume depletion, acute haemorrhage with shock from a bleeding gastric ulcer, acute RPN with or without ureteric obstruction, septicaemia, or the development of malignant hypertension; often these complications coexist. The clinical features of acute renal failure are characteristic and include oliguric renal failure and a severe systemic acidosis, often with a serum bicarbonate concentration of less than 10 mmol/l. In older patients, transient reversible reductions in GFR may result from the use of NSAIDs for the symptomatic relief of coexisting osteoarthritis. The features of this form of acute renal insufficiency are also characteristic and include retention of sodium, potassium, hydrogen ions and water, leading to oedema, systemic acidosis and hyperkalaemia, and hypertension which is associated with hyporeninaemia and hypoaldosteronism. This form of vasoconstrictive acute renal failure is related to suppression of the increased production of intrarenal vasodilator prostaglandins by NSAIDs in the presence of activated vasoconstrictive factors, such as angiotensin, catecholamines and vasopressin. It is exaggerated by sodium depletion, and withdrawal of the incriminating drug usually leads to resolution of the acute renal insufficiency.

Hypertension occurs in more than 60% and malignant hypertension in about 7% of patients with analgesic nephropathy. The major factor responsible for hypertension is probably a reduction in nephron population and an increase in total body exchangeable sodium. A small proportion of patients demonstrate the physiological paradox of sodium depletion and severe hypertension. Activation of the renin–angiotensin system and loss of renal medullary vasodilator substances may be involved in this phenomenon. There is a high incidence of atheromatous renal artery stenosis or thrombosis in analgesic nephropathy. Renovascular disease may be unilateral or bilateral.

Approximately 20% of patients develop secondary gout, usually when the GFR falls below 60 ml/min per 1.73 m^2 body surface area, and this appears to be more common in males.

Urinary tract infection, which may be silent, occurs in up to half the patients. It rarely, if ever, causes renal deterioration except by the development of mixed infection staghorn calculi or septicaemia, which may be precipitated by instrumentation or obstruction in the presence of active urinary infection. Other factors contributing to stone formation are renal tubular epithelial celluria and necrotic papillary tissue which provide a nidus for calcium precipitation, urinary stasis, and secondary renal tubular acidosis. Sterile pyuria is very common and may be related to covert infection, renal calculi or renal tubular epithelial celluria.

Up to 40% of patients develop mild to moderate proteinuria (up to 3 g/24 h). The incidence of proteinuria increases with declining GFR and more than 90% of patients have significant proteinuria when the GFR is less than 10 ml/min per 1.73 m^2 body surface area. The proteinuria is mixed glomerular and tubular.

Haematuria in analgesic nephropathy is usually related to cystitis with urinary tract infections, renal calculi, and continuing analgesic abuse, and less commonly to glomerular lesions, malignant hypertension, recent RPN or transitional cell tumours of the urothelium. The mean induction time of the carcinoma is approximately 20 years, and the average exposure time 17 years. It has been estimated that the risk of tumour development in analgesic abusers is increased by a factor of 89 for ureteric tumours, 77 for renal pelvic tumours and 7 for bladder tumours. Cigarette smoking appears to contribute to the risk of tumour development.

Ureteric obstruction may be caused by necrotic papillary tissue, calculi or a ureteric stricture, and should be suspected if a patient has renal pain and colic. However, obstructive uropathy may be silent and the only indication of obstruction may be unexplained deterioration in renal function. Ureteric obstruction in the presence of urinary tract inflection may lead to a life-threatening pyonephrosis.

Non-renal manifestations of the analgesic syndrome

Gastrointestinal manifestations

Dyspepsia is common in patients who abuse analgesics, especially aspirin-containing compounds, and about 35% have a gastric ulcer. The ulcer is characteristically large and prone to the usual complications of haemorrhage, perforation, pyloric obstruction, 'hour-glass' stricture and recurrence after gastric surgery. Abnormalities of liver function tests and relapsing pancreatitis have also been noted.

Haematological manifestations

Approximately 60–90% of patients have anaemia secondary to gastrointestinal bleeding or chronic renal failure. Mild cyanosis, when present, is due to met- and sulph-haemoglobinaemia and is related to p-phenetidine, a metabolite, and p-chloracetanilide, a contaminant of phenacetin. However, cyanosis has become extremely rare because of the introduction of purer forms of phenacetin and the exclusion or replacement of phenacetin in analgesic mixtures. The other forms of anaemia seen in analgesic nephropathy include a paracetamol-related haemolytic anaemia, refractory sideroblastic anaemia, and macrocytic and megaloblastic anaemia. About 10% of patients have a palpable spleen.

Neuropsychiatric manifestations

Headaches are the commonest reason given by patients for analgesic abuse, and usually have no organic basis. The headaches are partly due to caffeine withdrawal. Significant personality inadequacies such as excessive introversion and neuroticism have also been described in analgesic abusers. These personality traits, together with a background of disturbed family and social life, are reflected in an addictive syndrome which often includes purgative abuse, smoking, alcoholism and use of psychotropic drugs and sleeping tablets. The combination of analgesic nephropathy and laxative abuse has been described as 'laxan nephropathy'. Cessation of analgesic abuse often results in withdrawal symptoms which have been ascribed to the psychotropic effects of caffeine and perhaps phenacetin. Organic features also occur, and bizarre headaches, migraine, dementia, psychosis, hallucinations and reversible electro-encephalographic abnormalities have been described.

Cardiovascular manifestations

Hypertension in analgesic nephropathy has been described earlier. A prominent feature of analgesic nephropathy is severe premature atherosclerosis. This is reflected in a high incidence of ischaemic heart disease (in approximately one third of patients), cerebrovascular disease, peripheral vascular disease, renal artery stenosis, and poor vascular access in patients on maintenance dialysis for terminal renal failure. Cardiac valve annulus calcification is probably also a reflection of degenerative disease. The premature atherosclerosis is due to multiple factors, including longstanding hypertension, the hyperlipidaemia of chronic renal failure, and the oxidant effect of phenacetin on low density lipoproteins (LDL).

Pregnancy and gonadal manifestations

Analgesic nephropathy is associated with subfertility and an increased incidence of toxaemia of pregnancy. Postmaturity has been described in patients who continue to take analgesics during pregnancy, probably due to suppression of uterine prostaglandin synthesis. Although animal experiments suggest that aspirin may be teratogenic and may cause congenital malformations, there is no clinical evidence in support of these experimental findings.

Pigmentation

Prominent skin pigmentation is seen in some patients with analgesic nephropathy and is aggravated by uraemia and a sodium-wasting state. The brownish-black colour of necrotic papillae and the dark urine are due to pigment breakdown products of phenacetin. A golden-brown lipofuchsin-like pigment is widely distributed in the brain, heart,

joint cartilage (like ochronosis), kidney and lower urinary tract. Lipofuchsin is a highly oxidized polymer of unsaturated fatty acids and its accumulation in multiple organs is probably related to the oxidant effect of phenacetin.

Premature ageing

Patients with analgesic nephropathy may have a striking appearance of premature ageing. The premature atherosclerosis, the accumulation of wear-and-tear pigment (lipofuchsin) in various organs and the autopsy changes in the brain (consistent with presenile dementia), all suggest premature biological ageing.

Natural history of the analgesic syndrome (Fig. 14.4)

The analgesic abuse habit usually starts in adolescence and the early twenties. The gastric and obstetric manifestations tend to occur between 25 and 35 years of age. The renal manifestations are invariably seen after the age of 30 years and evolve over the subsequent 5–20 years. The vascular

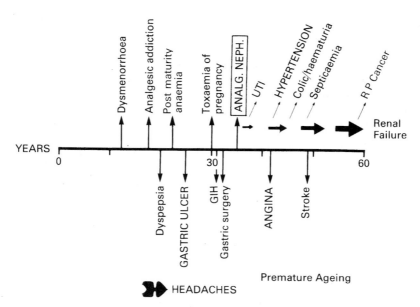

Fig. 14.4 Natural history of the analgesic syndrome. UTI — urinary tract infection; GIH — gastrointestinal haemorrhage. (Reproduced with permission from Nanra 1980)

Table 14.3 Relationship between renal function, radiology and biopsy abnormalities in analgesic nephropathy. (Reproduced with permission from Nanra et al 1978)

Reduced GFR	Impaired concentrating capacity	Impaired acidification	IVU		
			Reduced renal size	Calyceal abormality	CIN
–	+	–	–	–	–/+
+	+ +	+	–/+	+	+
+ +	+ + +	+ +RTA	+	+ +	+ +
+ + +	+ + + +	+ +RTA	+ +	–/+ (RPN in situ)	+ + +

GFR — glomerular filtration rate; IVU — intravenous urogram; CIN — chronic interstitial nephritis; RTA — renal tubular acidosis, RPN — renal papillary necrosis.

complications and transitional cell tumours of the urothelium are late manifestations and often occur after 50 years of age.

The presenting clinical manifestations of the analgesic syndrome change after cessation of analgesic abuse for 5–10 years. There is a reduction in the severity of renal failure, urine abnormalities, coronary artery disease, and anaemia, and a complete disappearance of malignant hypertension, gastric ulcer, and cyanosis. However, the patients are older and there is an increase in transitional cell carcinoma.

NSAID-associated analgesic syndrome

The NSAID-associated analgesic syndrome is similar to that seen in the analgesic abuse-associated analgesic syndrome after prolonged absence of analgesic abuse with a few significant differences; these are, absence of female predominance and urinary tract tumours, and milder degrees of renal insufficiency and urine abnormalities.

DIAGNOSIS

The diagnosis of analgesic nephropathy is based on a history of significant analgesic abuse and the demonstration of RPN or chronic interstitial nephritis. If renal radiology is non-diagnostic, the presence of a defect in renal concentrating capacity or chronic interstitial nephritis on renal biopsy is suggestive of analgesic nephropathy. A renal biopsy should also be considered if there is significant proteinuria. The relationship between renal function, renal radiology and renal biopsy abnormalities is summarized in Table 14.3.

Significant analgesic abuse is the total consumption of at least 2 kg aspirin or phenacetin in the form of an analgesic mixture. This quantity is usually achieved by an intake of five 'powders' a day for a minimum of 3 years. Since nephrotoxicity of analgesics is directly related to duration of intake and dose, an intake of one 'powder' a day for 15 years would also be sufficient to cause renal damage. Most patients, in fact, admit to taking larger quantities, 3–12 'powders' daily, for up to 20–30 years. The analgesics are either in tablet or powder form; the latter are favoured in some countries, e.g. Australia, and usually contain twice as much analgesics as tablets. Most patients attempt to conceal their habit; verification of abuse may require indirect approaches such as interviewing family members, questioning the patient about headaches and confronting the patient with evidence of analgesics in urine or serum. At the bedside, a positive urine Phenistix test usually indicates recent aspirin intake. The commonest given reason for analgesic abuse is headaches (more than 90% of patients). Others give non-specific aches and pains as the reason and some freely admit to a habit or a mood-lifting effect of analgesic mixtures.

RPN is usually demonstrated by typical calyceal changes on intravenous urography. Retrograde pyelography may be necessary if the definition of the calyces is poor because of reduced renal function. RPN may occasionally be confirmed by histological demonstration of necrotic papillary tissue in urine or if medullary

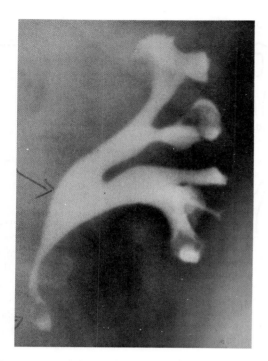

Fig. 14.5 Pyelogram of a patient with analgesic nephropathy. Note (from top to bottom) clubbed calyces, 'ring shadow', medullary cavity and papilla in ureter. (Reproduced with permission from Nanra 1983)

tissue is obtained on renal biopsy. In a patient with renal colic, tissue fragments should be carefully sought in urine and subjected to histological examination. Similarly, every effort should be made to collect possible necrotic tissue for histological examination during cystoscopy and retrograde ureteric catheterization.

The radiological changes of RPN may be of the papillary or medullary type. The calyceal abnormalities which are diagnostic of RPN are 'ring shadows' indicating complete papillary necrosis and separation from the medulla, calyceal extensions ('horns' or 'flares') due to partial papillary separation, medullary cavities ('match-stick sign') and medullary calcification (Fig. 14.5). The radiological types and stages of RPN are illustrated in Figure 14.6. In acute RPN the papillae may appear swollen. After separation and loss of necrotic papillae, the calyces appear clubbed. A shaggy appearance of the clubbed calyx suggests recent loss of a papilla, and in the chronic state

the clubbed calyx has a smooth outline. In a small proportion of patients with RPN in situ, no obvious calyceal abnormalities may be noted. However, careful examination of well-demonstrated calyces on intravenous urography or retrograde pyelography should reveal significant abnormalities. A filling defect in a calyx or the renal pelvis may indicate the presence of a renal pelvic carcinoma. It may be difficult to differentiate a tumour from a sloughed papilla, blood clot or radiolucent calculus. Characteristically, in a calyx, a transitional cell tumour tends to develop in the infundibulum opposite a papilla. Ultrasound examination of kidneys is less sensitive and specific than intravenous urograms in the diagnosis of RPN; in end-stage renal failure, ultrasonography may be useful — small echogenic kidneys, papillary calcification, and small intrarenal cysts are suggestive features of analgesic nephropathy.

RPN may also occur in other medical conditions, e.g. diabetes mellitus, sickle cell disease, obstructive uropathy, chronic alcoholism and renal amyloidosis, and less commonly in severe hyperbilirubinaemic states and in conditions associated with medullary ischaemia, such as graft rejection, vasculitis, malignant hypertension and renal medullary candidiasis. The radiological changes in these conditions may be indistinguishable from the RPN seen in analgesic nephropathy.

Radiologically, RPN in analgesic nephropathy should be differentiated from reflux nephropathy, chronic obstructive uropathy, a tuberculous medullary cavity, a calyceal diverticulum, medullary sponge kidney and medullary calcification from hypercalcaemic and hypercalciuric states. The most important differential diagnosis is between analgesic nephropathy and reflux nephropathy (Table 14.4).

The finding of characteristic capillary sclerosis and lipofuchsin-like pigment on examination of pathological specimens provides significant clues to an analgesic aetiology.

MANAGEMENT

Once the diagnosis of analgesic nephropathy is made, the patient must be reviewed carefully for

Papillary type of RPN

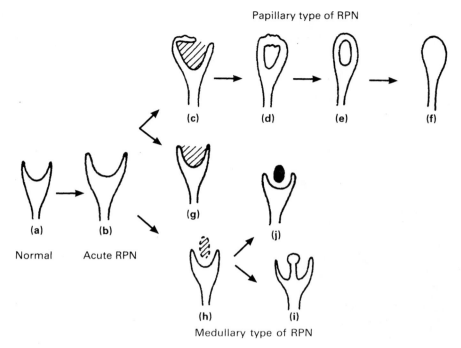

Medullary type of RPN

Fig. 14.6   The radiological types and stages of renal papillary necrosis (RPN). (**a**) Normal renal papilla. (**b**) Swollen papilla in acute RPN. Chronic RPN may be of the papillary (**c–g**) or the medullary (**h–j**) type. (**c**) Total RPN with 'flare' or horn. (**d**) 'Ring sign' with shaggy appearance suggesting recent separation of necrotic papilla. (**e**) 'Ring sign' with smooth appearance suggesting long-standing RPN. (**f**) Clubbed calyx remaining after passage of necrotic papilla. (**g**) Total RPN in situ. (**h**) Medullary type of RPN in situ. (**i**) 'Match stick' sign. (**j**) Papillary calcification. (Modified from Hare 1970)

evidence of other manifestations of the analgesic syndrome, and for complications of analgesic nephropathy and chronic renal failure, if the latter is present.

The treatment of chronic analgesic nephropathy requires careful attention to the following points.

1. Total avoidance of all NSAIDs. The single most essential aspect in the management of analgesic nephropathy is complete avoidance of all NSAIDs because almost all such drugs have significant acute and chronic nephrotoxic effects (see earlier). Regular intake of even small doses of individual analgesics such as aspirin and para-cetamol may be associated with progressive renal disease. Over 80% of patients with analgesic nephropathy stop analgesic abuse after medical counselling and the majority appear to lose their persistent headaches which were the major reason for analgesic abuse. It is essential that the long-term follow-up includes regular testing of blood and urine for evidence of continuing analgesic intake to identify patients who are at risk. The Phenistix (Ames) test is a simple and practical method of screening for salicylates in urine. Evidence of phenacetin and paracetamol intake may be obtained by laboratory screening for the metabolite p-aminophenol.

2. Maintenance of a high fluid intake. A fluid intake of greater than two litres daily ensures a high urine flow rate and affords significant protection against further renal damage and recurrent urinary tract infections.

3. Treatment of the manifestations and com-plications of analgesic nephropathy and the anal-gesic syndrome. Careful attention should be paid to all the manifestations of the analgesic syndrome (see earlier), particularly urinary tract infections, hypertension, sodium and water depletion, systemic acidosis, hyperuricaemia and secondary

Table 14.4 Differences between analgesis nephropathy and reflux nephropathy. (Reproduced with permission from Nanra 1983)

	Analgesic nephropathy	Reflux nephropathy
Clinical		
Age	Rare under 30 years	More common in children
Sex ratio	Female preponderance	Female preponderance
Childhood history	–	+/–
Peptic ulcer	+/–	–
Renal colic	+/–	–
Radiological		
Renal involvement	Bilateral	Unilateral/bilateral
Medullary calcification	35%	Rare
Calyceal abnormalities	All calyceal groups	Usually polar superior > inferior
Cortical scarring	+	+ + +
Compensatory hypertrophy	+/–	+ +
Reduction in size on serial IVUs	+	–
Dilatation of lower $\frac{1}{3}$ of ureter	–	+/–
Vesicoureteric reflux	–	+/–
Renal calculi	+/–	Rare

IVU—intravenous urogam

gout, hyperlipidaemia and renal osteodystrophy. Diuretics which may exaggerate sodium depletion and aggravate hyperuricaemia should be avoided or used with caution.

4. Careful long-term follow-up and regular review. Patients with chronic analgesic nephropathy should be regularly reviewed to allow early detection and management of serious complications. These include cardiovascular complications such as renal artery stenosis and thrombosis; cerebrovascular disease; ischaemic heart disease and peripheral vascular disease; silent obstructive uropathy which may lead to pyonephrosis; covert urinary tract infections and staghorn calculi; transitional cell carcinoma; and proteinuria.

Renovascular lesions should be suspected when blood pressure control is difficult, when antihypertensive requirements are high, when there is unexplained reduction in renal function or renal function deterioration with the use of angiotensin–converting enzyme inhibitors, or when acute malignant hypertension supervenes. Occasionally routine intravenous urography may suggest differential renal function or one 'non-functioning kidney'. Differences in renal size and abdominal bruits are usually not helpful. Renal duplex scanning, if available, is the most reliable non-invasive method for the detection of renovascular disease, with specificity and sensitivity greater than 95%. Renal perfusion scans and split isotope function studies are less reliable. The diagnosis of renal artery stenosis or thrombosis is confirmed by renal angiography. The functional significance of renal artery stenosis may be assessed by a pre- and post-captopril DTPA scan. The management of the renovascular lesion has to be planned for individual patients; the options available are continuation of medical therapy, dilation to the stenotic segment by balloon angioplasty, or direct surgical correction of the lesion by endarterectomy or a bypass procedure. Surgical management may be complicated by extensive atheromatous disease and may carry additional morbidity and mortality because of the presence of multi-organ complications, especially cardiovascular complications. Treatment of renal artery stenosis by nephrectomy should be avoided because of the serious loss of functioning renal tissue which may result in sudden deterioration in renal function and progression to terminal renal failure. The use of angiotensin-converting enzyme inhibitors in patients with unilateral renal artery stenosis is controversial. Angiotensin-converting enzyme inhibitors should be used with caution in the presence of bilateral renal parenchymal disease and should be avoided if there is bilateral renal artery stenosis because of the high risk of precipitating acute renal failure by reducing intrarenal angiotensin-dependent glomerular filtration.

The possibility of a urothelial tumour should be suspected if there is persistent isomorphic microscopic haematuria, or painless macroscopic haematuria. The investigations should include several examinations of urine for malignant cells and a comprehensive visualization of the urinary tract by intravenous urography, cystoscopy and retrograde pyelography. Urine cytology, in the hands of an experienced cytopathologist, is a simple and non-invasive test which, when positive for malignant cells, is almost diagnostic. False positive tests may occur when urine samples are collected directly from ureteric catheters. A renal pelvic carcinoma is usually treated by nephro-ureterectomy. In the presence of significant renal insufficiency, loss of one kidney may lead to a marked reduction in renal function and possible terminal renal failure.

In patients with persistent proteinuria, a renal biopsy should be considered if the proteinuria is predominantly glomerular and if proteinuria exceeds 2 g/day.

Acute renal failure in patients with analgesic nephropathy is a potentially fatal complication and requires urgent treatment by the following measures:

1. Rapid control of life-threatening complications such as hyperkalaemia, systemic acidosis and septicaemia.
2. Control of severe hypertension independently of intravascular volume depletion with drugs such as calcium channel blockers or sodium nitroprusside.
3. Establishment of an adequate urine flow by rapid volume expansion and parenteral diuretics such as frusemide and mannitol in appropriate dosage.
4. Use of acute dialysis if necessary.
5. Early exclusion of ureteric obstruction by ultrasound examination of the urinary tract and ureteric catheterization.

Obstructing papillae are frequently dislodged and fragmented by ureteric catheterization. Failure to do so may require extraction of the papilla by a Dormia basket during ureteric catheterization or by direct surgical intervention.

Urological procedures are frequently necessary in patients with analgesic nephropathy, and the common indications are diagnostic, unexplained reduction in renal function, renal colic, haematuria and persistent urinary tract infections.

COURSE AND PROGNOSIS

At the time of initial presentation, approximately 10% of patients with analgesic nephropathy have severe chronic renal failure, with GFR values below 10 ml/min per 1.73 m^2 body surface area, and usually require dialysis within six months. Of the remaining patients, within careful management, 20% show an improvement in GFR, 50% remain stable and 30% deteriorate. Those likely to deteriorate may be identified by the following adverse clinical markers:

1. Evidence of continued analgesic abuse
2. Suboptimal control of hypertension
3. Disproportionate hyperuricaemia and clinical secondary gout
4. Persistent proteinuria, especially tubular proteinuria
5. Reduced GFR at initial consultation, especially if less than 20 ml/min 1.73 m^2 body surface area.

Occasional patients develop acute irreversible reduction in GFR following malignant hypertension, nephrectomy for hydronephrosis, pyonephrosis, renal pelvic carcinoma or severe renovascular hypertension, and acute-on-chronic RPN associated with severe hypotension following complications such as gastrointestinal haemorrhage, acute pancreatitis or myocardial infarction.

The overall 5-year cumulative survival of patients with analgesic nephropathy is 70%. The common causes of mortality are ischaemic heart disease, cerebrovascular accidents, septicaemia and, in patients who are precluded from a renal replacement programme, uraemia. A transitional cell carcinoma carries a fairly poor prognosis and the 10-year survival is approximately 50%. Patients with analgesic nephropathy tend to fare relatively poorly during dialysis and post-transplantation because of the high incidence of vascular complications related to severe atherosclerosis.

REFERENCES AND RECOMMENDED READING

Burry A F 1967 The evolution of analgesic nephropathy. Nephron 5: 185–201

Dawborn J K, Fairley K F, Kincaid-Smith P, King W E 1966 The association of peptic ulceration, chronic renal disease and analgesic abuse. Quarterly Journal of Medicine 35: 69–83

Dubach U H, Rosner B, Strumer T 1991 An epidemiologic study of abuse of analgesic drugs. Effects of phenacetin and salicylate on mortality and cardiovascular morbidity (1968 to 1987). New England Journal of Medicine 324: 155–160

Duggin G G 1981 Mechanisms in the development of analgesic nephropathy. Kidney International 18: 553–561

Gault M H, Rudwal T C, Engles W D, Dossetor J B 1968 Syndrome associated with the abuse of analgesics. Annals of Internal Medicine 68: 906–925

Hare W S C 1970 The radiology of analgesic nephropathy. In: Kincaid-Smith P, Fairley K F (eds) Renal infection and renal scarring. Mercedes, Melbourne, p. 409

Kincaid-Smith P 1978 Analgesic nephropathy. Kidney International 13: 1–113

Mahony J F, Storey B G, lbanez R C, Stewart J H 1977 Analgesic abuse, renal parenchymal disease and carcinoma of the kidney or ureter. Australia and New Zealand Journal of Medicine 7: 463–469

Nanra R S 1980 Clinical and pathological aspects of analgesic nephropathy. British Journal of Clinical Pharmacology 10: 359S–368S

Nanra R S 1989 Analgesic-associated nephropathy. In: Massry S G, Glassock R J (eds) Textbook of nephrology, 2nd edn. Williams & Wilkins, Baltimore, p. 842

Nanra R S 1992 Papillary necrosis and analgesic abuse. In: Glassock R J (ed) Current therapy in nephrology and hypertension, 3rd edn. B C Decker, Mosby-Year Book, St Louis, p. 114

Nanra R S 1993 Analgesic-induced renal disease. In: Schrier R W, Gottschalk C W (Eds) Diseases of the kidney. 5th edn, Little Brown and Co., Boston p. 1104

Nanra R S, Taylor J S, de Leon A H, White K H 1978 Analgesic nephropathy: etiology, clinical syndrome, and clinicopathological correlations in Australia. Kidney International 13: 79–92

15. Reflux nephropathy

G. J. Becker

TERMINOLOGY

It was once thought that chronic tubulointerstitial nephritis was usually the result of chronic infection of the kidney, hence the term 'chronic pyelonephritis' was employed in situations where urine infection was associated with this histological appearance, particularly if renal scars were also found. This term still lingers in most general medical textbooks, though for many years nephrologists have preferred a nomenclature based more specifically on the causes of the renal damage, as in obstructive nephropathy (Ch. 28), analgesic nephropathy (Ch. 14) and reflux nephropathy. Reflux nephropathy is a common disease, characterized by coarse renal scars, and derives its name from our understanding of the pathogenesis of the disease, particularly with respect to the role of vesicoureteric reflux in infancy.

PATHOLOGY

Characteristically the renal scars consist of a deep cortical depression overlying a dilated 'clubbed' calyx (Fig. 15.1). One or both kidneys may be affected. The scars often affect the upper or lower poles (focal reflux nephropathy), but may also involve the lateral calyces or the whole kidney (generalized reflux nephropathy). This pattern of scarring can be explained by the genesis of the lesion, since each scar consists of one or more fibrotic contracted renal pyramids (see below). Compensatory hypertrophy occurs in the unaffected tissue, accentuating the irregular outline of the kidney.

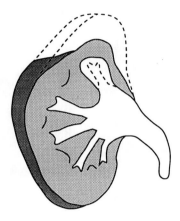

Fig. 15.1 Diagrammatic representation of typical upper polar reflux scarring

The microscopic appearance is of focal areas of chronic tubulointerstitial nephritis, with atrophy and dilatation of renal tubules and interstitial collagenous scarring with cellular infiltrates (Fig. 15.2). Periglomerular fibrosis is often prominent. Glomeruli may be affected by sclerotic changes affecting the whole glomerulus or segments (Fig. 15.3).

PATHOGENESIS OF RENAL SCARRING

The renal scars develop during infancy or early childhood. Three factors — vesicoureteric reflux (VUR), intra-renal reflux and urinary infection — combine to cause bacterial infection of one or more renal pyramids in the immature kidney. These areas of acute pyelonephritis then fail to grow, and instead contract and fibrose.

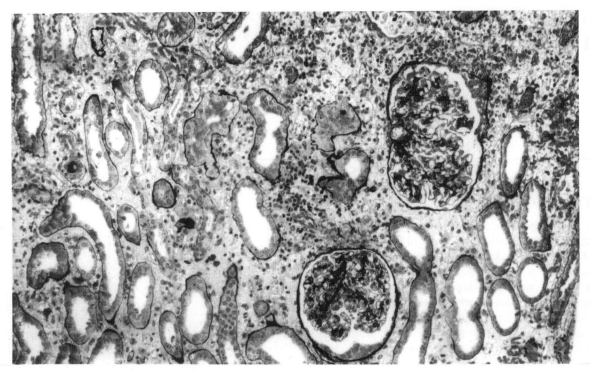

Fig. 15.2   Histological appearance in reflux nephropathy with chronic tubulointerstitial nephritis and tubular atrophy

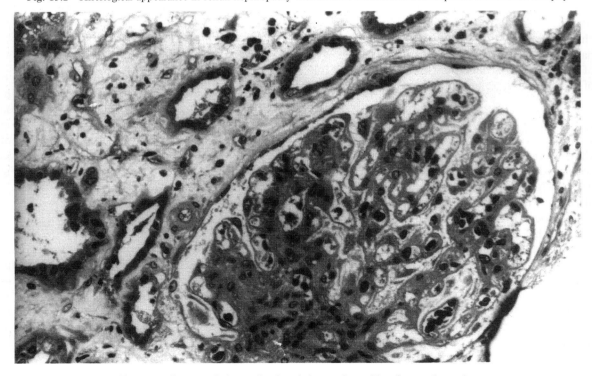

Fig. 15.3   Segmental glomerulosclerosis in a patient with reflux nephropathy

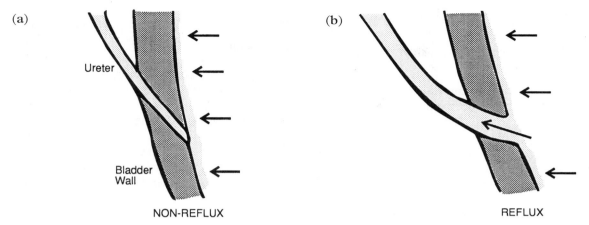

(a)

Ureter

Bladder
Wall

NON-REFLUX

(b)

REFLUX

Fig. 15.4 a, b Vesicoureteric junction. (a) In a normal, non-refluxing, vesicoureteric junction, the ureter has a long intramural tunnel and consequently the urine does not reflux up the ureter during voiding. (b) Congenital vesicoureteric reflux is associated with a short intramural tunnel, and often a wider ureteric orifice. Urine refluxes up the ureter on voiding

Vesicoureteric reflux

Normally, during micturition or at any other time when the pressure in the bladder exceeds that in the ureter, reflux of urine up the ureter is prevented by the presence of a valve mechanism at the vesicoureteric junction. The one-way valve effect depends on the oblique insertion of the ureter through the muscular bladder wall, resulting in a long intramural segment (Fig. 15.4a). In about 0.5% of neonates this mechanism is poorly developed. The tunnel is less oblique (Fig. 15.4b), and urine refluxes up the ureter, particularly during voiding. This can be detected by micturating cystography (Fig. 15.5), and through the cystoscope the ureteric orifice may be seen to be laterally placed and wider than normal. With growth the tunnel elongates, resulting in resolution of the reflux is most patients by adolescence, particularly if the reflux is only mild.

Family studies suggest that VUR is genetically determined, and it has been suggested that the inheritance follows a pattern of autosomal dominance with variable penetrance. The incidence of reflux in siblings of children with vesicoureteric reflux has been reported to be as high as 45%.

The severity of reflux can be graded according to the findings on micturating cystography (Fig. 15.6). The risk of renal scarring is proportional to the severity of reflux. It is rare for neonates

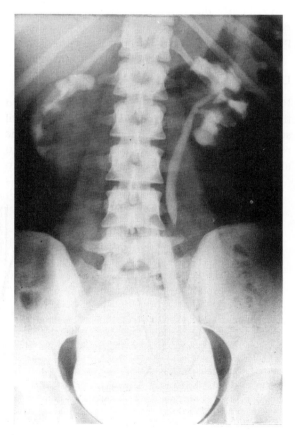

Fig. 15.5 Micturating cystogram showing radiocontrast which has been instilled through a urethral catheter refluxing up the ureter during voiding. Dilatation of the ureter and pelvis is associated

subsequently to develop scars unless the reflux is severe.

Intra-renal reflux

In some children radiocontrast can be demonstrated to reflux up the papillary ducts during micturating cystography. This intra-renal reflux is seen most commonly in the polar regions, where scars subsequently develop. Intra-renal reflux usually occurs into the compound polar papillae, where there are often gaping refluxing papillary duct orifices, unlike the slit-like non-refluxing orifices usually seen in simple papillae (Fig. 15.7). Accordingly, with severe VUR, urine can reflux into the renal substance in a distribution dictated by the presence of compound papillae. This subsequently determines the pattern of scarring. About 90% of kidneys have one or more compound papillae.

Urinary tract infection

Prospective studies in children have demonstrated that the usual initiating event leading to renal scarring is urinary tract infection. Vesicoureteric reflux can result in introduction of organisms into all areas affected by intra-renal reflux, leading to

local acute bacterial infection of the kidney with consequent scarring of the affected renal pyramid(s). This segment of the kidney then progresses to fibrous contracture, while the rest of the kidney grows normally or even hypertrophies; accordingly the depth of the scar increases as the child ages.

It has been suggested that this scarring occurs with the first one or two episodes of urine infection. Accordingly patients often already have renal scars when they present, and new scars are seen to develop infrequently in previously normal kidneys.

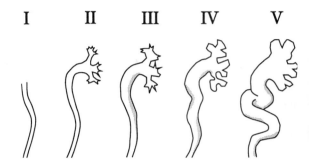

Fig. 15.6 Reflux grades I–V as defined in the International Reflux Study in Children. A grading from mild reflux affecting only ureter (grade I) to severe, with dilatation of the ureter and pelvis (grade V) is used in this study

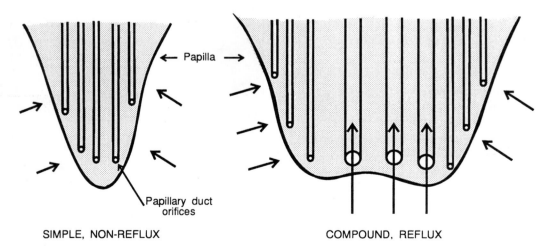

Fig. 15.7 A comparison of the simple non-refluxing papillary duct structure, with the compound, refluxing, papillary duct structure commonly found in the polar areas of kidneys. The simple non-reflux papilla has papillary duct orifices which are slit-like and do not allow reflux on voiding. The compound papillae have wide-open papillary duct orifices which allow urine to pass up into the papillae on voiding.

There are, however, some patients (particularly males) with typical reflux scarring but no past history suggestive of urine infection. In pigs, high pressure intra-renal reflux can lead to focal renal scarring, and it may be that sterile reflux can similarly damage kidneys in man. Another controversial possibility is that of 'congenital reflux nephropathy' whereby either intrauterine reflux, or coincidental malformation of the vesicoureteric junction and the kidney, might result in children being born with grossly malformed kidneys in association with reflux. Neither of these propositions is proven.

Irrespective of the relative contribution of reflux and urine infection it is clear that virtually all the renal scarring is fully developed by adolescence, and that the future progression of the disease is virtually independent of either factor; instead it depends mainly on the development of segmental glomerulosclerosis in the residual nephrons.

PREVALENCE

The exact prevalence of VUR and reflux nephropathy is difficult to determine. Though it appears that about 0.5% of neonates have vesicoureteric reflux, scarring occurs in only a small proportion of these children. In neonates reflux seems to occur with equal frequency in males and females, however subsequently females detected with reflux scarring outnumber males by a factor of at least 5 to 1.

1–2% of schoolgirls have bacteriuria, and of these 20–35% have VUR, again suggesting a prevalence of around 0.5%. Similarly studies in adult females, of whom 3–5% have bacteriuria, show that of these about 10–20% have renal scarring, suggesting a prevalence of reflux nephropathy in females of around 0.3–0.5%.

It must be emphasized that only a small proportion of children with reflux progress to reflux nephropathy.

CLINICAL FEATURES

Most patients present with urine infection, though pregnancy complications and features of renal damage such as hypertension, proteinuria or renal failure can also precipitate diagnosis. Males are particularly likely to present with features of renal damage.

Urine infection

Urinary tract infection is the most common clinical problem associated with vesicoureteric reflux and reflux nephropathy. With severe reflux, stasis due to the large volumes of refluxing urine is probably at least partially responsible for a predisposition to UTI, but in less severe cases the predisposition to bladder infection is probably coincidental (see Ch. 16).

In neonates urinary infection commonly manifests as fever and failure to thrive. In older patients the usual symptoms of dysuria, frequency, and acute pyelonephritis can occur. The first detected infection may occur in childhood or, in females, with sexual activity or pregnancy. In most patients infections are recurrent.

The commonest clinical picture is of a woman with a history of recurrent urine infections and scarred kidneys, who may go on to develop hypertension and renal failure.

Hypertension

Reflux nephropathy often causes hypertension. It is responsible for over 60% of severe hypertension in children. About 60% of adults with reflux nephropathy are hypertensive at presentation.

Proteinuria and renal failure

It is now obvious, at least in the adult, that late progression to renal failure occurs not because of ongoing reflux scarring, but because of the development of focal glomerulosclerosis (Fig. 15.3). The glomerular lesion is manifested by the presence of proteinuria. About 45% of adults with reflux nephropathy excrete more than 0.2 g of protein in the urine per 24 hours, and 20% more than 1 g/24 h. Proteinuria is more common in patients with impaired renal function, and there is a strong correlation between the presence and severity of proteinuria and renal prognosis.

Reflux nephropathy is the cause of renal failure in about 10% of patients commencing maintenance dialysis in Australasia and Europe, at a mean age of 30 years. This is the lowest mean age of commencing treatment among the common causes of chronic renal failure. The incidence of renal failure due to reflux nephropathy is approximately equal between the sexes.

Other clinical features

Less common features of reflux nephropathy include loin pain when voiding, childhood enuresis, and renal calculi. A family history is common, and other developmental abnormalities of the urinary tract, particularly duplex ureters, may be present. Though there are many bladder abnormalities, such as posterior urethral valves and neurogenic bladder, associated with both reflux and scarring, the precise relationship of the VUR to the scarring is often unclear, since urinary obstruction is usually also present.

Reflux nephropathy and pregnancy

The presence of renal scarring and a predisposition to urine infection has a significant influence on pregnancy. Attacks of acute pyelonephritis, pregnancy-induced hypertension, pre-eclampsia and fetal prematurity are all common complications of pregnancy in women with reflux nephropathy. In those with already impaired renal function acceleration of renal failure may occur.

DIAGNOSIS

Radiological appearance

The diagnosis of reflux nephropathy mainly depends on the demonstration of typical scarring by intravenous pyelography. Coarse cortical indentations are seen over dilated calyces. This can occur on all aspects of the kidney though the poles are most frequently affected. Hypertrophy of unaffected tissue occurs, and gross disparity in renal size is common. A wide variety of distortion of the kidneys can result, depending on the severity and distribution of the scars (Fig. 15.8).

The differential diagnoses include obstructive nephropathy in which the calyceal dilatation and cortical thinning is generalized (unless the obstruction has affected only part of the kidney), renal papillary necrosis (Ch. 14) where both kidneys are usually equally affected and the scarring is less coarse, vascular infarction of a pyramid when the calyx should not be clubbed, and renal tuberculosis where strictures are also usually seen.

Renal radionuclear imaging

Radionuclide imaging (Ch. 5) using compounds which are retained by the proximal tubule cells, such as ^{99m}Tc-labelled dimercaptosuccinic acid (DMSA), has been demonstrated to be a very sensitive way of detecting early scarring, or the areas of inflamed but not yet contracted tissue, in young children.

Micturating cystography and cystoscopy

The diagnosis can be confirmed by micturating cystography showing reflux (Fig. 15.5) or by cystoscopy where lateral gaping ureteric orifices may be seen. Since patient management is rarely altered by these tests they are not normally performed except in very young children or when surgery is contemplated.

Renal biopsy

Renal biopsy is usually not indicated in patients with reflux scarring. Occasionally a renal biopsy from a patient with an apparently normal intravenous pyelogram shows a histological picture similar to reflux nephropathy. Careful review of the IVP or a DMSA scan will often reveal subtle changes. The entity of 'non-scarred' reflux nephropathy diagnosed histologically remains controversial, but on theoretical grounds there is no reason that it should not occur since imaging techniques to show renal scars are moderately insensitive.

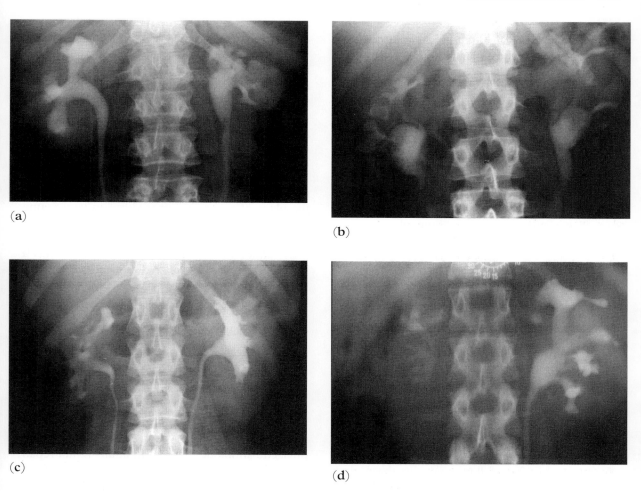

Fig. 15.8a–d   IVPs in reflux nephropathy.

Early screening for reflux

The early diagnosis of reflux in children is an area of great concern, since prevention of scarring is dependent on very early diagnosis. As yet a reliable non-invasive method for screening neonates is not available. Studies addressing the use of ultrasound of fetal kidneys in utero suggest that detection of renal pelvic dilatation may be useful in predicting severe reflux. Similarly ultrasound after birth can be helpful. Micturating cystography is an invasive and uncomfortable procedure and can only be currently justified in screening the children of parents with a strong history of familial reflux.

MANAGEMENT OF REFLUX NEPHROPATHY

The most important aspects of management are control of urine infection and hypertension. The place of anti-reflux surgery and of various manoeuvres to prevent progression are much more controversial.

Control of urine infection

Urine infection in early childhood is believed to be critical in the genesis of reflux scarring. Moreover throughout life it is the major cause of morbidity, at least in females.

In children with VUR or reflux nephropathy, prophylactic chemotherapy to prevent urine infection and regular surveillance for asymptomatic bacteriuria is recommended. Should urine infection occur it should be treated promptly, and eradication proven by follow-up urine culture. Most would recommend prophylactic antibiotic therapy until puberty or until reflux has been shown to have resolved.

It is no longer believed that recurrent urine infections in adults lead to significant permanent renal damage; however the morbidity of recurrent cystitis or pyelonephritis is sufficient to justify surveillance and appropriate treatment.

Control of hypertension

About 20% of children with reflux nephropathy become hypertensive, and the disease is the commonest cause of accelerated hypertension in children. Over 60% of adults with reflux scarring are hypertensive. Hypertension is a major risk factor, not only for cardiovascular disease, but also for subsequent renal functional decline. In particular, very rapid deterioration in function will occur if accelerated hypertension supervenes. Accordingly the blood pressure should be checked regularly, and treated appropriately. Adolescence is a particular time for concern, since many patients are lost from follow-up during this period, and re-present with severe hypertension and impaired renal function.

Anti-reflux surgery

Paradoxically, in this disease which occurs because of vesicoureteric reflux, there is little evidence that repair of the reflux alters the course of the disease.

Anti-reflux operations are usually based on re-inserting the ureter through a new, longer, intramural tunnel. Recently a variety of techniques whereby the tunnel is strengthened by the injection of material (e.g. polytetrafluoroethylene or collagen) around the ureteric orifice have been developed, allowing eradication of reflux by a less invasive cystoscopic approach.

Though it is clear that anti-reflux surgery is rarely indicated there is controversy relating to the place of anti-reflux procedures in very young children with severe reflux. Though two large-scale trials in children also treated by prophylactic antibiotics have been unable to show a reduction in scarring in the surgical cases, these trials are not yet complete and many paediatric urologists still recommend repair in this situation. Certainly, if compliance with prophylaxis against infection is likely to be a problem, surgery has a role to play.

In both adults and children anti-reflux procedures seem not to reduce the frequency of attacks of cystitis, however because attacks of clinical acute pyelonephritis are less common such a procedure may be indicated in patients with recurrent pyelonephritis not controllable by prophylactic antibiotic therapy. In adults reflux repair has no influence on the progression of renal failure and therefore should not be performed for this purpose.

RECOMMENDED READING

Arant B S 1991 Vesicoureteric reflux and renal injury. American Journal of Kidney Diseases 17: 491–511

Bailey R R 1973 The relationship of vesicoureteric reflux to urinary tract infection and chronic pyelonephritis — reflux nephropathy. Clinical Nephrology 1: 132–141

Becker G J 1985 Reflux nephropathy. Australian New Zealand Journal of Medicine 15: 668–675

Cardiff–Oxford Bacteriuria Study Group 1978 Sequelae of covert bacteriuria in schoolgirls. A four-year follow-up study. Lancet Vol 1: 889–893

Cotran R S 1982 Glomerulosclerosis in reflux nephropathy. Kidney International 21: 528–534

Edwards D, Normand I C S, Prescod N et al 1977 Disappearance of vesicoureteric reflux during long-term prophylaxis of urinary tract infection in children. British Medical Journal 2: 285–288

Ransley P G, Risdon P G 1979 The pathogenesis of reflux nephropathy. Controversy in Nephrology 16: 90–97

Rolleston G L, Maling J M J, Hodson C J 1974 Intrarenal reflux and the scarred kidney. Archives of Diseases in Children 49: 531–539

Torres V E, Velosa J A, Holley K E et al 1980 The progression of vesicoureteric reflux nephropathy. Annals of Internal Medicine 92: 776–786

White R H R, O'Donnell B 1990 Managemet of urinary tract infection and vesicoureteric reflux in children. British Medical Journal 300: 1391–1394

Zucchelli P, Gaggi R 1991 Reflux nephropathy in adults. Nephron 57: 2–9

16. Urinary tract infection

R. R. Bailey

INTRODUCTION

Urinary tract infections (UTI) are the commonest bacterial infections treated in general practice and are responsible for considerable morbidity, particularly for women in the sexually active age group. Infections in the urinary tract range from asymptomatic bacteriuria to severe sepsis, often with hospital-acquired organisms, affecting high-risk patients such as diabetics or those on immunosuppressive therapy.

DEFINITION

Apart from the outer one third of the female urethra, the urinary tract is normally sterile. UTI can be defined as a condition in which bacteria are multiplying within the urinary tract, regardless of bacterial count.

PATHOGENESIS

Urinary tract infections

Except in the first year of life and after the age of 60 years, UTI predominantly affect females. The entry of bacteria into the female bladder is facilitated by the short urethra and this explains, at least in part, the observation that recurrent symptomatic UTI frequently follow sexual intercourse. Even gentle massage of the vagina can lead to organisms being introduced into the bladder. In one study, 30% of sexual intercourse episodes resulted in a significant increase in the colony counts of bacteria in clean voided urine specimens. These increases in bacterial counts induced by intercourse were asymptomatic and transient.

Some workers feel that women whose external urethral meatus is pushed intravaginally during sexual intercourse are more prone to UTI. The direction of the hymenal scar may influence the orientation of a woman's urethral meatus during intercourse.

The presence of residual bladder urine is important in allowing an inoculum of bacteria to multiply within the urinary tract. The frequency of recurrences of UTI is increased in women with small but significant increases (1–10 ml) in the volume of residual urine. In many women this residual urine appears to stem simply from a bad bladder emptying habit. Some females with recurrent UTI have persistence of uninhibited infantile bladder contractions.

Many women using diaphragms for contraceptive purposes have an altered vaginal flora. Instead of the normal lactobacilli the vagina becomes invaded by enterobacterial organisms. This may explain why women using diaphragms have an increased prevalence of both symptomatic and asymptomatic *Escherichia coli* UTI compared with women using other methods, or no contraception. The presence of a diaphragm may alter the angle of the bladder neck and therefore affect bladder emptying. The additional use of a spermicide may also be important as available preparations encourage the growth of enterobacterial organisms. A cervical erosion may act as a continuing source of infection.

Infection due to two or more bacterial species, or to more than one serotype of *Esch. coli*, is uncommon. There are theoretical reasons why, in a dynamic system, UTI are invariably due to a single strain. Genuine mixed infection is most common in patients with multiple urinary calculi.

Esch. coli remains the predominant urinary tract pathogen, but as many as one quarter of symptomatic UTI in general practice are due to *Staphylococcus saprophyticus* (novobiocin-resistant coagulase-negative staphylococcus). The surface agglutinin of this pathogen appears to be a key determinant of virulence permitting it to colonize the urinary tract. The third commonest urinary tract pathogen in domiciliary UTI is *Proteus mirabilis*. This organism, and the other *Proteus species*, invariably involve the kidney, possibly because of their high motility or ability to adhere to the urothelium. *Proteus species* also have the ability to split urinary urea into ammonia, which by trapping hydrogen ions leads to an alkaline urine and the risk of stone formation. Other urinary tract pathogens, and those that are more frequently seen in hospitalized patients, include the *Proteus species* other than *mirabilis*, *Streptococcus faecalis*, *Klebsiella pneumoniae*, *Enterobacter sp*, *Acinetobacter sp*, *Pseudomonas aeruginosa* and *Serratia marcescens*.

The bacteria which produce a UTI are mainly derived from the patient's faecal flora. Some strains or serotypes of *Esch. coli* involved in UTI invade the kidneys more commonly than others. Furthermore, although strains of *Esch. coli* reach the bladder in proportion to their frequency in the faecal flora, strains rich in K antigen are more likely to succeed in subsequently invading the kidney. This is probably due to the inhibitory action of K antigens on phagocytosis and destruction by complement.

In the great majority of women with recurrent UTI the infecting organism is a new strain with each episode. Women who suffer recurrent UTI have a higher number of enterobacterial organisms in the introital region but this does not appear to be related to poor hygiene.

Esch. coli strains isolated from patients with acute pyelonephritis are frequently characterized by traits considered important for virulence. The strains belong to a limited number of O:K:H serotypes [i.e. combinations of lipopolysaccharide (O), capsular polysaccharide (K), and flagellar antigens (H)], they carry fimbrial adhesins, are resistant to killing by serum, and produce haemolysin.

There has been considerable research into the ability of urinary tract pathogens to adhere to urothelial cells. This ability has been attributed to both the degree of piliation of the bacteria and the increased number of receptor sites on the urothelial cells of women with a tendency to recurrent UTI. The receptor density on urothelial cells may be genetically determined and is higher in patients with UTI and renal parenchymal scarring than in healthy controls.

Bacterial adherence signifies the ability of an organism to bind to host cells, e.g. mucosal epithelial cells. In the urinary tract, adherence may increase bacterial virulence by several mechanisms. Attachment may promote persistence by reducing elimination at the time of micturition. In patients, however, most isolates that persist the longest are in those who have asymptomatic bacteriuria, i.e. lack adhesive capacity. Attachment helps to localize *Esch. coli* to the upper urinary tract as receptors for this organism are on epithelial cells of the ureter and renal pelvis as well as the lower urinary tract. In epidemiological studies, attaching *Esch. coli* are associated mainly with acute pyelonephritis. In addition attachment may promote inflammation, such as is characteristic of acute pyelonephritis.

An assessment has been made of the relation of certain glycolipids present in human urothelial cells and the pattern of variation among individuals of different blood groups and secretor status. Studies have shown that in adults the expression of these glycolipids is dependent on P and ABO blood group systems and on secretor status.

The adhesion of pyelonephritogenic strains of *Esch. coli* is often mediated by P fimbriae with specificity for glycosphingolipids corresponding to antigens of the P blood group system. P fimbriae mediate bacterial adherence to human epithelial cells via digalactoside-specific binding to the P blood group antigens which are expressed on cells throughout the urinary tract in P-positive individuals. *Esch. coli* from the urine of women with acute pyelonephritis express P fimbriae in nearly all cases. In contrast, less than 50% of *Esch. coli* from women with cystitis express P fimbriae.

Girls with acute pyelonephritis in the setting of vesicoureteric reflux have been reported to have a decreased likelihood of having *Esch. coli* with P fimbriae, as compared with girls without reflux. This suggests that adherence mediated by P fimbriae may be less important when the defences of the upper urinary tract are compromised by an anatomical or functional abnormality. A plausible interpretation of these findings is that a variety of functional and anatomical abnormalities in the urinary tract permit *Esch. coli* lacking P fimbriae to ascend the ureter, establish renal infection and cause subsequent bacteraemia. This is consistent with the findings that the proportion of strains that are P fimbriated is lowest in those patients with abnormalities of the upper urinary tract.

In contrast to normal patients where organisms causing *Esch. coli* urosepsis express P fimbriae in all cases and have minimal antibiotic resistance, infection in those patients with compromising urological or medical conditions is caused by organisms that lack P fimbriae and are resistant to multiple antibiotics. This suggests that, in contrast to the situation in normal patients, in those patients with urinary tract abnormalities, urinary tract instrumentation or medical illness non-P fimbriated *Esch. coli* may have access to the kidneys, be traumatically introduced into tissues as a result of urinary tract instrumentation or evade phagocytosis and result in bacteraemia.

Uncircumcised infant boys have more symptomatic UTI than those who are circumcised. Uncircumcised males who do not cleanse under the foreskin may have a potential source of infecting enterobacterial organisms. Healthy males secrete a potent antibacterial substance (possibly related to its zinc content) in their prostatic fluid, but in men with persistent or chronic bacterial prostatitis the gland seems incapable of eradicating the infection.

Homosexual males have a much higher incidence of symptomatic UTI than heterosexual males. UTI will be present in 5% of homosexually active men with acute urinary tract symptoms. These infections are invariably due to *Esch. coli* which have been shown on serotyping to be from the dominant strain in the stools. This patient group is at increased risk of UTI.

Human urine lacks both cellular and humoral defence mechanisms and it is therefore not surprising that it readily supports bacterial growth. The generation time of a particular bacterial strain in urine may be influenced by factors such as the pH, osmolality, concentration of urea or glucose, amino acid composition, the special properties of the urine in certain physiological situations (e.g. pregnancy) and the antibacterial properties of the urothelium.

Complement, lysozyme and antibody play a role in the bacteriolysis of Gram-negative bacteria. In some patients with infection of the upper urinary tract the infecting Gram-negative bacillus is sensitive to the bactericidal activity of normal serum but is not killed by the patient's own serum. In such patients, however, the serum is able to kill closely related bacterial strains. Serum has been shown to contain an antibacterial factor (a 7S globulin) specific for the homologous strain. Phagocytosis in urine is impaired because phagocytes are relatively ineffective in a hyperosmolar environment.

Although the ascending route is common for most UTI, there may also be haematogenous spread. There is little evidence of lymphatic spread of infection through the urinary tract.

Abacterial cystitis (urethral syndrome)

The aetiology of abacterial cystitis remains unknown, but is almost certainly multifactorial. In girls the syndrome may be due to a vulvitis or threadworm infection, while irritation from antiseptics, deodorants or bubble baths may be responsible in some women.

Most of the effort put into understanding this condition has gone towards establishing possible microbial causes. The balance of opinion is against a role for urethral colonization with lactobacilli and other lower genital tract commensals as these organisms are found just as frequently in healthy control women. Candidates for possible pathogens include infection with low numbers of aerobic organisms, or infection with *Chlamydia trachomatis*, *Neisseria gonorrhoeae*, *Trichomonas vaginalis* and *Herpes simplex* (types 1 and 2) as well as anaerobic organisms and other fastidious organisms such as *Gardnerella vaginalis* or *Ureaplasma urealyticum*.

Bacterial L-forms have also been suggested as a cause of abacterial cystitis, but they are extremely difficult to isolate. These osmotically fragile variants have lost their cell wall, either as a result of treatment with an antibiotic that interferes with cell wall synthesis (e.g. β-lactam antibiotics) or because of natural defence mechanisms. The hypertonicity of the renal medulla encourages their survival and once the antibiotic has been stopped the infectious agent reverts to its bacterial form. It is likely that this is the mechanism responsible for many true relapses of infection.

Many post-menopausal women who have problems with frequency, dysuria and urgency, but sterile urine, may be improved by treating their atrophic vaginitis (e.g. with dienoestrol 0.01% cream).

CLINICAL PRESENTATIONS

A patient with a UTI may present at one end of the clinical spectrum with a severe systemic illness or be completely asymptomatic at the other extreme.

Clinical presentations of urinary tract infections
1. Symptomatic
   Frequency–dysuria syndrome
      Bacterial cystitis
      Abacterial cystitis (urethral syndrome)
   Acute pyelonephritis
   Acute prostatitis
2. Covert (asymptomatic)

Symptomatic urinary tract infections

Symptoms may be referable to the lower urinary tract and include frequency, dysuria, urgency, strangury, initial or terminal haematuria and suprapubic discomfort. If bacteriuria is demonstrated this syndrome is referred to as *bacterial cystitis*. However, up to one third of women suffering from frequency and dysuria do not have bacteriuria. This has been termed the *urethral syndrome* or *abacterial cystitis* (the preferred term).

Some patients present with loin pain, tender kidneys, fever and rigors and may have a positive blood culture. This is the syndrome of *acute pyelonephritis*.

Males with *acute bacterial prostatitis* present with 'flu-like' symptoms, low backache, often few urinary tract symptoms and have a swollen tender prostate gland.

Urinary tract symptoms, especially those referable to the bladder and urethra, may not correlate with the site of infection.

A detailed physical examination is rarely beneficial but a distended bladder should be excluded. In the male it is important to do a rectal examination and to examine the genitalia, and in a woman to do a pelvic examination and view the cervix. Some women with UTI will also have a vaginal thrush infection, while others may have an associated cervicitis, often with enterobacterial organisms. These problems should be treated specifically, as they may be a focus for further ascending UTI.

Covert (asymptomatic) UTI

Patients are rarely completely asymptomatic when bacteriuria is present. However, they do not present to their general practitioners but come to attention when the urine is cultured for some other reason. They frequently admit to an odour to the urine and state that they are suspicious that there may be something wrong with the urinary tract.

Many different populations of healthy individuals have been screened for covert bacteriuria but, with the exception of pregnancy, there is no good evidence to support routine screening.

Neonates

In a Christchurch study 1% of 1460 neonates had covert bacteriuria. 11 of the 14 infected children were male and 8 were found to have vesicoureteric reflux. In some instances the bacteriuria cleared spontaneously.

Schoolchildren

In American schoolgirls aged 6–18 years the prevalence rate of covert bacteriuria was 1.2%, but only 0.03% for boys of the same age. A prevalence rate of 1% was also found among a series of

Christchurch girls who were leaving high school or starting university or nursing training. When these same girls returned for contraceptive advice to a student health clinic the prevalence rate had increased to almost 10%.

Non-pregnant women

Sexually active women screened for covert bacteriuria in many communities have shown a prevalence rate in the range of 3–10%. An American study demonstrated a 1.6% prevalence rate of bacteriuria amongst 3303 nuns. Of these, 2212 were under 45 years of age and for them the prevalence rate was only 0.6%, i.e. comparable to schoolgirls.

Pregnant women

The earliest populations screened were pregnant women, of whom usually 5–6% were found to have covert bacteriuria. The latter was not necessarily associated with pyuria. The reported rates varied from 2% in a private clinic in the United States to 18.5% in a report on urbanized New Zealand Maori women. The reasons for such a high prevalence rate in Maori women remains obscure.

In women with bacteriuria during pregnancy the reported incidence of acute pyelonephritis developing in the later stages of the pregnancy or the puerperium has been in the range of 15–40% (usually about 15–20%). In some early studies it was shown that women with bacteriuria in pregnancy were at an increased risk of developing pre-eclampsia, lowered fetal birth weight, shortened gestation interval, more congenital fetal defects, increased perinatal mortality, infected amniotic fluid and transference of the infection to the infant. Subsequent reports indicate that these risks are not as high as was initially thought.

About 20% (18–51%) of women with covert bacteriuria in pregnancy have a radiological abnormality of the urinary tract (e.g. reflux nephropathy, stones, pelviureteric obstruction, achalasia of the ureter, ureterocele) which may require surgery. The incidence of urinary tract abnormalities is similar in women with covert bacteriuria who are not pregnant. There is no evidence that the bacteriuria has been the cause of these lesions.

The elderly

Although the prevalence of covert bacteriuria is fairly constant in any given community the affected individuals are continually changing. Elderly, institutionalized women have a very high prevalence of asymptomatic bacteriuria. However, healthy elderly women and men both have a steeply increasing prevalence of bacteriuria with age.

CLASSIFICATION OF URINARY TRACT INFECTIONS

From a clinical and management point of view it is useful to classify UTI as uncomplicated or complicated. All UTI in males should be considered as complicated.

Classification of urinary tract infections
1. Uncomplicated
   Normal urinary tract
   Normal renal function
2. Complicated
   Abnormal urinary tract (e.g. calculi, vesicoureteric reflux, reflux nephropathy, analgesic nephropathy, obstruction, paraplegia, ileal conduit, atonic bladder, indwelling catheter, chronic prostatitis)
   Impaired host defences (e.g. neutropenia, immunosuppressive therapy, organ transplant recipient, diabetes mellitus)
   Impaired renal function
   Virulent organism (e.g. urease-producing *Proteus sp*, metastatic staphylococcal infection)
   All males

DIAGNOSIS

The diagnosis of a UTI can only be proven by culturing the urine. This may constitute a problem in clinical practice. Difficulties in the management of these infections make a careful follow-up of such patients essential. To ensure that follow-up is confined to patients who really are infected, an accurate bacteriological diagnosis is necessary. This policy must apply to infants, children and males. A case can be made, however, to withhold a urine culture in a woman in the sexually active age group who has an isolated episode of cystitis. It may be more cost-effective to treat the women with a single dose or a three-day course of treatment and only culture the urine if the symptoms do not resolve or recur shortly after completing treatment.

Midstream specimen

The most widely used method of obtaining urine for culture is the clean-catch midstream (MSU) technique. All variations of this method suffer from the disadvantage that some contamination of the specimen is inevitable in the female. As only 2% of normal women are able to void a completely sterile urine it is necessary to quantitate the bacterial content of the MSU specimen. Kass provided systematic statistical analyses of bacterial counts on urine in order to establish reliable criteria for separating contamination from true infection with Gram-negative bacilli. No corresponding data were produced for infections with Gram-positive cocci. These findings have been misinterpreted by many, even though it was stressed that it was necessary to accept several basic constraints when interpreting the results.

A single MSU specimen, with a bacterial colony count of $> 100\ 000/ml$ ($> 100 \times 10^6/1$), represents only an 80% confidence level in diagnosing a UTI in a female who is asymptomatic or has only mild lower urinary tract symptoms. This means that in this clinical context 20% of positive cultures are false positives and represent heavy contamination of the specimen. Such an error rate has been obtained under ideal conditions from populations of healthy, agile, cooperative young women attending special screening clinics. To ensure more accuracy in diagnosis multiple cultures of MSU specimens are necessary. A small number of women with sterile bladder urine persistently produce heavily contaminated MSUs. Such women carry large numbers of enterobacterial organisms in their introital region.

A bacterial count of $> 100\ 000$ colonies/ml ($> 100 \times 10^6/1$) in an MSU from a patient with acute pyelonephritis has a confidence limit exceeding 95%.

In women with marked frequency of micturition, or those infected with *Staphylococcus saprophyticus* the bacterial count may be low. Stamm et al demonstrated that if a woman has urinary tract symptoms and an MSU specimen has been collected and handled carefully then a single pathogen present in a count as low as 100/ml may indicate a UTI. A recent international working party has encouraged the use of a bacterial count of $> 1000/ml$ ($> 10^6/1$) of a potential pathogen in a symptomatic female as a diagnostic criterion, although there was some support for a figure of $> 10\ 000/ml$ ($> 10 \times 10^6 /1$).

In males, where there is a much reduced risk of contaminating a voided MSU specimen, a bacterial count of $>1000/ml$ ($> 10^6 /1$) of a pathogen has a very high confidence limit.

In general practice, hospital practice and in the majority of outpatient clinics there is usually no preparation of supervision of patients before or during the collection of MSU samples, and often an unacceptable delay in culturing the specimens. Special problems also exist in the collection of samples from infants and children, the elderly, bedridden or paraplegic patients, from women who are menstruating or who have a vaginal discharge, and from patients in the post-surgical or postpartum period. In infants and children the confidence limit for a single positive culture from an MSU, or from a specimen collected in an adhesive bag is less than 40%. For women in the puerperium, even with extremely careful urine collection, 30% of MSU cultures have been demonstrated to give false positive results.

Colony counting of MSU is laborious, but this has been simplified by the introduction of the quantitative loop, the filter-paper method and the many variations of the dip-inoculum method which are now commercially available. Chemical screening tests have proved generally unsatisfactory and many are too crude for individual patient examination. Some dipstick reagent strips now include the nitrite test or a test to detect leucocytes. If a patient has acute urinary tract symptoms, a positive nitrite test and the presence of pyuria then it is extremely likely that the urine is infected.

Symptomatic UTI are invariably accompanied by > 10 leucocytes/cmm (> $10 \times 10^6/1$) in uncentrifuged fresh urine. If contamination of the specimen can be excluded, this is evidence of an inflammatory (not necessarily infective) process. The leucocyte concentration gives an accurate assessment of the leucocyte excretion rate. Of women with asymptomatic bacteriuria only about one half will have > 10 leucocytes/cmm (> $10 \times 10^6/1$) in the urine. The presence of pyuria is therefore of no value as a screening procedure for detecting patients with bacteriuria. Similarly the presence of proteinuria is of no value in screening for bacteriuria. This point deserves emphasis because some laboratories will not culture the specimen unless proteinuria is detected or leucocytes are seen during a non-quantitative assessment.

Suprapubic aspirate

The technique of suprapubic aspiration (SPA) of the distended bladder has made the diagnosis of UTI much more rapid, efficient and accurate. Contamination of the specimen is avoided and this eliminates the extra work and inconvenience of doing multiple MSUs and the need for quantitative bacterial counts — any bacteria obtained by SPA can be regarded as significant. In most infected SPA specimens bacteria can be seen microscopically in a drop of unspun urine, and prompt treatment instituted. The technique of SPA is safe for all groups of patients, including infants and children, simpler than a venepuncture, quicker than obtaining a carefully collected MSU, readily acceptable to patients and easily performed by trained nurses. In addition there is no urgency about transporting the specimen to the laboratory. This technique must be used in order to appreciate its simplicity and obvious advantages but it is important to wait for a 'full' bladder.

In a study of asymptomatic women it was shown that > 100 000/ml (> $100 \times 10^6/1$) Gram-negative bacteria in an MSU were confirmed by SPA in 92%, and in 70% when the urine contained Gram-positive bacteria. When the MSU culture contained more than one bacterial species, the presence of infection was confirmed by SPA in only 11%. When there were 10 000–100 000/ml ($10–100 \times 10^6/1$) in the MSU the finding of Gram-negative bacteria indicated a UTI in 74%, but the presence of Gram-positive organisms was confirmed by SPA in only 30% and mixed organisms in 2%.

SPA should be used more widely in clinical practice.

Catheter specimen

There is little justification, except in unusual circumstances, for catheterizing the bladder specifically to obtain a specimen of urine for culture. Although such a specimen rarely leads to false positive results the technique may introduce bacteria into the bladder, and is uncomfortable and also time-consuming.

In elderly women, particularly those who are incapacitated, it is often difficult to obtain uncontaminated urine using the MSU technique and they may not be able to hold an adequate volume of urine in their bladder for SPA. In these circumstances the use of the Alexa bag catheter or a straight plastic catheter is recommended.

Prostatic specimens

When prostatic infection is suspected, localization of the UTI is required and the voided urine and expressed prostatic secretions (EPS) are partitioned. When the man has a full bladder, the glans penis is washed and then the first 5–10 ml of urine (VB_1 — voided bladder 1) is collected and cultured for 'urethral' organisms. An MSU specimen (VB_2), or a specimen obtained by SPA, will then define what organism is in the bladder. The prostate gland is then massaged and any EPS are cultured, followed by the first 5–10 ml of urine (VB_3) voided immediately after the massage. When a prostatic infection is present the EPS culture will be positive and the count in VB_3 will exceed that in VB_1. When VB_2 or an SPA is infected it indicates the existence of bladder bacteriuria, which may or may not be associated with a prostatic infection.

ESTABLISHING THE SITE OF INFECTION

Localization tests are a useful research tool but are not widely used and are of little clinical value.

Direct techniques

In 50% of patients with covert bacteriuria or bacterial cystitis the infection involves the upper urinary tract. A simple but laborious method of localization is the Fairley bladder washout test, which localizes the bacteriuria to either the upper or lower tract. Selective ureteric catheterization will identify the side of an upper tract infection. Percutaneous needling of the renal pelvis can also be used to localize the UTI to one kidney. Confirmed upper UTI requires more careful and intensive investigation, treatment, and subsequent follow-up.

Renal biopsy is of limited value because of the small sample of tissue obtained and the patchy nature of renal parenchymal infection.

Indirect techniques

In renal parenchymal infection the maximum concentrating ability of the kidneys may be impaired. This can be assessed by measuring urinary osmolality after overnight dehydration, after dehydration until there has been a 3% reduction in body weight, or following the administration of intranasal desmopressin. This defect is non-specific and reversible after the infection has been treated. In some patients with acute pyelonephritis there may also be a temporary reduction in glomerular filtration rate.

Serum antibody titres to the infecting organism, as measured by haemagglutination or direct bacterial agglutination using the patient's own organism as antigen, have not fulfilled expectations in identifying patients with renal parenchymal involvement. General correlations have been demonstrated between these antibody titres and defects in concentrating ability, but the results are variable and not sufficiently predictive to be of clinical value.

The antibody-coated bacteria technique was developed for differentiating the site of UTI. This technique uses direct immunofluorescence to detect antibody-coated bacteria in urine sediment on the basis that antibody-coated bacteria are found in the urine of patients with kidney infections but not in those with uncomplicated bladder infections. Unfortunately this test is technically difficult, time-consuming, difficult to standardize, very imprecise in the paediatric population, beset with false positive and false negative results and therefore of little clinical value.

The response to single-dose treatment (see below) may be a simple and practical clue to the site of infection, in that most patients with bladder infections respond whereas those with upper tract infections often do not.

TREATMENT

It is useful to consider UTI as uncomplicated or complicated, as the management is different.

Although it is somewhat controversial, and it may be inconvenient for both doctor and patient to withhold antimicrobial therapy until the results of urine culture and antibacterial sensitivity tests are known, we consider this to be ideal clinical practice. Only in a very ill patient should it be essential to start treatment before this information is available. Many general practitioners, however, feel under pressure to initiate antimicrobial therapy at the initial visit.

Even if an untreated patient loses her symptoms, the bacteriuria usually persists. The prescribing of an alkalinizing agent (e.g. Citravescent or Ural) alone does not eradicate the infection although it may temporarily alleviate lower urinary tract symptoms. The traditional advice to 'drink plenty' is a useful adjunct to antibacterial thereapy, principally because it results in more frequent bladder emptying. Although the administered drug will have its urinary concentration reduced in the presence of a diuresis, this is of little practical importance.

The management of women with abacterial cystitis is unsatisfactory, mainly because of ignorance regarding its aetiology. The symptoms invariably settle, however, over a period of 2–5 days and may be improved by a high fluid intake. Alkalinization of the urine is rarely of benefit. Antibacterial therapy seems to influence recovery in some of these women, particularly those with pyuria. There have been no controlled studies comparing the effects of antimicrobial treatment with placebo in women with abacterial cystitis.

Antimicrobial treatment regimens for UTI can be classified as:

1. Curative
2. Prophylactic or preventive
3. Suppressive.

Curative treatment

A major error in the treatment of UTI has been that most doctors have given too much drug for too long. The aim of treating a UTI should be to use the shortest course of the simplest, safest and cheapest antimicrobial agent that will eradicate the offending organisms. The possible side effects of the chosen drug should be weighed against the severity of the illness. There is now considerable evidence that a single oral dose of an antimicrobial agent is as effective as a conventional short course for the treatment of uncomplicated UTI. Single-dose therapy is associated with a lower incidence of side effects such as vaginal candidiasis and skin rash.

Most practitioners prefer to treat their patients when they first present rather than waiting 12–24 hours for a culture. Thus up to a third of the patients with the frequency–dysuria syndrome may be treated unnecessarily. At present there is no proof that antibacterial therapy actually influences the recovery from abacterial cystitis, although if given treatment these women appear to recover at a similar rate to those with bacterial cystitis.

Single-dose treatment

There has been considerable interest in the use of single-dose antibacterial therapy for treating UTI. The first drug evaluated in detail was amoxycillin given as a single 3 g oral dose which proved comparable to a 5-day course. A single oral dose of 1.92–2.88 g co-trimoxazole or 600 mg trimethoprim is more effective than amoxycillin and equivalent to a 3- to 5-day course of either preparation.

Although single doses of doxycycline, pivmecillinam, sulphamethizole, cefuroxime (intramuscularly), and netilmicin (intramuscularly) have been shown to be efficacious, with the exception of netilmicin they are less effective than cotrimoxazole or trimethoprim. A 600 mg dose of trimethoprim is the drug of choice for single-dose treatment, although a single dose of one of the new 4-quinolones has proven very effective, despite some doubt over their activity against *Staphylococcus saprophyticus*. A novel compound, fosfomycin trometamol in an oral dose of 3 g, has proved highly effective and has been marketed specifically for single-dose treatment of bacterial cystitis. Amoxycillin and the cephalosporins are no longer recommended in single-dose schedules.

Suggested drugs for single-dose oral treatment of uncomplicated urinary tract infections
Trimethoprim 600 mg
Co-trimoxazole 1.92 g
Norfloxacin 800 mg
Pefloxacin 800 mg
Ciprofloxacin 500 mg
Fosfomycin trometamol 3 g

It is recommended that single-dose therapy be considered as the initial treatment for all uncomplicated UTI in sexually active women, and also for girls who are known to have a radiologically normal urinary tract.

Advantages of single-dose antimicrobial therapy for the treatment of uncomplicated urinary tract infections
Simple
Effective
Cheap
Well tolerated
Preferred by patients
Assured compliance
Fewer side effects
Less risk of resistant organisms developing
Less hazard to fetus
Simple method of localizing site of infection
Indicator of the need for urinary tract investigation

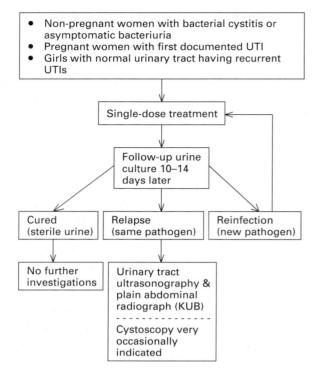

Fig. 16.1   A suggested scheme for the management of uncomplicated urinary tract infections

Short (3-day) course

An alternative to single-dose therapy for women with bacterial cystitis is a short course of treatment. Recent studies have clearly demonstrated that 3 days is sufficient.

One of the most popular antibiotics for the treatment of UTI has been amoxycillin, but unfortunately in many areas up to 30% of *Esch. coli* in the community and 50% in hospitals are now resistant to this drug. It is therefore a poor choice as a first-line drug before the drug sensitivity profile is known. Amoxycillin, however, remains the drug of choice for treating *Streptococcus faecalis*. The problem of resistance to amoxycillin has been addressed by combining it with clavulanic acid or sulbactam, β-lactamase inhibitors, which are resistant to some of the many β-lactamases produced by bacteria. A clavulanic acid-potentiated form of amoxycillin (Augmentin) has proved disappointing in some

clinical studies, with a slow clinical response, a high proportion of bacteriological relapses, and a troublesome side effect profile.

Co-trimoxazole is one of the most effective agents available for oral administration. This antibacterial combination, however, is a common cause of adverse drug reactions, most of which are related to the sulphamethoxazole component. Trimethoprim has also been formulated in combination with other sulphonamides with greater efficacy in the urinary tract. Numerous studies however, have shown trimethoprim to be just as effective as co-trimoxazole. It is also rational to use trimethoprim alone as, in the urinary tract, the antibacterial efficacy of this drug combination is almost entirely due to the trimethoprim component. In some centres, however, there is now an increasing resistance of *Esch. coli* to trimethoprim and co-trimoxazole.

Nitrofurantoin remains a valuable drug, although it is ineffective against *Proteus mirabilis*. Unfortunately many doctors continue to prescribe a dose of 100 mg every 6 hours, which frequently causes nausea or vomiting. Studies have shown equal effectiveness with a dose of 50 mg every 8 hours with minimal side effects. A macrocrystalline formulation of nitrofurantoin is associated with fewer gastrointestinal side effects.

Nalidixic acid is effective against most Gram-negative organisms but is ineffective against *Staphylococcus saprophyticus*, the second commonest pathogen in domiciliary practice. Unfortunately this drug is still recommended for use in a dose of 1 g 6-hourly, which has an unacceptably high incidence of unpleasant side effects. Comparative trials have shown a dose of 0.5 g every 8 hours to be just as effective and much better tolerated. Nalidixic acid is most bactericidal at a concentration equivalent to that obtained in urine after an 0.5 g dose. Oxolinic acid has similar disadvantages to nalidixic acid and should be used in a dose of 375 mg twice daily.

The use of nalidixic acid and oxolinic acid has now been largely superseded by an effective new generation of quinolones such as norfloxacin, enoxacin, ofloxacin, pefloxacin, ciprofloxacin, fleroxacin and lomefloxacin. These orally absorbed,

Table 16.1 Drug regimens for an oral 3-day course treatment for bacterial cystitis

Drug	Dose	Comment
Trimethoprim	300 mg q 24 h	An ideal agent
Co-trimoxazole	960 mg q 12 h	Should be replaced by trimethoprim alone
Nitrofurantoin	50 mg q 8 h	Not effective v *Proteus spp.*
Nalidixic acid	500 mg q 8 h	Not effective v *Staph. saprophyticus*
Oxolinic acid	375 mg q 12 h	No longer recommended
Norfloxacin	400 mg q 12 h	} Valuable newer agents
Ciprofloxacin	250 mg q 12 h	
Lomefloxacin	400 mg q 24 h	
Cephalexin	250 mg q 8 h	} Useful if renal insufficiency present
Cephradine	250 mg q 8 h	
Cefaclor	250 mg q 8 h	
Sulphamethizole	1 g q 8 h	Unfashionable
Pivmecillinam	200 mg q 8 h	
Amoxycillin	250 mg q 8 h	High incidence of resistance — useful for *Strep. faecalis*
Augmentin	500 mg amox/ 125 mg clavulanic acid q 12 h	Proving disappointing

broad-spectrum synthetic 4-quinolones are highly effective against a wide range of pathogens, including hospital-acquired organisms.

Cephalosporins, such as cephalexin, cephradine and cefaclor, remain effective drugs. The sulphonamides such as sulphamethizole have become unfashionable for the treatment of UTI, although they remain efficacious.

The recommendations in Table 16.1 apply only to patients with normal renal function. When renal function is impaired the renal handling of the drug must be known. Cephalexin is well proven in patients with all degrees of renal insufficiency.

Course of treatment for severe or complicated UTI

Patients with uncomplicated acute pyelonephritis should receive a 5-day course of treatment after a blood culture, preferably with at least one dose of a parenterally administered drug if vomiting is a problem. Many of these patients require hospitalization for rehydration, analgesia and parenteral antibiotics. A blood culture should be considered before antimicrobial treatment is started. Some clinicians still treat acute pyelonephritis for at least 2 weeks, but comparative studies have shown that this is not necessary.

For patients who are extremely ill the choice of drug now lies between an aminoglycoside, one of the new 4-quinolones or a β-lactam antibiotic. Drugs in the former group are still preferred until the sensitivity profile is known. Some clinicians prefer tobramycin to gentamicin, because of the reduced risk of nephrotoxicity. Netilmicin is a newer aminoglycoside with a reduced risk of nephrotoxicity and ototoxicity. However its use has been restricted because of its price. Amikacin should be retained for the treatment of resistant pathogens. These patients may have impaired renal function necessitating careful monitoring of both renal function and serum peak and trough concentrations of the drug. All patients, irrespective of their renal function, require a full loading dose of an aminoglycoside (e.g. 2.5–3.0 mg/kg). The normal maintenance dose of 1.0–1.5 mg/kg should be adjusted according to the measured or assessed creatinine clearance, and given at an increased interval. For the treatment of UTI this method is preferred to giving a smaller dose every 8 hours. For a rapid guide to dosage the creatinine clearance can be easily assessed at the bedside by using the variables of age, weight, sex and plasma creatinine in the Cockcroft–Gault formula (see Ch. 3).

There is no substitute, however, for monitoring the peak and trough (pre-dose) serum concentrations of the aminoglycosides every second or third day and even daily if treatment is extending beyond 5 days. Some clinicians prefer to individualize aminoglycoside dosage, based on measured pharmacokinetic parameters and computer predictions.

The aminoglycosides have been shown to be just as efficacious, easier to use and safer if the maintenance dose is given as a single daily dose rather than in divided doses.

The new 4-quinolones such as norfloxacin, ciprofloxacin and lomefloxacin are highly effective for the treatment of serious UTI and should rival the aminoglycosides as the drugs of choice. These broad-spectrum synthetic compounds are highly effective against a wide range of pathogens, including hospital-acquired organisms. In addition they are extremely efficacious in the treatment of prostatitis. Several of the drugs in this group are available in an intravenous formulation and after a few doses can be switched to tablets. This has enabled patients to be discharged from hospital earlier and thus reduce the costs of treating acute pyelonephritis.

There is an extensive list of β-lactam antibiotics, including the third and fourth generation cephalosporins, the semi-synthetic or ureido-penicillins, the monobactams, penems and the β-lactamase inhibitors. These antibiotics have not replaced the aminoglycosides, are being superseded by the 4-quinolones and have significant side effects, including skin rashes, vaginal candidiasis, coagulation disorders, diarrhoea, pseudomembranous colitis and renal failure. Cefazolin remains a useful drug for severe urinary tract sepsis, while ceftriaxone has proved the most effective of the newer β-lactam drugs and comparable to the aminoglycosides.

Prophylactic or preventive treatment

Many women have recurrent or closely spaced symptomatic UTI which cause considerable anxiety and much morbidity. This is a particular problem in young sexually active females. Many of these women benefit by ensuring that they always empty their bladder completely, particularly after intercourse. Some benefit may be obtained by applying an antiseptic cream (e.g. 0.5% cetrimide w/w) to the periurethral area before intercourse.

If these simple techniques fail, the pattern of recurrences can be interrupted by instituting prophylactic therapy after the urine has been sterilized. Nitrofurantoin in a dose of 50 mg taken last thing at night after the patient has emptied her bladder is highly effective, as is 100 mg of trimethoprim or 0.24 g of co-trimoxazole. There have been satisfactory results with a 1 g oral dose of hexamine hippurate and, in patients with renal insufficiency, 125 mg of cephalexin. Recent trials have shown that it is just as effective to give a dose on alternate nights or even three times a week. In some women a dose after intercourse is effective.

The excellent results with nitrofurantoin reflect the fact that the drug causes no alteration to the faecal flora. The development of resistant bacterial strains during the administration of nitrofurantoin is unknown. Trimethoprim may have advantages as a prophylactic agent because it is excreted partly through the vagina and thus eliminates a possible source of infecting pathogens.

Suppressive treatment

Some patients have gross urological abnormalities (e.g. urinary calculi, ileal conduit, chronic prostatitis, meningomyelocoele, neurogenic bladder) so that it is impossible to sterilize their urinary tract. In these patients the presence of an antimicrobial agent may prevent the bacteriuria from becoming a bacteraemia. If these patients are asymptomatic,

Table 16.2 Drug regimens for a parenteral 5-day course of treatment

Drug	Dose
Gentamicin Tobramycin * Netilmicin	Loading dose 2.5–3.0 mg/kg body weight; maintenance doses according to drug levels and renal function
Amikacin	Loading dose 15 mg/kg body weight; maintenance doses as above
Ciprofloxacin	100 mg q 12 h } Can be switched
Lomefloxacin	400 mg q 24 h } to oral formulation
Ceftriaxone	2 g q 24 h — very effective
Cefazolin	1 g q 8 h
Cephradine	1 g q 8 h
Ceftazidime	0.5–1.0 g q 12 h
Aztreonam	1 g q 12 h
Ipipenem/cilastin	500 mg/500 mg q 8 h
Amoxycillin	0.5–1 g q 8 h
Clavulanic acid/ amoxycillin	200 mg/1 g q 8 h

*5 mg/kg as a single daily dose is just as efficacious and less toxic

Table 16.3 Drug regimens for prophylactic therapy

Drug	Dose each night, alternate nights, 3 nights a week or after intercourse
Nitrofurantoin	50 mg
Trimethoprim	100 mg
Co-trimoxazole	0.24 g
Norfloxacin	200 mg
Cephalexin	125 mg — useful if renal insufficiency
Hexamine hippurate	1 g

however, they should be left untreated and attention given to maintaining a good fluid intake and to ensuring regular and complete bladder emptying. If antimicrobial therapy is given when these patients are asymptomatic bacterial resistance will develop. When the patient does become symptomatic there will then be no effective drugs left to use.

Special treatment problems

Men

Acute bacterial prostatitis generally responds very well to standard therapy. This is not always the case for chronic prostatitis. Men with recurrent bacteriuria frequently carry the infecting organism in their prostatic fluid. Careful segmental urine cultures are essential in making the diagnosis. Until recently there were few antimicrobial agents that could effectively cross non-inflamed prostatic epithelium from plasma into prostatic fluid, but long-term low-dose therapy (e.g. with nitrofurantoin, trimethoprim) could prevent the prostatic bacteria from initiating bacteriuria or even bacteraemia. However the new quinolones penetrate prostatic tissue and are now established as the drugs of choice for the management of bacterial prostatitis.

Covert bacteriuria in pregnancy

The initial treatment should be with a single dose or a 3-day course of an appropriate drug. Studies show that either a single 1.92 g dose of co-trimoxazole or a single 600 mg dose of trimethoprim is highly effective in treating women with covert bacteriuria *between 16 and 30 weeks gestation*. If bacteriuria returns after treatment the woman should be given a second course, or another single dose, and then started on prophylactic treatment in the form of a 50 mg dose of nitrofurantoin each night until the puerperium.

The women who have a recurrence of bacteriuria during pregnancy are most likely to have a urinary tract abnormality. Such women should have ultrasonography of the urinary tract and a plain abdominal radiograph after delivery.

Elderly women

The prevalence of bacteriuria rises with increasing age in women, with the lowest rate in those living independently and the highest in the elderly residents of long-stay geriatric wards. Community studies have shown that about one fifth of elderly women have bacteriuria. At the onset of a chronic debilitating illness and institutionalization the rate of bacteriuria in women rises rapidly, with frequencies of 25–50%.

It is widely believed, however, that although bacteriuria in the elderly may be related to mortality, it is more likely that the bacteriuria is a marker for other diseases that are the primary cause of the increased mortality rate rather than being the direct cause.

If elderly women with bacteriuria are asymptomatic they are best left untreated because of the high chance of inducing bacterial resistance. These women are often infected with some of the more unusual and resistant organisms.

At present, in the absence of obstructive uropathy, no convincing evidence exists to support the routine use of antimicrobial therapy for postmenopausal women with asymptomatic bacteriuria.

Symptomatic UTI (and not just smelly urine) should be treated in elderly patients of any age. The approach to treating symptomatic infections in the elderly should be no different to that for women in other age groups. It is important to note that in the elderly the symptoms may be atypical or non-specific (e.g. confusion, confined to bed, etc.).

The treatment of atrophic vaginitis should be given early consideration in elderly women with recurrent symptomatic UTI. It is correctable with the use of oral or topical oestrogen therapy. This promotes accumulation of glycogen by vaginal epithelial cells thus allowing the growth of *Lactobacillus spp.* and the production of lactic acid which causes a marked acidification of vaginal secretions with suppression of the vaginal growth of potential urinary pathogens.

If an elderly woman has an underlying urinary tract abnormality which definitely cannot be corrected (e.g. by relief of obstruction, or removal of a calculus or catheter) then bacteriuria, if asymptomatic, is best left untreated. Inappropriate treatment will lead rapidly to increasingly resistant pathogens.

Urinary catheters

Long-term indwelling urinary catheters should be avoided if at all possible. All such patients will have bacteriuria. The offending pathogen(s) will be resident in the biofilm lining the catheter. The latter is impermeable to antimicrobial agents. Catheters that are blocking up should be replaced but this need not be done routinely if the patient is asymptomatic and the urine is draining freely. These patients should receive a good fluid intake.

Catheter-acquired bacteriuria after short-term catheter use in women often becomes symptomatic. For those with lower urinary tract symptoms single-dose treatment is just as effective as a course of treatment.

In the non-institutional setting clean intermittent urethral catheterization constitutes a minimal risk since the introduction of bacteria rarely produces a serious infection. Intermittent catheterization has revolutionized the care of patients with spinal cord injury or disease and neurogenic bladders. The risk of UTI is greatly reduced by the absence of a chronic indwelling catheter and the periodic elimination of residual urine. With each catheterization, bacteria may be introduced into the urinary tract. However with good technique this risk is very low.

Acute papillary necrosis complicating acute pyelonephritis

Some patients, usually elderly, with severe acute pyelonephritis may develop acute renal papillary necrosis with complicating acute renal failure. This unusual complication may occur in diabetics, alcoholics and those consuming non-steroidal anti-inflammatory drugs. Elderly women who are ill with acute pyelonephritis should have these drugs temporarily discontinued, as well as the angiotensin-converting enzyme inhibitors.

FOLLOW-UP

Ideally a patient should be reviewed about 10–14 days after treatment and a further urine specimen should be obtained for culture. It was formerly suggested that 7 days would be an ideal time to assess cure, but some of the new antimicrobial agents (e.g. longer-acting quinolones) may be excreted in the urine for up to a week.

The early reappearance of the same bacterial species or the same serotype of *Esch. coli* suggests that the original pathogen was not eradicated and that the patient may require a longer period of treatment and further investigation. A genuine relapse will rarely occur if the urine is sterile 10–14 days after treatment.

Most recurrences, however, are reinfections with a different bacterial species. This is no reflection on the previous treatment and merely indicates the recurrent nature of the problem.

INVESTIGATION

Every infant, every child and every male should have urinary tract investigations undertaken following their first UTI. There should be no exception to this rule. In children under the age of 2 years a micturating (voiding) cystourethrogram should also be undertaken to exclude vesico-ureteric reflux. The latter investigation need not be done in older children if high quality organ imaging (e.g. intravenous urogram, DMSA scan or ultrasonography) has shown a normal upper urinary tract. It is also useful to measure the plasma creatinine concentration.

It is not cost-effective to undertake invasive investigations on young sexually active women with an ocasional attack of bacterial cystitis. If such a woman had no urinary tract problems as a child, has occasional UTI which respond rapidly to a single dose of an oral antimicrobial agent, and follow-up urine specimens show no microscopic haematuria and are sterile on culture it is safe to forgo any further investigations. If the woman has acute pyelonephritis or any unusual finding (e.g. persistent microscopic haematuria or persistent pyuria), then organ imaging (urinary tract ultrasonography and a plain abdominal radiograph) of the urinary tract (KUB) should be undertaken. Prompt surgical handling of urological lesions should be practised.

Cystoscopy in younger women has been over-used by urologists. In this large patient group cystoscopy rarely influences management. This investigation, however, should be considered in most males, in some older women, or if there is something unusual clinically, in the examination of the urine or in the response to treatment.

SIGNIFICANCE OF A URINARY TRACT INFECTION

Any UTI raises the question of whether it is a marker for some underlying urinary tract pathol-ogy. This applies particularly to infants and young children, because of the strong likelihood of there being a potentially damaging urinary tract abnor-mality. The most important of these is the presence of primary vesicoureteric reflux.

There are still many patients who are concerned that recurrent UTI may be progressively damaging their kidneys. There is now good evidence that infection in the context of a normal urinary tract is a benign condition and the patients should be reassured of this. However, infection in the presence of urinary tract obstruction, stones or gross vesicoureteric reflux may be damaging to the kidneys.

REFERENCES AND RECOMMENDED READING

Bailey R R (ed) 1983 Single dose therapy of urinary tract infections. ADIS Health Science Press, Sydney

Bailey R R 1992 Management of lower urinary tract infections. Drugs 45 (Suppl. 3): 139–144

Begg E J, Atkinson H C, Jeffery G M, Taylor N W 1989 Individualised aminoglycoside dosage based on pharmacokinetic analysis is superior to dosage based on physician intuition at achieving target plasma drug concentrations. British Journal of Clinical Pharmacology 28: 137–141

Boscia J A, Abrutyn E, Kaye D 1987 Asymptomatic bacteriuria in elderly persons: treat or do not treat? Annals of Internal Medicine 106: 764–765

Hooton T M, Hillier S, Johnson C, Roberts P L, Stamm W E 1991 *Escherichia coli* bacteriuria and contraceptive method. Journal of American Medical Association 265: 64–69

Kass E H, Svanborg Eden C (eds) 1989 Host-parasite interactions in urinary tract infections. University of Chicago Press, Chicago

Kunin C M (ed) 1987 Detection, prevention and management of urinary tract infections. Lea & Febiger, Philadelphia

Lipsky B A 1989 Urinary tract infections in men: epidemiology pathophysiology, diagnosis, and treatment. Annals of Internal Medicine 110: 138–150

Nicolle L E, Mayhew W J, Bryan L 1987 Prospective randomized comparison of therapy and no therapy for asymptomatic bacteriuria in elderly, institutionalized women. American Journal of Medicine 83: 27–33

Ohkoshi M, Naber K G 1992 International consensus discussion on clinical evaluation of drug efficacy in urinary tract infection. Infection 20 (Suppl. 3): S135–S242

Pims J M, Büller H R, Kuipjer E J, Tange R A, Speelman P 1993 Once versus thrice daily gentamicin in patients with serious infection. Lancet 341: 335–339

Privette M, Cade R, Peterson J, Mars D 1988 Prevention of recurrent urinary tract infections in postmenopausal women. Nephron 50: 24–27

Rubin R W, Bean T R Jr, Stamm W E 1992 An approach to evaluating anti bacterial agents in the treatment of urinary tract infection. Clinical Infectious Disorders 14 (Suppl. 2): S246–S251

Stamm W E, Counts G W, Running K R, Fihn S, Turck M, Holmes K K 1982 Diagnosis of coliform infection in acutely dysuric women. New England Journal of Medicine 307: 463–468

Stapleton A, Latham R H, Johnson C, Stamm W E 1990 Postcoital antimicrobial prophylaxis for recurrent urinary tract infection: a randomized, double-blind, placebo-controlled trial. Journal of American Medical Association 264: 703–706

17. Renal tubular disorders

A. Z. Györy

The majority of renal tubular disorders are genetically determined although acquired forms, especially those due to drugs, are being described with increasing frequency.

All causes of renal failure, whether acute or chronic, affect tubular function, but this chapter deals only with those which affect tubular function first and glomerular function secondarily, if at all. However, a number of metabolic disorders, especially among the acquired forms, cause both glomerular and specific tubular abnormalities (e.g. multiple myeloma).

Only the major abnormalities likely to be encountered in a large hospital population will be discussed here. For rare conditions, specialized textbooks should be consulted.

SPECIFIC ISOLATED DEFECTS OF TUBULAR TRANSPORT

Carbohydrate

Glycosuria

Glycosuria is defined as glucose in the urine in the presence of normal or only slightly elevated plasma glucose concentrations. Clinically it is unimportant, its only significance being in the differential diagnosis of diabetes mellitus and other tubular disorders with glycosuria.

Normally glucose does not appear in the urine until plasma concentrations reach 10 mmol/l (threshold). Maximum excretion is reached at plasma concentrations of 15 mmol/l (tubular maximum or T_m). Glycosuria is either due to a reduced tubular maximum capacity (type A), when threshold is reduced in so far as T_m is reduced, or to a reduced threshold (increased splay) with normal T_m (type B). In type A the total number of transport sites is reduced but they are otherwise normal, while in type B the total number of sites is normal but affinity for glucose is reduced. The abnormalities at the molecular level have not been determined.

Genetics. Inheritance is autosomal recessive in that parents of severely affected children have only a mild abnormality. A few families, however, have an autosomal dominant pattern where both parents and children are equally affected.

Clinical features. Glycosuria is usually persistent, but can be intermittent if blood glucose concentrations fall below threshold. The abnormality persists throughout life without symptoms, except under conditions of prolonged starvation where it can lead to hypoglycaemia, reduced extracellular fluid (ECF) volume and ketosis.

The differential diagnosis includes diabetes mellitus (where it is due to hyperglycaemia) but the two can occur together. It also occurs in the Fanconi syndrome (in which there are multiple tubular defects) and in the glucose–galactose malabsorption syndrome (a combined renal–jejunal defect) or with gluco-glycinuria and phosphate diabetes.

Diagnosis. Glucose in the urine must be demonstrated with the glucose oxidase method when plasma concentrations are below 7.5 mmol/l. Non-specific tests for reducing substances give positive readings with many other sugars and are unsatisfactory. Fasting blood glucose and glucose tolerance must also be determined to exclude coexisting diabetes mellitus. Chronic renal failure must be excluded, as this can occasionally cause glycosuria.

Treatment. No treatment is required.

Amino acids

Hartnup's disease

This condition is characterized by neutral amino-aciduria with a pellagra-like skin rash, cerebellar ataxia, psychotic illness, mental retardation, and the 'blue diaper' syndrome in infants.

The basic defect is an abnormality in renal tubular and intestinal transport of free neutral (monoamine and monocarboxylic) amino acids. Oligopeptides containing these, especially trypto-phan, are handled normally. The decreased re-absorption in the gut results in increased break-down by bacteria which in turn leads to increased amounts of indoles and indicans in both stool and urine. Tryptophan is needed for at least half the normal daily requirement of nicotinamide, so that non-absorption causes niacin deficiency. Indoles may inhibit nicotinamide synthesis, thus creating a vicious cycle.

The abnormality can affect all amino acids in the group or only individual members. In the 'blue diaper' syndrome the abnormality affects only tryptophan, leading to excess indigo dye excretion (blue colour).

Clinical features. The aminoaciduria is con-stant whereas the psychotic effects, which range from mild emotional instability to delirium, are episodic and variable and coincide with bouts of a pellagra-like red skin rash which is scaly on the exposed surfaces, sensitive to sunlight and can lead to blister formation. There is cerebellar ataxia and nystagmus without sensory loss which are worse when the skin rash is worse.

The condition improves with age.

Diagnosis. The normal total urinary amino nitrogen is less than 50 mg per day whereas in Hartnup's disease it is about 500 mg/day. A low urinary total amino nitrogen excludes the disease. Amino acid analysis reveals an increased excretion of alanine, serine, threonine, asparagine, glut-amine, valine, leucine, isoleucine, phenylalanine,

tyrosine, tryptophan, histidine and citrulline. Threonine, tyrosine, and histidine are grossly increased in the urine.

Patients with an increased indole acetic acid excretion should be further investigated. The differential diagnosis is from nutritional pellagra.

Treatment. Treatment consists of nicotin-amide 40–200 mg/day (or the acid form). A high protein diet is also beneficial. Monoamine oxidase inhibitors are contraindicated and sunlight should be avoided.

Cystinuria

This is a rare condition leading to excess secretion of cystine, ornithine, arginine and lysine (COAL) and the formation of cystine crystals and stones in the urine; renal failure develops as a complication of the stone disease.

The basic defect is an abnormality in the transport of COAL in renal tubules and the intestine. In the brush border all four have a common transport step whereas in the basolateral membranes the step for cystine is different, allowing it to accumulate in the cells. In the intestines ornithine rejection leads to an increase in putrescine excretion whereas lysine rejection in-creases cadaverine excretion in both faeces and urine.

Clinical features. Clinically, only cystine stone disease is of importance. It accounts for 1–3% of all stone disease. The stones are solitary or multiple and occasionally staghorn calculi are seen. Onset is between the first and fourth decade and the disease is more severe in males. The renal course is that of stone disease, with recurrent infection and renal failure due to secondary glomerular obstruction and destruction. Heterozy-gotes suffer from calcium oxalate stone disease rather than from cystine stones.

Diagnosis. Normally less than 130 μmol/day (11 μmol/mmol creatinine) of cystine is excreted per mg of creatinine. Affected homozygotes ex-crete more than 250 mg/mg creatinine and heterozygotes have an intermediate excretion rate. Solubility in urine is less than 1250 μmol/l.

Treatment. The aim is to reduce excretion and to increase solubility of cystine stones. The latter is achieved by increasing urine output to 2–4 l/day by increased intake of fluid. Alkalinization of urine to pH 7.5–8.0 with sodium bicarbonate must be checked with indicator paper.

In difficult cases, penicillamine can be used to decrease cystine excretion. Toxic effects of penicillamine are anaemia and loss of taste, which can be counteracted by oral zinc supplementation. Other toxic manifestations are fever, rash, haematuria with or without glomerulonephritis, nephrotic syndrome and agranulocytosis. Tiopronin (Thiola, α-Mercaptoproprionyl) may be tried in patients who show unacceptable reactions to d-penicillamine. Reactions to Tiopronin are similar to d-penicillamine, but less frequent.

Electrolytes

Renal tubular acidosis

Renal tubular acidosis (RTA) is defined as a systemic metabolic acidosis due to a specific tubular abnormality, usually out of proportion to any impairment of renal function which may be present.

Three basic types can be distinguished, each with a large number of individual causes: distal or classic RTA; proximal RTA or bicarbonate-wasting disease; and hyperkalaemic hypoammonuric RTA.

Distal RTA. Patients with distal RTA have a chronic hyperchloraemic systemic acidosis and a persistently alkaline urine (pH usually above 5.7; mean 6–6.8) and hypokalaemia. Renal function is relatively or entirely normal. Other manifestations include urolithiasis, urinary tract infections, nephrocalcinosis and osteomalacia. If the condition is untreated, chronic renal failure may develop.

An incomplete form of the disorder is often missed because these patients do not normally have systemic acidosis although the basic abnormality is present together with a persistently alkaline urine and urolithiasis. Patients with this incomplete renal tubular acidification defect (IRTAD) can usually excrete their daily acid load by virtue of an above average ammonia excretion in relation to urine pH (which is slightly lower after acid loading than in patients with RTA).

Aetiology of distal renal tubular acidosis

Primary
  Genetic
  Idiopathic
Complicating genetically transmitted systemic disease
  Ehlers–Danlos syndrome
  Hereditary elliptocytosis
  Medullary cystic disease
Autoimmune disease
  Hypergammaglobulinaemia
  Sjögren's syndrome
  Systemic lupus erythematosus
  Chronic active hepatitis
Nephrocalcinosis
  Primary hyperparathyroidism
  Vitamin D intoxication
  Idiopathic hypercalciuria
  Medullary sponge kidney
  Hypophosphatasia
Tubulointerstitial disease
  Obstructive uropathy (transient)
  Chronic pyelonephritis
  Renal transplantation
  Acute renal failure (transient)
Drugs and toxins
  Analgesic nephropathy
  Lithium
  Amphotericin B
  Cyclamate
  Toluene
  Ureterosigmoidostomy

Some patients with acquired forms of RTA can reduce pH to below 5.7, but not to the normal value of 5.2 or less. These patients do not develop systemic acidosis unless there is coexistent renal failure. The abnormality is only of academic importance in relation to secondary causes and should not be called RTA, but IRTAD.

Aetiology. Distal RTA may be primary or due to a variety of disorders, including autoimmune diseases, nephrocalcinosis and tubulointerstitial disease. It may also complicate genetically transmitted systemic disease or be drug-induced.

Basic abnormality. The normal kidney can reduce (acidify) urine pH to 5.2 or less when stressed maximally with an acid load (e.g. after ingestion of ammonium chloride). This is a function of the distal nephron and is abnormal in patients with distal RTA. Even severely acidotic patients cannot reduce urine pH to below 5.7–6.0. The precise transport abnormality has not been defined but is due either to reduced pump activity or to increased back diffusion of hydrogen ions, both of which result in reduced net hydrogen ion secretion. The normal daily production of hydrogen ions needing excretion by the kidney (approximately 1 mmol/kg per day in adults and 3 mmol/kg per day in children) can thus not be eliminated, leading to retention and systemic metabolic acidosis.

The excretion of both titratable acid and ammonium ions depends on the presence of an acid urine and is thus reduced in patients with distal RTA. Neither of these methods of acid excretion is in itself at fault in distal RTA. The reduced hydrogen ion excretion leads to a reduction in serum bicarbonate, which is replaced by chloride ions whose proximal tubular reabsorption is stimulated by both the acidosis and low tubular bicarbonate.

In patients with the incomplete form (IRTAD), urine pH can usually be lowered to 5.7, at which level sufficient titratable acid and ammonium ion excretion can be generated to balance endogenous acid generation. If the latter is increased for any reason (large protein intake) these patients will also manifest a systemic metabolic acidosis. In addition, in some patients with IRTAD it is not the lower urine pH but an above-normal ammonia production for any given urine pH that balances endogenous acid production.

Proximal tubular reclamation of filtered bicarbonate, which also depends on hydrogen ion secretion, is normal in both RTA and IRTAD.

All other manifestations of distal RTA and IRTAD are secondary abnormalities.

Genetics. Primary RTA is inherited as an autosomal dominant trait. RTA and IRTAD can occur in the same families.

Clinical features. The clinical features of RTA are summarized in Table 7.1. Of the 137 patients in this series, 46 (34%) were males and 91 (66%) females. The genetic and idiopathic types of the disease are usually discovered between the first and third decades of life.

Table 17.1 Clinical features of RTA in 137 patients

	Males (%)	Females (%)
Aetiology		
Familial	50	19
Idiopathic	39	56
IRTAD	6.5	2.3
Acquired	4.3	23.1
Presenting symptoms		
Hypokalaemia	13	31
Renal stones	24	23
Family investigation	35	9
Osteomalacia	11	15
Urinary tract infection	4	10
Nephrocalcinosis	6.5	1
Stunted growth	2	0
Accidental discovery	2	8
Unknown	2.5	3

IRTAD — incomplete renal tubular acidification defect

The hypokalaemia is the result of increased potassium secretion due to increased delivery of sodium to the distal nephron sites and secondary hyperaldosteronism due to a depletion in extracellular fluid volume following the sodium loss. If severe, it will lead to muscle paralysis and even rhabdomyolysis, respiratory arrest or cardiac arrhythmias. If prolonged, hypokalaemia will cause a renal concentrating defect resulting in polyuria and nocturia.

The medullary (and occasionally cortical) nephrocalcinosis and urolithiasis are the result of a combination of factors, the most important of which are the consistently alkaline urine pH, reduced urinary citrate excretion as a result of systemic acidosis and reduced magnesium excretion. RTA accounts for 5% of all stone disease. All the above factors reduce the solubility of calcium salts (carbonate, phosphate or oxalate) in the urine, leading to local precipitation. In about half the inherited cases there is also hypercalciuria. The nephrocalcinosis and urolithiasis and their inevitable complication of infection contribute to polyuria, nocturia and gradual nephron 'drop-out', leading to terminal renal failure if untreated.

Osteomalacia with bone pain and real or pseudo-fractures is a late complication and never occurs without at least one of the other complications, particularly nephrocalcinosis or urolithiasis. It is most likely the result of chronic systemic acidosis with hydrogen ion retention, which is then buffered by calcium liberation from bone and excretion of calcium salts.

Systemic acidosis also leads to hypophosphataemia and eventually secondary hyperparathyroidism. Elevated blood hydrogen ion concentration may also lead to reduced formation of 1,25-dihydroxycholecalciferol $(1,25(OH_2)D_3)$, thus contributing to the mild hypocalcaemia and osteomalacia.

If the acidaemia is severe, it can lead to depressed respiration with a resultant severe dyspnoea, dizziness or even coma. If severe enough, it also contributes to the reduction in glomerular function together with the reduced extracellular fluid volume; both are reversible causes of renal failure in RTA.

In IRTAD only urolithiasis and nephrocalcinosis have been reported.

In both RTA abd IRTAD of the inherited or idiopathic type the defect persists throughout life and spontaneous remission has not been reported. Even in the secondary forms, remission is rare, except in some of the drug-induced cases. If untreated, many patients go on to end-stage renal failure.

Diagnosis. The diagnosis should be suspected in any patient with a hyperchloraemic systemic metabolic acidosis, especially if associated with hypokalaemia, and should be seriously considered in patients with stone diseases.

For a definitive diagnosis, the following criteria must be met:

1. Urine pH above 5.2 (usually above pH 5.7 during systemic acid loading).
2. Systemic metabolic acidaemia must be demonstrated during the acid loading with NH4Cl 0.1 g/kg orally.
3. The urine for pH measurement must be free of urea-splitting organisms.

Distal RTA and IRTAD can be easily excluded with pH-sensitive paper if the pH of early morning urine specimens can be shown to have reached a value of 5.0.

The differential diagnosis includes other forms of systemic metabolic acidosis with hypokalaemia (usually the diarrhoeal syndromes) and proximal RTA. If during acid loading a fall of serum bicarbonate has been demonstrated but urine pH has not dropped to 5.2 units or below, proximal RTA is very unlikely and would have to be coexisting with distal RTA. A fall of 2–3 mmol/l in serum bicarbonate concentration is usual during acid loading.

Familial occurrence cannot be excluded in seemingly idiopathic cases unless acid loading tests are carried out because of the possibility of IRTAD in other family members.

Treatment. The aim of treatment is to correct the systemic acidosis and to maintain a normal acid–base balance. Initially care has to be taken not to worsen hypokalaemia or hypocalcaemia when instituting alkali therapy. In RTA, once hypokalaemia and hypocalcaemia have been corrected, sodium bicarbonate or Schohl's solution (1–2 mmol/kg per day of HCO_3 ions in adults and 2–3 mmol/kg per day in children) can be given on a long-term basis. Potassium supplementation is not needed once acidosis has been corrected. In patients with IRTAD and nephrocalcinosis or urolithiasis ethacrynic acid (which is able to reduce urine pH to normal values) 50–100 mg three times per week can be started. Alkalinization in these patients is useless and may worsen these complications. Hypokalaemia is not usually a problem. Infection and obstruction should be eradicated.

Proximal RTA. With proximal RTA there is also a systemic metabolic hyperchloraemic acidosis and persistently alkaline urine pH, but, in contradistinction to distal RTA, this is accompanied by marked bicarbonaturia. It is rarer than distal RTA and clinically indistinguishable from it, although some clues exist, i.e. a more severe systemic acidosis and an inconsistently alkaline urine pH.

An incomplete form has been described in one patient.

Aetiology. Many of the causes of proximal RTA result in multiple tubular defects, as in the Fanconi syndrome (FS).

Basic abnormality. The basic defect is an inability of the proximal tubules to pump enough hydrogen ions per unit time to reclaim all the filtered bicarbonate. Normally about 80% of all filtered bicarbonate is reabsorbed in the proximal tubules; in this disease it can be reduced to 50–60%, resulting in an increased delivery of bicarbonate ions to distal nephron sites. This increased delivery 'swamps' the capacity of the distal nephron to secrete hydrogen ions and thus some bicarbonate escapes into the urine. Since both titratable acid and ammonia 'trapping' can only occur in an 'acid' urine, the excess bicarbonate not only results in a direct loss of bicarbonate but also in the reduced formation of titratable acid and ammonia excretion in the distal nephron. Net acid excretion is therefore reduced once again and unable to balance the daily production. In addition, circulating (filtered) bicarbonate is also lost. The systemic acidosis in proximal RTA is thus more severe than in the distal type.

Once the serum bicarbonate concentration has been reduced to values where the filtered load equals the impaired proximal tubular hydrogen ion secretory capacity, all or most filtered bicarbonate will be reabsorbed so that none reaches the distal nephron, thus allowing normal urine pH (less than 5.2), tibratable acid and ammonia excretion. Now the endogenous acid load can be excreted and a new steady state is reached, but at the expense of a reduced serum bicarbonate concentration.

Genetics. The single defect has only been described in one family, in which inheritance was autosomal.

Clinical features. Proximal RTA usually occurs with other abnormalities of proximal tubular function, e.g. in the Fanconi syndrome.

There are insufficient idiopathic cases to formulate patterns of incidence.

The acidosis requires larger amounts of alkali supplementation than distal RTA. An important complication is hypokalaemia which, unlike in distal RTA, is made worse by correcting the acidosis. Hypokalaemia results from the increased leak of sodium bicarbonate to the distal nephron sites where the increased sodium delivery results in increased potassium excretion.

Nephrocalcinosis and urolithiasis can occur and are the result of the constantly alkaline urine. Osteomalacia is very rarely caused by proximal RTA although proximal RTA has been described as the result of bone disease.

The course of the acidosis in proximal RTA is variable, as is the pH of the urine, which can vary

---

Aetiology of proximal renal tubular acidosis

Primary single tubular defect
  Genetic (very rare)
  Idiopathic
  Transient in infants
Multiple tubular defects (Fanconi syndrome)
  Genetic
  Idiopathic
Genetically transmitted systemic disease
  Cystinosis (FS)
  Wilson's disease (FS)
  Fructose intolerance (FS)
Autoimmune disease
  Sjögren's syndrome
Chronic hypocalcaemia and secondary hyperparathyroidism
  Vitamin D deficiency or resistance (FS)
  Vitamin D dependency (FS)
Tubulointerstitial disease
  Medullary cystic disease (FS)
  Renal transplantation (FS)
Drugs and toxins
  Outdated tetracyclines (FS)
  Streptozotocin (FS)
  Lead (FS)
  Mercury (FS)
  Maleic acid (FS)
  Acetazolamide ingestion
  Sulfanilamide
Dysproteinaemic states
  Multiple myeloma (FS)
Other renal diseases
  Amyloidosis (FS)
  Nephrotic syndrome (FS)

---

from a normal value of pH 5 or less to 8.0 or above, depending on the bicarbonate load.

There is a primary transient form of the disease in infants, usually occurring below the age of 1 year and resulting in severe acidosis, failure to thrive, vomiting, dehydration and death if untreated. This is probably the form first described as RTA in the literature by both Lightwood and Butler in the mid 1930s. It usually becomes less severe as the child ages and disappears by the age of 3 or 4 years.

Distal RTA can also occur at this early age although not usually below the age of one.

Diagnosis. The diagnosis of proximal RTA rests on the demonstration of a reduced tubular maximum for bicarbonate (by the method of bicarbonate titration). This requires simultaneous arterial and urinary bicarbonate determinations, as the serum concentration is gradually increased from very low (acidotic) to above normal levels by bicarbonate infusion. The normal T_m is at or above 25 mmol/l but in proximal RTA it is usually below 18 mmol/l (at about 15 mmol/l).

A relatively simple test to differentiate proximal from distal RTA is to determine the pH of first morning specimens. A single finding of a pH of 5.0 or less excludes distal RTA. A pH above this, together with systemic acidosis and hypokalaemia, strongly suggests proximal RTA. The early morning test can be supplemented by acid loading (NH_4Cl 0.1 g/kg) last thing at night.

It is important to distinguish proximal RTA from the hyperkalaemic hypoammonuric type of RTA since in both minimum urine pH can be below 5.0.

Treatment. Alkali supplementation in the form of potassium bicarbonate is required to return serum bicarbonate concentrations to normal. Alkali requirements can be of the order of 3–10 mmol/kg per day and at times even higher, especially in small infants with the transient form.

The condition is rare, and because of insufficient experience it is not yet known what effect the very high alkaline urine pH produced by this therapy will have on nephrocalcinosis and urolithiasis. This is especially so in the Fanconi syndrome where, in spite of normal citrate excretion, nephrocalcinosis has occurred and further alkalinization of urine does not increase citrate excretion but makes urine pH more alkaline.

Hyperkalaemic hypoammonuric RTA. This is defined as a systemic hyperchloraemic metabolic acidosis with hyperkalaemia in the presence of relatively well preserved renal function, although in most cases studied so far some renal impairment was present.

The underlying defect in this relatively recently characterized group of diseases is not well defined. There is usually an inability of the tubules to respond to aldosterone—in which case plasma renin activity (PRA) is increased or normal depending or ECF volume—as well as lack of

---

Aetiology of hyperkalaemic hypoammonuric renal tubular acidosis

1. Deficient tubular response to mineralocorticoid (pseudohypoaldosteronism)
   a. Without salt wasting
   b. With salt wasting
      (i) Rare childhoon forms
      (ii) Adult forms with mild to moderate renal insufficiency, e.g.:
         Diabetic nephropathy
         Gouty nephropathy
         Chronic pyelonephritis
         Nephrosclerosis
      (iii) Drugs (potassium-sparing diuretics, non-steroidal anti-inflammatory drugs, β-blockers)
2. Hyporeninaemic hypoaldosteronism in some patients with adult salt-wasting pseudo-hypoaldosteronism (see above)
3. Mineralocorticoid deficiency
   a. Generalized adrenal cortical deficiency (Addison's disease, tumour, and enzyme defects)
   b. Isolated aldosterone deficiency with normal renin (familial, idiopathic or enzymatic defects)

---

aldosterone with or without reduced PRA. In hyporeninaemic hypoaldosteronism the abnormality is thought to be an inability of the kidney to respond normally to a reduction in ECF volume with an increase in renin secretion. However, some aldosterone secretory abnormality is also postulated since aldosterone does not respond to the elevated potassium levels.

The origin of the acidosis is a combination of a mildly reduced hydrogen ion secretion (either proximal or distal), intracellular shift of hydrogen ions due to the hyperkalaemia and reduced ammonia excretion.

Clinical features. The condition is usually completely asymptomatic unless hyperkalaemia is severe enough to cause cardiac arrhythmias.

The differential diagnosis includes other forms of RTA, although these usually demonstrate hypo- rather than hyperkalaemia. Primary adrenal cortical abnormalities must be excluded. Determination of PRA differentiates between the major forms.

Urine pH reaches normal minimal values of 5.2 or less when acidosis is present. Ammonia excretion is usually reduced, especially in relation to total acid secretion.

Diagnosis. This condition should be suspected if hyperkalaemia and systemic metabolic acidosis seem inappropriately high for the degree of renal impairment. Metabolic acidosis in chronic renal failure rarely occurs until the glomerular filtration rate has fallen to 20–30% of normal.

In group 1, aldosterone secretion and PRA are normal or elevated and PRA responds normally to postural stimulation. In group 2, both are low and PRA does not increase with assumption of the upright posture.

Minimum urine pH, while acidotic, must be 5.2 or lower and ammonia excretion is usually reduced.

Treatment. 9-α-Fluorocortisone administration in doses of 0.1–0.2 mg/day usually corrects the hyperkalaemia and systemic metabolic acidosis.

Therapy with β-blockers must be carefully monitored in these patients as it can exacerbate the hyperkalaemia.

Bartter's syndrome

This syndrome consists of hypokalaemia, systemic metabolic alkalosis, normotension with elevated aldosterone and renin secretion, and growth retardation in children.

The renal tubular defect is not known but the following have been suggested:

1. A primary defect in sodium (or chloride) reabsorption in early tubular segments (up to and including the thick ascending limbs of the loop of Henle) leading to an increased distal sodium load which stimulates potassium secretion and leads to a decrease in extracellular fluid volume and thus stimulation of aldosterone and renin secretion.

2. A primary potassium abnormality resulting in increased secretion. (Adrenalectomy does not entirely correct the abnormality.)

Genetics. An increase of familial incidence has been noted. Sex distribution is equal.

Clinical features. Onset is mainly in childhood, when it leads to growth retardation, but a late growth spurt usually results in normal height in adulthood. Patients present with weakness, polyuria, vomiting, constipation and muscle paralysis. Other manifestations of severe hypokalaemia may be present, e.g. muscle wasting, rhabdomyolysis and cardiac arrhythmias. Polyuria and nocturia (enuresis) are the result of a severe concentrating defect due to the primary abnormality complicated by hypokalaemia. Hypomagnesaemia has been reported. The condition is permanent.

Diagnosis. The diagnosis rests on the demonstration of potassium wasting (more than 20 mmol/day) in the presence of hypokalaemia with systemic metabolic alkalosis, elevated aldosterone excretion and increased plasma renin activity. Hyperplasia of the juxtaglomerular apparatus on renal biopsy confirms the diagnosis.

The differential diagnosis includes adrenal cortical tumours or ACTH-secreting carcinomas (in which blood pressure is usually elevated) and diuretic abuse. Cathartic abuse or villous papilloma of the colon also cause confusion, although in these cases urinary potassium excretion is low.

Treatment. The mainstay of therapy is lifelong potassium supplementation with or without aldosterone antagonists or potassium-sparing diuretics such as amiloride.

Various other treatments have been tried, in particular drugs which interfere with renal prostaglandin synthesis, such as indomethacin, aspirin and clinoril.

Magnesium supplementation is also very helpful.

Vitamin D resistant rickets (VDRR)

VDRR is predominantly a familial disorder and is characterized by short stature, genu valgum or varum, osteomalacia, hypophosphataemia, phosphaturia and hydroxyprolinuria.

The basic abnormality is a defect in proximal tubular and jejunal phosphate reabsorption, leading to phosphate loss in urine and reduced absorption from the gut. Reduced calcium absorption in the gut has been demonstrated in some patients, and defective renal conversion to the active $1,25(OH_2)D_3$ (type I) and target tissue defect (type II) have also been demonstrated. Bone is unmineralized with increased osteoid. The abnormality is permanent.

Genetics. The condition is transmitted by one X-linked dominant gene with a frequency of 1 in 25 000.

Clinical features. VDRR usually presents in childhood or adolescence although rare cases presenting in adulthood have been described. It is characterized by a reduced growth rate, short stature (normal trunk length), fractures and genu valgum or varum. Females have a less severe form. Tooth eruption may be delayed.

X-rays of bones show rachitic lesions in children and osteomalacia with pseudofractures in pelvis, lower extremities, ribs and scapulae in adults. The presenting symptoms in adults are bone pain and fractures or pseudofractures.

Diagnosis. In suspected individuals a low fasting serum phosphorus and phosphaturia are essential to make the diagnosis. The X-ray findings (see above) are corroborative evidence. Immunoreactive parathyroid hormone (iPTH) assays are usually slightly elevated in type I and markedly so in type II. Urinary cyclic AMP excretion and tubular maximum for phosphate are both increased.

The differential diagnosis includes simple vitamin D deficiency rickets or osteomalacia with markedly reduced serum calcium concentrations and persistently high iPTH, and pseudo-vitamin D deficiency rickets (PDR) which is inherited as a simple autosomal recessive trait characterized by hyponatraemia, mildly reduced or normal serum phosphorus concentration, renal tubular acidosis and aminoaciduria. PDR responds to vitamin D supplements without phosphate supplements, although requirements for the vitamin are 100 times higher than normal. In PDR, the proposed abnormality is reduced production of $1,25(OH)_2D_3$.

Treatment. Treatment requires very high doses of vitamin D (up to 500 000 units per day) together with phosphate supplements (1–4 g/day). 25-Hydroxycholecalciferol and $1,25(OH)_2D_3$ have a short half-life so that accidental overdoses and serious hypercalcaemia can be quickly corrected. Surgical intervention may be necessary.

Pseudohypoparathyroidism

This is a sex-linked dominantly inherited disease characterized by the typical physical findings of a round face, depressed nasal bridge, short thick neck, short stature with brachydactyly (especially of the metacarpal and metatarsal bones), hypocalcaemia, hyperphosphataemia and increased iPTH values. Serum alkaline phosphatase is normal.

The basic abnormality is end-organ (renal tubular) resistance to the action of PTH (a defective renal adenylate cyclase system).

The clinical manifestations are those of hypocalcaemia: tetany, muscle cramps, twitching and even convulsions. The average age of onset of symptoms is 8 years.

Treatment requires very high doses of vitamin D (up to 100 000 units) or active equivalents and calcium supplements to bring serum values to normal.

Water

Abnormalities of water excretion are probably the commonest abnormality of the exocrine function of the kidneys. Since water is not actively transported, most of these abnormalities are produced by alterations in membrane permeability to water, and all presently known derangements are mediated by the antidiuretic hormone (ADH)/ adenylcyclase–phosphodiesterase system and not primarily through membrane abnormalities.

There are two main groups of abnormalities, one resulting in excess loss of water, the other in an inability to excrete water. Most abnormalities are secondary rather than primarily of renal origin.

Excessive water loss — nephrogenic diabetes insipidus

In this condition the tubular segments responsible for concentrating the urine do not respond to circulating endogenous or exogenous ADH, resulting in polyuria, nocturia, polydipsia and hypernatraemia in most cases.

The condition may be hereditary, idiopathic, drug-induced or due to a variety of renal and other disorders.

Aetiology of nephrogenic diabetes insipidus
Hereditary
Congenital nephrogenic diabetes insipidus
Fabry's disease
Non-hereditary
Idiopathic
Cystic disease
Interstitial (medullary) nephropathy
Obstructive disease
Chronic renal failure
Electrolyte disorders
Hypokalaemia
Hypercalcaemia
Drugs
Diuretics
Lithium
Demeclocycline (tetracycline)
Methoxyflurane
Colchicine
Vinca alkaloids
Amphotericin B
Propoxyphene
Isophosphamide
Sulfonylureas
Glibenclamide (glyburide)
Tolazamide
Acetohexamide
Phenothiazines
Trifluoperazine
Chlorpromazine
Miscellaneous
Multiple myeloma
Amyloidosis
Sjögren's syndrome
Low protein intake

In the hereditary form and those drug-induced forms which have been investigated, the defect has been localized to the adenylate cyclase enzyme. This defect results in reduced formation of cyclic AMP. However, in many cases membrane defects (at either the receptor site for ADH or the effector site) preventing an increase in water permeability cannot be excluded with certainty. This latter possibility should be considered particularly in conditions such as chronic renal failure and multiple myeloma.

Other mechanisms, e.g. medullary 'washout' eliminating the high osmolality in the medulla, may

contribute to excessive water loss in patients with low protein intake and chronic renal failure. Osmotic diuresis, as occurs for example in the latter condition, preventing water equilibration across the collecting duct epithelium, may also contribute.

Genetics. The congenital form is rare and has a sex-linked dominant pattern of inheritance, with reduced and variable penetration in females.

Clinical features. The presenting symptoms are polyuria, polydypsia and dehydration although the polyuria is less (3–6 litres/day) than in central diabetes insipidus.

In the inherited form onset is in late infancy, presenting with dehydration, vomiting, fever and hypernatraemia. Hypernatraemia causes restlessness, ataxia, spasm, seizures and grand mal fits.

Because the polyuria is less severe than in the central form, if the thirst mechanism is intact and water is available, hypernatraemia may not be present and the diagnosis can be missed. However, nephrogenic diabetes insipidus of all varieties can lead to dehydration, hypotension and shock.

In hypercalcaemia (and more rarely hypokalaemia) profound polyuria with hypotension is common and the thirst mechanism seems to be impaired.

Diagnosis. The diagnosis rests on the demonstration of a lack of response to either endogenous ADH (following dehydration) or exogenous ADH (following injection of pitressin tannate in oil or nasal instillation of DDVAP).

Urine osmolality before ADH administration may be anywhere between 200 and 400 mosmol/kg, the latter especially if urine flow rates are less than 2 ml/min and glomerular filtration rate is reasonably preserved (more than 50 ml/min). An osmotic diuresis due to glucose or salt excretion must be excluded.

The rise in urine osmolality due to exogenous ADH must be less than 10%, although incomplete forms of the syndrome (rare) may produce a slightly greater rise.

The diagnosis is usually made by exclusion of central neurogenic causes of diabetes insipidus and after psychogenic polydypsia has been excluded. In central, or neurogenic diabetes insipidus (CDI), even after a 3–5% loss in body weight following dehydration, urine osmolality fails to rise but does so promptly following exogenous ADH administration. The differentiation from the incomplete form of CDI can be more difficult as urine osmolalities can reach values of 400–500 mosmol/kg in dehydration with exogenous ADH producing a rise greater than 10%.

Drug-induced NDI is diagnosed by excluding all other causes and preferably by rechallenge after cessation of the drug.

Treatment. There is no satisfactory drug therapy for CDI. Adequate free water ingestion (without salt) is the mainstay of therapy and this should be tailored to maintain normal blood pressure and serum sodium concentrations.

Thiazide diuretics have been advocated. They are said to act by producing volume depletion, which leads to increased proximal sodium and water reabsorption and thus reduced amounts of urine reaching the distal sites, but this explanation is unsatisfactory as patients are already dehydrated. Prostaglandin synthetase inhibitors have been tried.

Water retention

Water retention usually presents as an isolated biochemical finding of hyponatraemia or with central nervous system manifestations (see below).

There are many causes of hyponatraemia due to excess ADH secretion, but the renal tubular response in these is normal. Plasma ADH levels rise with age in relation to serum osmolality.

Aetiology. There are no known intrinsic renal abnormalities resulting in increased tubular sensitivity to endogenous ADH, and all the causes to be discussed are due to drugs.

Although the basic abnormality is not clearly defined, these drugs are thought to enhance sensitivity of the tubules to the action of ADH.

Clinical features. Clinically these drugs produce a varying degree of dilutional hyponatraemia and associated hypo-osomolality. The symptoms are due to hyponatraemia and cerebral oedema with irritability, disorientation, lethargy, twitching, nausea, seizures and even coma. The ECF volume is normal or increased. The hyponatraemia is

Drugs which increase sensitivity to ADH
Vasopressin
Oxytocin
Cyclophosphamide
Acetaminophen (paracetamol)
Indomethacin
Sulfonylureas (chlorpropamide, tolbutamide)

usually chronic, and, since mortality is about 10%, should be regarded as a serious complication, especially in the elderly. Acute hyponatraemia can have a mortality of 50%.

Diagnosis. The diagnosis of this syndrome of inappropriate urine concentration is made by demonstrating a urine osmolality which exceeds that of plasma by at lease 50 mosmol/kg while the plasma osmolality is low (usually around 250–270 mosmol/kg. If renal function is unimpaired, urine osmolality is usually between 400 and 700 mosmol/kg. In addition, normo- or hypervolaemia should be demonstrated. Haematocrit (packed cell volume), serum albumin, urea and creatinine values are normal or below normal; blood pressure is normal or high; tissue turgor is normal; and mucous membranes are moist. Measurement of plasma volume can be very helpful. Urine sodium concentrations are usually in the range of 20–30 mmol/l despite reduced serum values. Blood ADH values are low.

The differential diagnosis must include other causes of dilutional hyponatraemia and the syndrome of inappropriate ADH secretion, usually caused by ADH-secreting tumours, central nervous system disease, lung disease, or drugs such as nicotine, vincristine, clofibrate, carbamezapine (Tegretol), isoproterenol, morphine and barbiturates.

The differentiation of drugs which enhance ADH *activity* from those which enhance ADH *secretion* can be very difficult in the absence of blood ADH measurements. In the latter ADH is either normal or elevated in the presence of both hypo-osmolality and hypervolaemia — both of which should reduce ADH levels. In the absence of such a test the diagnosis can only be made by a careful history and examination to exclude the diseases and drugs known to cause inappropriate secretion by ADH.

A particular diagnostic dilemma is caused by diuretic therapy in the elderly, in whom even a single chlorothiazide tablet per day can result in serious hyponatraemia. The mechanism is thought to be an altered or reset volume-sensing mechanism, which even with a minimal reduction in ECF volume (of, say, 400 ml) will switch on both ADH secretion (or fail to suppress it in the face of hypo-osmolality) and proximal tubular sodium reabsorption. The latter results in excess sodium and water retention and reduced delivery to the diluting segments so that urine cannot be diluted and concentrating ability is impaired. Urine osmolality is usually around 350 mosmol/kg, with relatively low urine sodium excretion (less than 10 mmol/day). This leads to confusion with sodium depletional syndromes which are also caused by diuretics but where ECF volume is grossly reduced. Plasma volume and ADH measurements may also be helpful.

Treatment. Withdrawal of the drug is the treatment of choice. If this is not possible, demeclocycline 200–600 mg/day is effective treatment.

METABOLIC DISORDERS WITH COMPLEX DEFECTS OF TUBULAR FUNCTION

This group of disorders includes variable combinations of multiple proximal tubular abnormalities characterized by aminoaciduria, glycosuria, uricosuria, phosphaturia with hypophosphataemia and bicarbonate wastage, resulting in a systemic metabolic acidosis due to distal or proximal RTA. Osteomalacia is a frequent feature of this complex. In the absence of other systemic disease this is usually referred to as the Fanconi syndrome.

Fanconi syndrome

In a number of both the inherited and the acquired forms the condition is due to a deposition of abnormal amounts of metabolic products. The

---

Aetiology of Fanconi syndrome
Hereditary
  Primary inherited
  Cystinosis
  Wilson's disease
  Lowe's syndrome
  Fructose intolerance
  Tyrosinaemia
  Vitamin D dependent rickets (PDR)
  Galactosaemia
Acquired
  Multiple myeloma
  Amyloidosis
  Sjögren's syndrome
  Nephrotic syndrome
  Renal transplantation
  Vitamin D deficiency
Drugs
  Outdated tetracycline
  6-Mercaptopurine
  Methyl-5-chrome
  Lead
  Cadmium
  Mercury
  Gentamicin

---

precise molecular mechanism is undetermined. A typical swan neck deformity of the proximal tubules has been described in some cases.

The osteomalacia was thought to be caused by the hypophosphataemia but recent evidence indicates that there may also be lack of conversion of vitamin D to its active form ($1,25(OH)_2D_3$) in the kidneys.

Clinical features. In the inherited primary form, the clinical presentation in childhood is usually with renal tubular acidosis and hypokalaemia, muscle weakness, paralysis, nausea, vomiting, dehydration and failure to thrive. For as yet unexplained reasons, patients with the Fanconi syndrome and RTA do not seem to suffer from urolithiasis.

In adults, as well as in children, presentation can be with bone pain and fractures due to osteomalacia or rickets. In children the latter also leads to growth retardation.

The prognosis is generally very good if the underlying condition itself is not lethal.

Genetics. The primary form of FS (De Toni–Fanconi Debré) is inherited in an autosomal manner.

FS may occur in association with systemic disease: multiple myeloma, cystinosis, Sjögren's syndrome, paroxysmal nocturnal haemoglobinuria, or following heavy metal administration, outdated tetracycline or gentamicin.

Diagnosis. The coexistence of generalized aminoaciduria, glycosuria with normal blood glucose concentrations and phosphaturia with hypophosphataemia confirms the diagnosis.

Treatment. The proximal RTA has to be treatment with alkali supplements along the lines discussed above. The hypophosphataemia must be corrected with phosphate supplements and the osteomalacia or rickets with vitamin D or its more potent active forms.

Some of the inherited conditions resulting in FS are reversible. These are Wilson's disease, fructose intolerance and galactosaemia.

Cystinosis

An autosomal recessive disorder commonest in children, this is a storage disease of lysosomes, leading to the deposition of cystine crystals in several organs, including the kidneys. The precise defect causing the accumulation of cystine is not known.

In children, the disease is considered malignant, leading to rapidly progressive renal failure, Fanconi syndrome and rickets. In adults it is mostly benign although in those in whom the onset can be traced back to childhood renal failure may occur.

Diagnosis rests on the demonstration of cystine crystals in cornea, conjunctiva, bone marrow, lymph nodes, the kidney or leucocytes. Treatment is unsatisfactory. d-Penicillamine has been tried with some success but careful monitoring is needed because of its side effects. Renal transplantation is successful and cystine deposits do not recur in the transplanted kidney since the defect is at the cellular level and not due to the presence or absence of a circulatory factor.

Wilson's disease

Wilson's disease is characterized by the accumulation of copper in the renal cortex and other organs. It is inherited as an autosomal recessive trait. The abnormality is at least partially reversible if treated with the copper-chelating agent penicillamine. The Fanconi syndrome occurs, as do proximal and distal RTA.

Galactosaemia

Galactosaemia is a congenital disease inherited as an autosomal recessive trait. It is due to a deficiency in the enzyme galactose-1-phosphate uridyltransfererase, leading to accumulation of galactose-1-phosphate in cells. The clinical manifestations are cataracts, hepatosplenomegaly, aminoaciduria, growth failure and diarrhoea in very young infants. Hypoglycaemia may also be present. The diagnosis is made by demonstrating galactose in urine. Treatment is avoiding foods, such as milk, which contain galactose (lactose).

Hereditary fructose intolerance

Hereditary fructose intolerance presents with renal tubular acidosis of the proximal type and, rarely, urolithiasis. The abnormality is due to a deficiency of aldolase activity in the renal cortex and liver leading to fructose 1-phosphate accumulation and phosphate depletion. Ingestion of fructose-containing foods immediately leads to the Fanconi

---

Aetiology of oxalosis
Hereditary
Acquired
  Rhubarb gluttony or excessive ingestion of oxalate or oxalic acid
  Ethylene glycol (antifreeze) poisoning
  Pyridoxine (vitamin B$_6$) deficiency
  Cirrhosis of the liver
  Klinefelter's syndrome
  Renal tubular acidosis
  Sarcoidosis
  Ileal resection and ileostomy
  Excessive vitamin C ingestion

syndrome, bicarbonate wasting, hyperuricaemia and hypercalciuria. The latter can lead to urolithiasis and nephrocalcinosis if not recognized and treated. It is inherited in an autosomal recessive manner. Abstaining from fructose-containing foods cures the condition.

Oxalosis

Primary hyperoxaluria and oxalosis is a generalized metabolic disorder of oxalate-glyoxylate metabolism leading to an increased load of oxalate in the blood. Nephrocalcinosis, urolithiasis and chronic renal failure are the usual sequelae.

The basic abnormality in the hereditary form is a defect in the transaminase needed to convert glyoxylate to glycine, resulting in increased conversion to oxalate rather than glycine. The pathology is produced by deposition of calcium oxalate crystals in many tissues, including the renal tubules (both inside the cells and in the tubular lumen) leading to nephrocalcinosis, lithiasis and eventually glomerular destruction and end-stage renal failure.

Genetics. The disorder is inherited as an autosomal recessive trait in the majority of families although some exhibit a dominant pattern.

Clinical features. Onset of symptoms is usually between the ages of 2 and 10 years and life expectancy, although variable, is markedly re-

duced. The kidneys are small and contracted, and stone disease with obstruction and infection are the commonest complications.

Diagnosis. An unequivocal rise in urinary oxalate excretion must be demonstrated. Normally the amount of oxalate excreted is less than 45 mg/day (0.45 mmol/day) and the ratio of oxalate to creatinine (in mmol) should be less than 0.05. In oxalosis, excretion is between 100 and 400 mg/day while in the acquired forms it is usually just above normal. Demonstration of oxalate crystals in bone, testes, walls of veins, arteries and sites of tissue injury is very helpful when gross, but minor deposition can be found in patients not suffering from primary oxalosis.

Differentiating the primary from acquired forms can be difficult if the rise in oxalate excretion is equivocal. The primary form usually occurs in children and the acquired forms in adults.

Treatment. Treatment is not effective in the primary form although some alleviation of stone disease can be obtained by high magnesium and phosphate diets. Pyridoxine (vitamin B_6) should also be tried. Treatment with vitamin B_6 should also be tried in the secondary forms for 6–8 weeks before rechecking the urine for a reduced oxalate excretion, and before life-long therapy is instituted. Renal transplantation is of questionable value because of the rapid accumulation of oxalate crystals in the transplanted kidney.

RECOMMENDED READING

Andreoli T E, Grantham J J, Rector F C 1977 Disturbances in body fluid osmolality. American Physiological Society, Bethesda

Earley L E, Gottschalk C W 1979 Strauss and Welt's Diseases of the Kidney, 3rd edn. Little, Brown and Co, Boston

McKusick V A 1978 Mendelian inheritance in man, 5th edn. John Hopkins University Press, Baltimore

Stanbury J B, Syngaarden J B, Fredricksen D S 1982 The metabolic basis of inherited disease, 5th edn. McGraw Hill, Blakiston

18. Cystic renal disease

K. A. Douek   W. M. Bennett

INTRODUCTION

Cystic diseases of the kidney make up 12–14% of all renal diseases, and account for 10% of patients who require renal replacement therapy for end-stage renal failure. Cystic diseases are a diverse and heterogeneous group of disorders, with some entities being relatively common while others are rare. Cystic diseases can be hereditary, congenital, or acquired. Clinical manifestations are protean with some patients remaining asymtomatic while others experience significant morbidity. Cystic renal diseases may come to attention at any age and many patients have various extra-renal manifestations.

In the last decade there have been many advances in the pathogenesis, genetics, and diagnosis of cystic renal diseases. In this chapter the classification of cystic diseases, hypotheses of renal cyst development, and the diagnosis/treatment of the more common cystic diseases will be discussed.

Definitions

A *renal cyst* is an enclosed sac or segment of a nephron dilated to a diameter of 200 μm or more. A *cystic kidney* is a kidney containing 3 or more such cysts. *Cystic kidney disease* is a distinct clinical and pathological entity associated with cystic kidneys.

CLASSIFICATION OF RENAL CYSTIC DISORDERS

Renal cystic diseases include a number of distinct conditions which can be classified on the basis of

Table 18.1 Classification of common renal cystic disorders

I.	Polycystic kidney disease
	Autosomal dominant polycystic kidney disease
	Autosomal recessive polycystic kidney disease
II.	Renal medullary cysts
	Medullary cystic disease
	Medullary sponge kidney
III.	Acquired renal cystic disease
IV.	Renal cysts in hereditary syndromes
	von Hippel–Lindau disease
	Tuberous sclerosis
	Other
V.	Simple renal cysts
	Simple
	Multiple

aetiology, character of the cysts, cyst location, and renal pathology. Over a decade ago a classification system was developed, which has proven useful. It incorporates genetic, functional and radiographic information to provide a basis for clinicopathological correlations. Table 18.1 is an abridged, simplified version which includes the most common entities the physician will experience in clinical practice (for more complete classification, see Gardner & Bergen 1990).

PATHOGENESIS OF RENAL CYSTS

Renal cysts vary in size from microscopic to several centimetres in diameter. They can be simple or multiple. The majority arise as dilated segments of renal tubules. The epithelium lining the cyst cavity often maintains relatively normal transport of water and solutes. The electrolyte composition of the fluid filling these cysts usually reflects the origin and transport capacity of the lining epithelial cells defining the cysts as gradient (distal) or proximal (non-gradient). The majority of non-gradient cysts have epithelium that is so nondescript that the original nephron site of origin cannot be discerned.

Currently there are four major hypotheses proposed for the formation of renal cysts. None of these is mutually exclusive and it is likely that elements of all of them play a role in individual diseases.

A. Increased compliance of the tubular basement membrane. It has been proposed that a biochemical defect (which still remains to be defined), either genetic or acquired, leads to altered physical properties of the tubular basement membrane or abnormalities in cyst–matrix interactions, predisposing to cystic dilation. Animals exposed to diphenylthiazole, a chemical which alters the compliance of tubular basement membranes, develop renal cystic changes. The extrarenal involvement seen in autosomal dominant polycystic kidney disease suggests a generalized basement membrane abnormality.

B. Altered secretion. There is growing experimental evidence that there is reversal of net water and solute movement with influx instead of efflux from affected nephrons, creating cysts. Cyst fluid secretion can be induced in cystic epithelia in vitro by stimulation of cyclic AMP.

C. Intratubular obstruction. Obstruction to tubular output secondary to epithelial hyperplasia and micropolyps would cause an increase in intraluminal pressure with secondary dilation. Electron microscopic studies of cyst walls often show the presence of polypoid lesions. However, this theory does not explain the formation of cysts in extra-renal locations in autosomal dominant polycystic kidney diseases. It is also unlikely that massive cystic dilation would occur in the setting of a normal tubular basement membrane.

D. Proliferation. Abnormal epithelial cell growth and production of excessive basement membrane has been documented in various experimental models of cystic disease and in human cystic epithelia. Abnormal regulation of cell growth is likely in autosomal dominant polycystic kidney disease.

There are also local environmental factors such as renally produced cytokines or growth factors that may influence the development of cystic disease. For example, animals raised in a germ-free environment do not manifest chemically induced cystic disease. In many diseases the kidneys are involved asymmetrically suggesting that local or environmental factors may be necessary for abnormal gene products to be fully manifested in renal cyst formation.

POLYCYSTIC KIDNEY DISEASE

This term refers to two hereditary cystic diseases, autosomal recessive polycystic kidney disease and autosomal dominant polycystic kidney disease. They are distinct entities not only by their mode of inheritance but also by their clinical and pathological characteristics. Both types may occur in children, although autosomal recessive polycystic kidney disease more commonly manifests clinically in this age group. Cysts in autosomal dominant polycystic kidney disease can be demonstrated in utero although renal failure and other clinical symptoms do not present until the third or fourth decade.

Autosomal dominant polycystic kidney disease (ADPKD)

ADPKD is one of the most common genetic disorders. It is responsible for approximately 10% of patients with end-stage renal disease requiring dialysis or transplantation. It affects 1:400 to 1:1000 people and is found throughout the world at similar prevalence rates, although it may be lower in blacks. It is usually classified as a renal disease but its extra-renal manifestations are not only numerous, they also have considerable effects on morbidity and mortality.

Genetics. This disease is transmitted by autosomal dominant inheritance — 50% of offspring of an affected parent inherit the abnormal gene. Random cases from spontaneous mutations can occur. There is almost complete penetrance of the gene such that, at the age of 80, virtually 100% of the patients carrying the gene manifest some evidence of disease. There is however considerable variability in its expression, with some patients being completely asymptomatic with evidence of renal cysts only at autopsy, while others have considerable renal and extra-renal morbidity.

In 1985, a mutant gene for ADPKD was found to be closely linked to the α-globin gene locus on the short arm of chromosome 16. The gene itself has not been isolated and cloned. By gene linkage methods in informative families, affected individuals can be identified before cysts are detected by imaging techniques. Highly polymorphic genetic markers are useful in prenatal or preclinical diagnosis.

Not all ADPKD is linked to the PKD locus on chromosome 16 (called PKD-1). Other gene(s) on yet to be identified chromosome(s) may be responsible for approximately 5–10% of phenotypic PKD (called PKD-2). Unlinked ADPKD (PKD-2) is thought to be a more benign disease with milder and delayed renal failure.

The nature of the genetic defect(s) in ADPKD and how they cause renal and extra-renal manifestations of ADPKD is unknown at present.

Clinical manifestations. ADPKD is a systemic disease. Although the kidney manifests many of the important clinical signs and complications of the disease, there is frequently important cardiovascular, gastrointestinal and neurological involvement (Table 18.2).

1. Cardiovascular involvement. There is an increased incidence of valvular disease in patients with ADPKD. Mitral valve prolapse is the most common abnormality with approximately 30% of patients carrying the gene being affected versus 6% of family members without the gene. There may also be aortic and tricuspid valve incompetence. There is an increased prevalence of left ventricular hypertrophy, presumably secondary to hypertension. Aortic aneurysms and dissection can also occur.

Table 18.2 Extra-renal manifestations of ADPKD

Manifestation	Frequency
Hepatic cysts	75%
Diverticulosis	70%
Cardiac valvular disease	25%
Intracranial aneurysms	10%
Ovarian cysts	40%
Inguinal hernias	15%

2. Gastrointestinal involvement. Diverticulosis is more common in ADPKD patients than in age-matched controls. Complications including diverticulitis, bleeding and perforation with abscess formation may present major clinical problems.

Hepatic cysts are the most common extra-renal manifestation of ADPKD and occur in 30–40% of patients. They are typically multiple and measure up to several centimetres. The incidence tends to increase with age and the severity of renal involvement. Hormonal status probably has an influence, since women are more severely affected than men. Most are asymptomatic although large cysts can cause pain and rarely portal hypertension with its complications, oesophageal varices, splenomegaly and ascites. Hepatic cysts may become infected. Liver function is generally preserved.

Inguinal hernias, as well as pancreatic and splenic cysts, are common. The latter are generally clinically silent.

3. Neurological involvement. Neurological involvement is manifested primarily by intracranial aneurysms. The reported incidence is variable and has ranged anywhere from 0 to 41%, the true incidence being probably around 10%. This wide variability has been attributed to the type of detection methods used, as well as the population of patients. There is evidence to suggest that certain families with ADPKD have an increased susceptibility to intracranial aneurysms compared with other families with this disease. Subarachnoid haemorrhages are responsible for approximately 2% of deaths in ADPKD patients.

Renal manifestations. ADPKD is a systemic disease but nonetheless the kidney manifestations usually dominate the clinical disease and its complications. Renal, structural, functional and endocrine abnormalities develop.

1. Structural abnormalities. Less than 5% of all nephrons are involved in cyst formation. It is not known whether all potential cysts are present at birth, with increases in size and number with time, or whether there is continual cyst formation. Clinically, most patients will have no detectable cysts at birth, by childhood will have several small cysts, and then will develop obvious cysts during adult life. Kidneys in adults can be enormous, reaching up to 40 cm in length and over 8 kg in weight. There is an increase in the incidence of renal adenomas, but no convincing increase in the incidence of renal cell carcinomas.

2. Functional alterations. Renal concentrating ability is impaired secondary to the structural abnormalities associated with a decreased ability to respond to vasopressin. Renal acidification is less consistently abnormal, and as in other patients with severely impaired renal function there may be some salt wasting.

There is less information regarding the decline in GFR during the progression of ADPKD. By the age of 50 approximately 30% of individuals, and by the age of 73 approximately 50% of individuals, will develop end-stage renal disease. Many patients will live a normal lifespan without the need for dialysis or renal transplantation. There is considerable phenotypic variability and no way of predicting which individuals will develop end-stage renal disease. Certain factors have been associated with a worse renal outcome:

a. PKD-1 gene,
b. fetal onset,
c. male gender,
d. hypertension, and
e. large kidneys.

The critical unanswered question is what causes the renal insufficiency since less than 5% of all nephrons are affected by cystic change. Since over 90% of the nephrons remain unaffected, the few cystic nephrons exert some type of adverse effect on the remaining non-cystic nephrons, either through compression, hypertension or induction of interstitial inflammation.

3. Endocrine alterations. ADPKD patients tend to be less anaemic with maintained erythropoietin production compared to patients with other forms of end-stage renal disease and similar GFR. There is also increased renin secretion and this may contribute to the hypertension seen in these patients.

4. Renal complications. Haematuria, both gross and microscopic, is seen in greater than 50% of patients. Haematuria is thought to be secondary to cyst rupture into the renal pelvis, however infection, carcinoma and nephrolithiasis can also be aetiological factors.

One third of ADPKD patients have proteinuria, although usually not of nephrotic proportion. Nephrolithiasis is relatively common and due to calculi of all types.

Infections of the bladder, renal parenchyma and cysts present a problem not only because of their frequency but also because of the difficulty in treatment. Cyst infections in particular are difficult to treat because of poor penetration of most antibiotics across cyst walls. It is possible that infection may hasten the decline of renal function.

60% of patients will complain of abdominal, flank and/or back pain which may be very severe. Some patients experience abdominal fullness rather than pain which can interfere with eating by producing early satiety.

Hypertension is seen in approximately 60% of patients, often occurring prior to the development of renal insufficiency. As mentioned in the previous section, the renin–angiotensin system appears to be activated, probably secondary to renal ischaemia and structural changes within the kidney.

Pathogenesis. The same potential mechanisms reviewed in the first part of this chapter are applicable. The most attractive theory is the one implicating a generalized defect in the physical properties of the basement membrane causing an increase in its compliance along with abnormal growth regulation of renal tubular epithelium. This would explain both the renal and extra-renal manifestations.

Pathology. The kidneys in this disease tend to enlarge massively. In 20% of patients the involvement is asymmetrical. There are hundreds of cysts scattered diffusely throughout the cortex and medulla. They can measure anywhere from a few millimetres to 10–20 centimetres. Normal renal parenchyma often exists between the cystic areas but as the cysts enlarge normal renal tissue becomes crowded out so that the end-stage kidney has little recognizable renal tissue (Figs 18.1, 18.2).

Microscopically the cysts are directly connected to the renal tubules and are lined with normal-looking epithelium. Their origin — proximal or distal tubular — often can be distinguished by the chemical content of the cystic fluid. Hepatic,

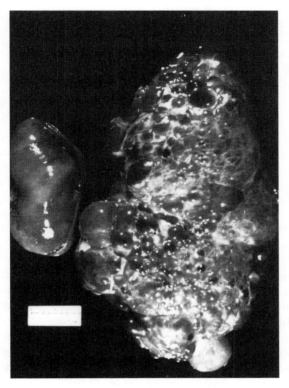

Fig. 18.1   A normal kidney and a polycystic kidney

cardiac and neurological involvement is common (see clinical manifestations).

Diagnosis. There is no definitive diagnostic test at this time; currently the diagnosis depends on demonstration of enlarged kidneys showing multiple cysts on ultrasound or CT scan (Fig. 18.3). A negative study in the first three decades of life does not exclude the presence of disease since it often takes cystic nephrons years to enlarge to detectable sizes.

Recently, gene linkage methods have been used for diagnostic purposes both prenatally and postnatally. Because the exact gene for ADPKD has not been isolated and cloned this test relies on markers on chromosome 16 flanking the ADPKD gene. These markers vary from family to family but they are the same in any one family. To make use of this test at least two clinically affected family members must be available. There is a 5% error rate. The availability of this test presents an ethical dilemma, especially prenatally, because not only do most patients with ADPKD lead full and productive lives, but the natural history of this disorder is variable from patient to patient. The test is of value in transplant donors who may be too young to have developed evidence of cystic disease, as well as in

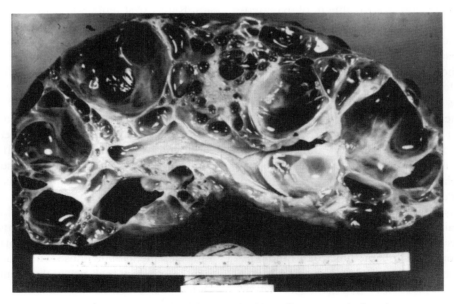

Fig. 18.2   Autosomal dominant polycystic kidney disease — sagittal section

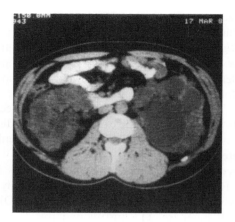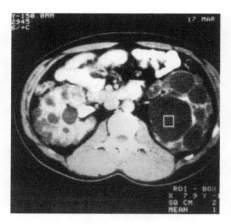

Fig. 18.3   Polycystic kidney disease — CT scan without contrast (left) and with contrast (right)

patients where management would be dictated by the knowledge of the gene status, for example in borderline hypertension in a family history of berry aneurysms. The risks and benefits of the DNA testing must be carefully explained to patients since there is no cure for this disease, only management of the complications.

Management. The most significant complication of this disorder is progressive renal failure and although this ultimate outcome is often not preventable, the progression of renal disease may be slowed by the aggressive treatment of hypertension, treatment of infections, and possibly dietary protein restriction. Once patients develop end-stage renal disease they require the same measures applied to other patients with chronic renal failure. With regard to renal replacement therapy, CAPD, haemodialysis and transplantation are all effective.

These patients, as described earlier, are highly susceptible to genitourinary infections. The renal parenchyma and/or cysts can be infected. It is important to avoid unnecessary urological instrumentation. Parenchymal infections respond to conventional antibiotics, however, in the case of cyst infections, drugs that penetrate cysts and are effective against urinary tract pathogens are needed. These antibiotics include chloramphenicol, trimethoprim–sulphamethoxazole, and the fluoroquinolone drugs, ciprofloxocin, and norfloxacin. If infection persists, surgical drainage may be required.

Occasionally patients develop haemorrhage into a cyst. This can usually be managed conservatively. Rarely angiography and embolization of the bleeding site is required.

Hypertension must be treated aggressively not only because it may accelerate deterioration of renal function but because it may increase the risk if intracerebral haemorrhage in ADPKD patients with berry aneurysms.

Abdominal and flank pain due to enlarging cysts can usually be managed with non-narcotic analgesics. Rarely cyst reduction, either by percutaneous or surgical drainage, is necessary in narcotic-dependent patients with severe persistent pain.

Hepatic cystic disease frequently occurs. This can be complicated by cyst infection which requires parenteral antibiotics and usually some form of surgical drainage. If portal hypertension occurs, hepatic cyst decompression may be useful.

If a heart murmur or click is detected, echocardiography is recommended. If a valvular abnormality is demonstrated, the usual guidelines for bacterial endocarditis prophylaxis should be implemented.

Routine screening for intracranial aneurysms is not recommended. However, patients who have a family history of intracranial haemorrhage, symptomatic patients, and those whose activities place them or others at high risk in the event of a rupture should be screened by CT scan or nuclear magnetic resonance for the presence of an aneurysm. Positive studies should be confirmed by angiogram and aneurysms treated by elective surgical repair if they are accessible and greater than 8–10 mm in size.

Autosomal recessive polycystic kidney disease (ARPKD)

This disease has also been called 'infantile polycystic disease', which is really a misnomer because although the onset is usually in infancy, the first clinical presentation may be in adulthood. The exact incidence is unknown but is estimated at anywhere from 1:10 000 to 1:40 000. There is a frequent association of cystic dilation of renal collecting ducts with varying degrees of hepatic fibrosis. The inheritance is autosomal recessive so heterozygotes are unaffected. Both sexes are involved equally. In a sibship of children from heterozygotes, each fetus has a 25% chance of being affected.

Pathology. The gross appearance shows the kidneys to be enlarged and normally shaped. Occasionally the kidneys can be so huge as to distend the abdominal cavity. There are even reports of individual kidneys being 10–12 times the normal weight. Pinpoint cysts corresponding to the ends of dilated cortical collecting tubules are visible on the capsular surface. The proportion of the kidney occupied by dilated tubules can range from as little as 10% to as much as 80%. The greater the extent of renal involvement by cysts, the more likely it is that the patient will manifest renal insufficiency.

The liver is the other major organ of involvement in this disease. The abnormality may vary from a slight increase in the number of biliary ducts with some portal fibrosis to many dilated and communicating biliary ducts surrounded by dense fibrous tissue. The hepatocytes themselves are normal and hepatic function is therefore rarely compromised. Hepatomegaly may occur at a later stage.

Other organs are seldom affected except for splenomegaly secondary to portal hypertension, and infrequently small pancreatic cysts.

Clinical presentation. Most patients afflicted with this disease present in infancy. Some cases may be suspected by fetal ultrasound while others are diagnosed at birth with huge flank masses that complicate delivery. If there is oligohydramnios secondary to renal dysfunction with minimal urine output in utero, the infants may be born with deep eye creases, a flat snubbed nose, micrognathia and large floppy low-set ears (Potter's syndrome). Contractures of the extremities may also be present. The main neonatal complication is pulmonary distress secondary to pulmonary hypoplasia from oligohydramnios. This is responsible for the majority of deaths that occur in early infancy. Hypertension is common as is some degree of renal insufficiency.

When there is oligohydramnios, renal function is likely to be severely compromised although these infants usually succumb to pulmonary insufficiency. However, many children will have a normal GFR. In them the major early and continuing abnormality is tubular dysfunction with impaired urinary concentrating ability, which can lead to dehydration. There may also be some distal renal tubular acidosis. The rate at which renal function is lost is highly variable, but the majority of those children surviving the first month of life do not develop severe renal insufficiency until later childhood or adolescence. Children who present with ARPKD later in childhood do so most often in conjunction with hepatic fibrosis and the complications of portal hypertension (variceal bleed or hepatosplenomegaly), or less commonly with the secondary effects of chronic renal insufficiency (anaemia, impaired growth, etc.).

Common complications other than hypertension are frequent urinary tract and cyst infections. Bacterial ascending cholangitis, although uncommon, can be fatal.

Diagnosis. The techniques of molecular biology that allow localization of the gene responsible for this disease are still in the preliminary stages. Ultrasound has replaced IVP as the primary diagnostic imaging tool, but even this technique is often too insensitive to pick up cysts. Ultrasound is most useful in the third trimester of pregnancy, as prior to that it lacks sensitivity. Diagnosis is usually suspected if hyperechoic large kidneys are seen, there is a small or non-visualized bladder and oligohydramnios. The cysts themselves are usually not visible. Less severe forms of ARPKD are likely to escape antenatal detection.

Prognosis and management. There is no cure for ARPKD. Treatment is directed at managing the complications. Mechanical ventilation may be required in the neonate. Infants and young children are at risk of dehydration, especially during intercurrent illnesses where there is an increase in insensible water loss. Bicarbonate may be required for renal tubular acidosis. Hypertension and urinary tract infections also need to be aggressively treated. For those who develop chronic renal failure, 1,25 dihydroxyvitamin D_3 and phosphate binders need to be used to prevent renal osteodystrophy. Erythropoietin is useful for anaemia, and most recently growth hormone has become available for clinical use. Dialysis and/or renal transplantation are required when symptomatic end-stage renal disease occurs, the latter being preferable as it offers definitive renal replacement therapy. With prolonged survival and accelerated growth and development, close monitoring for the complication of portal hypertension is required. Fever with abnormal liver function tests should lead to a high level of suspicion of cholangitis, which can be lethal.

In addition to the above significant medical problems, the psychosocial stresses in the child and family can be overwhelming; social support using a team approach is an integral part of management.

Survival of all but the most severely affected neonates who demonstrate pulmonary hypoplasia is possible. 15-year survival for those who survive beyond the first year is approximately 79%. Causes of death include renal failure, sepsis, hypertension and cardiac failure, bacterial cholangitis and portal hypertension.

Acquired renal cystic disease (ARCD)

ARCD is the development of multiple fluid-filled cysts in kidneys of patients with progressive renal disease who have no history of hereditary cystic disease.

Although first described in the 1840s, it was 'rediscovered' in the 1970s and has become an exceedingly common entity in dialysis patients, with 50–90% of patients who have been on dialysis for more than 5 years being affected. Men may be at slightly higher risk than women, and blacks are more frequently and severely affected than caucasians. Patient age, type of renal disease and dialysis modality have no influence on the epidemiology of this disease. Duration of renal failure is the major determinant of cyst formation. The importance of being aware of and recognizing this entity lies in the fact that ARCD is a premalignant state.

Pathology. This is a bilateral condition; small multiple cysts mostly less than 0.5 cm in size predominate in the renal cortex, although there may be involvement of the renal medulla. The kidneys often retain the markedly shrunken appearance characteristic ESRD, although they can increase in size and become quite large — this tends to be a late finding. This last characteristic can occasionally make it difficult to distinguish ACD from APKD. The fluid in the cysts can be clear or haemorrhagic. Occasionally there is renal epithelial hyperplasia with papillary projections, nuclear atypia and mitoses. It appears that there is a continuum between epithelial hyperplasia, adenomas and carcinoma.

No solid lesions or cysts are found in other solid organs in ARCD, in contrast to ADPKD.

Clinical manifestations. The majority of patients with ARCD are asymptomatic and ARCD is discovered during incidental abdominal ultrasound or CT scan imaging. Other common modes of presentation are gross haematuria, flank or abdominal pain, fever, palpable abdominal mass, retroperitoneal haemorrhage, nephrolithiasis, and manifestations of renal cell carcinoma.

Of these symptoms and signs the most serious complication is the development of renal cell carcinoma, whose incidence is 40 times that in the general population (Fig. 18.4). The incidence is higher in male patients and blacks. Further complicating matters, tumours are often clinically silent (86%). In patients on dialysis for more than 10 years, the incidence is 5%. The tumours tend to be multifocal and bilateral, and metastases are seen in approximately 20% of patients. It would appear that the development of carcinoma is a continuum and that the sequence of events is that

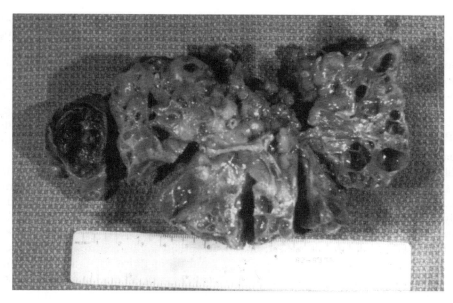

Fig. 18.4   Acquired renal cystic disease with evidence of renal cell carcinoma

of dysplasia → hyperplasia → adenoma → carcinoma.

Pathogenesis. There are many proposed theories but as with all cystic diseases the pathogenesis remains an enigma. Some have suggested that chemicals from the haemodialysis equipment may play a role, however this does not explain acquired cysts in patients on peritoneal dialysis or patients with longstanding renal insufficiency who have never been dialysed. Another proposed mechanism is tubular obstruction from fibrosis and/or calcification. The uraemic milieu seems to be the most important factor, and a retained metabolite acting as a renotropic hormone is probably the most plausible theory since it would explain the cyst involution seen in patients after transplant and would also explain recurrences observed with failure of the renal transplant.

Diagnosis. Imaging modalities used in diagnosing ARCD include ultrasound and CT scan, the latter being superior (especially when enhanced). Each cyst found on either ultrasound or CT is accompanied by 10–20 small undetectable cysts.

Management. Managing this entity has been difficult, not only because of its clinical quiescence but also because of its malignant potential. Thus it is not surprising that there is a lot of controversy surrounding the issue of whether it is cost-effective to screen all dialysis patients for renal carcinomas, and if so with what modality and how often. Many clinicians agree that patients treated by dialysis for more than 3 years should be screened for ARCD using sonographic examination or CT scans annually. However, because of the high cost of screening, some institutions examine only symptomatic patients.

It is noteworthy that following successful renal transplantation there is regression of acquired cysts in a relatively short period of time ($\frac{1}{4}$ to $\frac{1}{5}$ of their previous size within a month). Pre-existing renal tumours, adenomas and carcinomas, usually do not regress after transplantation but rather grow because of patients' immunosuppressed states. These patients should therefore be included in screening protocols, especially if there is graft failure over several years, since the renal allograft may acquire cysts and there may be an increase in the number of cysts in the remaining native kidneys.

Regardless of the detection protocol used, any renal cell carcinoma found that is more than 2 cm in diameter provides a strong indication for nephrectomy. Some have even suggested bilateral nephrectomies because of increased risk of malignancy in the other kidney.

The 5-year survival is approximately 35%, a value close to that for classic renal cell carcinoma.

Medullary sponge kidney (MSK)

MSK is a renal cystic disease characterized by the presence of dilated collecting ducts confined to the medulla. It is common disorder and is usually asymptomatic. Most cases are sporadic and it is most certainly a developmental defect. As it is generally asymptomatic the diagnosis is not usually made unless there are secondary complications. Thus the true incidence remains unknown, although it has been estimated to be approximately 1/5000 in the general population. There is no sexual or racial and probably no familial preponderance.

Pathology. There is usually normal kidney architecture unless there are secondary changes from complications. The only visible abnormality is marked spherical, oval or irregular enlargement of medullary and inner papillary portions of the collecting duct. The cysts usually measure 1–3 mm, and are bilateral in 70% of cases. They frequently contain densely radiopaque spherical concretions composed of apatite.

Clinical features. This is an asymptomatic disorder unless it is complicated by urolithiasis, infection and/or haematuria.

Stones occur probably because of a combination of hypercalciuria and stasis. MSK has been reported in 2–5% of patients with renal calculi.

Infection is a common occurrence as is haematuria (gross or microscopic). The latter is usually painless, recurrent and often unrelated to stones or infection. Because the defect is medullary there is most often a defective concentrating ability as well as renal tubular acidosis of the distal type. GFR tends to be preserved.

MSK may be associated with hemihypertrophy of the body. It is controversial whether there is an increased incidence of hyperparathyroidism.

Some patients with recurrent colic become narcotic-dependent.

Diagnosis. MSK is usually diagnosed as an incidental finding in patients undergoing IVP for a renal disorder, usually stones or infection. It has been estimated that 0.5% of IVPs will show MSK. There is a very characteristic image with radial or linear structures in papillae or cystic collections of contrast material in ectatic collecting ducts. Plain films show enlargement of one or both kidneys and the presence of variable numbers of radiopaque calculi.

Treatment. For most patients, MSK will be an incidental finding and no treatment is required except a yearly urinalysis and urine culture to exclude infection. Patients should be informed of the benign nature of this disease and of the possibility of haematuria, infections and forming stones. For those patients with nephrolithiasis the management is similar to that of other patients with stone disease. Active and progressive stone formation can nearly always be arrested by thiazides and is effective not only in patients with hypercalciuria but also those with normocalciuria. Infections need to be treated promptly. If there is systemic acidosis secondary to distal RTA, oral or parenteral bicarbonate salts should be given.

MSK has an excellent prognosis, end-stage renal disease is a very rare occurrence and when it occurs is because of recurrent urolithiasis and pyelonephritis.

Medullary cystic kidney disease (MCKD)

This is a rare disorder, most often seen in children or adolescents, which inevitably progresses to ESRD. Another condition, juvenile nephronophthisis, is similar histologically as well as clinically, except that it manifests itself at a later age. Whereas MCKD is an autosomal recessive disorder, this latter condition is inherited in an autosomal dominant fashion. Both of these conditions can occur sporadically. Because these disorders are so similar clinically, except for the differences discussed above, they are generally discussed as one entity.

MCKD is characterized by the presence of multiple cysts, arising from distal and collecting tubules and confined to the medulla and cortico-medullary junction. The kidneys are usually

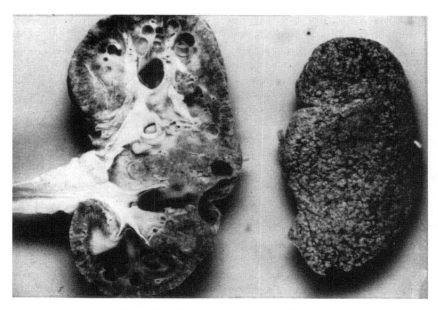

Fig. 18.5   Medullary cystic kidney disease

small bilaterally (Fig. 18.5). Microscopically there is interstitial fibrosis, tubular atrophy and glomerulosclerosis.

Clinically, patients usually present in the first or second decade of life with manifestations of chronic renal failure. There is frequently nocturia due to decreased concentrating ability and sodium wasting so that it is unusual for these patients to be hypertensive. The diagnosis should be suspected in patients who develop ESRD in childhood and have a positive family history. Excretory urography and renal biopsy may be used to make the diagnosis. There is no cure for this disorder and treatment is directed at managing the manifestations of chronic renal failure, including sodium therapy if there is a salt-wasting nephropathy.

Simple cysts

Simple cysts are the most common cystic abnormality encountered in human kidneys. They can be solitary or multiple and frequently increase with age, being rare in children and having a frequency of 30% in patients over the age of 40.

They can be unilateral or bilateral, usually spherical and unilocular, measuring 0.5–4 cm.

They are usually diagnosed during abdominal imaging for other purposes, although occasionally patients have presented with a palpable abdominal mass, haematuria after trauma, mild proteinuria, infection, or rarely hypertension. Further evaluation is deemed unnecessary unless the radiographic appearance suggests the possibility of malignancy — certain criteria are used to define this.

No treatment is required unless they become symptomatic.

Miscellaneous renal cystic disorders: tuberous sclerosis and von Hippel–Lindau disease

Tuberous sclerosis is inherited as an autosomal dominant disorder. It is manifested by variable mental retardation, seizures and characteristic skin lesions known as adenoma sebaceum. The lesions usually are most apparent in a butterfly distribution around the nose. Renal involvement can occur in the form of angiomyolipomas as well as multiple renal cysts, the latter being occasionally responsible for renal impairment and hypertension. Renal cell carcinoma can develop in these cysts.

Von Hippel–Lindau syndrome, also inherited in an autosomal dominant fashion, is defined as intracranial haemangioblastomas that occur in association with multiple systemic angiomas, especially retinal. The renal lesions of von Hippel–Lindau include cysts, haemangiomas and adenomas, as well as renal cell carcinoma. There is also an increased incidence of phaeochromocytoma in patients with von Hippel–Lindau syndrome.

REFERENCES AND RECOMMENDED READING

Gabow P A 1991 Polycystic kidney diseases. Seminars in Nephrology 11: 595–684

Gagnadoux N F, Habib R, Levy N et al 1989 Cystic renal diseases in children. Advances in Nephrology 18: 33–58

Gardner K D, Bergen J 1990 The cystic kidney. Kluwer Academic Publishers

Grantham J J, Slusher S L 1984 Management of renal cystic disorders. In: Suki W N, Massry S G (eds) Therapy of renal diseases and related disorders. Martinus Nijhoff Publishers, pp 383–404

Welling L W, Grantham J J 1991 Cystic and developmental diseases of the kidney. In: Brenner B M, Rector F C (eds) The kidney. W B Saunders, pp 1657–1694

19. Urinary calculi

B. T. Emmerson

INTRODUCTION

Calculi are a common cause of morbidity. Approximately 12% of males and 5% of females will have an episode of renal colic during their lifetime. Although much is known about their prophylaxis, this knowledge is often not utilized clinically in their prevention. The development of extracorporeal shock wave lithotripsy (ESWL) has simplified the management of established calculi but has not reduced the importance of prophylaxis.

COMPOSITION OF URINARY CALCULI

Over 60% of renal calculi consist principally of calcium oxalate, with or without the addition of calcium phosphate salts. Up to 20% may consist principally of calcium apatite or phosphates, and are usually radiopaque. Of the non-calcium-containing and therefore radiolucent calculi, the most important consist of uric acid (7%), magnesium ammonium phosphate (struvite — approximately 7%) and cystine (approximately 3%). The magnesium ammonium phosphate or struvite stones are caused by an infection with urea-splitting organisms, particularly Proteus and Pseudomonas, and these cause the production of ammonium and hydroxyl ions which raise the urine pH. Such stones are best regarded as infection stones.

PATHOGENETIC FACTORS

Calculi are rarely due to a single cause, but develop as a result of several abnormalities. Supersatura-tion of the crystal constituents at some time is essential for the formation of a calculus. The first step would be nucleation of a crystal (combination of soluble ions to form a solid phase), on the surface of which other crystals may be added. There are a variety of heterogeneous factors in urine which can inhibit this nucleation including citrate, protein and glycosaminoglycans. Normal urine is mostly supersaturated for calcium oxalate and this is maintained in solution by the presence of a variety of inhibitors of crystal formation and other factors which act by determining the retention of the crystal within the urinary tract and its subsequent growth. In general, however, crystal components would need to be present in abnormally high concentration and/or their solubility might be diminished by factors such as change in pH of the urine (Table 19.1). More than one factor may be present in one patient and, in a considerable proportion of patients, no cause is discernible.

Table 19.1 Some solutes responsible for the formation of urinary calculi

Solute	Reason for presence in excess	Reference
Calcium	Hypercalcaemic states	Pak 1991
Calcium	Hypercalciuric states	Lemann et al 1991
Oxalate	Malabsorptive states	Williams 1978
Uric acid	Hyperuricaemic states	Yu 1981
Uric acid	Hyperuricosuric states	Coe & Kavalach 1974
Cystine	Cystinuria	Dahlberg et al 1977
Xanthine	Xanthinuria	Frayha et al 1973
Dihydroxy-xanthine	Adenine phosphoribosyl-transferase deficiency	Van Acker et al 1977

Inadequate urine volume

Whatever other factors might be operating, renal calculi are preventable by an adequate urine volume. Although the normal urine volume is usually recorded as 1500 ml per 24 hours, a large proportion of normal subjects have urine volumes significantly and consistently less than one litre per 24 hours. It does not appear to be easy for a normal subject voluntarily to increase urine volume but it is nonetheless important to emphasize the dominant role urine volume has on the concentration of all urine constituents.

Abnormal concentrations of urine constituents

Of the normal components of urine, the concentrations of calcium, urate and oxalate are most important in determining crystal nucleation and calculus formation. Of metabolites, the concentration of which becomes abnormal (principally in genetic disease), one needs to consider urate cystine, xanthine and dihydroxyadenine.

Increased urinary acidity

The tendency to stone formation is mostly increased by increasing urinary acidity. A persistently low urine pH tends to increase calculus formation, particularly in relation to calcium oxalate and uric acid calculi. This tends to occur in some patients with gout (who have a reduced ammonia production by the kidney and increased excretion of titratable acid), and in chronic diarrhoeal states associated with metabolic acidosis due to intestinal alkali losses. These include ileal resection or disease, gastrectomy and ulcerative colitis.

Loss of inhibitors of crystallization

Citrate is an important constituent of urine which tends to complex calcium and reduce the tendency to crystallization of calcium salts. Citrate excretion is reduced in acidosis.

Familial and other factors

Urinary glycosaminoglycans prevent crystal growth by binding to the surface of calcium oxalate crystals. The formation of uric acid crystals may lead to calcium oxalate crystals orientating themselves on the surface of such a crystal to promote calculus formation. There is considerable interaction between all of these factors. A familial predisposition to the formation of calculi exists but, except when due to metabolic abnormalities leading to overproduction of metabolites, the extent to which this is inherited or is related to dietary habits is not clear.

Necrotic papillae may form a nidus for stone formation, which is thus a feature of analgesic nephropathy. 'Medullary sponge kidneys' are associated with renal stones.

SPECIFIC CONTRIBUTORY FACTORS

The most important of these are hypercalciuria, hyperuricosuria and hypocitraturia.

Hypercalciuria

This is seen in about 60% of stone patients. The cause comprises a broad spectrum of processes regulating calcium transport which appear largely to be genetically determined. The boundary between normals and hypercalciurics is not clearly defined. An arbitrary line is usually drawn at 7.5 mmol (300 mg) per 24 hours for males and 6.25 mmol per 24 hours for females, roughly equivalent to 0.1 mmol per kg per day. However, 8% of normal subjects without renal calculi excrete calcium in excess of these amounts. Several inhibitors of calcium crystallization, including citrate, pyrophosphate, magnesium and various polypeptides are present in urine but none has yet achieved diagnostic or therapeutic significance. High urinary calcium values may be associated with hypercalcaemia which, if found, needs to be investigated and treated in its own right. Patients with high urinary calcium values who are normocalcaemic are said to have 'idiopathic hypercalciuria'.

Two forms of hypercalciuria?

Two subsets of patients with hypercalciuria have been defined. 'Absorptive' hypercalciuria has been attributed to a primary increase in the jejunal absorption of calcium and is thought to be inherited. Although the serum calcium does not rise, some undefined signal appears to be transmitted to the kidney which results in an increase in urinary calcium excretion. Patients with 'absorptive' hypercalciuria cease to overexcrete calcium when the intestinal overabsorption is prevented (e.g. by a low calcium diet or by oral calcium-binding agents).

'Renal' hypercalciuria is believed to be due to a tubular defect, resulting in inadequate calcium reabsorption in the renal tubule with compensatory hyperabsorption of calcium of the gastrointestinal tract. Renal hypercalciuria, which is much less common than absorptive hypercalciuria, is not influenced by dietary manipulations. The distinction between the two forms is somewhat arbitrary and it may be difficult to decide which of them is present in a given patient, without special investigations. Even then, it may be difficult.

Hyperuricosuria

Uric acid calculi usually consist of pure uric acid. They are radiolucent and often contain an orange/yellow pigment. Occasionally there is some admixture of calcium oxalate or calcium phosphate. A small amount of uric acid may be present in a mixed calculus, especially if the urine is infected. Ammonium urate calculi affect malnourished children in tropical countries and usually form in the bladder and lower urinary tract.

Although uric acid calculi occur frequently in patients with gout, this association is not invariable and only about a quarter of patients with gout develop uric acid calculi. Conversely, only a quarter of patients with uric acid calculi suffer from gout, so the concordance between the two diseases is not high. The solubility of uric acid is about ten times greater at a pH of 7 than at a pH of 5. The pK_a of uric acid is 5.75, at which pH half is in the ionized form as urate and half in the un-ionized form as uric acid. Thus urines with a pH of less than 5.5 are often supersaturated with uric acid. Uric acid calculi are caused either by a high uric acid concentration in the urine or by a low urine pH.

The urinary uric acid concentration depends on urine volume as well as the rate of uric acid excretion. Urine volume, which is a prime determinant of the concentration of all urinary constituents, depends on fluid consumption and fluid loss from the body, which varies with climate, exercise and body temperature.

High uric acid excretion

In a stable metabolic state, urate elimination during any period must be equal to urate production. Two thirds of this urate is eliminated by the kidneys. Uric acid excretion is likely to be elevated in conditions associated with increased intrinsic production of urate or when there is a large quantity of diet-derived urate.

Intrinsic overproduction of urate occurs as the result of several mutations involving enzymes regulating purine synthesis and re-utilization. The Lesch–Nyhan syndrome (severe deficiency of hypoxanthine-guanine phosphoribosyltransferase — HGPRT) may present in infancy with the passage of yellow/orange gravel in the urine. Patients with partial HGPRT deficiency have no neurological abnormality but severe overexcretion of urate may be present for years prior to the development of either uric acid calculi or gout. Marrow overactivity secondary to myeloproliferative disorders, leukaemia or other neoplasms leads to urate overexcretion but not commonly to uric acid calculi.

Dietary factors (of which the patient may be unaware) frequently cause high urine urate values. Moderate amounts of high purine foods such as meat or yeast products, or large amounts of food with a moderate purine content, provide considerable urate loads which are largely eliminated by the kidneys. A high ethanol intake may lead to degradation of purine nucleotides and an increased urate production.

Hyperexcretion of urate may be present in association with low serum urate values in patients whose urate clearance is high. Thus the presence of a normal serum urate concentration does not exclude a high urine urate excretion, nor does an elevated serum urate concentration indicate a high urine urate — more often it would be secondary to a low urinary urate excretion. This occurs as a normal variant, in the presence of intrinsic tubular disease, or with uricosuric drugs. Increased urate clearance also occurs after the withdrawal of some drugs (e.g. diuretics) or the disappearance of a metabolite (such as lactate) which had previously been causing urate retention.

Reduced urine pH as a cause of uric acid calculi

Many patients with uric acid calculi have normal serum and urine urate concentrations. It has been suggested that some of these patients form stones because of persistently low urinary pH values. This in turn has been attributed to reduced ammonia production by the kidneys with an increase in the excretion of titratable acid. Reduced renal ammoniagenesis may be due to an intrinsic tubular defect, to renal insufficiency or to dietary factors.

Hypocitraturia

Citrate, an inhibitor of crystallization of calcium oxalate and phosphate, is one of the important calcium complexing agents in urine, a function it performs by reducing free calcium ion concentration. The main contributor to a lowered urinary citrate is systemic acidosis, which can be due either to renal tubular acidosis or to enteric diseases with chronic diarrhoea. In many cases, no cause for the low urinary citrate is apparent. Urinary citrates are regarded as reduced when they are less than 1.7 mmol/day, and diet may be an important determinant. Citrate excretion is normally greater in women, which may account for their lower prevalence of renal calculi.

Hyperoxaluria

Primary hyperoxaluria is a rare inherited metabolic disease caused by an enzyme deficiency. Enteric hyperoxaluria, on the other hand, is more common and results from excessive intestinal absorption of oxalate from the colon. It occurs in small bowel disease, malabsorption and after a jejuno-ileal bypass. A low dietary calcium may promote oxalate absorption because of reduced binding by calcium of dietary oxalate in the gut. There has been little study of the contribution of such dietary oxalate to oxalate calculus formation.

Renal tubular acidosis

This condition is characterized by a reduced ability to secrete hydrogen ions, particularly by way of the distal renal tubules. In the complete form, this results in a hyperchloraemic metabolic acidosis, which may be associated with hypercalciuria, hypocitraturia and nephrocalcinosis. In the incomplete form, these features may be mild and systemic acidosis may be only slight. The increased urinary alkalinity diminishes the solubility of calcium salts and increases the tendency to calculus formation. Such patients are thought to constitute approximately 3% of unselected stone formers.

Inflammatory bowel disorders

A range of chronic diarrhoeal diseases (such as Crohn's disease, ulcerative colitis, ileal resection and ileal disease) can lead to an increase in the intestinal elimination of water, bicarbonate and sodium and result in a concentrated urine with a lowered pH. Hypocitraturia and hyperoxaluria may also be present and the concentrated acid urine may also promote the formation of uric acid stones.

Specific components

The next three conditions reflect the situation where urine supersaturation occurs with a compound that is poorly soluble in the normal pH range and which, when normally present, is present in only small amounts.

Cystinuria

In this condition, which affects between 1% and 3% of stone formers, excessive amounts of cystine appear in the urine as a result of abnormal mucosal and tubular transport mechanisms for the dibasic amino acids. Cystinuria may be diagnosed by the 'benzene ring' shape of cystine crystals in urine, by the nitroprusside test or by the demonstration of excessive amounts of cystine in the urine.

At the usual urinary pH values, approximately 1.25 mmol (300 mg) of cystine are soluble in one litre. Homozygous cystinurics may excrete three times this amount daily. The frequency of homozygosity is approximately 1 in 10 000.

Xanthinuria

Xanthinuria is a rare metabolic disorder characterized by gross deficiency of xanthine oxidase, with a block in the metabolism of hypoxanthine to xanthine and of xanthine to uric acid. This leads to high values of urinary xanthine (up to 3 mmol/ 24 h) and hypoxanthine (up to 1 mmol/24 h) and low rates of urate production and excretion. Marked hypouricaemia is usually present. Less than 50 patients with xanthinuria have been described and only half of these suffered from xanthine calculi.

All patients treated with allopurinol develop partial xanthine oxidase deficiency. In the absence of abnormalities of purine metabolism, the increase in the excretion of xanthine and hypoxanthine is usually not sufficient to produce problems. However, xanthine calculi have been reported in a few patients with HGPRT deficiency who continue to overproduce purine metabolites after the administration of allopurinol.

Dihydroxyadenine calculi

2, 8-Dihydroxyadenine calculi are extremely rare. They are indistinguishable from uric acid calculi by the common chemical tests but are readily identified by means of uricase or infrared spectroscopy. Most cases have been diagnosed in young children but first attacks of renal colic due to dihydroxyadenine calculi have been reported in a few persons over 40 years of age, usually in association with renal disease.

Dihydroxyadenine calculi are invariably associated with a severe deficiency of the adenine re-utilization enzyme adenine phosphoribosyltransferase (APRT). Because of its imperfect re-utilization, adenine accumulates and is converted to 2,8-dihydroxyadenine by xanthine oxidase. The disorder is probably inherited as an autosomal recessive trait although dihydroxyadenine calculi have been reported in heterozygotes and in patients with partial deficiency of this enzyme. Inhibition of xanthine oxidase by allopurinol reduces the formation of dihydroxyadenine and the tendency to develop calculi.

PRESENTATION

Not all patients present with pain. Some urinary calculi are asymptomatic and are diagnosed incidentally during radiological examination. Others present with complications, such as obstruction or infection. However, the majority of patients with renal calculi present with pain, usually referred to as 'renal colic'.

'Colic'

Pain due to renal calculi may be distinguished by its sudden onset, its extreme severity and its radiation as well as by associated urinary symptoms. It is usually unilateral with localization of the pain in the loin, the groin or intermediate points. The pain lasts for hours rather than for minutes or days, and while there may be a continuous background of pain, there may also be bouts of increased severity during which the patient becomes pale and distressed. Associated urinary symptoms (sometimes not apparent at the time of initial presentation) include dysuria, discoloration of the urine, frank haematuria or the passage of solid material from the urethra.

There is a significant tendency for recurrence of renal colic and further episodes tend to occur in 14% within the first year, in 35% within 5 years and in about 50% within 10 years.

EVALUATION

The extent of investigation of a patient with calculus disease will depend upon the extent of the problem. However, a simple series of investigations should probably be undertaken in most

Table 19.2 Some useful tests in the investigation of patients with urinary calculi

Test	Yield
Serum calcium	Primary hyperparathyroidism
Serum uric acid	Hyperuricaemic states; xanthinuria
Serum creatinine	Current status of renal function
Urine calcium	'Idiopathic' hypercalciuria
Urine uric acid	Hyperuricosuric states
Nitroprusside test	Cystinuria
Urine pH	Tubular acidosis
Micro-urine	Crystals; infection
Stone analysis	Uric acid; cystine
Intravenous pyelography	Sponge kidney: presence of obstruction

patients because of the potential chronicity of the problem (Table 19.2). A history of predisposing factors should focus particularly upon a family history of calculi, on medications (including vitamins such as vitamin C and D), dietary aberrations, enteric disease, fluid intake and the presence of renal or other disease relevant to the formation of renal calculi.

INVESTIGATION

Stone analysis

Whilst of particular value in relation to uric acid and cystine calculi, knowledge of the chemical composition of any calculus is often of considerable value in planning appropriate therapy for the individual. Every effort should be made to analyse any stone which might become available or to find such a stone.

Micro-urine

Microscopic haematuria would support the diagnosis of calculus formation in patients with negative radiological findings. Sterile pyuria is a common finding in patients with renal stones and does not contribute to any specific diagnosis. The most important information is the demonstration of infection and the identification of the organism responsible. This is important for prognosis as well as for therapy. Hexagonal cystine crystals may be seen but the significance of calcium oxalate crystals is doubtful since some may be present in normal subjects. The presence and number of uric

acid crystals varies with urine pH, so that their presence is not of diagnostic significance.

Blood tests

Blood tests for calcium, phosphate, urate, creatinine and bicarbonate are justified. Hypercalcaemia is an important factor contributing to calculus formation. It should be managed by determining its cause, e.g. hyperparathyroidism, hypervitaminosis D, etc. It is essential that either a normal serum calcium be demonstrated or an abnormal serum calcium be investigated.

Mild hypophosphataemia is common in stone formers, but this test lacks discrimination and is not useful in distinguishing the various types of stone former. Plasma urate and creatinine concentrations are valuable in reflecting disorders of urate metabolism or of renal function. The presence of acidosis would imply the need to pursue its cause.

Pyelography and ultrasonography (see Ch. 5)

All patients with renal calculi require structural studies of the urinary tract, usually by intravenous pyelography. This may demonstrate uric acid or other radiolucent stones, may establish the diagnosis of sponge kidney or may indicate the need for surgical intervention.

Biochemical measurements of urine

Because of the simplicity of the test, and because of the potential long-term management implications of a renal calculus, at least one 24-hour collection of urine should be undertaken while the patient is maintaining his/her normal lifestyle. Each 24-hour urine should be analysed for its sodium, calcium, phosphate, urate and creatinine concentrations as well as to provide information about urine flow rate, acidity, and renal function.

Urine calcium

If urine calcium is increased, its cause can be investigated and treatment instigated towards restoring it to more appropriate levels. Its importance as a contributing factor has already been emphasized.

Urinary uric acid

The concentration and excretion rate of uric acid in the urine are more important parameters than the serum urate concentration. Hyperuricaemia in a patient with a renal calculus is not diagnostic of uric acid calculi, since the finding may be secondary to associated renal insufficiency, or be entirely unrelated to stone formation. The most useful investigation is the determination of the urinary urate excretion on the patient's usual diet. Studies on a purine-free diet are indicated only when genetic overproduction of urate is suspected. The 24-hour urine estimations not only provide information concerning the usual urine volume and the urate and creatinine clearances but are particularly valuable in estimating the total uric acid excretion and the uric acid concentration in the urine. During treatment, these latter two should be kept as low as possible.

Urine pH

The failure of urine pH to fall below 5.4 after oral administration of ammonium chloride is seen in a number of conditions apart from tubular acidosis. Proteus infections, hyperglobulinaemic states, the consumption of antacid preparations and noncompliance with instructions concerning the acid load, all lead to an apparent failure to acidify the urine. If these conditions are excluded, a urine pH of 5.5 or more will indicate failure of hydrogen ion excretion.

Urinary cystine

Although relatively rare, screening tests for increased urinary cystine excretion are simple and justify being used as a routine.

This comprises the basic series of investigations, which should probably be undertaken in each patient with a renal calculus. Further investigations are less frequently indicated. However, if recurrence of stones becomes a problem, further observations of the various abnormal parameters may be important, as well as the measurement of urinary oxalate and urinary citrate. If hypercalciuria persists and more calculi develop, further investigation can be undertaken to determine its cause by studies of fasting urinary calcium excretion (to demonstrate a renal leak of calcium), or the response to a calcium load (a greatly increased urine calcium suggests an absorptive hypercalciuria). Treatment can then be directed towards the appropriate cause.

TREATMENT

Appropriate treatment may follow directly from the results of investigation. In the absence of a specific cause, non-specific advice can be given as follows, and can be modified to suit individual patients.

High fluid intake

Fluid intake should be sufficient to achieve a urine volume of at least 2 litres per 24 hours and preferably greater. It is difficult for most patients to increase their fluid intake significantly; success in increasing urine flow rate usually requires the patient to measure and record urine volume for at least a 24-hour period each week until an adequate volume is being maintained. Measuring urine volume at regular intervals is one important reason for continuing to monitor patient progress.

Dietary modification

Since this is a chronic condition, with which the patient must live, any acceptable dietary modification can usually be of only modest degree. A moderate reduction of dietary sodium, calcium, protein and oxalate is generally recommended, although no comprehensive study to establish the beneficial effect of such dietary restriction on stone formation has been undertaken. However, the rationale is as follows. Since a high urinary sodium promotes renal calcium excretion, sodium excretion (and hence sodium intake) should be restricted to 100 mmol per day. Although a low calcium diet may result in increased oxalate absorption, a modest reduction of calcium intake by the restriction of high-calcium-containing foods to give an intake of about 1 g of calcium per day is usually recommended. This does not amount to calcium restriction but rather the avoidance of an excessively high calcium intake. Similarly, protein intake may be important in that it provides an acid load, promotes calcium excretion and, if it contains much purine, increases urinary urate. Since there is suggestive evidence that many patients with renal calculi are heavy consumers of meat proteins, a reduction of high meat consumption to a modest level is prudent. It is also customary to advise patients to avoid oxalate-rich foods such as spinach, rhubarb, tea, chocolate and vitamin C, but again it is excess which is to be moderated rather than a moderate level of consumption to be reduced. Thus, general dietary advice is given with the intention of minimizing excesses rather than promoting actual restriction of any dietary component.

Manipulation of urine pH

In view of the potential for many calculi to form at a low urine pH and for a deficiency of urine citrate to contribute to calculus formation, potassium citrate has been given and shown to reduce the risk of recurrence of calculi. This will correct any hypokalaemia, enhance citrate excretion and often reduce calcium excretion. The usual dose is 15–20 millimoles equivalents twice daily, although this can be doubled, and increased doses will be needed in the presence of acidosis.

Monitoring the progress of the patient, of recurrences and of the various risk factors will identify those who need more complex or more extensive therapy than the above. Any additional drug therapy would have to be prolonged and any such long-term therapy, which might have potential side effects, would need to be clearly justified. It would be directed against a specific urine constituent.

Treatment of hypercalciuria

Thiazide diuretics reduce calcium excretion and are effective in reducing recurrences of renal calculi in controlled trials in patients with idiopathic hypercalciuria. The usual dose would be hydrochlorothiazide 50 mg b.d, trichlormethiazide 4 mg a day or methylchlothiazide 2.5 mg a day. Should these fail to control the hypercalciuria or should the hypercalciuria recur despite treatment, cellulose phosphate (which reduces calcium absorption but may increase oxalate absorption) could be used for a time. This approach is rather empirical because theoretically the thiazide should be more effective for renal hypercalciuria whereas the cellulose phosphate should be more effective in absorptive hypercalciuria. The usual potential adverse effects of thiazide diuretics need to be watched for, although these may be slight if a low dose is sufficient.

Hyperuricosuria and allopurinol

In a stone former, the maximum desirable uric acid concentration in urine is 3 mmol/l (approximately 50 mg/100 ml) and the optimal 24-hour urinary uric acid excretion on a normal diet is less than 4 mmol (approximately 670 mg/24 h). Initially, uric acid stones can be managed with a high fluid intake, alkalinization of the urine and moderate dietary purine restriction. However, if the stones become recurrent, allopurinol in a dose of 300 mg per day should be used in patients with normal renal function. Since the commonest cause of a high urinary uric acid is a high nucleoprotein-containing diet, dietary modifications should be attempted, particularly in the early phases of treatment. However, the use of allopurinol in the treatment of recurrent uric acid calculi is well established and efficacious. The potential for side effects, particularly allergic ones, will still exist.

Most important, however, is the syndrome of hyperuricosuric calcium nephrolithiasis in which controlled trials have shown that patients with calcium oxalate calculi who are also hyperuricosuric have fewer recurrences during treatment with allopurinol. The precise mechanism of such prevention is poorly understood but is thought to relate to uric acid providing a nucleus for calcium oxalate crystal formation and attachment. Thus, allopurinol in a full dose of 300 mg per day is recommended in those patients with calcium oxalate calculi who remain hyperuricosuric after dietary modification.

The use of either allopurinol or thiazides in appropriate patients should reduce the risk of recurrence by almost a half. In all cases, monitoring to check progress of risk factors is desirable.

Treatment of specific causes of nephrolithiasis

The specific treatment of uric acid calculi with allopurinol has already been referred to. This drug reduces the production and thereby the excretion of uric acid and almost invariably brings the total excretion of uric acid and its concentration in urine down to levels which do not promote calculus formation.

In patients with dihydroxyadenine calculi, allopurinol is also useful to inhibit xanthine oxidase which is involved in the conversion of adenine to dihydroxyadenine.

Xanthine stones can only be helped by increasing the volume of urine. Raising urinary pH above 7 does not increase solubility.

Cystine calculi can often be prevented by a sufficiently high fluid intake with alkalinizing agents to bring the urine pH above 7.5 if possible. Cystine excretion may be reduced by a diet low in methionine and cysteine. Penicillamine therapy in doses up to 1.5 g per day will reduce the high urinary cystine concentrations, but the side effects of therapy may be a particular problem (chiefly in the form of sensitivity reactions which may affect the kidney, skin or bone marrow).

Antibiotic therapy

There is no general agreement about the management of patients with renal stones complicated by constant, symptomless infections. Such patients are usually submitted to surgery because the infection will continue while the calculus remains. However, if surgery is contraindicated or unsuccessful, it is reasonable not to give antibiotics unless the patient is febrile or has other local or general symptoms attributable to infection, or unless symptomatic infection occurs when antibiotics are withdrawn. If infection stones cannot be completely removed, acidification of the urine with methionine to reduce pH to less than 6 is desirable.

Indications for surgical intervention

The development of extracorporeal shock wave lithotripsy (ESWL) and other non-invasive procedures has radically altered the surgical management of urinary calculi. Open surgery is now usually indicated only in persisting calculi greater than 2 cm in diameter, and fewer than 5% of patients require surgery. Close liaison with the surgeon remains desirable in patients with persisting renal calculi which are not responding to medical therapy, or where obstruction or recurrent infection remains a problem.

REFERENCES AND RECOMMENDED READING

Brocks P, Dahl C, Wold H, Transbol I 1981 Do thiazides prevent recurrent idiopathic renal calcium stones? Lancet 2: 124–125

Buckalew V M 1989 Nephrolithiasis in renal tubular acidosis. Journal of Urology 141: 731–737

Coe F L 1981 Prevention of kidney stones. American Journal of Medicine 71: 514–516

Coe F L, Kavalach A G 1974 Hypercalciuria and hyperuricosuria in patients with calcium nephrolithiasis. New England Journal of Medicine 291: 1344–1350

Coe F, Parks J H 1990 Defenses of an unstable compromise: crystallization inhibitors and the kidney's role in mineral regulation. Kidney International 38: 625–631

Dahlberg P J, van den Berg C J, Kurtz S B, Wilson D W, Smith L H 1977 Clinical features and management of cystinuria. Mayo clinic Proceedings 52: 533–542

Fleisch H 1978 Inhibitors and promotors of stone formation. Kidney International 13: 361–371

Frayha R A, Salti I S, Abu-Haidar G I, Al-Khalidi W, Hemady K 1973 Hereditary xanthinuria and xanthine urolithiasis: an additional 3 cases. Journal of Urology 109: 871–873

Goldberg H, Grass L, Vogl R, Rapoport A, Oreopoulos D G 1989 Urine citrate and renal stone disease. Canadian Medical Association Journal 141: 217–221

Hosking D H, Erickson S B, van den Berg C J, Wilson D H, Smith L H 1983 The stone clinic effect in patients with idiopathic calcium urolithiasis. Journal of Urology 130: 1115–1118

Lavan J N, Neale F C, Posen S 1971 Urinary calculi. Clinical, biochemical and radiological studies in 619 patients. Medical Journal of Australia 2: 1049–1061

Lemann J Jr, Worcester E M, Gray R W 1991 Hypercalciuria and stones. American Journal of Kidney Diseases 17: 386–391

National Institutes of Health Consensus Development Conference on Prevention and Treatment of Kidney Stones. Bethesda, Maryland, March 28–30, 1988. Journal of Urology 1989 141: 705–808

Pak C Y 1991 Etiology and treatment of urolithiasis. American Journal of Kidney Diseases 18: 624–637

Pak C Y C, Fuller C 1986 Idiopathic hypocitraturic calcium-oxalate nephrolithiasis successfully treated with potassium citrate. Annals of Internal Medicine 104: 33–37

Pak C Y C, Holt 1976 Nucleation and growth of brushite and calcium oxalate in urine of stone-formers. Metabolism 25: 665–673

Pak C Y C, Britton F, Peterson R 1980 Ambulatory evaluation of nephrolithiasis. Classification, clinical presentation and diagnostic criteria. American Journal of Medicine 69: 19–30

Scott R, Paterson P J, Smith M, Mathieson A 1978 Reduction in urinary oxalate values by allopurinol. Urology 12: 212–214

Smith M J V 1977 Placebo versus allopurinol for renal calculi. Journal of Urology 117: 690–692

Uribarri J, Oh M S, Carroll H J 1989 The first kidney stone. Annals of Internal Medicine 111: 1006–1009

Van Acker K J, Simmonds H A, Polter C, Cameron J S 1977 Complete deficiency of adenine phosphoribosyltransferase. New England Journal of Medicine 296: 127–132

Williams H E 1978 Oxalic acid and the hyperoxaluric syndromes. Kidney International 13: 410–417

Wilson D M 1990 Clinical and laboratory evaluation of renal stone patients. Endocrinology and Metabolism Clinics of North America 19: 773–803

Yendt E G, Cohanim M 1978 Prevention of calcium stones with thiazide. Kidney International 13: 397–402

Yu T F 1981 Urolithiasis in hyperuricemia and gout. Journal of Urology 126: 424–450

Renal failure

20. Acute renal failure

Z. H. Endre

DEFINITIONS

A lack of understanding of the pathophysiology of acute renal failure (ARF) is partly responsible for the lack of improvement in overall mortality from ARF over the last 30 years despite major improvements in our supportive care delivery techniques including haemodialysis. It is certainly responsible for our difficulties in defining and classifying this condition. The following definitions will be employed in this chapter.

Clinical definition

ARF is a syndrome usually defined as *a rapid loss of renal function with accumulation of nitrogenous wastes* (measured as creatinine or urea). If renal function was normal prior to the onset of ARF, the hyperbolic relationship between plasma creatinine or urea and glomerular filtration (GFR) means that the diagnosis of ARF indicates that a loss of more than 50% of GFR has occurred. Lesser degrees of loss will elevate creatinine if GFR is already reduced. This latter syndrome of acute-on-chronic renal failure is probably far more frequent than is recognized, since minimal elevations of creatinine, which represent a background loss of 50% of renal function, are frequently not recognized. Although the majority of cases of ARF are characterized by oliguria, this definition includes the significant number who are non-oliguric, ranging from 10–50%. The causes of acute renal failure are usually classified into pre-renal, renal or post-renal and are shown in Table 20.1.

Table 20.1 Causes of acute renal failure

Cause	Precipitant
Pre-renal (reversible and irreversible)	
Hypovolaemic states	Haemorrhage, gastro-intestinal tract and third space losses
Reduced cardiac output	Cardiogenic shock
Systemic hypotension	Sepsis, hepatic failure, anti-hypertensives
Increased renovascular resistance	Hepatic failure, α-agonists
Decreased efferent arteriolar resistance	Non-steroidal anti-inflammatory drugs (NSAID), angiotensin-converting enzyme inhibitors (given with reduced effective plasma volume or renal artery stenosis)
Arterial or venous obstruction	Thrombosis, emboli
Rhabdomyolysis	
Intravascular haemolysis	
Renal	
Acute tubular necrosis (ATN)	Pre-renal causes and nephrotoxins
Acute cortical necrosis	Profound shock, especially with abruptio placentae
Glomerular disease	Rapidly progressive and post-infectious glomerulonephritis
Acute interstitial nephritis	Drugs, infection, myeloma, lymphoma, granuloma, uric acid
Small vessel disease	Vasculitis, toxaemia of pregnancy, haemolytic–uraemic syndrome, malignant hypertension
Post-renal	
Obstruction	Tumuors, bleeding, fibrosis, stones

Acute tubular necrosis (ATN)

'ATN' has outlasted alternative terms and appropriately focusses the pathophysiology of most of the clinical features of ARF back onto the renal tubule. Therefore ATN is used here to refer to *ARF due to nephrotoxins or to the pre-renal group of causes.*

Frequently, ARF is used in a more restricted sense to refer to the same rapid loss of renal function, but due only to the group of pre-renal vascular causes and to nephrotoxins. This restricted group is characterized by focal tubular necrosis in the case of vascular causes and to more generalized tubular necrosis when toxins are involved. More functionally descriptive titles, including vasomotor nephropathy and acute (intrinsic) renal failure, have been used to focus on the proposed pathophysiology within this restricted group. As suggested already, this duplication of terminology stems primarily from our ignorance of the pathophysiology of ARF. This uncertainty is increased by the common absence of renal biopsy material; even when it is available, biopsy appearances are frequently non-specific and unhelpful when the clinical diagnosis is made.

Table 20.2　The history in ARF

History	Possible diagnosis
Enuresis	Chronic renal disease, vesicoureteric reflux
Recent urinary tract infection	Obstructive uropathy, vesicoureteric reflux
Polyuria, nocturia	Chronic renal disease
Prostatism	Obstruction
Diabetes mellitus	Acute-on-chronic renal failure, acute pyelonephritis, papillary necrosis, chronic renal disease
Cardiac disease	Pre-renal ARF, nephrotoxic ATN
Recent trauma, surgery	Pre-renal ARF, ATN
Contrast media	Contrast nephropathy
Drugs, especially antibiotics, diuretics, antihypertensives ACE inhibitors and NSAIDs.	Nephrotoxic ATN, acute interstitial nephritis
Compound analgesics	Papillary necrosis, obstruction
Pain	Calculi, obstruction, acute pyelonephritis, cyst haemorrhage, rupture, infection

Reversible pre-renal acute renal failure

A further source of confusion in nomenclature is *the subgroup of ARF, which is reversed following the administration of fluids with or without diuretics.* This restricted group is often called 'pre-renal acute renal failure' or 'pre-renal azotaemia/uraemia' since most causes fall into the pre-renal group of causes of ARF, which result in diminished renal perfusion. The assumption is made that, untreated, this group will develop typical ATN. However, since the diagnosis of this subgroup is only conclusive in retrospect after reversal of the clinical signs, its true relationship to ATN must remain conjectural. For simplicity, this group will be referred to as 'reversible pre-renal ARF'. When the same group of causes leads to ARF, which is not immediately reversible, the syndrome will be referred to as ATN.

DIAGNOSIS

Virtually every case of acute renal failure requires urgent investigation to establish the aetiology and to allow urgent treatment of potentially reversible causes of ARF.

History

Important clues to the aetiology may be obtained by noting any symptoms and their duration (Table 20.2), a history of preceding renal disease (including childhood enuresis, calculi, recurrent urinary tract infection or prostatism), or of preceding systemic diseases with a high incidence of renal involvement (including diabetes mellitus, hypertension, cardiac failure and systemic lupus erythematosus). A full drug history must be taken. Drugs frequently associated with ARF are shown in Table 20.3. History or signs of recent trauma or surgery or of previous surgery or of previous surgery to the urogenital tract may provide further clinical pointers to the diagnosis and the likely aetiology.

Examination

A comprehensive physical examination is required to look for possible causes (Table 20.1) and

Table 20.3   Common causes of nephrotoxic ARF

Pre-renal ARF	Angiotensin-converting enzyme inhibitors, non-steroidal anti-inflammatory drugs, cyclosporin
Renal	
Acute interstitial nephritis	Antibiotics, diuretics, non-steroidal anti-inflammatory drugs
ATN	Cyclosporin, aminoglycosides, amphotericin B, radiocontrast agents
Post-renal	
Intratubular obstruction	Cell debris: aminoglycosides
	Crystals:
	urate (e.g. following cytotoxic treatment of malignancy)
	methotrexate (in high dose therapy)
	Papillae
Calculi	Triamterene

possible sequelae of ARF. The four simple questions shown in Table 20.4 can serve as a reminder to the causes of ARF. Pre-renal and post-renal causes are frequently rapidly reversible and should be excluded first. Critical features to assess are the state of hydration, blood pressure and pulse rate. Vaginal or rectal examination is essential to exclude the two commonest causes of post-renal obstruction in females and males, respectively pelvic neoplasm and prostatic hypertrophy. A distended bladder in the presence of oliguria or anuria clearly points to bladder outlet or urethral obstruction. Acute urinary tract obstruction is usually associated with some pain. Signs of previous urogenital tract surgery also point to obstruction.

Intrinsic renal disease may not be associated with any positive physical features. Frequently, a diagnosis of glomerulonephritis is suggested by the combination of an active urinary sediment with an unremarkable history or one of recent systemic or respiratory infection and equivocal clinical signs. or by signs only of the sequelae of oliguric renal failure. Features of the nephritic or nephrotic

Table 20.4   ARF — key diagnostic questions

1. Is renal function impaired?
2. Is renal blood flow impaired — arterial or venous?
3. Is there outflow obstruction?
4. Is there intrinsic renal disease?

syndromes give a clearer signal that the ARF is glomerular in origin. A recent onset of hypertension or the presence of malignant hypertension, the presence of a skin rash or nailfold haemorrhages or of arthralgia suggests glomerular or tubulointerstitial disease due to vasculitis or an allergic response, usually to drugs.

Investigation

Whilst the history and clinical signs alone may be suggestive, the diagnosis usually requires further biochemistry and imaging of the renal tract and may require renal biopsy. Even this is an oversimplification, since most cases of ARF are complex, often with multiple contributing factors, multiple organ damage and multiple sequelae. Such cases often arise in or end up in the intensive care unit and can be further complicated by the consequences of the transfusion of blood, fluids, drugs, peptic ulceration, gastrointestinal tract haemorrhage and nosocomial infection. A basic screening protocol, required for all patients suspected of having ARF, is given in Table 20.5. A flow chart for subsequent patient investigation is shown in Figure 20.1.

While most patients are oliguric an increasingly larger fraction (10–50%) have a normal or, less commonly, a greater than normal urine output; both latter groups are described as having 'polyuric' or 'non-oliguric' ARF. Anuria, effectively a urine volume of less than 200 ml per 24 hours, suggests urinary tract obstruction or renal cortical necrosis. Polyuric ARF is probably most frequent with nephrotoxic drugs, but can be present with any pre-renal or renal cause of ARF.

Table 20.5   ARF screen

Repeat serum biochemistry
Confirm elevated creatinine
Blood gases: if HCO_3 <20 mmol/l

Random urine for:
urinalysis: blood and protein
microscopy
culture
Na. osmolality, creatinine
Commence strict-fluid balance monitoring

Renal ultrasound
Radionuclide scan

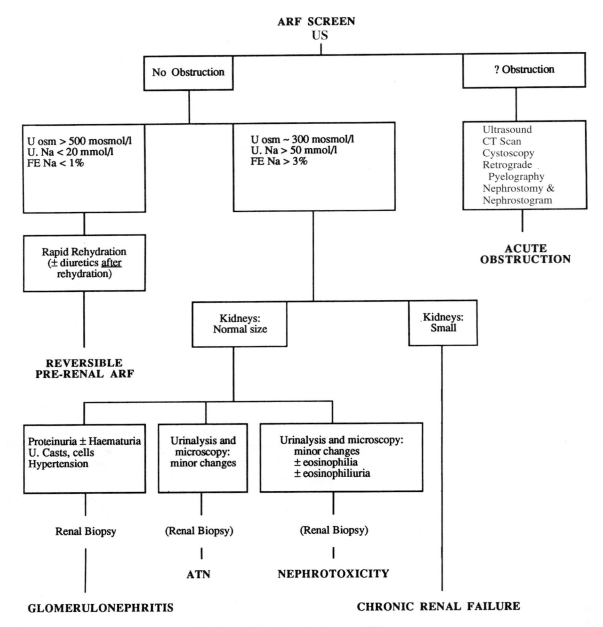

Fig. 20.1 Diagnostic algorithm in ARF

Imaging of the renal tract is usually essential, *but care must be taken not to harm further the injured kidneys.* Intravenous pyelograms, CT scan with contrast and other imaging modalities employing iodinated contrast agents (ionic and non-ionic) can all cause ARF. Contrast-induced ARF is more likely when background renal damage is already present. There is evidence that non-ionic contrast agents are just as likely to provoke ARF (contrast nephropathy) as ionic agents, and both are more likely to provoke ARF in the presence of underlying renal insufficiency, especially with concomitant diabetes mellitus where up to 100% of patients with a creatinine > 400 mmol/l will develop ARF. Associated risk factors include age, dehydration, previous evidence of contrast nephrotoxicity and hypoxia. The following sequence of imaging modalities is suggested:

1. Ultrasound
2. Radionuclide scan (^{99m}Tc-DTPA or ^{99m}Tc-DMSA depending on the likely aetiology of ARF)
3. CT scan without contrast
4. Cystoscopy and retrograde pyelography
5. Nephrostomy and pyelography.

This sequence is followed until sufficient anatomical information is obtained to exclude urinary tract and vascular obstruction.

MRI will become a useful adjunct in the future since contrast with iodinated agents is not necessary and because blood flow as well as anatomical structure can be visualized. CT scan is particularly useful where there is difficulty identifying one or both kidneys, when multiple radiopaque calculi are present and when very large or very small calculi are suspected. Abdominal and pelvic CT are essential when non-calculous ureteric, bladder or pelvic urethral obstruction has been diagnosed, since malignant causes of obstruction may be intraluminal, mural or extramural, MRI scans of this region may also be more helpful in the future, because of the greater visualization of soft tissues obtainable with the MRI technique. Where the integrity of the renal circulation is in doubt, radionuclide scan (^{99m}Tc-DTPA) is simple, safe and may help to exclude unilateral or bilateral ureteric obstruct. A ^{99m}Tc-DMSA scan is indicated where pyelonephritis and scarring are suspected. Where doubt persists regarding the patency of the urinary tract, cystoscopy and retrograde pyelography are mandatory. Care is required in interpreting pelvicalyceal structure from retrograde pyelography, since pseudoclubbing of the calyces may be artefactually and transiently in-duced by the pressure used to introduce contrast into the pelvicalyceal system.

DIFFERENTIAL DIAGNOSIS

The two common reversible causes of ARF are acute obstruction and reversible pre-renal ARF. *These two conditions must be excluded as a matter of urgency.* The extent of reversal following obstruction and the potential for pre-renal ARF to develop into ATN are both time-dependent. Investigations for both should proceed simultaneously. Obstruction is usually excluded by ultrasound examination. Occasionally, obstruction may occur without dilatation of the collecting system. This is more common in patients with extensive radiopaque calculi, with acute obstruction, with retroperitoneal fibrosis and with extensive infiltration of the ureter. Where doubt persists about the patency of the urinary tract, cystoscopy and retrograde pyelography remain essential. The remaining imaging modalities are outlined above. Reversible pre-renal ARF must be distinguished from other renal group causes of ARF (Table 20.1), particularly from ATN since this group has virtually the same aetiology. The flow chart in Figure 20.1 illustrates both the minimum set of investigations required in the assessment of ARF and an algorithm for achieving a diagnosis.

Urinary indices can help distinguish between the causes of ARF (Table 20.6). In patients with oliguria, preservation of parameters of normal tubular function is strong evidence against the intrinsic renal tubular damage seen in ATN. Normal indices for sodium reabsorption (urinary sodium less than 10–20 mmol/l) and maintenance of urinary concentrating ability (urinary osmolality greater than 500 mosmol/kg) suggest that renal failure and oliguria have followed the main pre-renal causes, namely hypotension, hypovolaemia or hypoperfusion. Rapid restoration of systemic blood pressure and circulating blood volume by intravenous fluids is indicated. In contrast, the finding of isosmolar urine (isosthenuria) and a high urinary sodium (greater than 40 mmol/l) suggests ATN and that only cautious fluid loading (under close monitoring of central venous pressure

Table 20.6   Typical urinary indices in ARF

	Reversible pre-renal ARF	Renal ARF		Post-renal ARF
		ATN*	Glomerulo-nephritis	
U osmolality (mosmol/kg)	> 500	< 400	> 500	< 400
U/P osmolality	> 1.3	< 1.1	> 1.3	1.1
U/P creatinine	> 40	< 20	> 40	< 20
U Na (mmol/l)	< 20	> 40	< 40	> 40
FE_{Na} (%)	< 1	> 1	< 1	> 1

* Typical values are shown for oliguric ATN. Diuretics increase U Na and FE_{Na}. In non-oliguric ATN values tend towards pre-renal ARF indicating some preservation of tubular function. In both oliguric and non-oliguric ATN due to circulatory failure, hepatic failure and burns, tubular function tends towards pre-renal values, especially with respect to U Na and FE_{Na}.

or pulmonary wedge pressure) or perhaps fluid restriction should be considered.

In many patients, these criteria provide little or no distinction between the various aetiologies of ARF and in some they may even be misleading. This is more likely if the patient is not very oliguric, if there is pre-existing renal, cardiac or hepatic disease or if diuretics have been administered. Somewhat more reliable is the refinement obtained by calculating the Urinary/Plasma osmolality ratio and especially the fractional sodium excretion (FE_{Na}):

$$FE_{Na} = (U_{Na}/P_{Na})/(U_{Cr})/P_{Cr}) \times 100$$

where U and P denote the urinary and plasma concentrations of sodium and creatinine. This equation is derived from the ratio of the sodium clearance ($U_{Na}V/P_{Na}$) to the GFR (measured as the creatinine clearance). Since the volume term (V) is identical if sodium and creatinine concentrations are measured on the same urine sample, there is no requirement for a timed or accurate measurement of the urine volume. Measurement of FE_{Na} therefore requires minimal extra effort compared to random urine and plasma electrolytes, provided a urinary creatinine concentration has been requested.

Determination of FE_{Na} may help considerably in the borderline cases cited and should be routinely done. Values of FE_{Na} less than 1% distinguish pre-renal and potentially reversible cases from patients with ATN where FE_{Na} is usually greater than 3%. The best example where this is regularly demonstrated is the hepatorenal syndrome. An $FE_{Na} < 1\%$ is usual in the early stages of this potentially reversible pre-renal cause of ARF, characterized by signs of increased renovascular resistance and retained tubular function. Exceptions to this general rule remain, particularly in non-oliguric ARF, in cases where renal function is changing rapidly and where nephrotoxins are involved. An $FE_{Na} < 1\%$ is also common in patients with marked intrarenal vasoconstriction and sodium retention. This is frequent with ATN due to burns, sepsis, radiocontrast, congestive cardiac failure and following NSAID ingestion, as well as ARF due to renovascular disease, acute glomerulonephritis and acute obstruction. An $FE_{Na} > 1.0\%$ can occur with pre-renal ARF in the presence of bicarbonaturia, underlying chronic renal failure or following diuretics.

Thus urinary indices often help support the distinction between reversible pre-renal ARF and ATN, but no index is 100% reliable. It is usually appropriate to combine the described diagnostic criteria (Fig. 20.1) with careful direct measurement of hydration and a fluid challenge. In many cases following the fluid challenge, intravenous loop diuretics will either provoke a diuresis or convert oliguric to polyuric ARF, and provide a further diagnostic clue as well as facilitate patient management.

Acute cortical necrosis is a subset of ATN where there is massive necrosis of both glomerular and tubular elements of the renal cortex and consequent virtual anuria. Necrosis may be patchy or bilateral and complete. This is now rare because of improved prenatal care and a decrease in incidence of its major cause, namely abruptio placentae, and because of aggressive management of postnatal haemorrhage. The diagnosis is now usually suspected where ATN fails to recover after 4–6 weeks. If positive a renal biopsy is definitive, however tissue sampling can allow the diagnosis to be missed where the condition is patchy. Renal angiography may then be diagnostic and will demonstrate patency of major renal vessels but failure to fill the interlobular arteries. Intravenous pyelography is seldom useful (and no longer indicated), but has occasionally shown a thin rim of viable cortex supplied by capsular vessels (the cortical rim sign). After some months, plain abdominal X-ray may show a thin calcified renal cortical margin ('egg shell' or 'tramline' calcification).

The remaining causes of ARF which must be distinguished from ATN are glomerular disease, acute interstitial nephritis and small vessel disease. While many of these are not rapidly reversible, *the same sense of urgency in establishing the diagnosis must remain even after obstruction and pre-renal causes of ARF have been excluded.* In many cases of glomerulonephritis and vasculitis leading to ARF, immunosuppressive therapy may arrest the disease process and sometimes allow partial recovery of renal function. Clearly, recovery is not possible once anatomical destruction of the glomeruli by the inflammatory process is complete. As well as urine microscopy, this group should be investigated for evidence of inflammatory activity with measurement of erythrocyte sedimentation, complement studies (C3 and C4 components), an antibody screen including anti-double-stranded DNA, ANCA and antiglomerular basement membrane antibodies. Clinical signs of an inflammatory process or simply of an active urinary sediment in the presence of normal-sized kidneys with no evidence for obstruction or pre-renal failure suggest the need for urgent renal biopsy. Clinical evidence of systemic disease such as lupus erythematosus or diabetes mellitus warrants appropriate additional investigations. In an individual, the presence of a multisystem disease may be compelling evidence that the disease is also responsible for ARF in that patient. However, specific and typical renal involvement must be verified for both diagnostic and prognostic reasons. Different patterns of renal involvement often suggest a different prognosis and require different management, for example with systemic lupus erythematosus. Furthermore, ATN not infrequently accompanies glomerulonephritis, particularly where the nephrotic syndrome has been over-vigorously treated with diuretics.

ARF due to acute interstitial nephritis is usually caused by drugs, especially non-steroidal anti-inflammatory drugs or the antibiotics ampicillin and cephalothin; these are suggested by an appropriate drug history. Drug-induced acute interstitial nephritis usually occurs within 15 days of exposure (range 2–44 days) with signs of an allergic reaction such as fever, rash or arthralgia (in 10–40%) and plasma eosinophilia (35–100%) and urinary eosinophilia (40–100%). These clinical features are absent in a substantial number of patients and the diagnosis is only realized from the histopathology. The most common pathology associated with drug-induced ARF remains ATN. However the management of ATN and acute interstitial nephritis are different. There is growing evidence from uncontrolled studies that steroids accelerate recovery in drug-induced acute interstitial nephritis. There is no indication for steroids in ATN. Renal biopsy is therefore warranted in any case of ARF where there is uncertainty regarding the aetiological diagnosis. Of the other causes of acute interstitial nephritis (Table 20.1), infection with direct or indirect renal involvement was previously most common and is suggested by an appropriate history. Infiltration with myeloma, lymphoma or granuloma may also not be suspected before renal biopsy.

PATHOGENESIS OF ATN

ARF is frequent and occurs in about 5% of hospitalized patients. ATN is the commonest cause of ARF and continues to have an average mortality of about 50% despite significant technical advances in supportive care and despite the potential for recovery to virtually normal renal function. Two factors impede our understanding of its pathogenesis and thus a rational therapeutic approach based on treating the disease process and not the symptoms of ATN.

The first is that renal 'ischaemia/hypoperfusion' is silent. Despite often clear-cut evidence of causation of a particular episode of ARF, the clinical diagnosis is always made retrospectively. The exact time of onset is rarely known and our understanding of pathogenesis of human ATN has been impaired, since the clue to the diagnosis has been the observation of an elevated creatinine or urea or the detection of oliguria. Both signs are secondary manifestations and require hours to days to elapse before confirmation is possible. This should be contrasted with the symptom of pain and the detection of ECG changes in patients with myocardial ischaemia, where the ease and clarity of diagnosis has facilitated rational evaluation and treatment strategies. Some potential exists for the early detection of renal ischaemia by non-invasive monitoring, e.g. with magnetic resonance spectroscopy (MRS). However, the application even of a suitable technique will still require clinical judgement of need. This will remain difficult in the typical asymptomatic and unpredicted low risk case.

The second factor is that a single pathogenetic mechanism for renal cell injury does not exist. In contrast, the functional changes in ATN are relatively uniform and have some relationship to severity of the precipitating insult. There are many initiating causes and many pathogenetic mechanisms of injury at the cellular level. Tracing the pathway of injury backwards from the final common state of renal dysfunction is difficult if not impossible and probably pointless. A great deal of early effort focussed on determining the cause of the reduction in GFR in ARF, partly since oliguria is such an obvious clinical manifestation. These studies have not provided a conclusive answer to the cause of oliguria and have often ignored the tubular injury accompanying the fall in GFR. In order to arrive at a therapeutically useful understanding of ARF, each injurious process needs to be characterized separately to gain insight into the pathogenetic mechanisms involved.

This discussion will focus only on the pathogenesis of ATN. For an analysis of other causes of ARF, the reader is encouraged to use the bibliography provided. Because of the obvious ethical and practical difficulties in investigating the pathophysiology of ATN in humans, most of the insights gained have come from animal studies, particularly in rats. There is a lack of obvious similarity of some experimental models of ARF to the presumed typical clinical causes. For example, the relevance of timed ischaemia induced by renal artery clamping to clinical renal hypoperfusion

secondary to systemic hypotension is uncertain because renal blood flow is rarely measured in humans with ARF and then only long after the precipitating insult. On the other hand the same experimental model replicates the injury to the kidney involved in certain surgical procedures such as aortic aneurysm repair and renal transplantation. Available evidence suggests that mechanisms found to be important in animal models of ARF are quite relevant to human ATN. This is fortunate since the heterogeneity and complexity of clinical ARF make it unlikely that clear insights could be gained from clinical studies alone.

Cellular mechanisms of ischaemic and hypoxic injury

Renal hypoperfusion is the most frequent diagnosed insult leading to ATN. Such hypoperfusion may occur in the absence of a profound fall in systemic hypotension. While cellular hypoxia and eventually anoxia will clearly follow ischaemia (no flow), low blood flow rather than cessation of flow is usually documented in the maintenance phase of ATN when most studies are necessarily undertaken. Hypoperfusion without cessation of flow can profoundly reduce regional oxygen delivery within the kidney (see Localization of ischaemic renal cell injury). An experimental equivalent for this injury is the induction of hypoxia during continued renal perfusion in vitro. In both ischaemic and hypoxic models the primary event initiating cellular injury is presumed to be cellular oxygen deficiency leading to inhibition of mitochondrial respiration. Subsequent mechanisms of cellular injury following ischaemia or hypoxia which have been studied include ATP depletion, sodium and calcium influx, intracellular acidosis, free radical associated injury, and injury to the cytoskeleton.

Through impaired mitochondrial oxidative phosphorylation, depletion of ATP is common to many injurious processes affecting renal cells. The sequelae of ATP depletion are shown in Figure 20.2. Changes in cell volume follow the rise in intracellular sodium and loss of potassium which accompanies inhibition of Na,K-ATPase. These

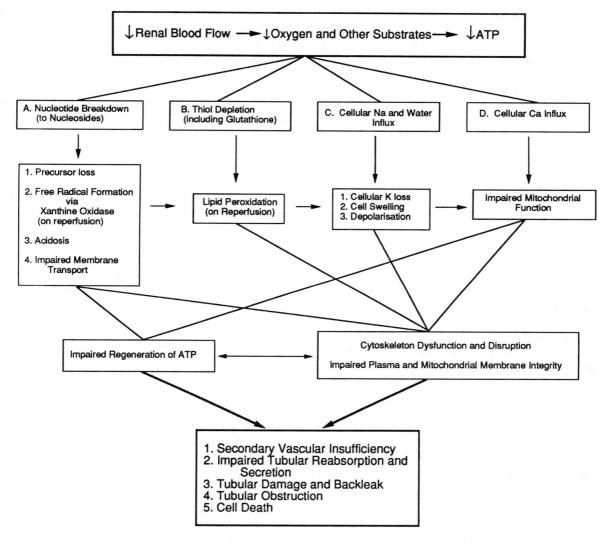

Fig. 20.2   Mechanisms of hypoxic and ischaemic renal cellular injury

sequelae occur in both tubular epithelial and vascular endothelial cells and are more marked in proximal than in distal tubular cells, probably because of both the greater cell ionic permeability and the lower capacity for anaerobic metabolism in proximal tubular cells. While these changes in cell volume are reversible, they may contribute to an increased vascular resistance and to reduced tubular flow rates. In the outer medulla this extra- to intracellular fluid shift may promote vascular congestion.

The influx of sodium will depolarize the cells and inhibit the transcellular transport of substances normally energized by the influx of sodium down its concentration gradient (i.e., the secondary active transport of urate, bicarbonate, phosphate, amino acids and glucose in the proximal tubule and of potassium in the distal tubule). Depolarization will also open voltage-dependent calcium channels leading to calcium entry. Cellular sodium influx will impair hydrogen ion efflux (via the Na/H-antiport) and calcium efflux (via

Na/Ca-exchanger, which may be reversed). Intracellular free calcium concentrations are also increased by release from mitochondria. With restoration of ATP levels, a greater than normal uptake of calcium into mitochondria occurs, which is ultimately deleterious to mitochondrial function. The raised cytosolic calcium activates phospholipases, phosphatases and proteases. Proteases convert xanthine dehydrogenase to xanthine oxidase, which may promote free radical injury (see below). In vascular smooth muscle cells, high calcium stimulates contraction and can raise renal vascular resistance. Pretreatment with calcium channel blockers reduces calcium entry to the cell, and provides significant protection against impairment of mitochondrial respiration. Calcium channel blockers have been shown to improve renal function both in experimental models of ARF and in the best defined human equivalent, namely transplantation of cadaver kidneys.

Intracellular acidosis occurs secondary to impaired hydrogen ion extrusion, to anaerobic dependence on glycolysis and to depletion of cellular buffering and because of ATP breakdown. There is evidence to suggest that this intracellular acidosis is protective rather than harmful under ischaemic conditions.

Cellular and intracellular membrane lipid peroxidation is postulated to occur secondary to free radical attack, although the extent of ATN injury due to this mechanism remains controversial. Renal ischaemia is associated with a reduction in the ATP-generating mitochondrial membrane surface area and with depletion of the endogenous free radical scavenging system comprising superoxide dismutase, catalase, glutathione peroxidase and glutathione reductase as well as of glutathione itself. In addition to the usual amounts produced as a by-product of normal metabolism, epithelial and endothelial cells and vascular polymorphonuclear leucocytes all have enzyme systems capable of generating large numbers of oxygen-derived free radicals under appropriate conditions. As indicated, ischaemia and calcium influx are activators of proteases which convert xanthine dehydrogenase to xanthine oxidase. Hypoxanthine accumulates from ATP degradation during ischae-

mia. The reintroduction of a supply of oxygen during reflow following ischaemia provides suitable substrates for a large burst of superoxide and hydrogen peroxide formation by the xanthine oxidase pathway. Some evidence for lipid peroxidation has been found but both this and the therapeutic window during which inhibition of xanthine oxidase by allopurinol or when exogenous free radical scavengers have been found to be of benefit are highly model dependent. The role of oxygen-derived free radicals in human ARF remains under investigation.

Integrity of the cytoskeleton appears to be essential for cell polarity, for the selective insertion of enzymes into particular membrane surfaces and for the transepithelial transport of most substances. ATP depletion disrupts the cytoskeleton and tight junctions. Recovery of renal cell transport function occurs with restoration of the cytoskeleton and cell polarity.

Localization of ischaemic renal cell injury

Different causes of renal ischaemic, hypoxic and toxic injury result in specific patterns of injury, with some cells reproducibly injured while other cells are not. Three main explanations for these patterns are apparent. Firstly, during the progressive reduction in renal oxygenation during hypoperfusion, some cells become hypoxic earlier than others so that they undergo both earlier and longer hypoxia. Secondly, some areas, especially the outer medulla of the kidney, appear to have prolonged vascular congestion indicating that restoration of blood flow is non-uniform in the kidney, with some areas suffering prolonged hypoxia while others are rapidly reperfused. Thirdly, some nephron segments and cell types are visibly more damaged than others, both in vivo and in vitro where identical conditions can be guaranteed. The first two groupings can be summarized as the selective onset and the selective relief of hypoxia, while the third reflects selective cellular susceptibility to hypoxic injury.

While the aetiology of post-ischaemic medullary vascular congestion is unclear, two major factors appear to contribute to selective regional hypoxia and to selective cellular vulnerability to hypoxia:

namely the heterogeneity of renal oxygenation and the heterogeneity of renal metabolism. Despite a high blood supply and low arteriovenous oxygen extraction, tissue Po_2 levels are low in renal cortex compared with venous blood.

The low Po_2 in both renal medulla and cortex is shunt limited. This shunt is not an anatomical shunt and is presumed to be due to diffusional arteriovenous shunting within the renal substance, in the vasa recta producing medullary hypoxia, and in undetermined preglomerular sites producing renal cortical hypoxia.

Renal metabolism is also remarkably heterogeneous. While substrate oxidation provides the cellular energy required to drive transepithelial transport processes, especially sodium transport and the transport of other species energized by sodium transport, the preferred substrates vary along the nephron. Proximal tubular cells receive substrates luminally from the glomerular filtrate and basolaterally from the postglomerular blood perfusing the peritubular capillary plexus. Cells of the distal nephron rely on the basolateral route, since most substrates have already been absorbed from the tubular fluid. Proximal tubular cells can oxidize substrates such as glutamine, α-ketoglutarate, glutamate, malate and succinate, and also generate glucose by gluconeogenesis. In contrast lactate can be used as a substrate by all nephron segments, while glucose is the preferred distal tubular substrate. Thus, highly specialized renal cells, often with specific substrate requirements, are responsible for a great deal of transport work but exist in an environment of borderline oxygen availability.

Patterns of injury in ATN reflect these regional and cellular metabolic differences and support the hypothesis that diffusional shunting of oxygen within the kidney maintains low tissue Po_2 levels which can in turn lead to necrosis with further reductions in total renal oxygen delivery during ischaemia or hypoperfusion.

The proximal tubule S3 segment is more susceptible to heavy metal injury. S1 and S2 segments are more sensitive to injury by cephalosporins and aminoglycosides. In contrast, distal tubular and collecting duct epithelium are relatively insensitive to toxic and ischaemic insults.

The apparently greater susceptibility of the S3 segment of proximal tubules to ischaemic, hypoxic and some types of toxic injury may have several causes. Anatomically, the location of this segment in the medullary rays suggests that the prevailing oxygen tension will be lower than in the cortical S1 and S2 segments, because of the diffusional shunting of oxygen already described. Additionally, post-ischaemic medullary 'hyperaemia', commonly seen in rat models of ARF, is actually due to vascular aggregation in the outer medulla and not to increased blood flow. This suggests that prolonged ischaemia may occur in this region despite relief of arterial obstruction. Thus selective relief of ischaemia may occur in the cortex where the S1 and S2 segments are located.

In contrast, a diversity of transport mechanisms, of binding and metabolism of toxins within the renal cell, allow nephrotoxin-specific patterns of injury to emerge. The most obvious mechanism is the capacity for normal transporters in proximal tubular cells to transport nephrotoxins into the cells, even to cytotoxic levels. For example, many cephalosporins are transported into the cell by the p-aminohippurate (PAH) carrier located in the basolateral membrane and unique to proximal tubular cells. As PAH transport is highest in the S2 segment, it is not surprising that this is where injury predominates in cephalosporin ATN. Cephalosporin nephrotoxicity is prevented by inhibitors of organic anion transport such as probenecid. Aminoglycosides also accumulate in this segment, but although they are transported across the basolateral membrane, the major uptake route is by binding to anionic phospholipids in brush border membrane and subsequent translocation into the cell. The basolateral route, however, allows binding of aminoglycosides to intracellular organelles which may represent the main mechanism for toxicity. In the medulla, many of these transport mechanisms are absent and the concentration of potential toxins probably depends on trapping by countercurrent diffusion.

MORPHOLOGY OF HUMAN ATN

Despite a profound reduction in GFR, the pathological features in clinical ATN are more subtle than in most experimental models. This feature, together with different methods of examining histological material (e.g, complete nephron dissection versus biopsy inspection) and earlier reliance on post-mortem material produced a variety of oversimplified and conflicting interpretations regarding the pathology of ATN. Our present understanding may be summarized as follows. ATN is characterized by the presence in small segments of an otherwise normal-appearing nephron of focal areas of necrosis of tubular cells with disruption of the underlying basement membrane (tubulorrhexis). Such areas of damage are scattered diffusely within the kidney. The most severe damage is usually found in the pars recta (S3) segment of the proximal tubule. Brush border effacement or thinning in proximal tubular segments is also observed, often in the absence of frank necrosis of the underlying cells. Hyaline casts containing Tamm–Horsfall protein are characteristically found within, and possibly obstruct, distal tubular segments. Such casts are pigmented in ARF following rhabdomyolysis and haemolysis. Glomeruli may show dilatation of Bowman's space. Interstitial inflammation and oedema are usually present. Brush border effacement and necrosis appear to be the only changes which distinguish recovered patients from those with ongoing ARF. Continuing necrosis may be seen after renal failure is established, particularly in non-oliguric patients. Mitotic figures indicating regeneration may be seen in the same regions as necrosis.

Since a single small area of necrosis (particularly as tubulorrhexis) can defunction an entire nephron, producing backleak of tubular fluid with or without associated obstruction of the nephron by casts, it is not surprising that the extent of frank necrosis is usually limited compared to the extent of loss of renal function, particularly the reduction in GFR. Sampling errors, produced by the restricted amount of biopsy material available, enhance the false impression of 'limited' tissue injury.

Nephrotoxic ATN also involves principally the proximal tubule, however tubulorrhexis is usually absent. With heavy metals, carbon tetrachloride and ethylene glycol, extensive proximal segments are usually damaged. However, most nephrotoxic ATN, including that associated with antibiotics and radiocontrast, shows milder and more focal lesions similar to ischaemic ATN. Aminoglycoside nephrotoxicity is classically associated with lamellar or myeloid bodies within proximal tubular lysosomes. Acute interstitial nephritis is associated with an inflammatory infiltrate in the renal interstitium as well as similar areas of necrosis involving proximal or distal tubular segments or both.

FUNCTIONAL CONSEQUENCES OF TUBULAR INJURY

Although ischaemic injury predominantly affects the proximal tubule, the functional sequelae of ATN usually demonstrate dysfunction of proximal and distal tubules including the thick ascending limb of Henle's loop (MTAL). Proximal injury is demonstrated by impaired tubular reabsorption of sodium, chloride and bicarbonate. This is usually observed clinically as an elevation of the urinary sodium concentration to above 40 mM and the FE_{Na} to over 3% (Table 20.6). MTAL injury is demonstrated by impaired diluting and concentrating ability and distal tubular damage by impaired urinary concentrating ability, particularly by unresponsiveness to ADH. The effects on potassium transport of injury to proximal segments is obscured clinically by distal tubular compensation and by the presence or absence of oliguria. Since Tamm–Horsfall protein is produced only by the MTAL, the detection of intratubular hyaline casts in ATN may reflect MTAL perturbation by local hypoxia.

Reduced GFR in ATN: the chicken or the egg?

Renal blood flow is reduced to 30–50% of normal in patients with ischaemic and toxic forms of ATN and is similarly reduced in the initial phase of many models of experimental ARF. In human ARF systemic hypotension is documented in less than 50% of post-surgical cases. While there is no doubt that critical hypoperfusion may be responsible for initiating ATN, it is not clear what role hypoperfusion has in the maintenance phase, during which GFR remains low. Even in the initial phase of ARF, GFR is usually disproportionately low compared to the modest reduction in renal blood flow observed. A number of factors have been postulated to be responsible for this reduced GFR: vascular factors — intrarenal vasoconstriction and/or a reduction in Kf (the ultrafiltration coefficient), and tubular factors — backleak of the glomerular filtrate across the damaged tubular epithelium, and/or intratubular obstruction.

There is little evidence for, and considerable evidence against a role for intrarenal vasoconstriction, whether generalized or confined to the afferent arteriole. Nor is there evidence for the theoretically potent combination of afferent arteriolar vasoconstriction and efferent arteriolar dilatation, which could simultaneously lower renal blood flow, raise renal vascular resistance and reduce GFR. A reduction in the glomerular filtration coefficient (Kf), which could arise from either a reduction in the capillary hydraulic conductivity (Lp) or in the filtering surface area as a result of mesangial contraction and increased glomerular vascular resistance, could lead to a fall in GFR. However, while direct evidence for a fall in Kf has been demonstrated in some experimental models, both physiological and ultrastructural evidence suggesting a fall in Kf is lacking in human ATN. In particular, when glomerular filtration is reduced by more than 50% in ATN, there is no evidence for activation of tubuloglomerular feedback leading to a reduction in glomerular filtration, although tubular damage leading to reduced proximal reabsorption and hence increased delivery of NaCl to the macula densa could theoretically activate such a mechanism. Thus, although a role for tubuloglomerular feedback in regulation of GFR under normal physiological conditions is well defined and although there is an attractive teleological argument that such a mechanism would preserve blood volume in the presence of impaired tubular reabsorption, tubuloglomerular feedback does not appear to be important in reducing GFR following renal hypoxia or ischaemia. Also against a major role for renal vasoconstriction is the observation that restoration of renal blood flow to normal levels by vasodilators does not restore renal function.

While decreased renal blood flow may not explain the reduction in GFR, the normally low prevailing renal tissue oxygen tension (see above) means that a much greater limitation of oxygen delivery will occur than that expected from the degree of impaired blood flow. This may at least account for the observation of continuing tubular damage in the presence of only a modest reduction in renal blood flow. Similarly, the experimentally observed release of potential local renal vasoconstrictors such as adenosine may be important in the further hypoxic exacerbation of tubular injury rather than as a primary cause of the reduction in GFR.

There is now considerable evidence both in experimental models of ARF and in human ATN that tubular damage may contribute to a decline in the observed GFR. Since radiocontrast nephrotoxicity could compound ischaemic ATN, intravenous pyelography is now usually avoided in ARF. However, previous experience with this technique demonstrated that the classic radiological finding in ATN was the presence of an early dense nephrogram *not* followed by a pyelogram. Consistent with the concept that glomerular filtration actually continues in ARF is the suggestion that a leaky tubular epithelium could lead to a reduction in observable GFR through backleak of the glomerular filtrate. Studies of the differential clearance of dextran molecules in severe human ATN following aortic and cardiac surgery have demonstrated both size-dependent backleak of up to 50% of the glomerular filtrate and delayed peak appearance of inulin in the urine suggesting intratubular obstruction. These findings confirm similar observations in experimental models of ATN and indicate that tubular damage in severe ATN is largely responsible for the loss of GFR.

CLINICAL COURSE OF ATN

The clinical course of ATN can be divided into three phases: an initiation phase, a maintenance phase, and a recovery (or polyuric) phase.

The initiation phase may last hours or days and is indistinguishable from reversible pre-renal ARF (see above). ATN is potentially preventable in this phase. The maintenance phase is the period during which GFR remains markedly depressed, usually below 5–10 ml/min, and usually lasts 1–2 weeks but sometimes up to 8 weeks. Continuation of the maintenance phase beyond 4–6 weeks raises the possibility of either irreversible ARF due to cortical necrosis or alternative causes of ARF which were originally excluded and which need reconsideration. Because of the very low GFR the maintenance phase is characterized by progressive accumulation of nitrogenous wastes and potassium and of metabolic acidosis and the clinical sequelae of these changes. The majority of patients in this phase are oliguric, however there has been a large increase in reporting of non-oliguric ATN, from less than 10% in early series to up to 50% of cases now. This change in the incidence of oliguria may reflect increased reporting of ATN and hence of milder cases, increased use of high doses of loop diuretics in the early management of ARF and an increasing incidence of nephrotoxic ATN which frequently non-oliguric. Although any cause of oliguric ATN can result in non-oliguric ARF, cases of ATN following cardiac surgery, burns and nephrotoxins are more frequently non-oliguric. Patients with non-oliguric ARF have fewer complications and require less dialysis. Even when dialysis-dependent, they are usually much easier to manage and have a mortality of about 25%, in contrast to oliguric ATN where the overall mortality remains 50%.

The recovery phase in oliguric patients is characterized by the return of urine flow to normal volumes or up to about 3 1/24 h. With careful fluid management in the maintenance phase, the massive diuresis seen previously with oliguric ARF is now uncommon and is also absent in non-oliguric ARF. Improvement in GFR with reversal of uraemia usually begins 24–48 hours after the onset of diuresis. In patients on dialysis the onset of changes in urine output may be less obvious and the onset of the recovery phase is marked by a stabilization or fall in creatinine and urea levels unrelated to dialysis. Recovery of tubular and glomerular function is initially asynchronous, with GFR improving rapidly over 1–2 weeks and then improving more slowly for up to 1 year. Tubular function recovers more slowly, and defects in concentrating ability and urinary acidification often persist for months or years.

COMPLICATIONS OF ATN

Metabolic complications include volume overload, hyerkalaemia, metabolic acidosis, hypocalcaemia, disproportionately rapid increases in urea in hypercatabolic patients and disproportionately rapid increases in creatinine, potassium, phosphate and urate in patients with ATN secondary to rhabdomyolysis. Volume overload (with the potential sequelae of peripheral and pulmonary oedema and hypertension) is the norm in oliguric renal failure. Even in non-oliguric cases, sodium and fluid intake must be managed carefully since the normal renal homeostatic responses to volume expansion are impaired.

Hyperkalaemia occurs consequent to a failure of potassium excretion (especially in oliguric cases), to intra- to extracellular shifts because of acidosis, to release of potassium from tissue catabolism, direct tissue trauma, sepsis and infection and from exogenous loading with potassium. Since even severe hyperkalaemia is usually asymptomatic, extreme vigilance is required in monitoring potassium levels which often change quite rapidly in ARF. The classic ECG changes of hyperkalaemia become manifest progressively at serum levels above 6.0 mmol/l. These are peaking of the T waves, shortening of the QT interval, prolongation of the PR interval, widening of the QRS complex and, eventually, cardiac arrest in diastole. These changes correlate poorly with actual serum levels and should not be relied upon.

Acidosis with reduced plasma bicarbonate levels results from failure of excretion of non-volatile acids and is therefore associated with an increased anion gap. Respiratory compensation may reduce the extent of the systemic acidosis at the expense of further bicarbonate depletion. Blood gas and pH measurement are essential when the serum bicarbonate level is < 15 mmol/l.

Hypocalcaemia is a frequent early complication of ARF, but is rarely symptomatic since the other complications of acidosis and hypermagnesaemia increase the free ionized fraction of calcium and also protect the myocardium. The possible causes of hypocalcaemia in ARF include hyper-phosphataemia, resistance to parathyroid hormone, low 25 and 1,25 vitamin D levels and, at least in the case of rhabdomyolysis, calcium influx into injured muscle cells. In the recovery phase, *hypercalcaemia* can occur, particularly in the rhabdomyolysis group, and may transiently require aggressive management.

Systemic complications of ATN include infection, disturbances of the cardiovascular, gastrointestinal tract, neurological and haematological systems and delayed wound healing. *Increased susceptibility to infection* occurs in uraemia, and infection remains the commonest cause of death in ARF. Respiratory system, urinary tract and wounds are the commonest infection sites. Prolonged catheterization of the bladder should be avoided if possible, particularly in oliguric patients. *Cardiovascular complications* are the second commonest cause of death in ARF and include pulmonary oedema (usually due to fluid overload), arrhythmias, hypertension and rarely pericarditis. *Gastrointestinal disturbances* are very common in acute uraemia, particularly anorexia, nausea and vomiting. Erosive ulceration may occur throughout the gastrointestinal tract and haemorrhage from such ulcers remains an important cause of death in ARF despite the widespread use of H_2-receptor antagonists. *Haematological disturbances* include anaemia and platelet dysfunction. Anaemia may result from haemorrhage, including that responsible for initiating ARF, or from inhibition of erythropoiesis if ARF is prolonged. Haemolysis and dilution may also contribute to anaemia. Platelet dysfunction is extremely common and usually improved by dialysis. Transient correction of platelet dysfunction can often be obtained with cryoprecipitate and with vasopressin (DDAVP). *Neurological disturbances* range from lethargy and asterixis, to stupor, seizures, coma and death in untreated uraemia.

MANAGEMENT

Prevention

Since the mortality of ATN remains high, it is essential that ATN be prevented wherever possi-

Table 20.7   Patients at high risk of ATN

Cardiac valve repair
Coronary bypass surgery
Aortic aneurysm repair
Transplantation of cadaver kidneys
Unavoidable exposure to nephrotoxins, including:
   radiocontrast agents
   antibiotics
   nephrotoxic antitumour drugs

ble. Three main prevention strategies are possible at present: fluid management, avoidance of nephrotoxins and the use of drugs which may prevent or modify the course of ARF.

Fluid management and maintenance of the circulating blood volume remains the primary strategy for prevention of ARF. While there is some evidence that the severity and duration of ATN are increased in salt-depleted animals and, conversely, that prior salt loading may decrease this severity, evidence in humans is limited. Prior blood volume expansion, at least with saline loading and perhaps with volume expanders remains a logical strategy in situations where ATN may be anticipated. These high risk situations are shown in Table 20.7.

Avoidance of nephrotoxins is clearly desirable but often ignored in the risk–benefit analysis of the investigations and treatments used for many conditions. Up to 30% of cases of ATN follow drug administration, particularly antibiotics and iodinated radiocontrast agents. As outlined (Investigations), the main risk factor predisposing to the development of ARF following any intravascular radiocontrast agent is the presence of underlying renal disease. In the presence of renal disease, diabetes mellitus is also a major risk factor. There is no evidence that newer non-ionic radiocontrast agents are less likely to induce ARF. Where potential benefits outweigh the risks, it is wise to ensure that patients with renal disease are well hydrated with normal saline prior to the injection of the radiocontrast agent.

While the frequency of ARF secondary to non-steroidal anti-inflammatory drugs is increasing steadily, antibiotics are the commonest nephrotoxins (Table 20.3) and usually cause reversible ATN or acute interstitial nephritis. Ampicillin has replaced methicillin as the most frequent β-lactam antibiotic cause of both pathologies. First generation cephalosporins, particularly cephalothin, remain the commonest nephrotoxins in the cephalosporin family. Cephalothin nephrotoxicity is synergistic with the aminoglycosides. The aminoglycosides, particularly gentamicin, remain a frequent cause of nephrotoxicity since the cheapness and therapeutic usefulness of gentamicin ensure its continued use. Fortunately, as with many iatrogenic forms of nephrotoxic damage, gentamicin nephrotoxicity is usually mild and reversible (in contrast to ototoxicity, which is irreversible). A common exception to this is tetracycline nephrotoxicity. With the exception of doxycycline, tetracyclines frequently cause irreversible elevations of creatinine. Amphotericin B produces dose-dependent and usually reversible elevation of serum creatinine. Finally, it should be remembered that diuretics, especially frusemide, may potentiate gentamicin and cephalosporin nephrotoxicity.

Drugs which may prevent or modify the course of ischaemic or nephrotoxic ATN include diuretics, calcium channel blockers, atrial natriuretic peptide, ATP and derivatives, scavengers of oxygen-derived free radicals, amino acids, dopamine and tri-iodothyronine. The place of these treatments remains to be established.

Diuretics, especially frusemide and mannitol, have been administered with some success in three clinical situations: in the prevention of ATN in high risk patients, in the reversal of early ATN or reversible pre-renal ARF (presumably by relieving tubular obstruction), and in the promotion of a diuresis in patients with established ATN (to simplify fluid management). As a prophylactic agent in experimental ARF, mannitol is more consistently successful than frusemide. Following the onset of ATN, there is little clinical or experimental evidence that either drug alters the course of the disease other than by facilitating fluid management. Nevertheless, diuretics are frequently tried. The potential risks of using diuretics in ARF should be remembered. Mannitol should be avoided in patients who already have signs of fluid overload because of the risk of pulmonary oedema, hyponatraemia and respiratory depression. Two groups of risks are associated with frusemide. Firstly, non-oliguric patients may become volume depleted, causing a worsening of ARF. The converse of this is that frusemide will often fail to promote a diuresis in the volume depleted patient. Secondly, frusemide potentiates both the vestibular and renal toxicity of gentamicin and cephalosporin nephrotoxicity. Diuretics have been used in all the high risk situations in Table 20.7. Benefit has been established only for the use of mannitol in crush injury and for surgery in jaundiced patients. The use of diuretics as prophylaxis is logical in the other high risk situations, but it is essential that adequate hydration is maintained before and after diuretic administration.

The clinical roles of the other drugs shown to modify experimental models of ischaemic and toxic ATN remain uncertain. To be effective, all, except ATP and its derivatives, require administration before the insult leading to ARF and they must often also be continued into the recovery phase. Because of the difficulty in predicting ARF, even in the high risk situations described, it has been difficult to assess the clinical value of these treatments. The one situation in which there is both a predictable and high incidence of ATN is in recipients of cadaver kidney transplants; 30–50% experience delayed commencement of renal function depending on the duration of warm and cold ischaemia prior to transplantation. This well-defined group require temporary dialysis after transplantation and have increased morbidity. Both calcium channel blockers and free radical scavengers have been modestly successful in reducing the incidence of ARF in this situation. However further studies are required, since even this group is quite heterogeneous and the optimum therapeutic time window differs for each treatment modality.

At present, the only therapy of benefit after the onset of ARF — the use of ATP and its derivatives and of inhibitors of ATP degradation — have unacceptable side effects. Thus, the only option in most cases of established ATN is to optimize supportive care in the maintenance and recovery phases.

Treatment of established ATN

Specific management is available for ARF associated with acute interstitial nephritis, vasculitis and some forms of glomerulonephritis. Urgent relief of obstruction is the definitive treatment for obstructive uropathy. No specific management is available for ischaemic and nephrotoxic ATN. However, there are 5 important non-specific therapeutic measures:

1. promotion of diuresis,
2. careful control of hydration, electrolytes and acid–base balance,
3. early diagnosis and treatment of infection,
4. optimization of nutritional status, and
5. early dialysis.

Diuretics and dopamine

Promotion of a diuresis is often possible with intravenous loop diuretics and with the low renal vasodilatory dose of dopamine (1–5 μg/kg/min). Such a diuresis is often beneficial, since it allows a liberalization of fluid management, optimized nutrition and a decreased need for dialysis. Although a single large dose of frusemide rarely promotes a sustained diuresis after more than 48 hours of ARF, regular administration of high doses (up to 100 mg hourly i.v.) will increase urine flow in the majority of patients. In some cases this is only effective in the presence of low dose dopamine infusion, although dopamine rarely promotes a diuresis after 24 hours of oliguria. Patients converted to non-oliguric renal failure may have an improved survival compared with non-responders, but, although such treatment is commonplace in the intensive care setting, data validating its efficacy is scanty and uncontrolled. It could be that diuretics and dopamine select out a group of patients with less severe injury. While the easier fluid management of patients induced to pass urine with loop diuretics and dopamine is probably sufficient justification, their use is not universally accepted. Practitioners must be mindful of the hazards of permanent deafness and the potentiation of antibiotic nephrotoxicity associated with this treatment.

Water and electrolyte balance

The usual abnormalities are overhydration, dilutional hyponatraemia and hyperkalaemia. The planned approach to avoiding these problems is sodium restriction plus daily fluid restriction to 400–500 ml plus the previous day's urine output. Hydration status must be assessed scrupulously and frequently. This includes clinical assessment, preferably with central venous pressure monitoring in the early phase, daily weighing and strict recording of fluid balance. Since body weight should drop by up to 0.5 kg per day because of protein and fat catabolism (which will produce an increase in body water), both a stable body weight and increasing body weight suggest volume expansion. Sodium intake is usually restricted to 40 mmol per day. Hyponatraemia is usually iatrogenic and can be corrected by restriction of free water intake.

Hyperkalaemia

Hyperkalaemia can be managed by restriction of intake to 40 mmol per day and the use of ion exchange resins as required — sodium polystyrene sulphonate (Resonium A™) 15–30 g three times per day. Hyperkalaemia greater than 6.0 is a medical emergency, for which the following treatments are available:

1. Calcium gluconate infusion, 1–3 ampoules of 10 g/dl solution over 3–5 min each with continuous ECG monitoring will reduce myocardial electrical irritability and reverse the ECG changes described above although serum potassium remains unaltered.
2. Infusion of 10% glucose intravenously, with or without supplementation with insulin (since glucose stimulates endogenous production), will promote a potassium shift into cells.
3. Sodium bicarbonate infusion (40–80 mmol, i.e. 50–100 ml of a 8.4 g/dl solution) over 1–2 hours will rapidly shift potassium into cells in exchange for hydrogen ions which are buffered by the bicarbonate.
4. Resonium A™, 15–30 g orally or rectally. By exchanging potassium for sodium in the gastrointestinal tract lumen this non-absorbable

ion exchange resin effectively but slowly controls mild elevations of potassium. Apart from dialysis, ion exchange resins are the only useful method of physically reducing total body potassium but take some time to act.

5. Dialysis will rapidly lower serum potassium levels and simultaneously lower total body potassium.

While glucose and insulin, bicarbonate and calcium gluconate infusion are extremely valuable, they provide only temporary safety since they do not reduce total body potassium. Once these infusions are ceased, serum potassium levels immediately begin to rise again through reversal of the extra- to intracellular shift. In addition, each of these methods adds to the fluid overload problem in oliguric patients. In summary, modest elevations of potassium (< 6.0 mmol/l) may be adequately treated with these methods in combination with Resonium A™. In non-oliguric patients loop diuretics may promote a further diuresis and assist with potassium removal. In oliguric patients with potassium levels > 6.5 mmol/l and fluid overload, urgent dialysis is indicated. In this group, the infusion of glucose and insulin, bicarbonate and calcium gluconate will protect the patient while preparing for dialysis.

Acidosis

Metabolic acidosis is minimized by dietary protein restriction but almost always requires treatment with oral sodium bicarbonate when the plasma bicarbonate level is less than 15 mmol/l. Sodium bicarbonate therapy inevitably increases sodium and water intake, with attendant risks of volume overload and hypertension. In addition, large oral doses of bicarbonate (> 6.0 g/day) are often not tolerated. Bicarbonate treatment of acidosis must therefore be undertaken cautiously.

Calcium, phosphate and magnesium

Hypocalcaemia in ARF requires treatment only when symptomatic. This is rare, presumably because the associated acidosis reduces calcium binding by albumin and increases the fraction of ionized calcium. Hypercalcaemia may occur in the recovery phase, especially in patients with ATN following rhabdomyolysis. This requires treatment. High fluid intake and frusemide are usually adequate. Occasional patients have resistant hypercalcaemia requiring treatment with diphosphonates. Hyperphosphataemia is treated with either aluminium hydroxide or calcium carbonate, both of which bind phosphate in the gastrointestinal tract and prevent absorption. Magnesium-containing compounds, such as most antacids, must be avoided in ARF because of the risk of hypermagnesaemia.

General supportive measures

Patients with ARF of any cause require meticulous monitoring to optimize their clinical status, to detect complications as early as possible and to facilitate renal recovery. The basic principles are summarized in Table 20.8.

Frequent changes in patient status are normal in the first days to weeks of established ATN. Such changes often reflect the development of complications, which must be systematically and repeatedly excluded. It is essential to monitor clinical status, especially haemodynamic status, serum biochemistry and haematological indices. The correct frequency ranges from several times daily at first, to daily, depending on the individual case. Dehydration will compromise renal blood flow, exacerbate renal injury and delay recovery. Fluid overload is often life threatening. Thus frequent, careful monitoring of haemodynamic status is essential. Since hydration is notoriously difficult to assess by inspection, central venous pressure monitoring is recommended for most patients until the patient comes into a well-defined equilibrium

Table 20.8   Monitoring patients with ATN

Clinical	Haemodynamic status: pulse, blood pressure, oedema, central venous pressure, fluid balance, weight
Biochemical	Serum electrolytes, creatinine and urea
Haematological	Haemoglobin, white cell count, platelet count
Bacteriological	Culture blood, urine, faeces and pus or drainage; swab skin, throat, wounds

fluid balance. However, care must be taken to recognize and treat vigorously the fluid overload and sepsis that may accompany the use of central venous lines. Daily or twice-daily measurement of electrolytes, creatinine and urea allows the early detection of electrolyte abnormalities and changes in renal function to be assessed from the rate of rise in creatinine. The rate of rise in the serum urea concentration also reflects the catabolic rate; very large and rapid increases in urea compared to creatinine levels may also be a sign of silent gastrointestinal tract bleeding.

Infection

The susceptibility to infection of patients with ARF cannot be overstated, since this complication occurs in up to 90% and is the single largest cause of death (in 30–70%). A high index of suspicion is required since patients with ARF may develop septicaemia without becoming febrile. Critical hypothermia may also occur and be overlooked if low-reading thermometers are not used to check patient temperature when readings of less than 35.5°C are obtained. The most common infections involve the urinary tract, septicaemia and respiratory tract. Wound infections, abdominal sepsis and infections related to medical implants such as catheters and intravenous cannulas bolster this large group. Consequently, urinary catheterization, vascular access and other sources of infection need to be discontinued as soon as they are no longer needed. The need for meticulous care of wounds, dressings, catheters and tubes cannot be overemphasized. The risk of infection is not reduced by frequent dialysis or by broad spectrum antibiotics.

Anaemia

Anaemia is common in ARF once the maintenance phase of ATN is established. Characteristically normocytic and normochromic, with the haemoglobin falling as low as 7.0 g/dl, the anaemia of ARF requires treatment infrequently and usually in the context of other problems such as ischaemic heart disease.

Drugs

All medications should be reviewed regularly. Stopping or reducing known nephrotoxins or drugs with systemic toxicity (for example, magnesium-containing antacids or aminoglycoside antibiotics,) when renal elimination is reduced is essential. Drugs which could reduce renal perfusion, such as antihypertensives and diuretics, also need to be reviewed regularly. The dose of such medications may need to be reduced in the pre-renal and established phases of ATN and may need to be increased again in the recovery phase.

Nutrition

Malnutrition plays a major role in the critically ill patient, including patients with ATN. While protein restriction may minimize uraemia and acidosis, it can compound malnutrition, especially in patients who are already hypercatabolic. The current general approach to nutrition in ATN is to institute dialysis early so that a relatively liberal protein intake can be encouraged. Adequate calories are necessary to minimize endogenous tissue catabolism and inhibit gluconeogenesis and starvation ketoacidosis. This will also limit the rate of increase in urea, potassium and titratable acids (phosphate and sulphate). This requires approximately 100 g carbohydrate per day orally or intravenously. Additional calories given as fat or carbohydrate will not appreciably further reduce catabolism. The intake of protein of high biological value should be at least 0.5 g/kg/day and up to 1.0 g/kg/day if the patient is on regular peritoneal dialysis where additional protein is required to replace dialytic losses. Dietary protein or parenteral amino acids minimize the breakdown of endogenous proteins, but do not reduce the need to excrete the waste products of protein metabolism. In some but not all studies, hyperalimentation with intravenous glucose and amino acids improved survival in patients with ATN. Central hyperalimentation of patients with ARF is complex and requires careful monitoring of blood volume, electrolytes, calcium, phosphorus, magnesium, osmolarity, liver function, acid–base balance and the coagulation profile. It also requires careful replacement of vitamins (C, B, K, D) and hormones (insulin for hyperglycaemia). Because of the fluid volumes and monitoring required, total parenteral nutrition is virtually impossible in patients with ARF unless they are on regular dialysis in an intensive care setting. Thus the principles of a minimum high calorie intake and of high quality protein intake are recommended, but total parenteral nutrition is not recommended except for critically ill patients in an intensive care unit.

Dialysis

Dialysis should be instituted whenever early signs of uraemia (anorexia, nausea, vomiting and occasionally pericarditis) are present or if fluid overload, electrolyte disorders or acidosis cannot be otherwise controlled. No specific value of creatinine or urea can be regarded as critical. Factors such as the rate of rise in creatinine and urea (in effect the extent of residual function combined with catabolic rate) and fluid and nutritional requirements must be evaluated in deciding the timing and type of dialysis. As a general principle it is usual to institute dialysis at much lower creatinine levels in acute renal failure than in chronic renal failure. Dialysis is also advised in hypercatabolic patients and in patients whose care is otherwise difficult to optimize. There is no proof from controlled prospective studies that patient survival is improved by early or intensive dialysis. However, ease of management including better maintenance of nutrition is probably adequate reason alone for the early institution of dialysis.

Conventional haemodialysis remains the most frequently used type of dialysis and is ideal for the haemodynamically stable, non-hypotensive patient. Peritoneal dialysis is also effective and is of particular value when haemodialysis is difficult due to problems with vascular access, hypotension or active haemorrhage. Peritoneal dialysis is probably less efficacious than haemodialysis in hypercatabolic patients, in patients with recent abdominal surgery or with undiagnosed abdominal disease. Continuous arteriovenous haemofiltration (CAVH), without or with concomitant dialysis (CAVHD), or continuous veno-venous filtration

(CAVVHD), are newer techniques which are safe, effective and often simpler alternatives to conventional haemodialysis. These are very effective in treating volume overload in haemodynamically unstable patients and useful in patients who are not hypercatabolic or hypotensive.

The recovery phase

Losses of sodium and potassium may be considerable in polyuric patients following oliguria. These require replacement and the patient's clinical progress must continue to be monitored regularly (Table 20.8) until biochemical and clinical recovery are both well advanced. Hypercalcaemia may occur and require treatment (see above). Recovery of some aspects of tubular function, such as acidification and concentrating mechanisms, may be delayed for months. Improvement in renal function may continue for up to 12 months after an episode of ATN.

PROGNOSIS

Renal function

Functional recovery and patient survival following ARF depend on the underlying cause and probably on the severity of renal injury. Functional recovery in patients with ATN following a prerenal cause generally occurs quickly. Relief of obstruction in patients with post-renal ARF usually corrects the uraemia rapidly although a small number progress to renal damage of the ATN type as a result of prolonged obstruction. Patients with ARF due to glomerular disease usually survive either with recovery of renal function or require renal replacement therapy, depending on the type of glomerulonephritis and any underlying disease.

The majority of patients who survive an episode of ATN recover clinically normal renal function and are clinically normal. Subclinical defects of tubular function and renal histology may be present. Varying degrees of interstitial fibrosis and tubular atrophy are seen in renal biopsies from patients with residual dysfunction or those who progress to chronic renal failure. Elevated blood pressures are found in a minority. Patients with renal cortical necrosis usually fail to recover renal function unless necrosis is incomplete; some of the latter show partial recovery followed by progressive loss of renal function.

Patient survival

The main prognostic factors affecting outcome are the underlying cause of ARF, the number and severity of pre-existing and complicating illnesses, the severity of ATN, and the age of the patient.

A clear overview of prognosis and treatment is hampered by the heterogeneity of causes of ARF, the clinical settings, variations in assessment methodologies and in patient characteristics. Considering only a single cause in a relatively homogeneous population, namely post-traumatic ATN in combat troops, the mortality declined from 90% in World War 2 to 65% in the Korean War with the introduction of haemodialysis. Mortality rates did not fall further in the Vietnam War despite improvements in resuscitation, evacuation and dialysis procedures. It has been suggested that improved resuscitation selected out more severely injured patients, who then survived and developed ATN, while the less severely injured were prevented from developing ATN.

Overall mortality rates have remained at around 50% for over thirty years. About 60% of all cases of ATN occur in a surgical setting, while 40% occur in a medical setting. Mortality is highest in the surgical group (~60%), lowest in obstetric patients (10–20 %) and intermediate in patients with ATN due to a 'medical' cause including nephrotoxins (~40 %). In obstetric patients, ARF is now rare, with most series since the early 1970s reporting no obstetric cases. Pre-existing illnesses affecting outcome adversely include heart disease, renal disease and neoplastic disease. Complicating illnesses such as acute cardiac disease, sepsis and gastrointestinal haemorrhage are all associated with a higher mortality. Finally the acute clinical setting is an important predictor of outcome with multiple organ failure, especially associated respiratory failure, hypotension, jaundice, acute pancreatitis and central nervous system depression all associated with poorer survival. Although age did not independently predict outcome in some studies, in most, patients under 40 have a better prognosis than elderly patients.

Non-oliguric ATN of any cause has a significantly lower mortality (~ 25%) than the oliguric variety. Reporting of this group has increased considerably, presumably because of an increase in the use of nephrotoxic drugs and because of increased detection of ARF on the basis of multiphasic screening. The better survival figures in this group suggest less parenchymal damage, as discussed earlier.

Thus, the persistent high overall mortality of ARF appears to be a consequence of more severe disease occurring in a clinical setting where multiple clinical problems already exist or complicate the illness.

THE FUTURE

There is little to suggest that the prevalence of ARF will change in the immediate future. Milder forms may be recognized because of increased awareness and by multiphasic biochemical screening. An increasing incidence of nephrotoxic ATN may be anticipated, particularly associated with non-steroidal anti-inflammatory drugs, antibiotics, radiocontrast agents and cytotoxic drugs. The severity of ATN in this group is varied. Despite improvements in resuscitation techniques, the incidence of more severe forms of ATN is likely to continue to increase because of the rise in the number of surgical procedures, particularly cardiovascular surgery, and because such procedures are more frequently undertaken in the elderly and in patients with multiple pre-existing diseases.

An improvement in functional and clinical outcome depends on a better understanding of the pathophysiology of ATN. Significant advances are occurring in this area. More immediately applicable are approaches to prevention, which range from critical awareness and prehydration to the use of drugs to prevent or reduce renal injury in high risk patients.

REFERENCES AND RECOMMENDED READING

Endre Z H, Ratcliffe P J, Ferguson D J, Tange J D, Radda G K, Ledingham J G G 1989 Erythrocytes alter the pattern of renal hypoxic injury: predominance of proximal tubular injury with moderate hypoxia. Clinical Science 76: 19–29

Myers B D, Moran S M 1986 Haemodynamically mediated acute renal failure. New England Journal of Medicine 314: 97–105

Rasmussen H H, Pitt E A, Ibels L S, McNeil D R 1985 Prediction of outcome in acute renal failure by discriminant analysis of clinical variables. Archives of Internal Medicine 145: 2015–2018

SUGGESTED FURTHER READING

Bihari D, Neild G 1990 Acute renal failure in the intensive therapy unit. Springer-Verlag, London

Brenner B M, Lazarus J M 1988 Acute renal failure. Churchill Livingstone, New York

Endre Z H, Iaina A 1989 Renal nuclear magnetic resonance. Renal physiology and biochemistry, Vol 12, No. 3. Karger, Basel

Solez K, Racusen L C 1990 Acute renal failure. Marcel Dekker, New York

Seldin D W, Giebisch G 1992 The kidney: physiology and pathophysiology. Raven Press, New York

21. Drugs and the kidney

W. M. Bennett

DRUG NEPHROTOXICITY

Therapeutic agents may be associated with a variety of clinical syndromes in nephrology. Acute renal failure, chronic renal failure, renal glomerular disease and a variety of fluid and electrolyte disorders may be produced by drugs. Since drug-induced disease is frequently reversible, it is important to consider this category of disease in the differential diagnosis of many clinical disorders.

Acute renal failure

Drugs are aetiological agents in acute renal failure in 10–30% of cases. The complex nature of the clinical settings in acutely ill patients makes a precise designation difficult. However, in patients with acute renal dysfunction and preservation of urine flow rates of more than 20 ml/h (non-oliguric acute renal failure) toxins were implicated in 30% in one recent large series. In this section the main features of common toxin-induced acute renal failure will be summarized.

Aminoglycoside antibiotics

These widely used antibiotics find clinical applicability in the management of serious infections in patients who often have severe underlying illness. In prospective studies, 10–25% of patients develop significant deterioration of renal function, which is usually manifested as non-oliguric acute renal failure. In most cases the renal failure reverses spontaneously when the drug is discontinued. However, an occasional oliguric patient will re-

quire dialysis support. Isolated proximal tubular dysfunction presenting as resistant hypocalcaemia, hypomagnesaemia and hypokalaemia, particularly in children, has also been noted. This tubular syndrome is most likely produced by aminoglycoside-induced renal magnesium wasting. Patchy proximal tubular necrosis has been observed in conjunction with aminoglycoside induced acute renal failure. On electron microscopy, proximal tubular cells show evidence of increased autophagocytosis and increased numbers of lysosomes. Many lysosomes contain whorled 'myelin-like' material referred to as myeloid bodies. These structures are thought to represent cell membrane phospholipids which accumulate because of inhibition of phospholipases by the aminoglycosides.

The relative nephrotoxicity of the commonly used aminoglycosides is generally related to the number of free amino groups on the drug molecule. Thus, neomycin, which has six free amino groups, is so nephrotoxic that parenteral use has been abandoned, while streptomycin, with only two free amino groups, has little or no nephrotoxic potential. Double blind randomized trials have suggested that gentamicin is more nephrotoxic than tobramycin or amikacin.

The pathophysiology of aminoglycoside nephrotoxicity has not been completely elucidated. Pharmacokinetic studies have demonstrated significant renal cortical drug accumulation. These cationic drugs are transported across both the apical and basolateral cell surfaces. However, the bulk of reabsorption takes place by pinocytosis across the luminal membrane. Aminoglycosides accumulate within lysosomes. Cell death may be due to lysosomal dysfunction, interference with mitochondrial respiration or damage to cell membrane ionic pumps.

Experimentally, nephrotoxicity can be modified by high sodium and calcium intake. In clinical practice it seems prudent to base drug dosage on pre-existing renal function, with careful attention to extracellular fluid volume and calcium status. Renal function should be monitored at least every 48 hours. Unfortunately, maintenance of 'therapeutic' drug concentrations in blood does not preclude development of significant nephrotoxicity. Blood levels should be used to ensure antibacterial efficacy since there is considerable interpatient variability in serum concentrations to a given dose based on body weight.

Cephalosporins

The older cephalosporin derivative cephaloridine regularly produces oliguric acute renal failure due to proximal tubular necrosis when given in doses of more than 6 g per day. The newer second and third generation cephalosporin derivatives are relatively free of nephrotoxicity. Congeners which accumulate within proximal tubular cells, such as cephaloglycine and cephaloridine, are most likely to produce nephrotoxicity in experimental animals. The few isolated cases which have been reported are most likely due to idiosyncratic or allergic mechanisms. When cephalosporins are administered in combination with aminoglycosides, nephrotoxicity appears to be increased. Clinicians should be aware that cephalosporins, particularly cefoxitin, may falsely elevate serum creatinine concentrations as measured by autoanalyzer methodology, producing 'pseudo' acute renal failure. Since renal function is not truly depressed, blood urea nitrogen levels do not change.

Tetracyclines

In patients with pre-existing renal disease tetracyclines may produce worsening azotaemia and acidosis due to drug-induced catabolism. However, reversible non-oliguric acute renal failure has also been observed, particularly in patients with cirrhosis of the liver treated with demeclocycline. If a tetracycline must be prescribed for a patient with renal disease, doxycycline is preferable since it has less antianabolic effect.

Amphotericin B

If amphotericin B is given in doses exceeding 3–5 g on a cumulative basis, nephrotoxic effects are inevitable. Patients with pre-existing renal disease or extracellular fluid volume depletion are particularly susceptible. Abnormalities of the urinary sediment and moderate proteinuria are early manifestations of nephrotoxicity. Hypokalaemia, distal renal tubular acidosis and impaired concentrating ability usually precede the development of frank renal failure. When acute uraemia is present, proximal tubular necrosis can be demonstrated on biopsy. Permanent depression of renal function may develop with repeated courses of amphotericin B. Saline loading, sodium bicarbonate and mannitol have all been advocated to modify amphotericin B nephrotoxicity, but no studies in man have yet conclusively demonstrated the benefits of such an approach. In addition to frequent urine sediment examinations, acid–base status, serum potassium and serum creatinine should be monitored every 48–72 hours. If toxicity occurs, dosage may be reduced or the drug administered every 48 hours.

Sulphonamides, penicillins and rifampicin

Soluble sulphonamide derivatives seldom cause acute renal failure by producing intrarenal crystallization. Most nephrotoxic reactions are due to allergic reactions or hypersensitivity mechanisms. Although antibiotics most commonly result in these reactions, it should be remembered that most diuretics, (including thiazides and frusemide) have molecular structural similarities to sulfonamides.

The highly effective combination of sulphamethoxazole and trimethoprim (co-trimoxazole) has been associated with elevations in serum creatinine. Trimethoprim and creatinine compete for organic base secretory sites in the proximal tubule, accounting for this phenomenom. Since glomerular filtration rate does not change it is unlikely that such creatinine rises represent drug nephrotoxicity. Fatal multisystem toxicity does occur with sulphonamides, probably due to immunological factors.

The clinical constellation of fever, pruritic morbiliform skin rash, eosinophilia, proteinuria, haematuria and non-oliguric renal failure may occur from five days to three weeks after administration of any penicillin or sulphonamide derivative. Eosinophiluria is often a clue to the diagnosis when systemic symptoms are minimal or absent. Renal biopsies show interstitial nephritis with infiltration of mononuclear cells and eosinophils. Although the immunopathogenesis is uncertain, in some cases it is related to the production of anti-tubular basement membrane antibodies. In difficult cases increased uptake of gallium-67 by the kidney 48 hours after isotope injection supports the diagnosis of acute interstitial inflammation. Discontinuation of the offending agent is usually associated with improvement in renal function although in some patients functional impairment persists. Most nephrologists recommend a 6–10 day course of prednisone 60 mg per day with rapid tapering although its value has not been tested in controlled trials. Other drugs rarely associated with a similar syndrome are cimetidine, cephalosporins, allopurinol and phenytoin.

Rifampicin has been associated with acute renal failure in patients receiving intermittent treatment with this drug for tuberculosis. Patients usually present with fever, chills, lumbar pain, myalgia, and nausea and vomiting. The urine sediment reveals microscopic haematuria, proteinuria and granular casts. Oliguria and uraemia may be severe enough to require dialysis. Since this syndrome may develop even if the first administration of rifampicin was a single dose, repeated courses of this drug should be avoided. In some patients anti-rifampicin antibodies can be demonstrated. Renal biopsy shows acute tubular necrosis, interstitial oedema and round cell inflammation.

Radiographic contrast media

In several large series, iodinated radiographic constrast media are the second most frequent cause of acute renal failure behind aminoglycoside antibiotics. Patients at particular risk are those with pre-existing renal dysfunction, insulin-dependent diabetics, and the elderly. The incidence of contrast nephropathy in diabetic patients with pre-existing renal insufficiency is at least 75%. This constitutes a relative contraindication to such radiographic investigations in this high risk group. Furthermore, some of these patients have some irreversible loss of function. Patients with multiple myeloma and other dysproteinaemic states are also at high risk.

The clinical features of this acute nephrotoxic reaction range in severity from a transient asymptomatic deterioration in renal function to oliguric renal failure requiring dialysis. Renal dysfunction usually begins within 24 hours of exposure. Serum creatinine peaks on the fourth or fifth day, with spontaneous improvement and returns to baseline in approximately two weeks. Oliguria occurs in patients who are dehydrated before the radiographic procedure. When urine output decreases, the decline usually is transient, returning to normal in a few days. There are no specific urinary sediment changes. However, fractional sodium excretion is low in patients with oliguria, in contrast to the high values noted in patients with other causes of oliguric renal failure. A persistent nephrogram on an abdominal X-ray supports the diagnosis of contrast nephropathy. The best treatment is prevention. Patients at high risk should be identified and adequate hydration assured by intravenous fluid therapy before and during dye administration. The dose of contrast medium should be as small as possible and repeat studies should be avoided. In high-risk subjects, 250 ml of 20% mannitol within one hour of the procedure may minimize the severity of nephrotoxicity. The pathogenesis of contrast nephropathy is poorly understood. Direct tubular toxicity, renal ischaemia, intrarenal precipitation of Tamm-Horsfall mucoprotein and hypersensitivity mechanisms have been proposed.

Cancer chemotherapeutic and immunosuppressive drugs

Hyperuricaemia and increased urinary uric acid excretion accompany chemotherapy when rapid cell lysis releases a large pool of nucleic acids which are metabolized to uric acid. Intrarenal obstruction by the poorly soluble uric acid crystals occurs in distal tubules and collecting ducts, resulting in oliguric renal failure. Preventive measures such as intravenous hydration to maintain a high urine flow rate and alkalinization by sodium bicarbonate to maintain urine pH above 7.0 may be useful. Allopurinol, a xanthine oxidase inhibitor, in doses of 300–600 mg per day is an effective means of preventing hyperuricaemia associated with tumour cell lysis. Patients with rapidly proliferating tumours or large tumour burdens (especially those with haematological neoplasms) are at particular risk, as are patients with pre-existing renal disease. When oliguric renal failure occurs, early haemodialysis is indicated for the management of metabolic disturbances resulting from release of intracellular ions such as potassium and phosphate as well as for removal of uric acid. Allopurinol should be initiated or continued to reduce uric acid production. Renal failure usually resolves in 4–7 days with these measures.

Cisplatin is a useful chemotherapeutic agent which demonstrates dose-dependent nephrotoxicity. Repeated courses of 50 mg/m^2 administered either as a single dose or spread over several days will result in nephrotoxicity in most patients. With a single dose the dysfunction is mild and reversible but with repeated courses the nephrotoxicity can be permanent. The drug is excreted predominantly by the kidneys, and platinum is detectable in the urine for weeks after a single dose. The cis-isomer is nephrotoxic but the transconfiguration of the molecule is without chemotherapeutic efficacy or renal toxicity. Cisplatin reduces sulfhydryl groups in the proximal tubular cells of experimental animals and, analogous to other heavy metals, such as mercury, probably inhibits key intracellular enzymes important for cellular integrity. Clinically, rises in blood urea nitrogen (BUN) and creatinine are the usual manifestations of nephrotoxicity. Some studies have shown increased urinary excretion of small molecular weight proteins such as β_2-microglobulin before a fall in glomerular filtration rate. Pathological examination of patients with cisplatin nephrotoxicity reveals proximal and distal tubular necrosis.

Interestingly, cisplatin produces renal magnesium wasting particularly in children, occasionally resulting in hypocalcaemia and tetany. Patients with pre-existing renal dysfunction and those receiving aminoglycoside antibiotics are at increased risk. The nephrotoxicity of cisplatin can be minimized by maintaining urine flow rates of 100 ml/hour by induction of a saline or mannitol diuresis.

The use of high dose methotrexate regimens (50–250 mg/kg) has resulted in a higher incidence of nephrotoxicity than occurred with conventional chronic low dose regimens. The parent drug and its insoluble metabolite 7-hydroxymethotrexate are secreted into the renal tubule where they precipitate in a fashion analogous to uric acid. The incidence of renal failure can be reduced by brisk alkaline diuresis during drug administration. Renal failure is usually transient, spontaneous recovery occurring within two to three weeks. During the period of renal failure the patient is at increased risk of myelosuppressive and adverse gastrointestinal reactions. Clearance of methotrexate by haemodialysis or peritoneal dialysis is poor.

Cyclosporin A is a promising new drug with potent immunosuppressive properties which has the potential for widespread use in solid organ transplantation. Dose-related, reversible acute tubular toxicity has been reported during use in renal transplantation. Ultimate organ function is probably not compromised although the drug may be difficult to administer to patients with post-transplant acute tubular necrosis. Monitoring of blood levels to a desired therapeutic window allowing safer treatment awaits further experience. Recently, severe renal failure due to glomerular thrombosis and tubular injury has been noted in recipients of bone marrow transplants.

Fluorinated anaesthetic agents

The useful anaesthetic agents methoxyflurane and enflurane are metabolized by the liver to inorganic fluoride and oxalic acid. Patients who undergo prolonged anaesthesia with these agents may develop non-oliguric renal failure. Renal function usually recovers completely although some patients never return to baseline levels. Microscopic examination of the kidney reveals deposition of calcium oxalate crystals within tubular lumens and renal interstitium. Chronic interstitial fibrosis may be a consequence of previous methoxyflurane-induced acute renal failure. Enflurane is less quantitatively biotransformed to fluoride and thus causes renal failure much less frequently. Experimentally, elevated inorganic fluoride concentrations lead to non-oliguric renal failure with proximal tubular necrosis, although oxalate deposition is not noted. Inorganic fluoride injections also produce vasopressin-induced polyuria. Previous exposure to the anaesthetic or drugs which enhance liver microsomal defluorination increases nephrotoxic potential. Anaesthesia should be at the lowest concentration for the shortest time possible, with careful attention to postoperative fluid replacement.

Miscellaneous agents

Acetaminophen (paracetamol) overdoses are becoming more frequent. Although fulminant hepatic necrosis usually dominates the clinical picture, renal failure has been noted without severe liver injury. Within a few hours of overdose nausea, vomiting and profuse diaphoresis are common. Hepatic dysfunction and oliguria become evident between 24 and 48 hours. Serum urea is low compared to creatinine because of the liver destruction. The prognosis depends on the extent of liver disease. If the patient survives the first few days, haemodialysis support is often necessary. The hepatic damage is due to bioactivation of the drug to a highly reactive metabolite. Reduced glutathione is important in preferential binding of the reactive metabolite and prevention of its covalent binding to tissue macromolecules. The microsomal enzyme system which controls hepatic drug oxidation is present in renal cortex as well as in the liver, suggesting a common mechanism for renal tubular necrosis. Compared to the liver, the renal cortex has plentiful stores of glutathione, perhaps explaining the relative resistance of renal tubular cells to damage.

Acute renal failure is common after ingestion of ethylene glycol. Tissue damage is due to calcium oxalate deposition. Characteristically the patient presents comatose, with oliguric renal failure and an anion gap metabolic acidosis. Early haemodialysis with removal of ethylene glycol and inhibition of ethylene glycol conversion to oxalate via glycoaldehyde by use of ethyl alcohol are indicated. The latter provides an alternate substrate for alcohol dehydrogenase, the enzyme involved in the metabolism of ethylene glycol.

Non-steroidal anti-inflammatory drugs

A large number of non-steroidal anti-inflammatory or aspirin-like drugs have recently become available for clinical use. Deterioration in renal function may occur by a number of mechanisms. Because of the prostaglandin inhibition produced by these compounds, patients requiring prostaglandins for preservation of renal blood flow are at risk when treated with these compounds. Examples include patients with cirrhosis of the liver, congestive heart failure, low sodium diets or chronic renal disease. Usually such patients have decreases in urine output and sodium excretion associated temporally with the institution of non-steroidal drugs. Azotaemia results, but is rapidly reversible when the drug is discontinued. Allergic interstitial nephritis causing acute renal failure with and without massive proteinuria has also been reported. The mechanism of the nephrotic range proteinuria is speculative, but it is known that prostaglandin E_2 and prostacyclin have inhibitory effects on T lymphocytes. Since interstitial infiltrates in the kidneys in these cases are of a T-cell origin, it is possible that prostaglandin inhibition allows release of lymphokines of T-cell origin which alter glomerular permeability to protein. Finally, several cases of papillary necrosis have been reported with non-salicylate, non-steroidal anti-inflammatory drugs. Renal function should be closely monitored in patients receiving any of this growing list of compounds.

Chronic renal failure

The best-known example of chronic renal failure associated with drugs is analgesic abuse nephropathy. Other toxic exposures may also produce chronic renal failure. For example, industrial or environmental exposure to cadmium leads to proximal tubular dysfunction with chronic interstitial nephritis evident on pathological examination of renal tissue. The binding of the metal to proximal tubular cells causes tubular proteinuria and aminoaciduria. Despite the high incidence of renal involvement with prolonged exposure, progression to frank renal failure is rare.

Exposure to lead may also result in chronic nephropathy. Emmerson has suggested, based on a meticulous follow-up of 400 children with acute lead poisoning, that chronically scarred kidneys are frequent sequelae to excessive exposure. Two unique aspects of chronic lead nephropathy are the high frequency of gout and hypertension, with blunted activity of the renin–angiotensin system. Histologically, acute damage in lead nephropathy primarily involves the proximal tubular cells. Characteristic eosinophilic intranuclear inclusion bodies are noted which may not persist beyond the first year of industrial exposure. The inclusion bodies are probably lead–protein complexes. By the time chronic renal failure supervenes, pathological changes are non-specific, with glomerulosclerosis, interstitial nephritis and nephrosclerosis as prominent features. The EDTA mobilization test performed by collecting urine for 48–72 hours after two doses of calcium disodium edetate parenterally 12 hours apart indicates an excessive body burden of lead if more than 650 µg are recovered.

Renal glomerular disease

Some drug-induced disease may present clinically as proteinuria or nephrotic syndrome. In the course of gold therapy for rheumatoid arthritis, 1–3% of patients develop proteinuria. Some even demonstrate a full-blown nephrotic syndrome with oedema, hypoalbuminaemia and hyperlipoproteinaemia. Clinical manifestations usually regress within a few months after the drug is discontinued. Renal pathology is often indistinguishable from idiopathic membranous nephropathy with granular deposition of IgG and IgM along glomerular capillary walls. Complement deposition has also been noted in some cases. Other heavy metals (mercury, bismuth, thalium), anticonvulsants, heroin and penicillamine have been associated with similar nephropathy. The recently released antihypertensive agent captopril has been implicated as a cause of proteinuria, although renal biopsies of kidneys from hypertensive patients treated with other drugs also show a high prevalence of glomerular abnormalities.

Drug-induced fluid and electrolyte disorders

Several common drugs may impair renal water excretion and lead to hyponatraemia. Narcotics, clofibrate, carbamazepine and vincristine cause central antidiuretic hormone (ADH) release. Cyclophosphamide probably causes hyponatraemia by simulating ADH action at renal cell receptor sites. Hypoglycaemic drugs and a variety of prostaglandin inhibiting non-steroidal anti-inflammatory drugs potentiate the cellular action of ADH. Drugs may also impair renal concentrating mechanisms, causing polyuria and nephrogenic diabetes insipidus. Lithium, fluorides and demeclocycline are the best-described clinical examples.

DRUG PRESCRIBING IN RENAL INSUFFICIENCY

Most drugs and their metabolites are fully or partially excreted by the kidney; therefore drug regimens often need to be adjusted in order to provide safe yet effective treatment for patients with renal insufficiency. In addition, the marked alterations produced in the biochemical and physiological milieu by uraemia may impair other organ systems, such as the liver, which are involved in drug metabolism. The following deals with practical aspects of administering drugs to patients with reduced renal function, including those requiring dialysis. More detailed discussions of this subject can be found in several recent reviews.

Pharmacokinetics and normal renal function

Onset, intensity and duration of pharmacological action of any drug are largely related to its concentration in blood or plasma. Pharmacokinetics is the study of factors that influence drug concentration in the plasma, i.e. drug absorption (bioavailability), distribution in body fluids, and elimination.

Bioavailability

Bioavailability is defined as the relative amount of administered drug that reaches the systemic circulation and the rate at which this occurs. It is usually determined by measuring the appearance rate and the peak level of a drug in the plasma after a single dose, whether administered parenterally or orally. Since more than 80% of drugs are administered orally, bioavailability is largely related to gastrointestinal absorption.

Since most orally administered drugs gain access to the circulation through the portal venous system, the absorbed drug is exposed to the liver during its first pass through the body. Any hepatic metabolism of the drug during this first pass will decrease bioavailability. This has been termed the 'first-past effect'. Some drugs are subject to an extensive first-pass effect. Depending on any alteration in hepatic metabolism caused by disease, bioavailability of a drug may increase or decrease because of an altered first-pass effect.

Effects of renal failure on bioavailability. There is little information in the influence of impaired renal function per se on drug bioavailability. Patients with renal disease may have several causes of delayed gastric emptying that could affect drug absorption. Perhaps the commonest cause of prolonged gastric emptying in renal patients is the use of aluminum-containing antacids. Aluminum slows gastric motility, resulting in poor absorption of isoniazid and other drugs. The consequent

---

Drugs subject to extensive first-pass effect
Imipramine
Pethidine (meperidine)
Phenacetin
Propranolol
Lignocaine
Pentazocine
Dextropropoxyphene napsylate
Terbutaline

---

constipation is often treated with the stool softener, docusate sodium, which may further retard gastric emptying. Antacids may also form non-absorbable chelation complexes with concurrently administered drugs, resulting in poor bioavailability. Digoxin and tetracyclines seem particularly susceptible to this effect. Because the effects of antacids on drug bioavailability are multiple and variable, it seems prudent to administer drugs at least one-half to one hour before antacid ingestion to ensure consistent absorption and therapeutic effect.

Distribution

Once absorbed, a drug is distributed from the blood throughout the body tissues. This is a reversible process that continues until the drug concentrations in plasma and tissue are equal. At this point of distribution equilibrium, any change in the plasma concentration reflects a similar change in the tissue concentration of the drug. This relationship is expressed as the drug's volume of distribution (V_d):

$$V_d = \frac{\text{amount of drug in the body}}{\text{plasma concentration}} \quad (1)$$

V_d is not an anatomical volume, but the volume in which the drug appears to distribute with a concentration equal to that in plasma. The V_d is useful for calculating the amount of drug in the body when plasma concentration is known or in predicting the plasma concentration after a given dose.

The V_d of a drug is primarily determined by its lipid solubility (and ability to penetrate tissues) and its degree of protein binding. For drugs preferentially bound to plasma protein, the apparent V_d is usually small and approximates the plasma volume. As drug protein binding decreases, however, the apparent V_d can be expected to increase. Drugs that are extensively bound to extravascular tissues may have an apparent V_d many times larger than total body water. Digoxin, for example, has an apparent V_d of 760 litres in a 70 kg man. The fraction of drug bound to plasma protein is retained in the vascular space and is not available for tissue distribution. Bound drug lacks pharmacological effects. The degree of protein binding has a significant impact on pharmacological effect. If protein binding decreases, more unbound or active drug is available for distribution and the intensity of pharmacological effect may be greater than expected for any given plasma concentration. Values indicating therapeutic plasma concentrations should be adjusted downward in this situation.

Effects of renal failure on drug distribution. Distribution of a drug in the body depends primarily on its lipid solubility and degree of binding to plasma proteins. The protein-binding capacity of many drugs is less in uraemic patients than in normal subjects (Table 21.1). This impairment is roughly proportional to the severity of renal failure. Because only the unbound (free) drug fraction is pharmacologically active, patients with renal failure may achieve a pharmacological effect at relatively lower total plasma concentrations than non-uraemic patients. This is best documented with phenytoin which, because of decreased binding in uraemia, achieves a therapeutic effect at lower 'total' plasma phenytoin levels. The 'free' plasma drug levels, however, are normal or increased.

Table 21.1 Plasma protein binding of some common drugs in uraemia

Acidic drugs	Basic drugs
Decreased	
Barbiturates	Diazepam
Cephalosporins	Morphine
Clofibrate	Triamterene
Cloxacillin	
Dicloxacillin	
Diazoxide	
Frusemide	
Penicillin G	
Phenylbutazone	
Phenytoin	
Salicylate	
Sulphadimidine	
Valproate	
Warfarin	
Not affected	
Indomethacin	Chloramphenicol
	Dapsone
	Desipramine
	Propranolol
	Quinidine
	Trimethoprim

The exact mechanism of decreased plasma protein binding in uraemia is unknown. Hypoalbuminaemia can contribute to decreased protein binding in uraemia, but cannot fully explain it. Most investigators believe that the protein-binding defect in uraemia is best explained by competitive displacement of drugs from their albumin binding sites by endogenous substances accumulating in renal failure. The nature of this binding inhibitor has been clarified in recent studies. Dilution of uraemic plasma causes a rise in the protein binding of warfarin and phenytoin, an effect dependent on the extent of dilution. Furthermore, acidification of uraemic plasma followed by charcoal dialysis or anion-exchange resin perfusion restores drug binding to normal, whereas acidification has no effect. In addition, a substance eluted from charcoal or unchanged resin, or extracted from organic solvent, will inhibit protein binding in normal human plasma in a dose-dependent fashion. Whatever the nature of this substance, it appears unique to the uraemic state, as successful renal transplantation corrects the protein-binding defect.

Pharmacokinetic consequences and clinical significance of decreased drug protein binding in uraemia are difficult to predict. An increase in the fraction of 'free' or unbound drug will increase the apparent V_d and may augment the pharmacologic effect of any given dose. Since most drug assays measure the total (bound and unbound) drug in plasma, the 'therapeutic concentration' may need downward adjustment. This cannot always be used to predict dosage requirements, however, since drug elimination (hepatic or renal) may vary with the level of free drug. For example, there is no difference in steady state free phenytoin concentrations despite decreased drug binding because total drug clearance actually increases. Therefore the dosage of phenytoin does not need to be adjusted in patients with uraemia.

Elimination

Once distributed throughout the body, the plasma concentration of a drug (and the amount of drug in the body) declines exponentially. The rate of drug elimination (E) is proportional to the amount of drug in the body. This can be characterized by an elimination rate constant (β), and is expressed as:

$$E = \beta \times \text{amount of drug in the body} \qquad (2)$$

Since equation 1 relates the amount of drug in the body to the plasma concentration and the V_d:

$$E = \beta \times V_d \times \text{plasma concentration} \qquad (3)$$

Just as with the clearance of creatinine, the clearance (C) of any substance (drug) is equal to its rate of elimination divided by its midpoint plasma concentration. Thus, dividing both sides of equation 3 by the plasma concentration gives:

$$C = \beta \times V_d \qquad (4)$$

In clinical practice, the rate of drug removal is more commonly expressed as the elimination half-life ($T_{\frac{1}{2}}$), i.e. the time required for the amount of drug to decrease by 50%. Assuming first-order kinetics:

$$T_{\frac{1}{2}} = 0.693/\beta \qquad (5)$$

Combining equations (4) and (5) yields:

$$T_{\frac{1}{2}} = \frac{0.693 \times V_d}{C} \qquad (6)$$

Thus, the half-life for any drug depends on its clearance and V_d (dependent on lipid solubility and protein binding). For a given clearance, the larger the V_d the longer the half-life. The length of time required for its virtually complete elimination from the body can be predicted from the half-life of a drug. After one half-life, 50% of the initial amount remains; after a second half-life, 25%; after a third, 12.5%; and after a fourth, 6.25%. After a fifth half-life, only 3% of the initial amount is left. It takes four to five half-lives until a drug is almost completely eliminated from the body.

For most drugs, body clearance is determined by metabolic clearance (biotransformation) and renal excretion. Total body clearance can be expressed as the composite of renal and hepatic drug clearances: $C_{total} = C_{renal} + C_{hepatic}$. Reduction of either of these parameters will prolong the half-life.

Metabolism (biotransformation)

Metabolic transformation is the biochemical conversion of a drug to another chemical form. This occurs mainly in the liver. This enzymatic conversion usually results in drug metabolites that are more polar and less lipid-soluble than the parent compound, thus enchancing renal excretion. By this process the liver contributes to the elimination (clearance) of many drugs.

The metabolites resulting from hepatic biotransformation may differ from the parent drug with respect to disposition and pharmacological effect. Most metabolites are less pharmacologically active than the parent compound, but several commonly prescribed drugs produce metabolites with significant pharmacological activity. Some of these are listed in Table 21.2. Interruption of the further degradation (by enzyme inhibition) or excretion of these active metabolites may result in an augmented pharmacological effect.

Effects of renal failure on drug elimination

The most obvious pharmacokinetic aberration of renal failure is decreased elimination of a drug. Most importantly, this relates to drugs exclusively excreted unchanged by the kidney. Renal failure may also have a significant impact on drugs cleared by hepatic biotransformation by affecting the rate of metabolism or the excretion of active metabolites.

Hepatic metabolism. The processes of drug oxidation, reduction, acetylation, ester hydrolysis and formation of drug conjugates are affected at various rates by uraemia. In general, oxidative metabolism is normal in renal failure. The clearance of many drugs eliminated by reduction and hydrolysis is slowed in uraemic patients. Acetylation rates may be normal or decreased, but formation of glycine, sulphate and glucuronide conjugates is usually normal.

Accumulation of active metabolites. Metabolites of certain drugs may be pharmacologically active. If these metabolites are normally excreted in the urine, or if they are further biotransformed by a process inhibited by uraemia, they may accumulate in the patient with renal failure. The high

Table 21.2 Commonly prescribed drugs metabolized to active compounds

Parent compound	Active metabolite	Significance
Acetohexamide	l-Hydroxyhexamide	May cause hypoglycaemia due to accumulation in renal failure
Adriamycin	Adriamycinol	Similar antitumour and toxic activity
Allopurinol	Oxypurinol	May precipitate renal stones
Cephalothin	Desacetylcephalothin	
Cefapirin	Desacetylcefapirin	
Chlorpropamide	2-Hydroxychlorpropamide	
Clofibrate	Chlorophenoxyisobutyric acid	May cause rhabdomyolysis
Daunorubicin	Daunorubicinol	Similar antitumour and toxic activity
Diazepam	Oxazepam	Can contribute to 'uraemic' encepthalopathy
Flurazepam	N-desalkyl-flurazepam	Can contribute to 'ureamic' encephalopathy
Imipramine	Despiramine	
Meperidine (pethidine)	Normeperidine	Can cause seizures
Phenacetin	Acetaminophen (paracetamol)	
Phenylbutazone	Oxyphenbutazone	
Prednisone	Methylprednisolone	
Primidone	Phenobarbitone	
Procainamide	N-acetylprocainamide	Accumulates due to long half-life
Rifampin (Rifampicin)	Desacetylrifampicin	
Succinylcholine (suxamethonium) chloride	Succinylmonocholine	May cause muscle paralysis

incidence of adverse drug reactions in patients with renal failure might be explained, in part, by the accumulation of these active drug metabolites.

Normeperidine, the metabolite of meperidine (pethidine), has less analgesic but more convulsant properties. This metabolite, which gradually accumulates with repeated dosage in renal failure, may account for central nervous system irritability and seizures in such patients.

The active metabolite of procainamide, N-acetylprocainamide, may accumulate in renal failure since it is excreted unchanged in the urine. This metabolite shows similar potency to the parent compound but with a very long half-life, making quinidine a more practical oral anti-arrhythmic for patients with renal failure.

Chlorophenoxyisobutyric acid may be responsible for the hypolipidaemic effects of its parent drug, clofibrate. Accumulation of this metabolite in renal failure may cause rhabdomyolysis. Dosage modification and serial evaluation of serum creatine phosphokinase are necessary when administering this drug to patients with renal failure.

Oxipurinol, a metabolite of allopurinol, contributes to the therapeutic inhibition of xanthine oxidase. Accumulation of this metabolite in pa-tients with renal failure may account for the increased incidence of side effects with allopurinol. It may also contribute to the formation of renal stones in patients with mild to moderate renal insufficiency.

Occasionally, administration of methyldopa causes prolonged severe hypotension in patients with renal failure. While this may be related to accumulation of the methyl-O-sulphate metabolite, it more likely reflects the effect of alpha-methyl noradrenaline in the central nervous system.

Renal excretion

Most drugs are cleared in part by renal excretion. Even when drug elimination involves mainly hepatic metabolism, drug metabolites are often excreted by the kidneys. As with the clearance of creatinine, renal clearance of a drug or its metabolite is the amount of drug excreted over time ($U_{drug} \times V$) divided by the plasma concentration. (U is the concentration of the cleared substance in the urine and V the rate of urinary secretion). Renal excretion of a drug (or its metabolite) is a composite of three processes: glomerular filtration, tubular secretion, and tubular reabsorption.

Tubular drug secretion is mediated by active transport processes that show some degree of structural specificity. Generally, two types of transport systems are present, one for organic acids and one for organic bases. Tubular reabsorption of drugs is usually a passive process characterized by the principles that govern passive absorption of drugs from the intestinal tract. It is dependent on the tubular concentration and lipid solubility of a drug and on urinary pH. For both weak acids and weak bases, the non-ionized fraction of the drug is more readily reabsorbed than the ionized form. For weak acids (pK_a 3.0–7.5), as urine pH increases, the ionized fraction increases, decreasing reabsorption and enhancing renal clearance. Alkalinization of urine is used to increase renal elimination of salicylates. The ionized fraction and renal excretion of a weak base (pK_a 7.5–10.5) increase as urine pH falls. High rates of urine flow may increase renal excretion by decreasing tubular drug concentration and/or the contact time necessary for passive reabsorption.

The extent to which renal failure influences drug elimination depends on the proportion of the drug excreted unchanged in the urine and on the pharmacological activity and renal excretion of drug metabolites. For drugs with little or no renal excretion, the half-life is relatively constant over a wide range of renal function. Such a drug would obviously require little dosage adjustment in renal failure. For a drug cleared essentially unchanged in the urine, the half-life increases as renal function declines. Typically, the drug half-life increases slowly until the creatinine clearance approaches approximately 30 ml/min; further reductions in creatinine clearance are associated with markedly increased half-life. The effect of renal insufficiency on half-life is greater for drugs predominantly (50% or more) excreted unchanged and in patients whose renal function is less than half of normal. Since the half-life of drugs excreted by the kidneys usually correlates with the serum creatinine and creatinine clearance, these renal function tests usually provide an estimate of the degree of dosage adjustment necessary to maintain safe yet efficacious plasma levels.

DOSAGES FOR IMPAIRED RENAL FUNCTION

If drug accumulation and resultant toxicity are to be avoided in the patients with impaired renal function, dosage modifications are often necessary. Because it takes four to five half-lives to reach a steady state drug concentration in the plasma, the initial loading dose is rarely adjusted in renal failure. For example, the half-life of digoxin in patients with severely impaired renal function may be 100 hours rather than the usual 24–36 hours. It would therefore take approximately 400 hours (16–17 days) to reach therapeutic plasma levels of digoxin without an initial loading dose. For this reason, patients with renal failure require the usual loading dose for most drugs.

Most dosage adjustments in patients with renal disease are made by altering either the size or the frequency of the maintenance dose. It remains unclear which method is best. For drugs with a large therapeutic index, either method is probably satisfactory. Lengthening the dosing interval causes wider swings in plasma concentration, resulting in periods of potentially toxic levels alternating with periods of subtherapeutic levels. For a drug whose half-life is prolonged from two to four times by renal failure, the time during which blood levels are below a theoretical therapeutic level may be significantly prolonged. This may be of particular importance for drugs with a short half-life (many antibiotics). Wide swings in blood levels may be overcome by administering a smaller maintenance dose than normal but at the normal dosing interval, allowing more constant blood levels. This method has the advantage of being safe but may fail to reach therapeutic levels. Increasing the maintenance dose in this setting may overcome the problem, but poses a new risk of drug accumulation and toxicity. Regardless of the approach used to modify drug dosage in patients with renal failure, it is important to know which drugs require adjustment and the degree of adjustment necessary. Specific information regarding a large number of drugs has recently been reviewed. Table 21.3 give some of this information for commonly prescribed antibiotics. Adjustment method I stands for lengthening the dosing interval

Table 21.3 Dosing guidelines for common antimicrobial agents in renal failure

Drug	Major excretion routes	Normal dose internal (hours)	Method	> 50	10–50	<10	Removal by dialysis	Toxicity and remarks
					GFR (ml/min)			
Antifungal drugs								
Amphotericin B	Non-renal	24	I	24	24	24[a]	No (H)	Nephrotoxic, renal tubular acidosis, hypokalaemia, nephrogenic diabetes insipidus, renal failure. Hepatic dysfunction, marrow suppression more common in azotaemic patients
Flucytosine	Renal	6	I	6	12–24	24–48	Yes[b] (H, P)	
Antituberculous drugs								
Ethambutol	Renal	24	I	24	24–36	48	Yes (H, P)	Decreased visual acuity, peripheral neuritis.
Isoniazid	Hepatic (renal)	24	D	No change	No change	66–100	Yes (H, P)	Genetic variation in hepatic acetylation.
Rifampicin	Hepatic	24	D	No change	No change	No change	?No	May cause acute renal failure (toxic or immunological)
Aminoglycoside antibiotics								All agents in this group are nephrotoxic and ototoxic; rarely cause respiratory paralysis. Usual loading doses are needed in renal failure patients. Blood levels best guide to therapy
Amikacin	Renal	8–12	I	12–18	24–36	36–48	Yes (H, P)	
Gentamicin	Renal	8	D	75–100	50–75	25–50	Yes (H, P)[c]	Concurrent administration of penicillins may result in subtherapeutic blood levels
			I	8–12	12–24	24–48		
Tobramycin	Renal	8	D	75–100	50–75	25–50	Yes (H, P)[d]	
			I	8–12	12–24	24–48		
Cephalosporins								All agents in this group may be nephrotoxic in combination with aminoglycoside antibiotics, diuretics and volume depletion
Cephazolin	Renal	8	I	8	12	24–48	Yes (H)	
			D	100	50	25	No (P)	Ineffective for urinary infections when GFR < 10 ml/min
Cephalothin	Renal (hepatic)	6	I	6	6	8–12	Yes (H, P)[c]	Nephrotoxicity rare when given alone; ineffective for urinary infections when GFR <20 ml/min. May spuriously elevate serum creatinine. Serum sickness, haematological abnormalities more likely when GFR descreased
Cephalexin	Renal	6	I	6	6	6–12[f]	Yes (H, P)	
Cefapirin	Renal (hepatic)	6	I	6	6	12	Yes (H)	
Cephradine	Renal	6	D	100	50	25	Yes (H, P)	

Drug	Route of elimination	t½ (h)	Method	Dose/interval (mild)	(moderate)	(severe)	Removed by dialysis	Remarks
Chloramphenicol	Hepatic (renal)	6	D	No change	No change	No change	Yes (H)	Ineffective for treating urinary tract infections when GFR < 40 ml/min
Clindamycin	Hepatic (renal)	6–8	D	No change	No change	No change	No (P)	Pseudomembranous enterocolitis may cause volume depletion
Erythromycin	Hepatic	6	D	No change	No change	No change	No (H, P)	May be ototoxic in renal failure
Nitrofurantoin	Renal	8	D	No change[g]	No change[g]	avoid[g]	?No (H, P)	Peripheral sensory neuropathy due to accumulation of metabolites
Penicillins								Agents in this group may cause allergic interstitial nephritis; seizures and coagulopathy may occur at high blood levels
Amoxicillin	Renal	8	I	6	6–12	12–16[h]	Yes (H); No (P)	
Ampicillin	Renal (hepatic)	6	I	6	6–12	12–16[i]	Yes (H); No (P)	
Carbenicillin	Renal (hepatic)	4	I	8–12	12–24	24–48[k]	Yes (H, P)	Hypersthenia reported
			D	75	50	25[k]		
Dicloxacillin	Renal (hepatic)	6	I	No change	No change	No change	No (H)	
Naficillin	Hepatic	6	I	No change	No change	No change	No (H)	High serum levels and coagulopathy may occur with combined hepatic and renal dysfunction.
Penicillin G	Renal (hepatic)	8	D	100	75	25–50	Yes (H)	An upper limit of 4–6 million units/day is suggested in severe renal failure; potassium salt has 1.7 mmol/million units.
			I	8	8–12	12–18		
Ticarcillin	Renal	4–6	D	75	50	25	Yes (H, P)	Same remarks as carbenicillin
			I	8–12	12–24	24–28		
Sulphamethoxazole-trimethoprim	Renal	12	I	12	18	24	Yes (H)	May cause increase in serum creatinine < 2 mg/dl; may achieve adequate urine concentration in patient with low GFR using normal doses
Sulfisoxazole (sulphafurazole)	Renal	6	I	6	8–12	18–24	Yes (H, P)	Rare crystalluria
Tetracyclines								Tetracyclines may potentiate acidosis, increase catabolism, raise serum phosphate and BUN; phosphate binders may retard absorption; not useful for urinary infection if GFR < 20 ml/min

Doxycycline	Renal (hepatic)	12	I	12–18	18–24		No (H, P)	Probable group drug of choice for extrarenal infections but not useful for urinary infection if GFR < 20 ml/min
Minocycline	Hepatic	12	I	18–24	24–36		No (H, P)	Acute interstitial nephritis reported. Can be used for extrarenal infection but not useful for urinary infection if GFR < 20 ml/min
Vancomycin	Renal	24	I	24–72	72–240	240	No (H, P)	Best guide to therapy is serum level before next dose. Ototoxic at levels of 80–100 µg/ml

GFR = glomerular filtration rate; I = interval extension (data units are hours between maintenance doses); D = dose reduction (data units are percent of usual maintenance dose); H = haemodialysis; P = peritoneal dialysis.

a Ineffective for renal parenchymal infection.
b Dose of 20–30 mg/kg needed after haemodialysis.
c May add 4–5 mg/l of peritoneal dialysate to obtain adequate serum levels.
d May add 4–5 mg/l of peritoneal dialysate to obtain adequate serum levels.
e May be added to peritoneal dialysate in desired serum dialysate concentration (20 µg/ml).
f Need usual doses to treat urinary tract infections.
g Ineffective when GFR < 20–30 ml/min.
h Normal doses needed to treat urinary infections.
i Normal doses needed to treat urinary infections; contains sodium 3 mmol/g; adverse reactions more common in renal failure.
k May inactivate aminoglycosides; may be ineffective to treat urinary infections with GFR < 15 ml/min; acidosis at high blood levels; contains sodium 4.7 mmol/g; hypokalaemic alkalosis.

and adjustment method D for decreasing the dose by the percentage indicated. For example, for a glomerular filtration rate of less than 10 ml/min one can give gentamicin by the dosing adjustment method D (25% every 8 hours) or by the interval method I (full dose every 48 hours). Such recommendations, however, are only approximations and must be accompanied by careful monitoring of the patient, particularly for signs of unexpected drug toxicity.

UNIQUE PHARMACOLOGICAL PROBLEMS IN PATIENTS WITH RENAL INSUFFICIENCY

Treatment of urinary tract infections

Treatment of urinary tract infections in a patient with renal failure may be difficult. With impaired ability to filter, transport and concentrate, optimal urinary antibiotic levels may not be achieved. Subtherapeutic levels have been demonstrated in the urine and renal parenchyma of patients in whom gentamicin was prescribed in doses adjusted for renal insufficiency. Despite adequate serum levels, urinary infection was not eradicated in some patients. These studies suggest that gentamicin (and probably other aminoglycoside antibiotics) may not be effective in the treatment of urinary tract infections in patients with severe renal functional impairment.

Oral penicillins and cephalosporins given in ordinary dosages to uraemic patients result in only modest accumulation in the serum and adequate concentrations in the urine. In patient with severe renal failure, bacteriological cure of both upper and lower urinary tract infections has been demonstrated with ampicillin prescribed in the same dosage as in non-uraemic subjects. Beneficial therapeutic effects of these drugs may be due to active tubular secretion resulting in high urinary levels. Therapeutic urinary concentrations of sulphonamides can be achieved in the urine of uraemic subjects provided ordinary doses are administered. When given in combination, trimethoprim and sulphamethoxazole exceeded minimum inhibitory concentrations of urinary pathogens, resulting in bacteriological cure.

Aggravation of the uraemic state

The physician is often faced with the problem of differentiating progressive renal disease and the uraemic syndrome from preventable drug side effects. Corticosteroids and tetracyclines may elevate the blood urea nitrogen level. The nausea, vomiting and diarrhoea often attributed to uraemia may be produced by several drugs, including allopurinol, antacids, aspirin and other non-steroidal anti-inflammatory agents. Qualitative platelet defects produced by aspirin, dipyridamole and sulphinpyrazone may mimic uraemic bleeding. A drop in haematocrit (packed cell volume) in a patient with renal failure should trigger a close examination of the patient's medication list. Bone marrow suppression occurs with many drugs; azathioprine, chlorambucil and cyclophosphamide are commonly used by nephrologists. Cephalosporins and methyldopa may cause haemolysis. Salicylates and other non-steroidal agents may produce gastrointestinal blood loss, and folic acid deficiency may be seen with triamterene or trimethoprim–sulphamethoxazole.

Differentiation of uraemia from drug toxicity is probably most difficult when evaluating the neurological aspects of ureamia. Central nervous system depression by phenobarbitone or magnesium intoxication may often be interpreted as metabolic encephalopathy. Metabolites of diazepam and flurazepam may accumulate in renal failure, producing a similar clinical picture. A metabolite of nitrofurantoin is implicated as causing a peripheral neuropathy similar so that seen with uraemia. Generalized seizures in severely uraemic individuals may be produced by high doses of penicillin or the meperidine (pethidine) metabolite, normeperidine.

Laboratory abnormalities

Uraemia may alter a variety of laboratory determinations, but may also modify the effects of drugs on laboratory tests. For example, high levels of direct bilirubin in dialysis patients are often related to an effect of propranolol metabolites on the autoanalyzer determination of bilirubin. Several drugs may interfere with serum creatinine determi-

> **Drugs that increase serum creatinine value independent of renal function**
> *By interference with tubular secretion of creatinine*
> Acetohexamide
> Cephalosporins
> Cimetidine
> Trimethoprim
> *By interference with laboratory determination of creatinine*
> Ascorbic acid
> Sulphobromophthalein
> Levodopa
> Phenylsulphonphthalein
> *p*-Aminohippurate

nation by either spuriously raising its concentration or by interfering with tubular secretion of creatinine. Any of these drugs may elevate the serum creatinine independent of renal function. A similar effect (laboratory artefact) has been demonstrated with acetoacetate, acetone and glucose, which could account for some of the cases of renal transplant 'pseudorejection' often seen in patients with poor diabetic control.

Adjustments for haemodialysis or peritoneal dialysis

In patients with renal failure who are undergoing dialysis, adjustments must be made for drug losses or physiological changes induced by the procedure. Drugs that are effectively removed by clinical haemodialysis usually have a molecular weight of less than 500. The driving force in haemodialysis is the concentration gradient of unbound drug between plasma water and dialysate. As protein binding of the drug increases, dialysis clearance decreases. Semisynthetic penicillins which bind to protein to more than 90% are poorly removed by dialysis. Propranolol, despite its molecular weight of only 260, is not dialysable because of its high degree of protein binding. In addition to protein binding and molecular size, removal of a drug during dialysis depends on the type of artificial kidney used. Most clinically used dialysers have cuprophan or cellulose membranes, which have similar characteristics. In general,

> **Common drugs requiring supplemental dosage after haemodialysis**
> 1. Antibiotics
>   Aminoglycosides
>   Streptomycin
>   Kanamycin
>   Gentamicin
>   Tobramycin
>   Amikacin
>   Cephalosporins
>   Cephalothin
>   Cephalexin
>   Cefapirin
>   Cephazolin
>   Cephradine
>   Penicillins
>   Penicillin
>   Ampicillin
>   Carbenicillin
>   Amoxicillin
>   Ticarcillin
>   Chloramphenicol
> 2. Antifungal agents
>   Flucytosine (5-fluorocytosine)
> 3. Antituberculous drugs
>   Ethambutol
>   Isoniazid
>   Cycloserine
> 4. Anti-infective agents
>   Metronidazole
>   Quinine
>   Sulfisoxazole (sulphafurazole)
>   Trimethoprim–sulphamethoxazole
> 5. Analgesics
>   Acetylsalicylic acid
>   Acetaminophen (paracetamol)
> 6. Sedatives, hypnotics and tranquillizers
>   Phenobarbitone
>   Lithium carbonate
> 7. Cardiovascular drugs
>   Procainamide
>   Methyldopa
>   Diazoxide
>   Sodium nitroprusside
> 8. Miscellaneous
>   5-Fluorouracil
>   Cyclophosphamide
>   Azathioprine
>   Primidone
>   Gallamine

Common drugs requiring supplemental dosage after peritoneal dialysis

1. Antimicrobial agents
   Amikacin
   Cephalexin
   Cephalothin
   Ethambutol
   Flucytosine
   Gentamicin
   Kanamycin
   Streptomycin★
   Sulphamethoxazole–trimethoprim★
   Sulfisoxazole (sulphafurazole)
   Ticarcillin
   Tobramycin
2. Analgesics
   Acetylsalicylic acid
3. Anti-arrhythmic agents
   Procainamide★
   Quinidine
4. Antihypertensive agents
   Methyldopa
   Nitroprusside
5. Neurological agents
   Diphenylhydantoin (phenytoin)
   Gallamine
6. Sedatives, hypnotics, tranquillizers
   Lithium carbonate
   Meprobamate
   Phenobarbitone
7. Miscellaneous
   Aminophylline★

★ In vivo data are lacking but indirect evidence strongly supports placing the drug in this category.

regularly scheduled drug doses should be given after dialysis to minimize removal. For drugs with significant removal it is best to replace a full maintenance dose after dialysis. Since haemodynamic factors and various other patient variables make precise adjustments difficult in clinical situations, it is best to check serum levels before the next regularly scheduled dose. A serum level measured immediatley after dialysis may not accurately reflect the total body burden since equilibration from intracellular pools may occur for several hours. There has been a recent resurgence of interest in chronic peritoneal dialysis, which has widespread patient and physician acceptance. Because of the relatively large surface area available for transfer, the peritoneal membrane is five to ten times more permeable to large molecular weight solutes than clinically used haemodialysis membranes.

RECOMMENDED READING

Anderson R J, Linas S L, Berns A L, 1977 Non oliguric acute renal failure. New England Journal of Medicine 296: 1123–1128
Anderson R J, Bennett W M, Gambertoglio J G, Schrier R W 1981 Fate of drugs in renal failure. In: Brenner B, Rector F (eds) The kidney. W B Saunders, Philadelphia, p 2659–2708
Bennet W M, Plamp C E, Porter G A 1977 Drug related syndromes in clinical nephrology. Annals of Internal Medicine 87: 582–590
Bennett W M 1981 Antibiotic-induced acute renal failure. Seminars in Nephrology 1: 43–50
Bennett W M 1983 Aminoglycoside nephrotoxicity. Nephron 35; 73–77
Bennett W M et al 1983 Drug prescribing in renal failure: dosing guidelines for adults. American Journal of Kidney Diseases 2: 155–193
Berglund F, Killander J, Pompeius R 1975 The effect of trimethoprim sulfamethoxazole on the renal excretion of creatinine in man. Journal of Urology 114: 802–808
Captopril Collaborative Study Group 1982 Does captopril cause renal damage in hypertensive patients? Lancet 1: 988–990
Depner T A, Gulyassy P F, 1980 Plasma protein binding in uremia: extraction and characterization of an inhibitor. Kidney International 18: 86–94
Durham S R, Bignell A H, Wise R 1979 Interference of cefoxitin in the creatinine estimation and its clinical relevance. Journal of Clinical Pathology 32: 1148–1151
Emmerson B T 1973 Chronic lead nephropathy. Kidney International 4: 1–5
Goodwin J S, Webb D R 1981 Regulation of the immune response by prostaglandins. Immunology Series 14: 99–135
Harkonen S, Kjellstrand C 1981 Contrast nephropathy. American Journal of Nephrology 1: 69–77
Kleinecht D, Kanfer A, Morel-Maroger L 1978 Immunologically mediated drug-induced acute renal failure. Contributions to Nephrology 10: 42–52
Linton A L, Clark W F, Dreidger A A, Turnbull D I, Lindsay R M 1980 Acute interstitial nephritis due to drugs. Annals of Internal Medicine 93: 735–741
Porter G A, Bennett W M 1980 Nephrotoxin-induced acute renal failure. In: Brenner B, Stein J H (eds) Acute renal failure. Churchill Livingstone, New York, p 123–162
Samuels B, Lee J C, Engleman E P, Hopper J 1977 Membranous nephropathy in patients with rheumatoid arthritis: relationship to gold therapy. Medicine 57: 319–327
Schilsky R L, 1982 Renal and metabolic toxicities of cancer chemotherapy. Seminars in Oncology 9: 75–83
Schulman H, Striker G, Deeg H G, Kennedy M, Storb R, Thomas E D 1981 Nephrotoxicity of cyclosporin A after

allogeneic marrow transplantation. New England Journal of Medicine 305: 1392–1395

Shils M E 1963 Renal disease and the metabolic effects of tetracycline. Annals of Internal Medicine 58: 389–408

Smith C R, Baughman K L, Edwards C Q, Rogers J F, Leitman P S 1977 Controlled comparison of amikacin and gentamicin. New England Journal of Medicine 296: 349–353

Smith C R, Lipsky J J, Laskin O L, Hellman D B, Mellits E D, Longstreth J, Leitman P S 1980 Double blind comparison of the nephrotoxicity and auditory toxicity of gentamicin and tobramycin. New England Journal of Medicine 302: 1106–1109

Sobel A, Heslan J M, Branellec A, Lagrue B 1981 Vascular permeability factor produced by lymphocytes of patients with nephrotic syndrome. Advances in Nephrology 10: 315–322

Takacs F J, Tomkiewicz Z M, Merrill J P 1963 Amphotericin B nephrotoxicity with irreversible renal failure. Annals of Internal Medicine 59: 716–724

Torres V E 1982 Present and future of nonsteroidal anti-inflammatory drugs in nephrology. Mayo Clinical Proceedings 57: 389–393

Tune B M 1975 Relationship between the transport and toxicity of cephalosporins in the kidney. Journal of Infectious Diseases 132: 189–194

Weiss R B, Poster D S 1982 The renal toxicity of cancer chemotherapeutic agents. Cancer Treatment Reviews 9: 37–56

Whelton A, Walker W G 1974 Intrarenal antibiotic distribution in health and disease. Kidney International 6: 131–137

22. Chronic renal failure

J. K. Dawborn

DEFINITION

Chronic renal damage causing more than 50% loss of renal function. This definition is chosen arbitrarily because it can be defined by measurement of glomerular filtration rate and because it appears that after 50% loss of renal function, renal damage and its consequences are likely to progress.

INTRODUCTION

Dialysis and transplantation have extended the life of patients with chronic renal failure and stimulated great interest in pathogenesis and treatment. Research in both animal models and patients has produced a large volume of literature and a bewildering array of data. Earlier detection and the ready availability of treatment have resulted in the disappearance of the clinical syndrome of terminal uraemia as it was previously known. Features such as peripheral neuropathy, haemorrhage and uncontrolled hypertension are virtually eliminated; others, such as renal bone disease and the complications of prolonged hypertension, are more common. The latter are accentuated in dialysis patients and some new problems have arisen, for example trace metal poisoning (from impurities in dialysis feed water) and dialysis-related amyloidosis. In general, the therapeutic problems of chronic renal failure extend into the period when patients receive dialysis, although with some change in emphasis. However, problems which arise strictly as a result of dialysis treatment will not be dealt with here.

AETIOLOGY AND CLINICAL PRESENTATION

The Australian and New Zealand Dialysis and Transplant Registry shows that approximately 55 patients per million population enter end-stage renal failure programmes each year. The cause of primary renal disease in these patients reflects that in patients with chronic renal failure. Approximately one third of patients suffer from glomerulonephritis, between 3 and 16% from analgesic nephropathy (depending on local conditions), 14% from diabetes mellitus and approximately 8% from polycystic kidneys, reflux nephropathy or hypertension. Miscellaneous conditions (obstructive uropathy, interstitial nephritis, amyloid disease, multiple myeloma, familial nephritis, etc.) and those of uncertain aetiology make up the balance.

Over half the patients entering our chronic renal failure programme initially present with hypertension. Approximately 80% were hypertensive when starting dialysis and almost all patients had more than a trace of protein on urine testing. This emphasizes the importance of investigating renal function in hypertension, particularly in any patient with proteinuria. Approximately 20% of patients present with symptoms of uraemia, usually tiredness and lethargy associated with anaemia or with anorexia, nausea and vomiting, often precipitated by an intercurrent infection and sometimes aggravated by tetracycline therapy. Asymptomatic chronic renal failure may be discovered as a result of examination during pregnancy or an intercurrent illness, for insurance or superannuation, or during investigation of drug toxicity to which patients with chronic renal failure are prone. A common symptom is the restless legs syndrome, which may cause the patient significant distress. Less common modes of presentation include muscle weakness or bone pain due to osteomalacia or spontaneous fracture in patients with severe hyperparathyroidism. Overt neuropathy is uncommon although autonomic neuropathy may be seen in patients with amyloid disease or diabetes. Patients may present with features of acute renal failure if complications such as infection, fluid imbalance or drug toxicity supervene. Immediate dialysis may be necessary while the diagnosis is being resolved. Under these circumstances simple investigations may reveal abnormalities which indicate an underlying chronic process, e.g. a relatively large urine volume, an inactive urinary sediment and small kidneys on plain X-ray or ultrasound. Untreated, severe renal failure may be complicated by pericardial effusion with tamponade. Such patients are usually hypotensive despite an elevated jugular venous pressure and hypotension may be aggravated by volume depletion if dialysis is instituted. The classic signs of pericardial tamponade are rarely present. It is important to recognize this sequence of events, which requires volume repletion and urgent pericardial aspiration.

Presentation of chronic renal failure
Hypertension
Urinary abnormality
Anaemia
Acute renal failure due to:
  infection
  dehydration
  drug toxicity
Uraemia
  Malaise, lethargy
  Anorexia, weight loss
  Nocturia
  Volume overload
  Pericarditis
  Pericardial tamponade
  Osteomalacia
  Bone fracture
  Restless legs

BIOCHEMICAL ASSESSMENT

The severity of renal failure is reflected in the plasma creatinine concentration. However interpretation of renal function on the basis of the plasma creatinine is made difficult by biological variability, differences in age, sex and body size and the fact that the plasma creatinine does not begin to rise until there is about 50% loss of renal function. If symptoms are more severe than indicated by the plasma creatinine, e.g. in patients with unusually low creatinine production such as an older or smaller patient, then some measurement of glomerular filtration rate is necessary. Problems of accurate urine collection detract from the routine clinical use of creatinine clearance as a measure of renal function; an isotopic measurement of GFR based on serial plasma sampling may be preferable. The reciprocal of the plasma creatinine (1/CR) is a useful tool in following changes in renal function in individual patients. Reciprocal plots magnify early changes which may otherwise be overlooked and the progressive changes are usually linear in patients with uncomplicated renal failure (Fig. 22.1). Reciprocal plots may be a guide to prognosis, and alterations in slope may indicate additional factors influencing the rate of progression.

The urine volume and plasma sodium and potassium concentration are usually normal in patients with stable chronic renal failure but both hyponatraemia and hyperkalaemia may on occasions require correction. Hyperphosphataemia, mild acidosis and hypercalcaemia are common, and anaemia (haemoglobin < 10 g/dl) is almost always present.

PATHOPHYSIOLOGY OF CHRONIC RENAL FAILURE

The hallmark of chronic renal failure is a reduction of glomerular filtration rate. This reflects decreased nephron mass and decreased overall excretory capacity. For substances which are handled predominantly by filtration (e.g. creatinine and, to a lesser extent, urea) metabolic balance is maintained by a compensatory increase in plasma concentration. However, renal tubules

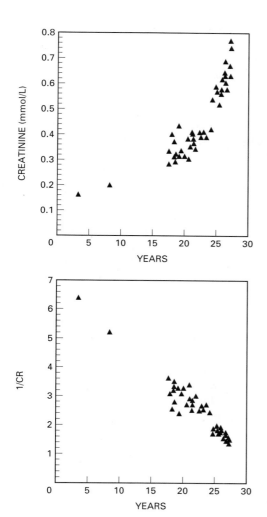

Fig. 22.1 A plot of plasma creatinine (Cr) and 1/CRv time in a patient with reflux nephropathy. Reciprocal plots magnify early changes in function and are usually linear allowing extrapolation to estimate prognosis.

Altered renal function in chronic renal failure
Reduced excretory capacity
Retained metabolites
Overperfusion of remaining nephrons
Reduced flexibility
Tubular adaptation
Reduced hormonal and metabolic function
Trade-off effects

---

tions. Thus metabolic balance is maintained but patients are vulnerable to overload if these tubular functions are stressed further, particularly in therapeutic situations. Examples include water intoxication, volume overload (e.g. acute pulmonary oedema from excess sodium retention) and hyperkalaemia.

Sodium and water

The kidney retains some regulatory ability with regard to sodium and water excretion. Decreased nephron mass, overperfusion of the remaining nephrons and excessive regulatory demands in patients with chronic renal failure lead to decreased flexibility of response and a tendency to both overload and depletion in certain clinical situations. The changes in sodium reabsorption required to maintain sodium balance in a patient with stable chronic renal failure after a reduction in GFR to 5 litres per day are shown in Table 22.1. Balance is achieved by an increase in the excretion fraction of sodium from 0.7% in normal patients to 14% in chronic renal failure. Doubling the sodium intake in a normal patient will lead to a transient expansion of extracellular volume (ECV) and an increase in blood pressure, producing a further 0.7% sodium excretion until balance is achieved. A similar adaptation in patients with chronic renal failure requires excretion of a further 14% of the filtered sodium. It is quite remarkable that the same stimulus in a patient with chronic

have the capacity to adapt to the increased solute load per nephron, and for substances such as sodium, phosphate, potassium and hydrogen ions the rise in plasma concentration is blunted by mobilizing spare capacity of these tubular func-

Table 22.1 Adaptation of sodium excretion following a decrease in glomerular filtration rate (GFR) in a patient with a sodium intake of 100 mmol/day

GFR (l/24 h)	Plasma Na$^+$ (mmol/l)	Filtered Na$^+$ (mmol/24 h)	Na$^+$ excretion (mmol/24 h)	Na$^+$ reabsorption (mmol/24 h)	(% filtered)
100	140	14 000	100	13 900	99.3
5	140	700	100	600	86.0

renal failure could achieve such a large change in tubular sodium transport and it is not surprising that this may be done at the expense of some permanent increase in blood pressure and extracellular volume. On the other hand, if the sodium intake is rapidly reduced to 10 mmol/day, a patient with chronic renal failure must reabsorb 99% of filtered sodium to remain in balance. It is likely that this degree of sodium (and water) reabsorption will be prevented by the increased filtered load of urea and non-reabsorbable anions and in any event could not be achieved without an unacceptable fall in the urine flow, with consequent retention of other substances which are partly flow-dependent such as potassium and urea. Sodium conservation is more efficient if sufficient time is given for adaptation.

Potassium

Potassium balance is achieved by a marked increase in potassium secretion per nephron, aided by an increase in urine flow rate and in the delivery of sodium and non-reabsorbable anions to the distal nephron which favours potassium ion exchange and excretion. Regulatory mechanisms affecting potassium excretion are probably stimulated by changes in plasma and intracellular potassium and hydrogen ion concentration. In advanced renal failure potassium excretion exceeds filtered potassium but plasma potassium is often normal. However, hyperkalaemia may occur suddenly if distal mechanisms for potassium excretion are compromised by a reduction in urine flow rate or sodium delivery. Some older patients and diabetics have a defect in aldosterone production and are more prone to hyperkalaemia. The same is true in patients who are given potassium-sparing diuretics which block distal potassium transfer and are potentially very dangerous in renal failure. Hyperkalaemia may be aggravated by acidosis, which causes potassium to shift out of cells into the extracellular fluid, or by an increase in endogenous or exogenous potassium load.

Intact nephron hypothesis

The similarity of adaptive processes in kidneys with predominantly glomerular or predominantly tubular damage has given rise to the concept of glomerulotubular balance. Despite considerable structural heterogeneity there remains a basic orderliness of function so that residual nephrons retain a predictable, definable and organized pattern of response. Thus it was demonstrated that in humans and animals with unilateral kidney damage, kidney functions such as free water and sodium reabsorption remained normal in each kidney if allowance was made for the reduction in GFR. However, in animal models, if the normal kidney was removed, the damaged kidney developed a defect in urine concentration and sodium conservation similar to that seen in chronic renal failure, regardless of the nature of the underlying kidney damage. These defects were attributed to an increase in solute load in an otherwise normally functioning nephron.

Despite this common mechanism, patients with conditions such as analgesic nephropathy or medullary sponge kidney, in which there is predominantly tubular damage, may show an early defect in concentration or acidification and a greater tendency to sodium loss. This is presumably due to direct interference with specific tubular functions in addition to overperfusion of the nephron and is an expression of anatomical heterogeneity of damage to the nephron. Factors such as anaemia, hypoproteinaemia, acidosis and hyperparathyroidism may also have independent effects on tubular function.

Hydrogen ions

As GFR falls, metabolic acidosis develops and by providing a stimulus to hydrogen ion secretion enables the diseased kidney to achieve a balance between hydrogen ion production and excretion. Until the GFR falls below 20 ml per minute the defect in hydrogen ion secretion is usually well compensated; after this a progressive fall in plasma bicarbonate becomes apparent. The changes in hydrogen ion excretion occur in the context of an increased solute and phosphate load. The same factors which impair proximal sodium reabsorption may cause an increased distal delivery of bicarbonate, with some urinary loss of bicarbonate, and failure to fully utilize other urinary buffers and to achieve maximal urinary acidification until a new steady state is reached. Hydrogen ion balance is achieved largely by increased renal ammonia production. The rate at which acidosis develops depends on protein intake (hydrogen ion load), urinary phosphate (buffer) excretion and the rate of nephron loss, which also determines the rate of adaptation. Persistent metabolic acidosis also causes gradual reduction of bone carbonate buffers and loss of calcium from bone.

Trade-off

It is apparent that maintenance of relatively normal ion balance in renal failure is achieved at some cost to the individual, e.g. hypertension, increased extracellular volume and decreased bone mineral, as outlined above. The price paid for renal compensation has been termed 'trade-off' and is more apparent the more complex the derangement of regulatory processes. The most discussed example is that involving the phosphate control system in which phosphate balance is maintained at the cost of hyperparathyroidism. Phosphate balance in chronic renal failure is maintained by a progressive reduction in tubular reabsorption of phosphate, similar to that which occurs for sodium. As GFR falls, the percentage of filtered phosphate which is reabsorbed falls from 90% to 15% or less. This is achieved by an increased secretion of parathyroid hormone (PTH), by direct effects of phosphate retention and possibly by other mechanisms. Reduced reabsorption of phosphate lowers plasma phosphate but improved phosphate balance is accompanied by a permanent increase in the level of PTH. This sequence of events is supported by experimental data showing a marked reduction in secondary hyperparathyroidism if dietary phosphate is reduced. Apart from its effect on bone, increased levels of parathyroid hormone may affect sodium and acid–base balance and produce toxic effects on other organ systems, either directly or through alterations in tissue calcium levels. Similar trade-off effects occur with other regulatory systems and in some situations disturbed regulatory processes may lead to toxic effects without any beneficial trade-off.

Uraemic toxins

The role of uraemic toxins in the pathogenesis of uraemia has been debated for many years. The extra-renal manifestations of uraemia dominate the clinical picture and virtually all organs are affected. It is tempting to attribute such widespread changes to some or all of the numerous metabolic products which accumulate in renal failure. This is particularly so when the introduction of a low protein diet or dialysis can cause symptomatic improvement coincident with a reduction in some of these metabolites. While this certainly points to protein metabolites and dialysable substances as being partly responsible for the uraemic syndrome, it should be remembered that dietary counselling and dialysis may have other effects, including improved nutrition and electrolyte status, which might explain part of their benefit. The list of potential toxins includes ions, protein metabolic products, hormones and unidentified 'middle molecules'. While it is difficult to incriminate specific toxins, it is equally difficult to deny that there may be ill-effects from a combination of substances acting over a prolonged period of time. The potential toxic effects of sodium, potassium water and hydrogen ions are undeniable and most would agree that urea or protein metabolites as a group produce some of the symptoms of uraemia. However, methodological difficulties have beset attempts to accurately measure plasma levels of such substances as guanidines and phenols, and there has been a lack of meaningful test systems which could demonstrate unequivocal toxic effects at the levels which are presumed to occur in renal failure. The effect of toxins may also be mediated indirectly by interference with enzyme or receptor function or in other ways interfering with metabolic or regulatory mechanisms. Such effects may be very difficult to demonstrate.

Some reference should be made to the middle molecule hypothesis which has stimulated so much research over the last decade. This concept arose from an appreciation of the therapeutic effectiveness of peritoneal dialysis despite its relative inefficiency in removing small molecules and of the importance of small amounts of residual renal function in preventing neuropathy and other complications of uraemia. It was postulated that these middle molecules (MW 500–1500) were toxic, poorly removed by conventional dialysis membranes, and cleared relatively well by a small number of remaining nephrons. However, dialysis schedules which favour retention of middle molecules are not necessarily harmful. It is possible that the size of the middle molecule has been overestimated. Efforts to isolate and test middle molecules have many problems and at present our knowledge is insufficient to assess their importance. Small molecule removal and other factors such as good nutrition, regular physical activity and the rate of ultrafiltration are also clearly important in improving symptoms of uraemia.

Progression of renal failure

The rate of progression of renal failure will vary depending on the severity of the underlying disease and the success of treatment. However there are many situations in which the underlying disease process appears to be quiescent but renal failure progresses nonetheless. Since a normal solitary kidney does not appear to be at risk, loss of more than 50% of renal function may be necessary before progressive glomerular sclerosis occurs. This may not be reflected in an obviously abnormal plasma creatinine level, and compensatory hypertrophy of the remaining nephrons may increase the GFR to 60 or 70% of normal. A great deal of interest has been shown in the common factors which lead to progressive loss of renal function which, when represented as a reciprocal creatinine plot, is often linear. Break points in such a plot are a valuable indication that some extra factor has intervened to influence the rate of progression and may be correctable (Fig. 22.2).

There is a considerable amount of experimental evidence that a high protein intake will accelerate glomerular sclerosis and renal failure. However clinical studies of the effect of protein restriction in slowing the rate of progression of chronic renal failure are more difficult to interpret. Few of the studies are controlled and most rely on demonstrating a change in the slope of reciprocal creatinine plots. While this is a useful clinical tool it may not be sufficiently specific or sensitive for

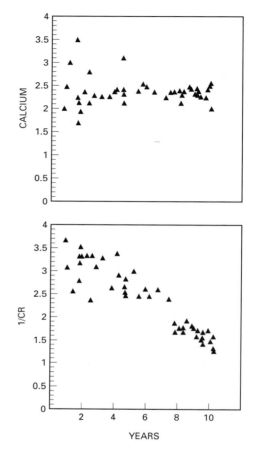

Fig. 22.2 Linear progression of renal failure with temporary and reversible deterioration due to hypercalcaemia associated with calcium carbonate therapy.

such studies. Bergstrom has shown similar improvement in patients who regularly attend a renal clinic but are given no nutritional advice. The place of protein restriction in slowing progression of renal failure is not clear at the present time. If there is benefit much of this may be due to associated changes in phosphate or mineral balance, improved blood pressure control, altered lipid metabolism or other factors. (See list). In many trials and certainly in clinical practice compliance with protein restriction is very variable and there is concern about excessive protein restriction, particularly in children and in the elderly.

Progressive renal impairment — Possible contributing factors
Hypertension
Hyperphosphataemia
Hypermetabolism
Solute overload
Hyperlipidaemia
Hyperparathyroidism
Hyperoxalaemia
Hyperuricaemia
Metabolic acidosis
Hormone imbalance
Lack of exercise
Drug toxicity
Disease progression

EXTRA-RENAL MANIFESTATIONS OF CHRONIC RENAL FAILURE

Anaemia

In a group of chronic renal failure patients entering our dialysis programme plasma haemoglobin varied from 5.7–12.5 g/dl (mean 8.7). Anaemia is usually normocytic and normochromic with some variation in shape of the red cells and few reticulocytes. The bone marrow is inappropriately normocellular, in contrast to the hypercellular marrow of patients with a comparable degree of anaemia and normal renal function. Marrow iron turnover is depressed and plasma erythropoietin levels are inappropriately low. The bone marrow response to erythropoietin is also impaired. Red cell half-life is reduced; since normal cells have a reduced half-life in uraemic plasma this defect is probably due to a circulating toxin. Some patients with renal failure have normal haemoglobin levels (particularly patients with polycystic kidney disease) and a haemoglobin level of less than 9 g/dl should not be accepted as being due to renal failure. Other common causes of anaemia should be investigated, particularly iron deficiency.

A relative lack of erythropoietin is the major factor in the anaemia of renal failure. This glycoprotein hormone is produced in the renal cortex in response to signals from a renal oxygen sensor, probably a haem protein. Normally, at a haematocrit of less than 20% the plasma erythropoietin level increases 100 fold. In renal failure the level of erythropoietin is normal or only slightly raised despite comparable anaemia. Although there is a poor response to chronic anaemia, uraemic patients may produce erythropoietin and increase their haemoglobin in response to a reduction in oxygen saturation (e.g. at high altitude). A similar response may be seen in renal failure patients with acute hepatitis, possibly due to the production of erythropoetin by the liver. For these reasons it has been suggested that the low erythropoietin levels in chronic renal failure may be related to suppression of erythropoietin production rather than loss of EPO-producing capacity. The sensitivity of the oxygen-sensing mechanism may be impaired.

The response of patients with chronic renal failure to the therapeutic use of recombinant human erythropoietin is usually excellent. Lack of response usually indicates iron deficiency or intercurrent infection. The improvement in symptoms is so striking that it is now believed that a large part of the uraemic syndrome is due to anaemia. Patients experience a rapid improvement in well-being and physical and mental function with quite modest improvement in their anaemia. Objective improvement may be demonstrated in cardiac output, cerebral function and bleeding diathesis without any detrimental effect on renal function, although there may be an associated increase in

---

Recombinant human erythropoietin
Indication:
   Symptomatic anaemia
Contraindications:
   Uncontrolled hypertension
   Epilepsy
   Correctable cause of anaemia
Use:
   Target haemoglobin 9–11 g/dl
   Dose 50–100 u/kg/wk
   Subcutaneous or intravenous route
Failure to respond:
   Iron deficiency (ferritin < 100 µg/l)
   Infection
Side-effects:
   Hypertension
   Convulsions
   Hyperkalaemia
   Hyperphosphataemia

---

blood pressure. A rapid rise in haematocrit may be a risk factor for hypertension in this patient population. Increased well-being and the consequent improvement in appetite may lead to some difficulty controlling plasma potassium, phosphate or uric acid concentration and these aspects should be carefully monitored.

Most patients respond to a relatively low dose of erythropoietin, e.g. 50–100 u/kg per week, preferably given subcutaneously. A plasma haemoglobin of 10–11 g/dl can usually be achieved in 6–8 weeks and maintained with a dose of 50–75 u/kg/week. Higher target haemoglobin levels are not necessary, require a higher dose of erythropoietin and may cause an increase in undesirable side effects such as hypertension, headache, arthralgia and oedema. Treatment should probably be reserved for patients with debilitating symptoms and/or haemoglobin of less than 10 g/dl. However as erythropoietin becomes more readily available it would not be unreasonable to normalize the haemoglobin levels in all patients with chronic renal failure. If this is done a close watch should be kept for some of the more serious complications of advanced uraemia, such as pericarditis, which have become less common since the ready availability of dialysis but may reappear if amelioration of uraemic symptoms leads to delay in the institution of dialysis.

Bleeding diathesis

In advanced renal failure bleeding time may be prolonged because of defective release of platelet factor III. Platelet aggregation, platelet adhesiveness, prothrombin consumption and prostaglandin release may all be reduced, and may contribute to skin and mucosal bleeding and the predisposition to haemorrhagic pericarditis. The prolonged bleeding time may be improved by dialysis or by correction of anaemia. Even partial correction of renal anaemia by erythropoietin is enough to normalize bleeding time. Bleeding time can also be corrected by infusion of blood or cryoprecipitate, or by the administration of desmopressin (DDAVP) or oestrogens. DDAVP is a vasopressin analogue capable of releasing factor VIII and von Willebrand factor; 0.3 mg/kg given

subcutaneously or intravenously (in 50 ml saline over 30 min) will improve the bleeding time in chronic renal failure patients for up to 4 hours and this is associated with increased factor VIII activity. Conjugated oestrogens will also normalize the bleeding time in uraemia for a period of 2–5 days. The effect of cryoprecipitate, DDAVP and oestrogens in improving the bleeding defect of uraemia has drawn attention to abnormalities in factor VIII and related clotting factors. Although the exact mechanism of action is not understood these various agents can be used to correct the bleeding defect of uraemia prior to surgery or invasive procedures.

Renal bone disease

The pathogenesis of renal bone disease is illustrated in Figure 22.3. The sequence of events by which phosphate retention leads to hypocalcaemia and hyperparathyroidism has been described earlier. The second major factor contributing to hypocalcaemia and renal bone disease is an absolute or relative deficiency of 1,25-dihydroxycholecalciferol, the active metabolite of vitamin D. Vitamin D_3 is hydroxylated to 25-hydroxyvitamin D_3 in the liver. Regulation of 25-hydroxyvitamin D_3 levels is normal in renal failure although patients who have reduced levels through malnutrition or other reasons are more likely to develop osteomalacia. The kidney regulates the further metabolism of 25-hydroxyvitamin D_3 by hydroxylation either to 1,25-dihydroxyvitamin D_3, which is a potent stimulus to calcium absorption, or to other less active metabolites. Normally renal hydroxylation of vitamin D is modulated according to the calcium and phosphorus needs of the body, but in renal failure deficiency of 1,25-dihydroxyvitamin D_3 causes impaired intestinal calcium absorption, hypocalcaemia, hypocalciuria and skeletal resistance to PTH (altered calcium set point for PTH regulation). The dual effects of hyperphosphataemia and lack of 1,25-dihydroxyvitamin D_3 by lowering plasma ionized calcium provide a stimulus for hyperparathyroidism. Conversely, in both experimental and clinical situations control of plasma phosphate levels and the administration of 1,25-dihydroxyvitamin D_3 effectively

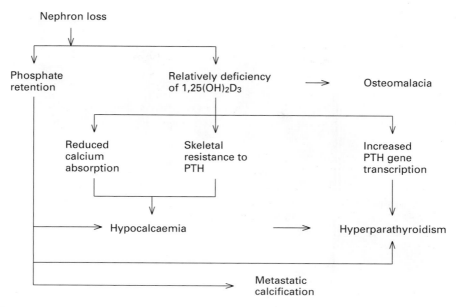

Fig. 22.3   Events leading to hypocalcaemia, renal bone disease and metastatic calcification. PTH — parathyroid hormone

prevent the development of hyperparathyroidism. Deficiency of 1,25-dihydroxyvitamin D_3 may also allow increased PTH gene transcription and increase PTH production by a direct effect on the parathyroid gland.

Deficiency of vitamin D metabolites is also an important cause of impaired bone mineralization in renal failure, and most patients with osteomalacia due to renal failure respond well to vitamin D therapy. However, the incidence of osteomalacia in renal failure patients varies considerably in different parts of the world and is relatively uncommon in Australia. In those patients who develop early and severe symptomatic osteomalacia it is likely that poor nutrition, lack of sunlight, chronic acidosis, hypophosphataemia or other factors also contribute to the mineralization defect. Most patients with chronic renal failure of more than a few years duration have histological evidence of bone disease. Those with predominantly hyperparathyroidism show areas of bone resorption, increased numbers of osteoblasts, marrow fibrosis and increased osteoid. The osteoid is usually lined by osteoblasts, and double tetracycline labelling (on two occasions at 3-week intervals) demonstrates extensive labelling and widely separate lines of uptake indicative of rapid bone turnover. Such active osteoid is typical of hyperparathyroidism and does not indicate coexistent osteomalacia (Fig. 22.4a). Patients with osteomalacia show increased lamellar osteoid seams usually not lined by large osteoblasts, and tetracycline labelling indicates slow bone turnover (Fig. 22.4b). Many patients have a combination of these features, with hyperparathyroidism the predominant change.

The diagnosis of established bone disease is not difficult. Overt hyperparathyroidism is indicated by hypocalcaemia, hyperphosphataemia, an elevated alkaline phosphatase level and subperiosteal bone resorption which can be seen on magnified X-rays of the hands (Fig. 22.5). In some patients with severe hyperparathyroidism the plasma calcium is normal or raised. This may be referred to as tertiary hyperparathyroidism but does not imply the presence of an autonomous adenoma. In most cases it is due to a very large gland mass and failure to suppress PTH secretion at normal plasma calcium levels. Hypercalcaemia can also be iatrogenic, due to the use of calcium carbonate as a phosphate-binding agent or to 1,25-dihydroxyvitamin D_3.

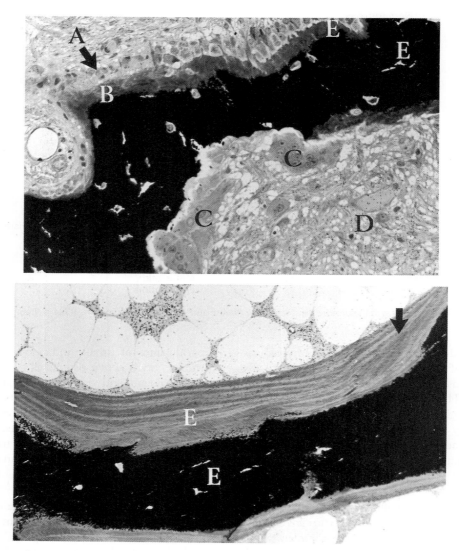

Fig. 22.4 Histological changes in renal bone disease. (**a**) Hyperparathyroidism showing osteoid seams of woven form lined by osteoblasts and, opposite, bone resorption with large plump multinucleated osteoclasts and adjacent marrow fibrosis (undecalcified sections). (**b**) Osteomalacia with wide lamellar osteoid seams (arrow) lacking prominent lining osteoblasts. Note the marked light/dark contrast. **A** — palaside of cells; **B** — non-lamellar structure; **C** — large fleshy cells; **D** — stringy texture; **E** — light/dark contrast. (von Kossa chlorazole blue × 250. Reproduced by courtesy of Dr. J M Xipell.)

Parathyroid hormone levels are usually markedly raised. Although some of this is due to circulating biologically inactive PTH metabolites, most assays now measure only biologically active PTH 1–84. There may be evidence of bone erosion at other joint surfaces, including the outer end of clavicles and the symphysis pubis. Areas of increased bone density may be seen, particularly in the skull and spine, and there may be vascular calcification, although these are late manifestations. By the time subperiosteal bone resorption is radiologically apparent, the histological changes of hyperparathyroidism are quite advanced. Early diagnosis therefore rests on the measurement of

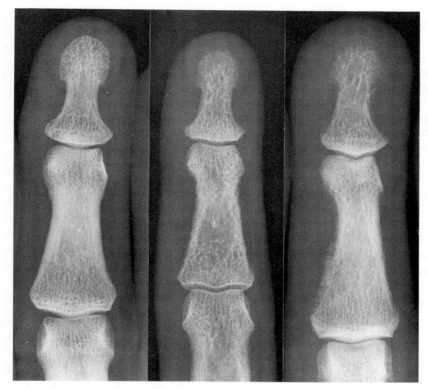

Fig. 22.5 Radiological changes of hyperparathyroidism in the hands. The normal finger (left) has well-demarcated thick cortex and the tufts are well outlined. Note the parallel bone structure. In moderate (centre) and severe (right) hyperparathyroidism there is progressive loss of cortical bone, resulting in first an irregular and then a fuzzy outline, with subperiosteal erosion seen best in the shaft of the middle phalanx and the tuft of the distal phalanx. Note also the disrupted bone lattice.

parathyroid hormone levels and, if necessary, confirmation by bone biopsy. Similarly, by the time patients present with symptoms of osteomalacia (muscle weakness, bone pain) or radiological changes the condition is far advanced. Biopsy of patients with an elevated alkaline phosphatase but no radiological evidence of hyperparathyroidism may uncover early cases of osteomalacia or mixed bone disease. A radioisotope bone scan may be useful in demonstrating microfractures. Patients on dialysis sometimes develop severe osteomalacia which is characterized by normocalcaemia, relentless progression, fractures, and resistance to vitamin D therapy. This is most uncommon before the institution of dialysis and has been attributed to accumulation of aluminium at the mineralization surface from contamination of the water

supply or from aluminium in the form of phosphate-binding gels.

Soft tissue calcification is usually only seen in patients with uncontrolled hyperphosphataemia. Calcification in the conjunctiva causes conjunctival irritation, and around joints an acute inflammatory response which simulates gout. Vascular calcification in the small vessels of the hand usually indicates severe and prolonged hyperparathyroidism. Extensive soft tissue calcification, pulmonary calcification and ischaemic necrosis of vessels are fortunately very uncommon.

Metabolic and endocrine disturbances

The ready availability of immunoassay and its application to renal failure has shown increased plasma levels of a large number of peptide hormones, including insulin, gastrin, glucagon, growth hormone, prolactin, luteinizing hormone (LH), follicle-stimulating hormone (FSH) and neurotensin. Increased levels of hormone may be due to persistent direct stimulation of regulatory mechanisms, indirect stimulation through reduced end-organ responsiveness, or decreased hormone catabolism. In many cases all three mechanisms are involved. Persistently elevated hormone levels may also imply interference with feedback control loops involving for instance the pituitary gland. Other hormone levels are reduced, for example erythropoietin, 1,25-dihydroxycholecalciferol and testosterone, because of destruction of hormone-forming cells or their suppression by uraemia. The clinical importance of these changes varies. Three hormonal abnormalities which warrant some discussion are those of thyroid hormone, sex hormones and insulin.

Thyroid function

Thyroid function is usually normal in patients with chronic renal failure although there may be clinical features and abnormalities of thyroid hormone which mimic hypothyroidism. There is an increased incidence of goitre, levels of protein-bound iodine are low, and decreased total (and sometimes free) thyroxine (T_4), tri-iodothyronine (T_3) and free thyroxine index have been reported. Although variable, it appears that the plasma concentration of thyroid hormones (particularly T_3) decreases progressively with increased duration of renal failure or dialysis. The major abnormality appears to be reduced peripheral conversion of T_4 to T_3 but there may also be alterations in intrathyroidal iodine regulation, T_4 release and thyroid–pituitary interaction. Plasma binding of T_4 and T_3 is usually normal although this may be altered by certain drugs such as androgens, β-adrenoreceptor-blocking agents and heparin. Because of these abnormalities the diagnosis of hypothyroidism in patients with chronic renal failure should be based on clinical criteria and measurements of thyroid-stimulating hormone (TSH), which should be high in patients with hypothyroidism but is usually normal in chronic renal failure.

Gonadal function

Infertility, menstrual abnormality, decreased libido and impotence are common in chronic renal failure. Gynaecomastia may occur in male patients but is more common in those undergoing dialysis.

Many young and active male patients maintain potency but impotence is common in the sick or elderly and its incidence increases with the duration of renal failure. Many factors contribute to this including anxiety, depression, poor nutrition and antihypertensive drugs. Many male patients are also infertile. Plasma testosterone levels are reduced and the levels of LH and prolactin are usually elevated. FSH is often elevated in patients with impaired spermatogenesis. It appears that testosterone production by Leydig cells is suppressed by uraemia and the cells may be resistant to the action of LH. There may also be an abnormality in the negative feedback effect of testosterone on the hypothalamus. All these hormone abnormalities are improved by renal transplantation. It is said that there may be an improvement in sexual function after treatment of secondary hyperparathyroidism. Testosterone replacement or stimulation of the hypothalamic–pituitary axis with clomiphene does not appear to have any beneficial clinical effect.

Many women with chronic renal failure have amenorrhoea or oligomenorrhoea and there is often reduced fertility. Furthermore, patients with advanced uraemia who become pregnant have a much higher risk of abortion or premature delivery, and contraceptive advice is necessary for women of childbearing age. Oestrogen and progesterone levels are often low but the level of gonadotropins varies. As in the male, there appears to be a combination of depressed end-organ function and defective hypothalamic–pituitary feedback. Normal fertility usually returns in young women after renal transplantation.

Insulin and glucose intolerance

Mild glucose intolerance is common in renal failure and although it is of little clinical importance this abnormality of carbohydrate metabolism has been extensively studied. Investigations have shown an increased basal insulin level, peripheral resistance to insulin, an impaired hypoglycaemic response to infused insulin and an increased and prolonged insulin response to glucose. Insulin degradation by the kidney and liver is decreased. All these abnormalities improve with dialysis and this may be partly due to improved nutrition and correction of potassium depletion and acidosis. Insulin requirements may decrease in diabetic patients as renal failure worsens.

Lipid metabolism

Atherosclerosis is a common cause of death in chronic renal failure patients but its incidence has not been definitely shown to be increased. Prolonged and persistent hypertension is certainly a predisposing factor but changes in lipid metabolism may play a role. The main abnormality of lipid metabolism is hypertriglyceridaemia associated with an increase in very low density lipoproteins (VLDL). This has been attributed to suppression of lipase activity. High density lipoproteins (HDL) are usually low but return to normal after successful renal transplantation. The situation in chronic renal failure resembles type 4 hyperlipoproteinaemia (as seen in diabetes, obesity and patients with an increased alcohol intake) and may be aggravated by certain drugs, such as androgens, and by excessive dietary carbohydrate. Hypercholesterolaemia is less common except in patients with nephrotic syndrome or coexistent vascular diseases. The abnormalities of lipid metabolism may be related to disorders of insulin production and degradation. Treatment is based on encouraging regular exercise and avoidance of excess carbohydrate and drugs which may aggravate hypertriglyceridaemia. Hypertriglyceridaemia may respond to Gemfibrosil, which fortunately has a low incidence of side effects. Associated hypercholesterolaemia can be treated with $HMGC_OA$ reductase inhibitors; however the incidence of side effects, particularly gout and myalgia, is increased and low doses are advised.

Nitrogen metabolism

Changes in nitrogen balance include those due to uraemia, to associated malnutrition, to changes in intestinal nitrogen breakdown and to dialysis. It is difficult to separate these different effects. Unnecessarily restrictive diets may lead to protein energy malnutrition, and emphasis should be placed on high-quality nutrition with ample essential amino acids, energy and vitamins but some restriction of total protein, carbohydrate and phosphate intake. There appears to be a decrease in the ratio of essential to non-essential amino acids and this may be corrected by dietary supplements of essential amino acids, including tyrosine and histidine, or keto acids. Such an approach is indicated in advanced uraemia, particularly if nausea limits intake through natural sources or if dialysis is not feasible.

It has been suggested that patients with chronic renal failure can re-utilize urea to synthesize protein but the quantities involved are too small to be of practical significance. The normal molar ratio of plasma urea to creatinine is approximately 30:1. Higher levels suggest an increased intake of non-essential amino acids through diet, gastrointestinal bleeding or increased catabolism, for example due to infection or steroids. It is said that creatinine production may be reduced in uraemia and this may occur if there is marked muscle wasting. However, a reduction in creatinine excretion may also be due to changes in diet or to further breakdown of creatinine to guanidines and other metabolites in the gut or elsewhere.

Immunological disorders

An increased tendency to infection and reduced ability to heal wounds has been recognized for many years but is of little clinical importance in well-nourished patients. There are defects in both antibody production and cellular response to antigen and in various aspects of leucocyte activity. Patients with chronic renal failure have an increased likelihood of becoming virus carriers, particularly of hepatitis B and cytomegalovirus, and have an increased incidence of cancer, both possibly related to immunological incompetence.

There is often a decreased response to vaccination which may therefore be less effective.

Cardiovascular system

Cardiovascular complications in uraemia are most commonly due to hypertension or extracellular volume expansion. Control of these plays a vital role in conservative management and is associated with a significantly better prognosis. Extracellular volume expansion is important in the pathophysiology of hypertension but is also a compensatory mechanism which depresses proximal tubular solute reabsorption. A primary objective in treatment is to maintain sodium balance by adjusting sodium intake to excretion and by avoiding sudden changes in extracellular volume, which may compromise renal function. Most hypertensive patients with chronic renal failure require antihypertensive drug therapy and blood pressure can be controlled by standard drug regimes.

Heart failure may be caused by uncontrolled sodium retention and aggravated by anaemia, pre-existing coronary disease, hypertension and other metabolic derangements associated with uraemia, such as chronic elevation of parathyroid hormone and catecholamines. Fluid overload may also cause functional aortic insufficiency. Early diastolic murmurs require careful evaluation but do not often indicate organic valve disease and may disappear after the correction of hypertension and fluid overload. There are occasional patients with gross cardiomegaly which is not explained by the above factors and the term 'uraemic cardiomyopathy' has been coined. However, this should not be taken to imply a common cause or recognized aetiology. The term 'uraemic retinopathy' has similarly been used but the changes seen are mostly due to hypertension and arteriosclerosis, with occasional patients showing retinopathy due to cerebral oedema, anaemia, retinal vein thrombosis and other complications.

In advanced uraemia, uraemic pericarditis may cause retrosternal pain, fever and a friction rub. This may be relieved by indomethacin but persistent pericarditis is debilitating and the risk of haemorrhage is always present. Small pericardial effusions are often seen on echocardiography, possibly associated with inadequate control of extracellular volume. Pericarditis or a radiologically detectable effusion is usually an indication for aggressive dialysis with reduction in extracellular volume. However, dialysis may precipitate cardiac tamponade (e.g. due to heparin) or volume depletion. Hypotension without a corresponding fall in jugular venous pressure is the common mode of presentation of cardiac tamponade. The classic signs of pericardial effusion and compression are usually not present but volume repletion and drainage of the pericardium should not be delayed on this account. Although echocardiography and other techniques can be used to define left ventricular function and assess the presence of pericardial fluid, appropriate management still rests on a rapid clinical assessment of their significance.

Central nervous system

Early treatment has made overt neurological manifestations of uraemia relatively uncommon. However, many patients experience slowing of mental function, poor memory, apathy and a reduced attention span, particularly if renal failure progresses fairly rapidly. A number of studies point to a defect in the reticular activating system, which is responsible for maintaining an optimal level of arousal and affects the assimilation and processing of new information. Asterixis and myoclonic jerks are common in advanced uraemia and the latter may be a prelude to generalized convulsions. Electroencephalographic changes parallel clinical symptoms and include generalized slowing and disorganization with bursts of slow waves and spiking.

Epileptic convulsions are most commonly due to hypertension and cerebral oedema, and indicate the need for urgent investigation and treatment, including correction of uraemia, volume overload and electrolyte imbalance. Incidental causes of fitting, such as subdural haematoma, subarachnoid or intracerebral haemorrhage (e.g. associated with intracerebral aneurysm) and intracerebral lesions such as abscess or tumour, should be considered if there are localizing signs or if epilepsy persists after control of uraemia. Convulsions can also sometimes be brought about by treatment, e.g. by rapid correction of electrolyte abnormalities or excessive fluid removal. Underlying personality traits may be accentuated and occasionally acute psychoses are seen. However, it is important to exclude other causes of toxic psychosis, such as drug poisoning and septicaemia, which may coexist with uraemia. Although overt peripheral neuropathy is uncommon, loss of ankle jerks, restless legs and paraesthesia may be associated with subclinical neuropathy and it is often possible to demonstrate reduction in nerve conduction velocity. However, provided nutrition is good and dialysis is instituted before clinical deterioration is apparent, it is unusual for either peripheral or autonomic neuropathy to progress. Evidence of overt neuropathy should bring to mind the possibilities of drug intoxication, diabetes, amyloid disease or polyarteritis nodosa. Similarly, although uraemic myopathy has been described, overt muscle weakness is more commonly due to osteomalacia.

CONSERVATIVE MANAGEMENT OF CHRONIC RENAL FAILURE

Despite the success of dialysis and renal transplantation there is no doubt that most patients are better off without these forms of treatment even if renal function is quite markedly impaired. There is every reason to assess such patients thoroughly and to supervise their management with a view to delaying progression of renal failure and treating any reversible complications. Treatment of the underlying condition is of paramount importance and is dealt with under the appropriate headings elsewhere. Practical examples where dramatic changes in prognosis can be made are the treatment of malignant hypertension, cessation of analgesics in patients with analgesic nephropathy, relief of obstruction and the treatment of such conditions as systemic lupus erythematosus, Goodpasture's syndrome and Wegener's granulomatosis. Even after chronic renal failure is established there is still much to be done to preserve renal function and improve the lifestyle of patients nearing end-stage renal failure. The most important aspects of conservative treatment are:

1. supervision and self-care
2. control of hypertension
3. maintenance of good nutrition
4. maintenance of fluid and electrolyte balance
5. prevention and treatment of bone disease.

Supervision and self-care

Patients with chronic renal failure should be involved in their own care as soon as possible. They should understand the cause of their disease, the anticipated rate of progression of renal failure and the things they can do to influence this. For patients with a good prognosis it may be sufficient to emphasize the importance of blood pressure control, good nutrition and sodium balance. As renal failure progresses, the need for phosphate control should be explained, as should the importance of reporting any symptoms such as headache, vomiting and fever which may indicate or lead to a complication. If the need for dialysis is anticipated, the patient should be warned well in advance in order to make any necessary adjustments at work or at home. The need for an access device should be explained and at this stage it is desirable for patients to be transferred to a renal failure clinic where they can get to know the various medical and paramedical personnel and meet other patients in the same predicament. Patients should understand the reason why they are taking drugs and, depending on their intelligence and motivation, be allowed to discuss the effect of treatment on blood pressure, weight or the levels of urea and phosphate. They should also understand the importance of limiting their drug treatment to those drugs which are clearly indicated and essential. Unfortunately some patients are reticent about learning the facts of their illness and doctors may be too busy to keep them adequately informed. However, in the long run, well-educated patients usually comply much better with prescribed regimens and require fewer consultations.

Control of hypertension

Progression of established renal failure may be delayed by control of hypertension. With few exceptions, the treatment of hypertension in chronic renal failure is the same as that in non-uraemic hypertensive individuals. Although a number of antihypertensive drugs are excreted by the kidney, their use is simplified by the fact that there is a defined therapeutic end-point, i.e. control of blood pressure, which together with the presence of side effects determines the dose used. The normal indications and contraindications for individual drugs apply but the aims of blood pressure control should be more stringent in patients with renal impairment. There are some differences in the use of diuretics. The sodium requirements of patients with chronic renal failure vary and need to be established individually for each patient. The majority of patients with chronic renal failure are hypertensive and require moderate sodium restriction (50–70 mmol/day) or a diuretic. Potassium-sparing diuretics should not be used because of the dangers of hyperkalaemia. If an increase in sodium excretion is required, it is usually necessary to use more potent loop diuretics. Patients should be encouraged to weigh themselves regularly and report excessive weight loss or gain. Those who are normotensive do not need sodium restriction; in fact, some normotensive patients require supplementation with either sodium chloride or sodium bicarbonate or both. This is particularly so if relatively minor intercurrent illnesses cause salt depletion as a result of decreased appetite and sodium intake or gastrointestinal losses. Clearly, any patient may develop salt depletion if gastrointestinal losses are severe, and immediate repletion is necessary. However, these patients do not require continued salt supplementation.

Nutrition

Good nutrition remains a cornerstone in the conservative management of chronic renal failure and the emphasis should be on the positive aspects of nutrition rather than an unnecessarily restricted diet. A reduced protein intake can relieve symptoms such as anorexia, nausea and vomiting, and reduce the load of hydrogen ion, sulphate, phosphate and potassium which the kidney has to excrete. Many patients have extremely poor dietary habits and badly need education as to the nutritional value of various foods. Moreover, dietary intake may be decreased by anorexia and leave the patient at risk of chronic malnutrition. There is some evidence that continued high solute loads contribute to loss of renal function in patients with established renal failure. Considering the high protein intake in most Western countries there seems to be good cause for avoiding an excessively large protein intake and ensuring adequate amounts of essential amino acids. Patients require 0.8 g/kg of protein a day, with a high proportion of protein of high biological value. It may be important, particularly in children, to supplement the diet with essential amino acids or keto acids in order to prevent nitrogen wasting and promote adequate growth. Adequate calories must be provided in the form of carbohydrate or fat to meet total energy requirements, bearing in mind that an excessively high carbohydrate intake may aggravate hypertriglyceridaemia. B-group vitamins and folate may be provided on a daily basis although deficiency is uncommon. Dietary education should begin as soon as the diagnosis of chronic renal failure is made. Early reduction of dietary protein and phosphate may delay the onset and progression of uraemia. If necessary, the adequacy of protein intake can be assessed by serial measurements of serum albumin or transferrin.

Dietary requirements alter after patients start dialysis treatment and again after renal transplantation. For instance, patients on peritoneal dialysis require a higher protein intake to replace peritoneal losses and usually restriction of carbohydrate to compensate for peritoneal glucose absorption. Changes in dietary management can be confusing to the patient if not adequately explained. A most important principle throughout the whole course of chronic renal failure, dialysis and transplantation is to make sure the patient has a balanced nutritious diet, and any restrictions should be made within this context. Good long-term nutritional advice requires the help of a skilled professional nutritionist.

Fluid and electrolyte balance

Regular review of blood pressure, weight and the state of hydration is necessary and should be more frequent as renal failure progresses. It is good practice to establish a routine of daily weighing and to teach patients the importance of maintaining sodium balance and reporting any intercurrent illness, fluctuation in weight or unusual symptoms. Temporary electrolyte imbalance may worsen quite rapidly if unattended and it often saves time to admit patients to hospital to have this corrected. There is no virtue in advising an increased fluid intake and patients should be encouraged simply to drink to satisfy their thirst. Sodium intake should be adjusted to need but there is no benefit in increasing sodium intake while giving large doses of potent diuretics. This regimen has little effect on overall renal function and makes the patients far more susceptible to salt depletion if sodium intake is reduced for some reason. Plasma sodium, potassium, bicarbonate, calcium and phosphate concentrations should be regularly monitored in addition to parameters of renal function. Changes in plasma sodium, potassium and bicarbonate usually reflect alterations in diet or fluid intake which may need correction. The control of plasma phosphate within normal limits is an important part of the prevention of renal bone disease. However, there is also evidence that hyperphosphataemia accelerates loss of renal function, probably by the deposition of calcium phosphate salts in the kidney. This is an added reason for maintaining normal levels of plasma phosphate from the time of diagnosis. Although specific measures are not usually taken to correct acidosis, the use of calcium carbonate as a phosphate-binding agent in the early stages will help to do this, and supplements of sodium bicarbonate can be used provided this does not cause sodium retention or aggravate hypertension.

Prevention and treatment of bone disease

Although bone biopsy is necessary to accurately define the type and extent of bone disease it is an unpleasant procedure and the histological techniques are demanding. In practice many patients can be treated without recourse to biopsy. Without treatment, hyperparathyroidism progresses at a variable rate. However, if the plasma phosphate and calcium are maintained in the normal range, this may be prevented. It should be possible to control the plasma phosphate with a combination of diet modification (phosphate intake 600–800 mg/24 h) and phosphate-binding agents, but frequently these measures are not introduced early enough. If the patient is hypocalcaemic, calcium carbonate can be given in a dose of 3–6 g daily with meals. Most physicians avoid aluminium hydroxide because of the problems of aluminium absorption. In some circumstances small doses (2–3 g daily) may be justified and aluminium absorption can be minimized by giving it with the main meals. Magnesium hydroxide is a poor phosphate binder; Ca salts of amino acids and dialysed whey protein are expensive. Calcium acetate is more effective than calcium carbonate and may cause less hypercalcaemia but it has an unpleasant taste. With all phosphate-binding agents compliance is a problem.

Some patients are particularly prone to hypercalcaemia when calcium salts are prescribed as phosphate binders and this limits their use and effectiveness (see Fig. 22.2). Regular monitoring of plasma calcium is essential. A few patients remain hypocalcaemic and the question arises whether one should add vitamin D analogues to improve gastrointestinal calcium absorption or directly suppress PTH secretion. The major problem is the risk of inadvertent hypercalcaemia and the possibility of further renal damage. If there is no biochemical or radiological evidence of bone disease the risk of 1,25-dihydroxyvitamin D therapy may outweigh the benefit. Vitamin D therapy is certainly indicated where there are radiological changes of hyperparathyroidism or symptomatic osteomalacia. However, this represents a rather late stage of the disease. The aim of treatment should be to return the alkaline phosphatase to normal without inducing hypercalcaemia. The safest vitamin D preparation is 1,25-dihydroxyvitamin D_3 or a synthetic analogue which acts rapidly and the effect of which will subside quickly if the drug is withdrawn. However, it is still necessary to monitor the plasma calcium regularly and to reduce the dose of vitamin D as the plasma alkaline phosphatase falls. There may be benefit in giving 1,25-dihydroxyvitamin D_3 in larger doses on an intermittent basis. There are also analogues such as 22 oxa-calcitriol which may directly suppress PTH secretion without stimulating calcium absorption. Further developments in this area can be expected.

Once end-stage renal failure is reached, the risk of further loss of renal function is of less concern. In such patients low dose vitamin D therapy may be warranted even in the absence of radiological or biochemical evidence of bone disease in order to delay progression of bone disease, particularly if renal transplantation is unlikely. Treatment can then be directed to normalizing PTH levels, which requires more aggressive treatment.

Subtotal parathyroidectomy should be reserved for patients with severe hyperparathyroidism in whom phosphate control and vitamin D are ineffective or produce hypercalcaemia. The operation is very successful in the hands of experienced surgeons and the major problem is postoperative hypocalcaemia. This can be reduced with pre-operative vitamin D therapy but most patients with a plasma alkaline phosphatase more than twice normal also require intravenous calcium supplements given by infusion into a large vein, preferably by a central venous catheter. After an initial period of rapid calcium replacement, plasma calcium can usually be controlled with oral vitamin D and calcium supplements. These may be necessary for some months after surgery, depending on the severity of the bone disease. There is usually an immediate improvement in symptoms of bone pain and itching and a more gradual mineralization of bone. Radiological areas of erosion disappear but areas of increased mineralization, such as may be seen in the spine or skull, sometimes increase in density. It has been claimed that anaemia, impotence, cardiac function and other clinical parameters may also be improved after treatment of hyperparathyroidism. Continued low dose vitamin D therapy is advisable to delay recurrence.

Osteomalacia in patients with chronic renal failure should be diagnosed by bone biopsy, as radiological changes occur late in the course of the disease. Most patients respond rapidly to vitamin D therapy but continued treatment is necessary and the same dangers of vitamin D therapy apply. In dialysis patients a vitamin D resistant form of osteomalacia, characterized by hypercalcaemia, may occur and has been attributed to aluminium deposition in bone. One such case has been reported in a patient prior to commencing dialysis. These patients often progress with multiple fractures and incapacitating pain but respond to renal transplantation or treatment with desferrioxamine and vitamin D.

MANAGEMENT OF COMPLICATIONS

Patients with chronic renal failure may develop complications which alter the course of the disease but many of these are reversible. Examples include acute urinary infection, septicaemia, urinary tract obstruction, gastrointestinal haemorrhage, dehydration or fluid overload with associated acute electrolyte disturbances and drug toxicity. Some of these are dealt with under the appropriate headings. These complications may be the cause of the patient's initial presentation and their correction often leads to improvement which can be maintained over many years. Patients with established chronic renal failure should be encouraged to report any change in health since relatively minor intercurrent illnesses may upset the delicate balance of compensated renal failure. For instance, vomiting may be expected to cause volume depletion but at the same time the patient's medications are often not taken and a vicious cycle of events is established which leads to progressive deterioration. If such patients are admitted to hospital, this deterioration can be prevented by intravenous fluid replacement, the use of parenteral medications and, sometimes, short periods of dialysis.

Drug intoxication is a common problem. Almost all drugs or their metabolites are excreted by the kidney and chronic renal failure is a common cause of drug toxicity. No drug should be given without a definite therapeutic indication and knowledge of how the drug is handled in renal failure (see Ch. 3). The prescription of anti-nausea drugs is usually unjustified and the patient would be better served by a reduction in protein intake and investigation of other possible causes of nausea, such as water intoxication, drug overdose or ulcer. Similarly, patients should be encouraged to avoid regular use of sedatives. Adding drug-related symptoms to the symptoms of uraemia does not improve the patient's well-being.

DIALYSIS

The decision as to when a patient should start dialysis is somewhat arbitrary. Dialysis should be started as soon as the patient's quality of life becomes unacceptable. In those who are fully employed, it is usual to start when work becomes too much for them. Diabetic patients are usually recommended to start dialysis earlier because of the increasing incidence of retinal complications in the later stages of renal failure. However these complications should be avoided by control of hypertension and regular attention to proliferative retinal lesions. Most patients are unable to cope well with a creatinine clearance below 5 ml/min but some continue to deny symptoms well beyond this point. It may be acceptable to delay dialysis, provided they remain asymptomatic. However, such patients are more likely to develop serious complications such as pericarditis, cardiac tamponade and peripheral neuropathy. These problems can mostly be avoided by regular consultation and patient education.

RECOMMENDED READING

Bergstrom J 1989 Is chronic renal disease always progressive? Contribution to Nephrology 75: 60–67

Bricker N S 1972 On the pathogenesis of the uremic state, an exposition of the 'trade-off hypothesis'. New England Journal of Medicine 286 (20): 1093–1099

El Nahas A M, J P Wight 1991 The management of chronic renal failure: 10 unanswered questions. Quarterly Journal of Medicine, New Series 1991 294: 799–809

Fouque D, Laville, M, Boissel J P, Clifflet R, Labweuw M, Zech P Y 1992 Controlled low protein diets in chronic renal insufficiency. Meta-analysis, British Medical Journal 304: 216–220

Fourner A, Drucke T, Moriniere P, Zingraff J, Bondailleiz B, Achaard J M 1991 The new treatments of hyperparathyroidism secondary to renal insufficiency. Advances in Nephrology 21: 235–306

The US Recombinant Human Erythropoietin Pre-dialysis Study Group 1991 Double blind, placebo-controlled study of the therapeutic use of recombinant human erythropoietin for anaemia associated with chronic renal failure in pre-dialysis patients. American Journal of Kidney Disease 18 (1): 50–59

23. Dialysis

D. C. H. Harris   J. H. Stewart

INTRODUCTION

The aim of treatment by dialysis is to replace all the lost functions of the natural kidneys, as far as this is possible, using artificial means.

The elements of dialysis

In dialysis (Fig. 23.1) blood is brought into contact, through a semipermeable membrane, with a physiological solution of electrolytes to which dextrose, or rarely other nutrients, has been added (the dialysate). Transfer of molelcules between blood and dialysate is governed by differences in concentration (diffusion) and/or pressure (convection).

For any particular molecular species the rate of *diffusive transfer* depends on its concentration gradient across the membrane, its delivery to (blood flow) or from (dialysate flow) the site of transfer, and the effective area and permeability of the membrane. The permeability of the membrane depends on the size of the molecular species and intrinsic properties of the membrane. Also to be taken into account are resistances to diffusion at the blood and dialysate surfaces of the membrane;

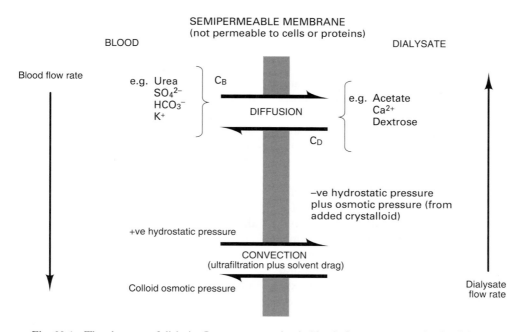

Fig. 23.1 The elements of dialysis. C_B — concentration in blood; C_D — concentration in dialysate

these are reduced by increasing their respective flow rates (see Fig. 23.7).

In the case of *convective transfer*, in which there is a net flow of water usually from blood to dialysate (ultrafiltration), dissolved molecules transfer by virtue of hydrostatic and osmotic pressure gradients (transmembrane pressure — TMP). TMP may be increased by reducing dialysate hydrostatic pressure with a dialysate pump located downstream from the membrane, or by increasing hydrostatic pressure in the blood compartment with a blood pump located upstream. The effective area and hydraulic permeability of the membrane also regulate the rate of convection. In general, increasing molecular diameter is less of a barrier to convective than to diffusive transfer.

Replacement of kidney function

The natural kidney performs both excretory and regulatory functions. *Excretion* is achieved by glomerular filtration (e.g. end-products of nitrogen metabolism, phosphate, salt, water) or tubular secretion (e.g. potassium, acid). For the most part the molecular species involved are small (molecular weight less than 500), hydrophilic and not highly bound to plasma proteins.

The *regulatory* activity of the kidney is rather more complex, the principal elements being tubular reabsorption (which also prevents wastage of salt, water and those essential nutrients and minerals which have small, hydrophilic molecules), and the release or activation of hormones.

By utilizing both diffusive and convective transfer, dialysis can perform most of the excretory functions of the kidney, and the addition to dialysate of solutes in carefully regulated concentrations can substitute effectively for renal tubular reabsorption. In practice this is possible for electrolytes and dextrose (see Fig. 23.1) but not yet for amino acids. Renal hormones with only paracrine or autocrine activity (e.g. renin, prostaglandins) are not required in the absence of natural kidney function, while others (1,25-dihydroxyvitamin D_3, erythropoietin) can be replaced exogenously.

DIALYSIS TECHNIQUES

Peritoneal dialysis

In this form of dialysis the peritoneum (including the walls of its capillaries) acts as the semipermeable membrane (with an effective surface area about the same as body surface area in an adult), its capillary bed delivers blood (at approximately 70 ml/min) to the dialysis site, and dialysate is run into the peritoneal cavity through a catheter inserted across the anterior abdominal wall (Nolph 1988).

Access

The catheter most widely used is made of *silicone rubber* and has two velour cuffs of polyethylene terephthalate around its proximal half, and rows of tiny side holes along its distal half. It is inserted in the operating theatre under local or general anaesthesia (Fig. 23.2), with the tip positioned in the rectovesical pouch. The deeper of the two cuffs is attached to the parietal peritoneum in a midline or paramedian position, and the proximal portion of the catheter is then drawn through a subcutaneous tunnel so that the second cuff lies inside the exit wound, which is sited above and medial to the anterior superior iliac spine and which should point downwards to reduce local infection.

In an emergency, a stiffer *polytetrafluoroethylene* (PTFE) catheter may be introduced blindly into the peritoneal cavity (previously filled with 2 litres of dialysate), passing it over a metal stylus by way of a stab wound through the skin and linea alba about 3 cm below the umbilicus. Its tip should also be directed into the rectovesical pouch. The risks of intra-abdominal trauma due to the stiffness of the catheter, and of infection due to almost unavoidable dialysate leakage, limit its use to 2–3 days.

Composition of the dialysate (Table 23.1)

The concentrations of potassium, magnesium, and usually sodium, are deliberately less than in normal extracellular fluid so as to encourage their removal,

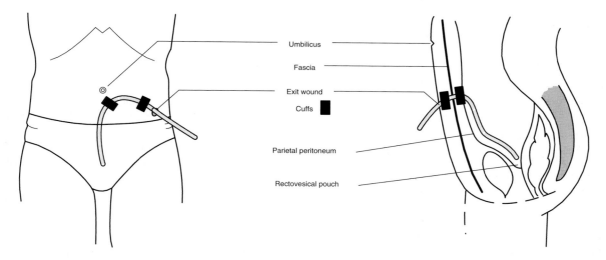

Fig. 23.2 The silicon rubber peritoneal catheter in situ

while that of calcium may be high in order to overcome the failure of intestinal absorption, or low to allow the prescription of calcium-containing phosphate binders (see below).

The physiological buffer bicarbonate cannot be used because in its presence dextrose solutions caramelize when sterilized by heat. Lactate, which is metabolized to pyruvate and then to acetyl CoA (predominantly in the liver), performs its buffering action by incorporating a hydrogen ion in the latter reaction. Thus, lactic acidosis may occur during peritoneal dialysis in a patient with liver failure. Since water transfers across the peritoneal membrane faster than simple sugars, convective transfer (ultrafiltration) can be regulated in peritoneal dialysis by varying the concentration of dextrose added to the dialysis solution. However, the amount of water removed in this way is limited by the gradual diffusive transfer of dextrose from dialysate into blood, with consequent loss of the

Table 23.1 Typical composition of dialysate solutions

	Plasma water* (mmol/l)	Peritoneal dialysis (mmol/l)	Conventional haemodialysis (mmol/l)	'Bicarbonate' haemodialysis (mmol/1)
Cations				
Sodium	152	132	137	140
Potassium	5	—	1.0	1.0
Calcium	1.3	1.75	1.65	1.5
Magnesium	0.6	0.25	0.25	0.5
Anions				
Chloride	110	96	101.8	106
Lactate	—	40	—	—
Acetate	—	—	40	4
Bicarbonate	29	—	—	35
Dextrose	6	28, 76, 126, 215	11	—

* Approximately 7% higher than total plasma concentrations because of volume occupied by protein and lipid macromolecules. That portion bound to plasma proteins is ignored (e.g. calcium). Low-calcium solutions are available also to permit the use of calcium-containing phosphate binders.

osmotic gradient. Hence fluid removal is favoured by relatively short dwell times ($\frac{1}{2}$–2 hours) while, because of plasma oncotic pressure, net transfer of water into the patient is a likely result of long dwell times (4–8 hours) even when high-dextrose solutions are used.

Delivery of dialysate

The filling and emptying of the peritoneal cavity may be performed manually or by using an automated cycling machine. In the *manual* method, a collapsible polyvinyl chloride (PVC) bag of sterile dialysate (0.5–3.0 litres) is connected to the abdominal catheter by about 1.5 m of PVC tubing and suspended about 1 m above the abdomen. The clamp is removed to allow dialysate (with the chill removed) to run into the abdomen by gravity at a rate of about 300 ml/min. If the patient is ambulant, the empty bag may be rolled up and tucked in his belt or a pocket. At the end of the dwell time, drainage is effected by lowering the bag to floor level, and the fluid is siphoned out at a rate of 100–200 ml/min. The bag of spent dialysate is detached and replaced by a fresh bag, either by the patient himself or by an attendant. Peritonitis is the main complication, and is usually due to touch contamination of the connection between the dialysate bag and the PVC tubing. Other complications include catheter exit site and tunnel infections, and incomplete or slow emptying of dialysate. Confinement to bed, constipation and peritoneal inflammation all interfere with free drainage of peritoneal dialysis fluid, as does incorrect siting of the catheter or its envelopment by omentum.

Cyclers automatically deliver into the abdomen (by gravity) a preset volume of dialysate which is warmed to 38°C. After the selected dwell time (usually 20–120 min), during which the next batch of fresh dialysate is measured and warmed, the clamps are switched to permit drainage, also for a set time (usually 10–20 min). The cycler may be loaded with as much as 50 litres of dialysis solution to provide a reservoir of fresh dialysate, while spent fluid drains into a single large container. The net gain or loss of fluid is the difference in weight of fluid entering and leaving the peritoneal cavity.

Efficacy

Peritoneal dialysis provides small molecule (e.g. urea) clearances of some 60 litres per week (approx 6 ml/min), only a little less than haemodialysis, and its continuous nature avoids the peaks of the latter; it alleviates symptoms as well as haemodialysis. The greater permeability of the peritoneal membrane allows relatively free diffusive transfer of larger molecular species. To the extent that this encourages the elimination of intermediate molecular weight uraemic metabolites, the so-called middle molecules (see Ch. 22), this may be desirable, but some of the small plasma proteins may be lost in this way by transudation. A far more serious *protein loss* occurs by exudation if there is peritoneal inflammation, whether caused by infection or chemical irritation.

Another advantage of peritoneal dialysis is that *residual renal function* may be preserved better due to the absence of the nephrotoxic cytokine release and hypotension which characterize haemodialysis treatment; thus clinically important clearance of water, salt and larger molecules is retained. Even though peritoneal permeability and histology may change with time, peritoneal adhesions and sclerosis are rare if chemical sclerosants (acetate, chlorhexidine) are avoided, and peritonitis is treated promptly.

Haemodialysis

In haemodialysis, the second and more frequently used form of dialysis therapy, molecular transfer between blood and dialysate is effected outside the body in a disposable dialyser which houses a synthetic semipermeable membrane. A machine, which together with the dialyser is called an artificial kidney, prepares and checks the dialysate, and circulates both dialysate and blood through the dialyser (Fig. 23.4).

The dialyser

The semipermeable membrane is a polymer, usually regenerated cellulose, but cellulose acetate, polycarbonate, polymethylmethacrylate and polyacrylonitrile are used. In the majority of dialysers, the membrane is drawn into 5000–20 000 *hollow fibres* of 5–50 μm wall thickness, 100–200 μm internal diameter and up to 20 cm length. Blood passes along these capillaries while dialysate is circulated around and between them. Less commonly, the membrane is arranged as *parallel plates*. Dialysate flows in the opposite direction (countercurrent) to blood flow (see Fig. 23.1). The effective surface area of the membrane ranges from 0.3 m² (suitable for infants) to 1.6 m² (suitable for large or hypercatabolic patients).

The extracorporeal blood circuit

Anticoagulated blood is pumped form the patient through the dialyser and returned to the patient's venous system. Access to the circulation, anticoagulation, and the monitoring of blood circulation outside the body will be described in turn.

Access. The simplest and most satisfactory access is provided by subcutaneous forearm veins which have been 'arterialized' by means of a surgically created (Brescia–Cimono) *fistula* between the radial artery and the cephalic vein (usually side-to-side) in the lower third of the forearm (Fig. 23.3, Chapman & Allen 1988). After 1–2 months, the walls of the run-off veins will have thickened sufficiently to permit repeated insertion of two widebore (14–16 gauge) needles or cannulas, the lower for withdrawal and the upper for return of blood. When either the radial or the ulnar artery is significantly narrowed the Brescia–Cimino fistula should not be created as there would be insufficient arterial flow for both the shunt and the hand. This method of access is also denied to patients with poorly developed or thrombosed forearm veins; for this reason, venous cannulation and arterial puncture at this site should be avoided in patients with renal disease.

A subcutaneously placed loop of autologous *saphenous vein*, inserted between the brachial or radial artery and the cephalic or antecubital veins (end-to-side), is the preferred alternative (Fig. 23.3). A conduit of *expanded microporous PTFE* may be used in the same site or in the front of the thigh between the superficial femoral artery and vein.

For transient renal failure, or when haemodialysis is required before a more permanent means of access has been established, *PTFE* or *polyurethane catheters* are inserted percutaneously, using the Seldinger technique, either into the iliac vein via the femoral vein or into the superior vena cava via the subclavian vein. These catheters carry a risk of infection (endocarditis). Whereas haemostasis is easier with the femoral approach, its use is limited because the patient is confined to bed.

Anticoagulation. Although the materials used in the extracorporeal blood circuit generally have acceptable biocompatibility, an anticoagulant, virtually always *heparin*, is necessary. A loading dose of 500–4000 units is injected into the venous access cannulas three minutes before switching on the blood pump, and heparin is then continued as an infusion of 600–3000 units/h until about half an hour before the end of dialysis. Mathematical modelling can be used to determine the optimum loading dose and infusion rate of heparin for each patient.

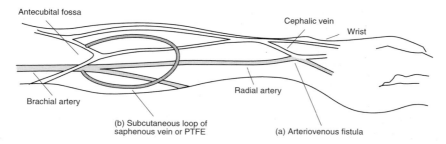

Fig. 23.3 Anterior view of a semipronated forearm showing the preferred sites for (a) direct arteriovenous anastomosis and (b) the alternative subcutaneous arteriovenous loop for vascular access for haemodialysis. PTFE — polytetrafluoroethylene

Low molecular weight heparin, which has anti-factor X but not anti-factor II activity, is gradually replacing standard heparin because of its longer duration of action (a bolus injection of 5000 units is effective for 4 h), and because it carries less risk of bleeding.

Monitoring the extracorporeal blood circuit (Fig. 23.4). Blood is pumped through the dialyser at rates of 150–500 ml/min, usually by means of an occlusive roller pump, but a non-occlusive pump, which has the advantage of not requiring pressure monitoring (see below), may be used.

Pressure monitors are sited proximal to the blood pump to ensure that filling is sufficient to maintain the desired flow, and between the dialyser and the return cannula to protect against obstruction to return flow. A bubble trap at the same point is monitored by an ultrasonic air and foam detector to warn against excessive air accumulation which may occur either by suction through a break in the low-pressure segment before the pump, or by transfer across the dialyser membrane from inadequately de-gassed dialysate. Activation of any of these monitors automatically stops the blood pump and clamps the line returning blood to the patient.

Dialysate preparation and delivery

In conventional 'single pass' haemodialysis (Fig. 23.4), dialysate is prepared by mixing a concentrated solution of electrolytes and sometimes dextrose (the concentrate) with purified water in the proportion of 1:34 using mechanically or electronically linked pumps in parallel. Before being mixed with the concentrate, the water is heated under negative pressure to remove dissolved gases, and then warmed to 38°C (see Table 23.1).

Because calcium and magnesium carbonate would precipitate from a bicarbonate-containing concentrate, acetate is used as the buffer. Alternatively two separate concentrate solutions and a third proportioning pump can be used. Acetate depresses myocardial contractility and is a vasodilator, and so may cause hypotension during

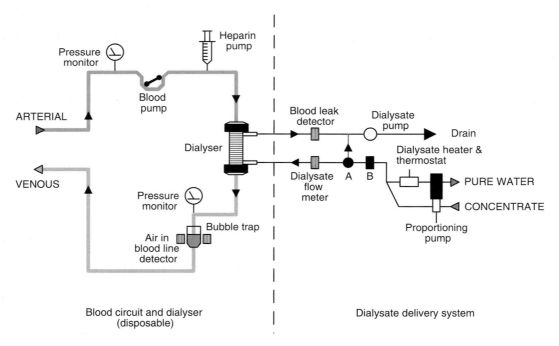

Fig. 23.4 The blood and dialysate circuits of a conventional single pass artificial kidney. A — dialysate bypass valve; B — conductivity and temperature monitors

dialysis. The use of non-physiological buffer anions (e.g. acetate, lactate) uncouples oxidative phosphorylation, causing intracellular accumulation of acid and phosphate. The resultant chronic metabolic acidosis and hyperphosphataemia might be overcome by using graded high-chloride followed by high-bicarbonate dialysate.

After mixing, the temperature and concentration (electrical conductivity) of the dialysate are checked, and it is then delivered to the dialyser at 500 ml/min. Rupture of the dialysis membrane is monitored by a blood leak detector (turbidometer) sited beyond the dialyser. Activation of these monitors switches the dialysate directly to drain and arrests the blood circuit.

Water purification

In order to avoid acute toxicity (e.g. fever, vomiting or haemolysis), or cumulative poisoning (e.g. vitamin D resistant osteomalacia, dementia related to aluminium; Table 23.3), raw tap water must be purified as shown in Figure 23.5.

Sorbent regeneration of dialysate

An alternative to the continuous preparation of fresh dialysate is its regeneration by passage through a sorbent-containing cartridge. This cartridge contains several layers, which remove heavy metals and oxidants, convert urea to ammonium,

and exchange cations for sodium and hydrogen, and anions for acetate. Calcium and magnesium are added by constant infusion to the regenerated dialysate before it is returned to a 5 litre reservoir for recycling to the dialyser.

This system can be operated independently of a continuous supply of pure water, is readily transportable, and permits individualization of the dialysis regimen, but it has a number of technical shortcomings which limit its efficacy.

Other modes of extracorporeal blood treatment

In *haemofiltration* plasma is subjected to a high rate of ultrafiltration using highly permeable membranes of cellulose or its esters, or of polyamides. Sterile replacement fluid (Ringer's lactate or a similar preparation) is infused either before (predilution) or after (postdilution) the filter. Since the filtration process mimics glomerular function, while fluid infusion is analogous to tubular reabsorption, the process is more physiological than conventional dialysis; it is also well tolerated even by fragile or ill patients. Disadvantages are the cost of the replacement fluid (which may be reduced by producing it on-line), and currently a ceiling of some 80 ml/min on the rate of filtration unless two filters are used.

Haemofiltration and haemodialysis may be used continuously, either separately or together, for

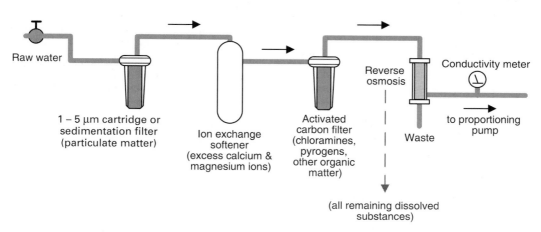

Fig. 23.5 A standard purification system for water for haemodialysis. A deionizer may replace the softener and reverse osmosis, or be added as a final step. Substances removed at each stage are bracketed

replacement of renal function, using disposable, technically simple equipment (e.g. CVVHD — *continuous venovenous haemodialysis*; CAVH — *continuous arteriovenous haemofiltration*; CAVHD, CVVH). Venovenous circuits avoid the danger of arterial catheterization, but a blood pump is necessary. In continuous haemofiltration convective clearances are equivalent to the filtrate produced; this usually is up to 10 ml/min, but may be double this with a blood pump, predilution or negative pressure applied to the filtrate. Continuous haemodialysis may be added to haemofiltration (so-called haemodiafiltration) by running dialysate fluid at one litre per hour countercurrent to blood on the opposite side of the dialysis membrane, resulting in urea clearances of up to 40 ml/min even when systemic blood pressure is low (Harris 1990, Fig. 23.6)

A system similar to that of haemofiltration may be used for plasma separation (*plasma filtration*) as an alternative to plasma exchange using centrifugation, in the treatment of such conditions as rapidly progressive glomerulonephritis and myeloma. The membrane is of polypropylene (pore size 0.5–0.6 μm) which permits the passage of macromolecules.

Haemoperfusion, in which blood is brought into contact with a binding agent (activated charcoal, ion-exchange resin), can be used in the treatment of some drug intoxications, but has been abandoned for treatment of renal failure because there is no known chemical which will remove urea and the method cannot be used to remove excess water and salt. Haemoperfusion may be complicated by thrombocytopenia, leucopenia or hypocalcaemia.

CLINICAL DIALYSIS

Indications for dialysis

Most dialysis is given for renal failure, but this or a related mode of treatment has been employed for poisoning, liver failure or plasmapheresis.

Preventive dialysis

When time and facilities permit, dialysis is started well in advance of the appearance of uraemic toxicity. Thus, in acute or acute-on-chronic renal failure, treatment is begun as soon as it is clear that kidney function will not recover promptly in response to a combination of specific treatment for the precipitating factor(s) and general measures to restore arterial perfusion of the kidneys.

In chronic renal failure the decision to start regular dialysis treatments is made as soon as the patient is no longer able to continue in his normal routine despite proper conservative management. This rarely happens until the glomerular filtration rate has fallen below 0.2 ml/s but may be necessitated by uncontrollable hypertension, fluid retention or hyperparathyroidism rather than by uraemia.

Emergency dialysis

There are times when dialysis must be given without delay, especially when oliguria is complicated by *pulmonary oedema*. Similarly, prompt dialysis is indicated when significant uraemic toxicity, e.g. hyperkalaemia, acidosis, encephalopathy or bleeding, is accompanied by overhydration or persistent oliguria, either of which limits the volume of intravenous fluid that might otherwise be given to correct the abnormality. *Hyperkalaemia* is the most acute and dangerous biochemical manifestation of renal failure. Effective emergency treatment, either by intravenous infusion of dextrose, bicarbonate or calcium (see Ch. 20), or by dialysis, is mandatory when there is widening of the QRS complex of the ECG (more than 0.11 s in any chest lead or more than 0.10 s in any limb lead), prolongation of the P–R interval beyond 0.20 s, skeletal or smooth muscle paralysis, or when the serum potassium is more than 7.0 mmol/l or is likely to rise above that level as a result of tissue breakdown (e.g. rhabdomyolysis, tumour lysis syndrome, gastrointestinal bleeding) or poor tissue perfusion (lactic acidosis).

Similarly, the need for emergency dialysis for overhydration, acidosis or other clinical manifestations of uraemia must take into account not only the current condition of the patient, but also the likely clinical course in the forthcoming 24 hours.

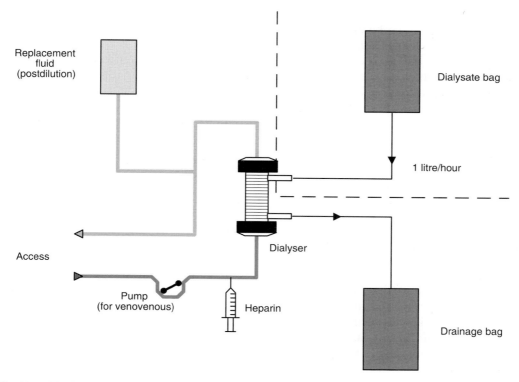

Fig. 23.6 The blood and dialysate circuits for continuous haemodiafiltration. A blood pump is necessary if access is venovenous. Replacement fluid may also be given prior to the dialyser (predilution). If the dialysate flow is interrupted (top right) clearance will occur only by haemofiltration (convection)

Poisoning

Haemodialysis, intermittent and continuous, can remove drugs with a low volume of distribution (less than 1 l/kg), molecular weight (less than 500 daltons with conventional membranes, higher with more porous membranes), plasma protein binding (less than 30%) and rate of natural elimination ($T_{1/2}$ more than 24 h), and blood concentration clearly above the toxic threshold. Such drugs include acetylsalicylic acid or salicylates, long-acting barbiturates, lithium, ethylene glycol, ethanol or methanol, bromides, and thiocyanate.

Sorbent haemoperfusion, in practice almost always using activated charcoal, is more efficient than haemodialysis in removing lipid-soluble and protein-bound drugs such as short- and medium-acting barbiturates, carbamazepine, salicylates and theophylline. It has been used for acute liver failure, but its efficacy is now doubted.

Objectives of dialysis

It is neither possible nor necessary to replace the whole of natural renal function by dialysis. Indeed, some of the regulatory functions of the kidney — such as promotion of erythropoiesis and control of carbohydrate and lipid metabolism, and the as yet poorly understood endocrine dysfunction which is responsible for loss of libido, impotence and infertility — are not influenced perceptibly by even the best dialysis regimens. Moreover, the glomerular filtration barrier is freely permeable to molecules up to about 20 000 daltons, whereas the permeability of most dialysis membranes falls markedly for molecules over 200 daltons. The only uraemic metabolite of intermediate molecular weight (200–20 000 daltons) known to be clinically significant is β_2-microglobulin (see below) but it seems likely that failure to eliminate substances of this class may be responsible for some long-term uraemic toxicity. To the extent that it is achievable, however, both the volume and the composition of extracellular fluid, and thereby of the intracellular fluid, should be kept within normal limits by dialysis itself in order to minimize the need for adjuvant therapy.

Fluid volume

Salt and water are equally important in determining body fluid status, as an increment in extracellular sodium chloride will, by its osmotic effect, cause thirst which almost inevitably will be quenched by drinking. Since total elimination of salt from the diet is not possible, fluid intake almost always exceeds fluid loss between dialyses; the accumulated excess, which should be no more than 2 litres, must be removed by ultrafiltration. The presence of either arterial hypertension (the most sensitive indicator of an expanded intravascular fluid compartment except when there is significant myocardial damage or antihypertensive drugs are being taken), or a raised jugular venous pressure, demonstrates the need for ultrafiltration.

Minor degrees of underhydration are more difficult to detect, but are suggested by postural hypotension, lability of blood pressure during dialysis (especially when ultrafiltration is attempted), weakness, loss of appetite, and a reduction in urinary output, which is a sensitive indicator of hydration status even at this level of renal function. When there is doubt, the effect on the arterial and venous pressures of giving additional fluid should be tested judiciously.

Fluid composition

The completeness with which body fluid composition is corrected by dialysis depends partly on clearance, which reflects the excretory role of the kidney, and partly on the chemical composition of the dialysate, by which certain of the regulatory functions of the kidney may be imitated. In this latter respect, it is the concentrations of buffer (acetate, lactate or bicarbonate) and calcium, and the osmolarity of the dialysate which are most important.

In the usually employed maintenance dialysis regimens, the weekly clearance of small molecular weight uraemic toxins is one tenth to one fifth of normal glomerular filtration rate. This is approximately the removal rate required to match natural renal elimination of potassium, magnesium, inorganic phosphate and urate. It is not difficult, therefore, to maintain plasma concentrations of the electrolytes, including bicarbonate, calcium and phosphate, always within or close to the normal range. There is no need to check plasma chemistry more often than every 3 months in maintenance dialysis, provided the patient is stable and clinically well, but measurements daily, or at least several times per week, are required in acute renal failure and hypercatabolic states.

In the case of substances such as urea and creatinine which are excreted more or less exclusively by glomerular filtration, dialytic removal cannot match that by healthy kidneys except during the period of a haemodialysis treatment itself, and so between treatments their concentration in body fluids rises to some 5–15 times normal. Because uraemic metabolites in this class seem to be relatively non-toxic, clinical manifestations of their accumulation are both slow to develop and difficult to detect. Indeed, there is no sensitive or reliable test (clinical or laboratory) which can be used to ensure that sufficient dialysis is being given to prevent delayed toxicity from this source.

Adequacy of dialysis

The best measurement currently available to monitor adequacy of dialysis is derived from the kinetics of generation and removal of urea, which resembles most known or putative uraemic toxins in being an end-product of protein catabolism and having a small, freely permeable molecule (Levine & Bernard 1990). Clinical evidence suggests that the amount of dialysis given should be sufficient to keep blood urea concentrations constantly below 30 mmol/l (averaging 15–20 mmol/l) when the dietary intake of protein, in a patient who is in a steady state, is about 1g/kg body weight per day.

This method of assessing the adequacy of dialysis ignores the potential toxicity of larger molecular species, which are better removed by peritoneal dialysis and haemofiltration than haemodialysis, and the fluctuation of uraemic toxins which characterizes intermittent dialysis.

The technical factors which most influence the amount of haemodialysis exchange are the blood flow (especially for low molecular weight metabolites; Fig. 23.7), the area of the membrane and the duration of dialysis (especially for larger molecules).

Dialysis regimens

In planning the management of a patient receiving dialysis, the most important decisions concern the type (haemo- or peritoneal) and amount of treatment and, for maintenance dialysis, where it will be done.

Maintenance haemodialysis

In stable end-stage renal failure when there are no unusual metabolic demands, haemodialysis treatments of 3–6 hours duration are employed 2–3 times a week. The amount of dialysis may be varied according to the size of the patient, his dietary intake of protein and the biochemistry of predialysis plasma.

The rate of ultrafiltration is adjusted so that fluid removal equals the accumulation since the previous dialysis (measured by weight gain). Additional adjustments are made if the patient is judged to be either over- or underhydrated before dialysis. Fluid removal may be predicted from the known performance characteristics of the dialyser used, calculated precisely by continuous monitoring of body weight, or measured directly.

Most dialysis centres teach their patients how to set up, check and run their artificial kidneys and to insert their own vascular cannulas, so that only a minimum of assistance and supervision will be required once the training period of 2–4 months is completed. Patients may then have treatment at home, for which they will be lent the equipment and given surgical supplies and solutions. If home treatment is impracticable for want of a willing helper, the patient can transfer to a self-care centre

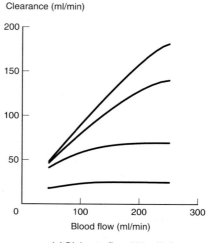

(a) Dialysate flow 200 ml/min

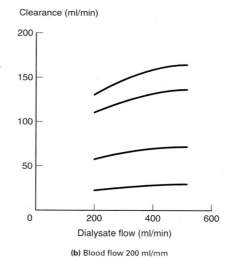

(b) Blood flow 200 ml/mm

Fig. 23.7   Clearance as a function of (a) blood and (b) dialysate flow rates in a conventional hollow fibre dialyser with regenerated cellulose membrane

away from the busy clinical atmosphere of a hospital renal unit.

For the majority of patients, renal physicians prefer home treatment, as this promotes independence and rehabilitation, and costs less. However, placing an artificial kidney in a home may exacerbate tensions within a family already dislocated by the effects of serious chronic disability. Because of the help required with treatment, it also accentuates the dependent status of the patient within the family, especially undesirable in the case of adolescents and unmarried adults.

25–30% of Australian maintenance haemodialysis patients are currently treated at home, and nearly the same number in self-care centres.

Maintenance peritoneal dialysis

This form of treatment may be used continuously or intermittently. *Continuous ambulatory peritoneal dialysis (CAPD)* involves three to five exchanges of 1–3 litres of dialysate every day. The exchanges, which are made by the patient, each take 30–45 minutes and are spaced either evenly throughout waking hours or to accommodate the normal daily activities.

For *intermittent peritoneal dialysis (CCPD —* continuous cycling peritoneal dialysis) a cycler is employed to give either 6–8 exchanges every night (for patients at home) or a total of 40–60 exchanges per week in two or three sessions in hospital. *Tidal peritoneal dialysis* can increase clearances by 10–20% by halting dialysate drainage before the abdominal cavity is empty, thus ensuring continuous blood–dialysate exchange. Intermittent treatment is employed in less than 5% of patients on maintenance peritoneal dialysis.

Fluid removal is regulated by the dialysate dextrose concentration, which may be varied between 28 and 215 mmol/1, and to a lesser extent by the dwell time.

Dialysis in acute renal failure

The amount of dialysis must be increased if the catabolic rate is high, as is usually the case in acute renal failure, after renal transplantation, or when maintenance dialysis is complicated by sepsis, bleeding or surgery. In peritoneal dialysis, higher clearances may be achieved by using a cycler to give tidal dialysis continuously. Haemodialysis is given every day or continuously. Blood urea should be kept below 30–35 mmol/l and hydration state must be monitored by weighing at least once daily or, in the more critically ill patient, by measuring central venous or pulmonary artery wedge pressure. Continuous haemodialysis is technically simpler than intermittent dialysis, and is the usual modality in intensive care units.

Choice of dialysis regimen

The efficacy of peritoneal dialysis is barely adequate to cater for normal metabolic demands, and both the daily loss of up to 10 g of protein and 3 g of amino acids into the dialysate and uptake of 100–200 g of simple sugar from the dialysate adversely affect nutritional status. Peritoneal dialysis is precluded by recent abdominal inflammation, trauma or operation, and because it reduces both vital capacity and lung compliance it is contraindicated in patients with severe pulmonary disease. Moreover, sooner or later peritoneal dialysis has to be suspended in nearly all patients because of recurrent peritonitis, antibiotic-resistant infection (staphylococcal, pseudomonal, fungal) or adhesions.

However, peritoneal dialysis can be used continuously, thus minimizing the need for dietary restrictions (fluid, salt, potassium) and phosphate binders. Because blood loss is avoided, haemoglobin levels are higher than when haemodialysis is employed. As there is no contact between blood and artificial dialysis membranes, the acute toxicity resulting from this source of bioincompatibility is avoided (Table 23.3). The facilities required for, and techniques used in, continuous ambulatory peritoneal dialysis are simpler than those of haemodialysis, making it more feasible for domiciliary treatment.

Continuous peritoneal dialysis is especially suitable for children, in whom the peritoneal cavity is large relative to body bulk, and for diabetics, in whom addition of insulin to the peritoneal dialysate provides a continuous means of blood sugar control and minimizes the threat of intraocular haemorrhage, which may occur as a result of giving heparin for haemodialysis. Also it is well tolerated by the majority of elderly patients who, if they have cardiovascular disease, may be unduly prone to symptomatic hypotension or angina during haemodialysis treatments. In Australia about one third of patients receiving maintenance dialysis, and perhaps one quarter receiving acute dialysis, are treated by the peritoneal method.

Unlike peritoneal dialysis, continuous haemodialysis can only be used for the treatment of acute renal failure and poisoning. In these circumstances, it has the advantages over intermittent therapy of avoiding osmotic disequilibrium (resulting from rapid removal of urea from extracellular space and the resultant movement of water into the intracellular compartment) and its clinical sequelae (raised intracranial pressure), and of keeping serum urea below 20 mmol/l even in hypercatabolic patients. Its disadvantage is the necessity for continuous anticoagulation.

Adjuvant therapy (see Table 23.2)

Erythropoietin, given intravenously or subcutaneously to patients with haemoglobin less than 80 g/l or symptomatic anaemia, is used to maximize rehabilitation and reduce the risk of sensitization against foreign antigens in transfused blood (which may reduce the chance of renal transplantation — Ch. 24). Resistance to erythropoietin may result from deficient iron stores (low serum ferritin), reduced iron availability (low transferrin saturation), excess interleukin 1 in sepsis or chronic inflammation, aluminium accumulation, hyperparathyroidism, or the presence of an unrelated cause for anaemia. Many patients require concomitant iron replacement (oral or parenteral). Side effects, which include hypertension, thrombosis of

vascular access and (rarely) seizures, are not common if the haemoglobin level is raised only to about 100 g/l.

Complications (see Table 23.3)

Bioincompatibility arises from interaction of blood with a synthetic dialysis membrane, or with a contaminant or unphysiological constituent (in practice, only the buffer anion) of dialysate. This may result in activation of the coagulation or the complement cascade, or release from platelets or leucocytes of cytokines, mediators of inflammation or vasoactive substances. The most important immediate consequences are transient hypoxaemia due to pulmonary sequestration of granulocytes caused by complement activation (especially with cellulosic membranes, and not occurring when dialysers are re-used); uncoupling of oxidative phosphorylation by the exposure of intracellular fluid to unphysiological anions resulting in intracellular accumulation of inorganic phosphate and hydrogen ions; and fever caused by the release of interleukin 1 when monocytes are exposed to acetate, pyrogens or bioincompatible membranes.

Amyloidosis is a recently recognized complication which occurs in at least 10% of patients who have been on haemodialysis for more than 10 years. The deposits consist of transformed β_2-microglobulin, whose production is increased by the release of cytokines such as interleukin 1, and whose clearance is much less with synthetic than

Table 23.2 Adjuvant treatment for dialysis patients

Indication	Treatment
Phosphate ↑	$CaCO_3$, $Al(OH)_3$, MgO, (approx. 1 g orally with meals)
Parathyroid hormone ↑	Increase dialysate calcium; phosphate binders; $1,25(OH)_2$ vitamin D (as calcitriol)
Water, sodium and potassium ↑	Restrict dietary intake (ion-exchange resins rarely required for hyperkalaemia)
Water-solution vitamins ↓ (especially C, B_6, folate)	Nutritious diet (oral supplements rarely required)
Iron (serum ferritin, transferrin saturation) ↓	Check for blood loss; oral iron
Haemoglobin ↓	Erythropoietin (or transfusion)
Renin ↑	β-blocker or ACE inhibitor
Normal alimentation not possible (especially if hypercatabolic)	Parenteral nutrition with 1.5–2.5 litres per day of 25–40% dextrose, 4% amino acid solution; electrolytes, trace elements and vitamins as required
All long-term patients (prevention of atherosclerosis)	Physical exercise; no smoking; high fibre, low saturated fat, low sugar diet

Table 23.3 Complications of dialysis therapy

Complication	Cause (s)
Haemodialysis and haemofiltration	
Accidents during haemodialysis	
Air embolism	Break in blood circuit before pump
Blood loss	Break in blood circuit after pump
Thrombosis in blood circuit	Insufficient heparin, hypercoagulable state
Haemolysis in dialyser	Overheated or hypo-osmolar dialysate
Symptoms occurring during haemodialysis (hypotension, vomiting, headache, fever)	Rapid ultrafiltration and/or rapid decrease in ECF osmolarity; acetate transfer from dialysate; contamination of dialysate with pyrogens, formaldehyde, trace metals, etc.; complement activation by dialysis membranes
'Trace-element' toxicity	
Haemolysis	Cu, Zn, NO_2, chloramines
Encephalopathy, anaemia	Al
Vitamin D resistant osteomalacia	Al, ?F
Hepatic fibrosis	Fe, ?Cu
Intradialytic fever	Zn, Cu, Ni
Amyloidosis (peri-articular)	Reduced natural clearance and increased production of β_2-microglobulin
Viral hepatitis (B; C)	Transfusion of infected blood/blood products, cross-infection within dialysis unit (unusual)
Vascular access	
Bacterial infection	Nearly always *Staph. aureus*
Thrombosis	Stenosis, erythropoietin
Peritoneal dialysis	
Incomplete drainage of dialysate	Catheter tip not in rectovesical pouch; occlusion of catheter holes by fibrin, omentum or adhesions; loculation of fluid (e.g. in hernial sac)
Cachexia	Protein loss into peritoneal dialysate
Obesity	Uptake of dextrose from dialysate
Infection	
Abdominal catheter tunnel	Nearly always *Staph. aureus*
Peritoneum	Contamination of dialysate, most often *Staph. epidermidis*; also Gram-negative, fungi
Any form of dialysis	
Pericarditis, ascites, asterixis, impaired neuromuscular coordination and cerebration	Insufficient dialysis
Peripheral neuropathy, cachexia	Inadequate nutrition, insufficient dialysis
Hypertension, pulmonary congestion	Overhydration, excessive salt intake
Pruritus, metastatic calcification, osteitis fibrosa	Hyperphosphataemia, hyperparathyroidism
Accelerated atherogenesis	Hypertension, smoking, abnormal lipid and carbohydrate metabolism, reduced physical activity

with the natural glomerular membrane due to its size (MW 11 800 daltons). Dialysis-related amyloidosis is characterized by carpal tunnel syndrome, and painful accumulation of amyloid around large joints causing erosions and cysts in the bone ends.

Secondary hyperparathyroidism, in part, may be a long-term consequence of unphysiological dialysate buffer anion which causes inorganic phosphate to be retained in the intracellular fluid compartment during haemodialysis treatments, preventing its effective removal.

Results

Acute renal failure

Generally it may be said that the standard of dialysis therapy in properly constituted renal and intensive care units is now so good that outcome is influenced only to a minor degree by the presence of renal failure itself, or by dialysis-related complications, although this is difficult to demonstrate due to the changing pattern of cases. When acute renal failure results from extensive trauma, sepsis or a grave surgical condition, mortality is high because it is only in the most severe instances that renal shut-down persists when modern resuscitative measures are employed (see Ch. 20). Death results usually from the primary condition, or from a complication of it such as sepsis or haemorrhage.

Dialysis can be used to permit adequate nutrition, and in the case of continuous haemo-diafiltration to remove endogenous toxins which have been implicated in the cardiopulmonary dysfunction of multiorgan failure. Acute cardiovascular instability and hypoxia (due in part to complement activation and the pulmonary sequestration of granulocytes) may be lessened by the use of more biocompatible membranes.

End-stage renal failure

The 3-year mortality is approximately 25% in non-diabetic haemodialysis patients under 55 years of age, and more in diabetics, older patients and those on CAPD. Just over half of the deaths are cardiovascular, resulting mainly from myocardial or cerebral infarction, cardiac arrest (hyperkalaemic or ischaemic) or intracranial haemorrhage (ANZDATA 1991).

Some 25% of all dialysis patients return to full-time work, school or domestic duties, and the same number are not fit to work; the remainder work part-time or are unable to find work. On average 1–2 weeks are spent in hospital each year for treatment of medical or surgical complications, most often in relation to vascular access.

One can be less precise about the quality of life enjoyed by these patients. Social life and physical recreation are limited both by the time spent on treatment and by the debilitating effect of anaemia, a problem which is alleviated by erythropoietin. Male patients often are impotent and female patients lack libido. Loss of income and out-of-the-ordinary expenditure frequently lead to a reduction in the standard of living. Added to these are the everpresent spectre of death and anxieties about transplantation; it is therefore not surprising that dissatisfaction, neurosis, anti-social behaviour and depression are common, not only in the patients themselves but also in their families.

Despite this, many, perhaps a majority, lead happy and productive lives.

Some 5% of maintenance dialysis patients do not want a kidney graft and a further 50% are ruled unfit for transplantation (e.g. because of age, ischaemic heart disease, widespread atheroma, bronchiectasis, cancer, peritoneal infection, chronic active hepatitis). For some 10% of dialysis patients, the presence of circulating cytotoxic antibodies, representing sensitization to transplantation antigens by transfusion, pregnancy or a previous graft, is a significant barrier to finding a compatible kidney donor.

TRENDS AND PROSPECTS

Medical

Although the incidence of irreversible renal failure is falling, improving clinical expertise and technology mean that more of those who present now can be treated successfully. There are no absolute contraindications to dialysis, and the major relative contraindications (age, systemic disease such as diabetes and atherosclerosis, significant organ dysfunction) are not individually barriers to acceptance into renal replacement programmes. As a result, the annual rate of entry of Australian patients has risen from 28 (in 1972) to 55 (in 1990) per million of total population, half being over 55 years of age. This, together with the relatively static rate of successful transplantation and an improving life expectancy on dialysis, means that by 1990 there were about 170 Australian dialysis patients per million of total population, compared to 28 per million in 1972.

Technical

The major obstacles to achieving the ultimate objective in this field, i.e. a continuously functioning, wearable artificial kidney, are the lack of sufficiently thrombo-resistant materials to obviate the need for continuous systemic anticoagulation, which would be hazardous, and the lack of sorbents which will concentrate from blood all uraemic metabolites, including urea. Removal of excess salt and water will be possible in such a system by using a highly permeable membrane for ultrafiltration, and either arterial pressure or a tiny mechanical pump.

The other major obstacle is *bioincompatibility* of the dialysis membrane and of unphysiological constituents of dialysis fluid. It is doubtful if the full extent of the immediate and long-term conse-quences of bioincompatibility have been recog-nized. Certainly the search for more compatible membranes and solutions will continue. At the present time, peritoneal dialysis has the advantage over extracorporeal haemodialysis of minimal exposure to foreign materials.

REFERENCES AND RECOMMENDED READING

ANZDATA Report, Disney A P S (ed) 1991 Australia and New Zealand Dialysis and Transplant Registry. Adelaide, South Australia

Basile C, Drüeke T 1989 Dialysis membrane biocompatibility. Nephron 52: 113–118

Chapman J R, Allen R D 1988 Dialysis and Transplantation. In: Morris P J (ed) Kidney Transplantation. W B Saunders, Philadelphia, pp 42–55

Editorial 1991 Dialysis amyloidosis. Lancet 338: 349–350

Fleming S J, Foreman K, Shanley K, Mihrshahi R, Siskind V 1991 Dialyzer reprocessing with renalin. American Journal of Nephrology 11: 27–31

Hakim R M 1990 Assessing the adequacy of dialysis. Kidney International 27: 822–832

Harris D C H 1990 Acute renal replacement — which treatment is best? Australian and New Zealand Journal of Medicine 20: 197–200

Levine J, Bernard D B 1990 The role of urea kinetic modeling, TAC urea, and Kt/V in achieving optimal dialysis: a critical appraisal. American Journal of Kidney Disease 15: 285–301

Nolph K D 1988 Comparison of continuous ambulatory peritoneal dialysis and haemodialysis. Kidney International 33: S123–S131

Pond S M 1991 Extracorporeal techniques in the treatment of poisoned patients. Medical Journal of Australia 154: 617–622

Schaefer R M, Horl W H, Massry S G 1989 Treatment of renal anaemia with recombinant human erythropoietin. American Journal of Nephrology 9: 353–362

Twardowski Z J 1989 New approaches to intermittent peritoneal dialysis therapies. In: Nolph K (ed) Peritoneal dialysis, 3rd ed. Kluwer, Dordrecht

Veech R L 1988 The untoward effects of the anions of dialysis fluid. Kidney International 34: 587–597

24. Transplantation

J. R. Chapman,   A. G. R. Sheil

INTRODUCTION

Transplantation of the kidney began in 1933 as an attempt to treat the otherwise fatal condition of acute renal failure. Yu Yu Voronoy transplanted a blood group incompatible kidney, damaged irretrievably by warm ischaemia and without the benefit of immunosuppression. The first person to have had his life prolonged by renal transplantation was one of nine patients transplanted in Boston between 1953 and 1954. This clinical programme was stimulated not only by the concept that renal transplantation could cure an otherwise fatal disease, but also by progress in experimental transplantation created by Medawar and his colleagues during the 1940s.

The first successful renal transplant was between identical twin brothers on December 23rd, 1954. Monozygotic twin transplants were the only true successes until the advent of azathioprine and prednisolone immunosuppression in 1961. The twin transplants were uniformly successful, and those with normal renal function returned to normal health and fertility. To achieve the same result between genetically dissimilar donors and recipients has been the goal for renal transplant programmes.

During the 1960s both transplantation and dialysis became practical options for the treatment of end-stage renal failure, each with its advantages and disadvantages. The two technologies developed as complementary techniques such that patients with end-stage renal failure now have a choice of treatment options. The majority of patients usually require more than one treatment modality during their lifetime, since only a few will receive a transplant before the need for dialysis, and most are placed on the transplant waiting list (Table 24.1). Transplantation is generally the preferred treatment, based upon the resulting improved quality of life, and also because it is a less expensive option than dialysis. Capital investment in haemodialysis equipment can be kept in check when active transplant programmes permit continued acceptance of new patients. In Australia, Scandinavia and the United Kingdom, 50% or more of patients alive with end-stage renal failure have functioning renal transplants, while in some countries this percentage is as low as 10%.

The single most significant limitation on transplantation is the number of kidneys donated, either by living related or cadaver donors. Living related donors usually provide only 10–15% of kidneys transplanted. Consequently transplant programmes rely heavily on the altruism of brain-dead cadaver donors and their families. While previously most cadaver kidneys came from

Table 24.1 Percentage of patients awaiting renal transplantation in Australia, March 1991, by age. (Data supplied by the ANZDATA registry.)

Age	Number of patients	Percentage of those on dialysis
0 −4	4	80
5 −14	18	86
15−24	105	77
25−34	205	74
35−44	275	71
45−54	314	60
55−64	250	33
65−74	62	9
Total	1233	

individuals sustaining head injuries in motor vehicle accidents, road safety campaigns have had a significant impact on reducing the number of fatalities with the result that most transplant programmes are now retrieving more kidneys from elderly donors dying from spontaneous intracerebral haemorrhage. When it is sought, consent to donation is withheld on up to 50% of occasions. There also remains, in many countries, a considerable barrier within the medical profession to seeking consent from potential donor families. Because of inadequate numbers of donor organs, some countries have inverted the presumption that consent to donation is needed and established legislation that all citizens are organ donors unless they have specifically opted-out by signing an appropriate document. Whether the 'opt-out' system itself or the publicity that surrounds advertising the opt-out mechanism has improved donor rates is uncertain. However, countries with opt-out legislation have higher donor rates than those without.

IMMUNE RESPONSE TO TRANSPLANTATION

The unmodified response to transplantation of tissue from one individual to another results in highly effective destruction of the grafted tissue unless the donor and recipient are genetically identical. It is widely held to be an unintended consequence of the general defence mechanisms aimed at preventing the invasion of an organism by others.

The fundamental interaction in allograft rejection is between a major histocompatibility complex (MHC) molecule on the target donor cell and a receptor on the host's T lymphocytes (Fig. 24.1). The T cell receptor is a surface-bound structure generated from a series of alternative genes in a manner analogous to immunoglobulins. Each clone of T cells thus has a T cell receptor gene rearrangement from which is derived its unique surface receptor. There are a very large number of possible gene rearrangements and thus possible receptor specificities. During maturation T cells undergo a process of selection in the thymus which ensures first that circulating T cells bind to the individual's own MHC molecules and second that they do not recognize the individual's own (autologous) protein antigens.

The MHC molecules are the most complex and polymorphic antigen system known to man. The genes for the MHC are on the short arm of chromosome 6 and have been grouped into class I, class II and class III genes. An abbreviated version of the MHC gene segment is shown in Figure 24.2. The molecules derived from the class I and II genes are termed human leucocyte antigens (HLA). The basic structure of all HLA molecules

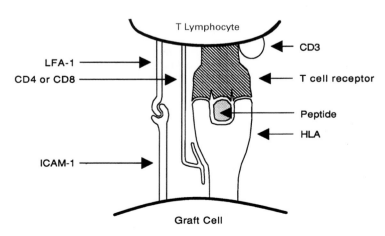

Fig. 24.1 Diagrammatic representation of the molecular interaction between a T lymphocyte and its target cell on the graft

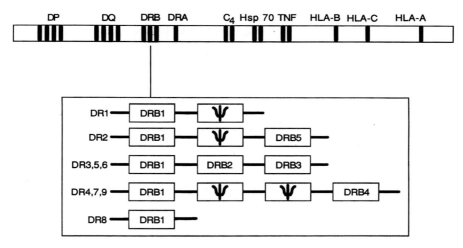

Fig. 24.2 Schematic representation of the major histocompatibility complex on the short arm of chromosome 6, showing the relative positions of the genes for the HLA molecules: class I genes HLA A, B, C; class II genes HLA DP, DQ, DRB and DRA; Class III genes including C4, heat shock protein 70 (Hsp70) and tumour necrosis factor (TNF). In the inset are shown the different gene arrangements observed in different HLA DR types, including the presence of pseudogenes which have no known expressed product (Ψ)

presents a standard molecular surface to the T cell receptor but with a cleft between two alpha helices within which peptide antigens are bound (Fig. 24.1). In this way, for example, a peptide from an influenza virus infecting a cell may be presented on the cell surface for detection by T cell clones that can bind to that particular combination of HLA and peptide and destroy the infected cell. Killing of the cell is 'restricted' both by the particular HLA molecule and by the peptide sequence of the influenza strain.

It has been shown experimentally that a surprisingly high proportion of circulating T cells will bind to HLA molecules from a foreign individual. Why this should occur is not yet certain, but it seems likely that a T cell receptor capable of binding self HLA + foreign peptide, can also bind foreign HLA + foreign peptide, if the HLA differences are not too great and binding to the foreign peptide is strong. Whatever the explanation, T cell recognition of an allograft leads to a cascade of immune effector cells and molecules which are recruited to destroy the graft (Fig. 24.3). The interaction between the T lymphocyte and the antigen-presenting cell has two prerequisites: the first is MHC-peptide/T lymphocyte receptor bind-

ing as detailed in Figure 24.1, while the second is a soluble signal in the form of interleukin 1 (IL-1). Subsequent interactions between the cellular components of the immune system utilize similar chemical signals called lymphokines. These serve to stimulate local cellular responses to the graft and to create an amplifying cascade of cells directed at graft rejection. A further effect of such mediators as tumour necrosis factor and interferon is to increase expression of cell surface molecules which provide non-antigen-specific adhesion factors for migrating lymphocytes.

RECIPIENTS

Ideal recipients for renal transplants are relatively young, with no coexisting systemic disease, and with renal failure which has progressed to the stage where dialysis will be required within months. There are, however, few ideal recipients; first because the majority of patients with renal failure are over 40 years of age, second because uraemia is usually associated with systemic disease such as coronary artery disease, and third, because of the long waiting lists for transplantation in most countries, almost all patients will have started

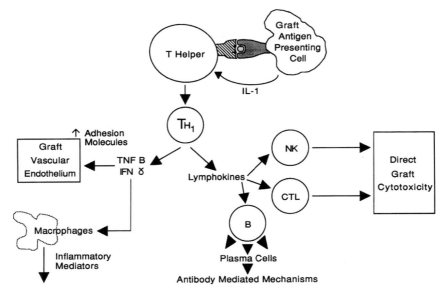

Fig. 24.3 A summary of the major effector mechanisms for allograft rejection, demonstrating the central role of the T helper cell and its interaction with a graft antigen-presenting cell. Production of lymphokines, tumour necrosis factor β and interferon-γ lead to a cascade of effector mechanisms involving macrophages, B lymphocytes (B), cytotoxic T lymphocytes (CTL) and natural killer cells (NK)

dialysis before a kidney becomes available. Thus many recipients are far from ideal, the decision for each individual being based upon age, type of renal disease, coexisting diseases and psychological and social factors.

Age

Most centres accept patients from birth to 60 years of age. Very young patients present considerable technical surgical and medical challenges. Over the age of 60 years the chance of cardiovascular and cerebrovascular disease increases, such that elderly patients are less frequently accepted for transplantation, particularly because kidney transplants are such a rare resource.

Renal disease

The diseases that lead to end-stage renal failure in Australia are shown in Table 24.2. The majority of these have little direct implication for acceptance, though polycystic kidneys are occasionally so large that nephrectomy is needed to enable renal

transplantation. Patients with analgesic nephropathy cause concern because of a high incidence of ischaemic heart disease and peptic ulceration. Congenital bladder abnormalities such as those seen with the 'prune belly syndrome' need urological assessment to determine whether or not

Table 24.2 Causes of renal failure for patients requiring treatment in Australia for the first time during 1990. (Data supplied by the ANZDATA Registry.)

Primary renal disease	no.	%
Glomerulonephritis	342	36
Diabetic nephropathy	135	14
Analgesic nephropathy	100	11
Polycystic kidney disease	75	8
Hypertension	78	8
Reflux nephropathy	62	7
Miscellaneous	96	10
Uncertain	58	6
Total	946	

Miscellaneous causes: interstitial nephritis, lead nephropathy, renal tuberculosis, sarcoid, radiation induced, congenital urological abnormalities, medullary cystic disease, calculi, cystinosis, gout, oxalosis, amyloid, myeloma, renal cell carcinoma, transitional cell carcinoma, haemolytic–uraemic syndrome, trauma.

Table 24.3   Causes of recurrent renal disease in renal allografts. (Data from Mathew T H 1991 Transplantation Reviews 5: 31–45.)

Disease		Frequency of recurrence	Graft loss
Focal segmental glomerulosclerosis		30%	Common and rapid
Membranous GN		10%	Progressive disease
Mesangiocapillary	type I GN	20%–30%	Progressive disease
	type II GN	95%	Rare
IgA nephropathy		50%	Rare
Henoch–Schönlein purpura		80%	Occasional
Goodpasture's (anti-GBM)		Depends on antibody status	
Systemic lupus erythematosus		1%	Occasional
Wegener's granulomatosis		Uncertain	Cyclophosphamide
Haemolytic–uraemic syndrome		50%	Rapid
Scleroderma		Uncertain	
Diabetes type I		100%	Slowly progressive
Oxalosis		90%	Common and rapid
Amyloidosis		33%	Occasional, progressive
Cystinosis		5%	Rare
Sickle cell anaemia		Uncertain	Uncertain
Monoclonal gammopathy		Uncertain	Uncertain

alternative urinary drainage via an ileal conduit is needed. Recurrence of the patient's original renal disease occurs in a number of types of glomerulonephritis and in some metabolic disorders (Table 24.3). Goodpasture's syndrome does not recur if antiglomerular basement membrane antibodies have been absent for a year. Primary hyperoxaluria will recur unless the metabolic defect is treated with a simultaneous liver transplant.

Coexisting disease

Myocardial infarction is the single commonest cause of death in patients with renal failure. All patients with cardiac symptoms need investigation and some require definitive surgery before transplantation. Centres vary in their policies for investigation of asymptomatic patients, and routine coronary angiography is recommended by some.

Malignancy should be excluded. Transplantation in patients with known previous malignancy carries a definite threat of recurrence. Most groups delay transplantation for at least two years from the time of initial treatment of the cancer because those who remain cancer-free after this interval have a low risk of recurrence.

Infection is a major problem in immunosuppressed patients and it is unwise to transplant in the face of any current infection. Potential sites of chronic infection should be sought, such as pulmonary tuberculosis and bronchiectasis. The former does not contraindicate transplantation if it has been treated effectively beforehand. Isoniazid is used for the first six months following operation. Bronchiectasis on the other hand, if widespread and severe, presents a relative contraindication. Dental caries and abscesses should receive appropriate treatment. Peritonitis in patients using CAPD must be checked for in the dialysate drained immediately pre-operatively.

Many uraemic patients have arteriosclerosis. Femoral and iliac arterial disease may not only threaten limbs but make the transplant arterial reconstruction difficult or occasionally impossible. Cerebrovascular disease may threaten perioperative stroke. Duplex ultrasound of the peripheral arterial tree has thus become a routine investigation in many centres.

Diabetes mellitus

Diabetic patients present a significant challenge to transplant clinicians. Not only do many have atherosclerosis as described above, but these patients may also have microangiopathy, surgically untreatable coronary artery disease, retinopathy, peripheral neuropathy, sympathetic neuropathy and increased susceptibility to infection. It is only in carefully selected diabetics that it is possible to match the success rates achieved for non-diabetics in terms of both patient and graft survival. In this selected group there is a case for considering combined pancreas and renal transplantation, in an attempt to prevent further progression of the secondary complications of diabetes.

Psychological and social factors

With improvement in transplant success rates one of the remaining preventable causes of graft loss is non-compliance with immunosuppressive medication. It is possible to predict some patients in whom this problem will occur. Patients who have not experienced dialysis, especially those who are young or unintelligent, and who are thus unable to compare life with immunosuppression and life on dialysis may make an unwise choice. Facial appearance may be considerably altered by the combination of corticosteroid and cyclosporin, causing considerable distress and non-compliance, especially in younger females. Errors in taking the prescribed dose occur in patients unable to read or to speak the local language, mandating care in prescription advice and use of predispensed medication containers for some patients. Capsules of cyclosporin are more easily assessed by blind patients than the liquid formulation.

Blood transfusion

In the experimental laboratory, rats can accept kidney transplants without immunosuppression provided they have previously received blood from the same donor. The clinical situation is much more complex, but even so, there is a recorded improvement in outcome in patients transfused before transplantation compared with those not. This was first observed definitively in the early 1970s, at a time when the policy was to avoid blood transfusion because of the risk of sensitization to HLA antigens. Many randomized controlled trials soon confirmed the original observations, with improvement in 1-year graft survival of the order of 10–15%. During the 1980s however, largely because of advances in immunosuppression, graft survival in untransfused patients improved steadily such that the difference is now 5% or less. The policy of routine pre-transplant blood transfusion, implemented during the 1970s, has thus largely been abandoned. Some Australian centres still transfuse 1–3 units of blood to patients on the transplant waiting list who are at low risk of becoming sensitized (males and nulliparous females), but not to multiparous patients who have a 15% chance of becoming highly sensitized. The need for repeated transfusion has become rare with use of erythropoietin, but in those who need blood for clinical reasons a leucocyte filter reduces the risk of sensitization.

MATCHING DONORS AND RECIPIENTS

Matching donors and recipients has the aim of ensuring the best chance of a successful outcome of transplantation. That is, the recipient receives a kidney which has the best chance of success while at the same time the best use is made of the donor's altruistic donation. Conflict with these simple aims arises because the shortage of donor kidneys dictates that those available must be used even when the level of matching is poor. Further, some patients may have to wait many years, or indeed may never be allocated a kidney, unless some weight is given to other factors such as the patient's age and length of time on the waiting list.

Blood group

Blood group compatibility is an essential prerequisite for cadaveric renal transplantation. Occasional living donor transplants have been performed successfully across incompatible blood groups, but only after extensive preparation of the recipients with splenectomy and plasmapheresis. Most centres also restrict the use of blood group 'O' kidneys to 'O' and 'B' patients, since the effect of permitting transplantation from 'O' donors to 'A' patients (though compatible and successful) would be to double the waiting time for 'O' patients compared with 'A'. Rhesus and minor blood groups do not affect transplant outcome.

Crossmatch

Preformed antibodies to donor HLA antigens in the recipient's serum at the time of transplantation result in hyperacute rejection, with loss of the graft during the first 1–24 hours. In the most extreme situation the graft turns blue and becomes infarcted soon after the surgeon releases the arterial clamps at the completion of the vascular anastomoses.

Antibody to donor HLA can be detected by the crossmatch test, which is an essential prerequisite for transplantation. Incubation of the recipient's serum with donor lymphocytes is followed by addition of rabbit complement and a dye such as eosin, to detect cells which have been lysed. Donor T and B lymphocytes express HLA class I antigens (HLA A, B, C) but only a small proportion of activated T cells express class II molecules (HLA DR, DQ) which are normally present on B lymphocytes and cells specialized for antigen presentation (e.g dendritic cells, Langerhans' giant cells, macrophages). Thus a positive T cell crossmatch implies that the recipient has antibody directed at donor HLA A, B, or C. In many centres the crossmatch is performed not only with T lymphocytes, but also with separated B lymphocytes to detect antibody to class II antigens. There is, however, disagreement over whether or not a positive B cell crossmatch represents a contraindication to transplantation. False positive T and B cell crossmatches may occur in patients with autoreactive cytotoxic antibodies, which are especially common in patients with systemic lupus erythematosus.

Tissue type

Since the HLA molecules define, for the immune system, the difference between self and non-self, matching of the donor and recipient HLA should theoretically prevent rejection. The situation which proves this contention is where the recipient and donor are identical (monozygotic) twins.

Inheritance of HLA occurs in 'haplotypes', with the HLAA, B, C, DR, DQ antigens from one chromosome inherited en bloc from each parent. The implications for living related transplantation

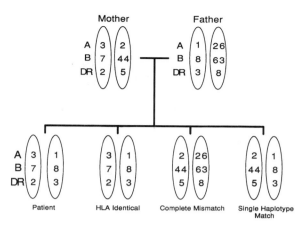

Fig. 24.4   Inheritance of the HLA genotype in a family where one child requires a renal transplant. There are four children in the family, one of whom is HLA identical having inherited the same haplotypes as the patient, one is completely mismatched having inherited the alternative haplotyes from both parents, and one has inherited the same haplotype as the patient from the father (HLA A1, B8, DR3), but the alternative haplotype from the mother. There is a 25% chance of a sibling being HLA identical, 25% of being completely mismatched, and 50% of being a one haplotype match with the haplotype from either mother or father.

are shown in Figure 24.4, where it can be seen that the patient is a 'one haplotype match' with each parent. The siblings may be one of three possible degrees of match with the patient: HLA identical, having inherited both of the same haplotypes; a one haplotype match, having inherited either the same paternal or maternal haplotype; or completely mismatched. Graft survival of living related transplants is stratified by the degree of match. Long-term results of HLA identical grafts reported to the UCLA Registry show that 70% function for at least 10 years, compared with 47% for one haplotype matches and 31% for cadaver donor grafts.

Matching for tissue type in cadaveric transplantation is hampered by the enormous diversity in the HLA system. There are, in most populations, up to 20 HLA A, and 40 HLA B antigens, while the diversity at class II increases with the accuracy of the typing methodology used. Serological tissue typing relies upon antibodies produced as a result of pregnancy, blood transfusion or transplantation. These reagents are found by screening serum samples from large numbers of volunteers against cells of known tissue type. This method uses the same test as the cross-match and detects the cell surface HLA molecules. It is also possible to define the gene sequence for an individual's HLA region by means of molecular genetic techniques. Although precise, these methods are currently impractical for transplantation. However, techniques which examine particularly important sections of gene sequence for HLA DR and DQ, using either restriction fragment length polymorphism (RFLP) or oligonucleotides and the polymerase chain reaction (PCR), may soon be applicable.

With serological tests for matching, HLA B and DR have been shown to have the greatest impact upon graft outcome. Data from the international Collaborative Transplant Study (CTS) show that there is a 20% improvement in 5-year cadaver graft outcome from matching (68% for HLA A, B, DR identical; 48% HLA A, B, DR mismatched). Retrospective analysis of matching for HLA DR using the RFLP technique has shown that the outcome of genetically matched but unrelated grafts equals the results from living related grafts.

While many countries, including Australia, use HLA matching for graft allocation, the genetic diversity of the HLA region prevents most patients from receiving an HLA identical graft.

Highly sensitized patients and regrafts

While the success rates for first transplants have improved to the point where acute rejection is an uncommon cause of graft loss, this is not true for recipients of second grafts who have lost their first graft or who have developed multiple anti-HLA antibodies. Patients who have rejected their first graft within a month have only a 40% chance of success with the second. Highly sensitized patients may have cytotoxic antibodies that cause a positive crossmatch with 99% of prospective donors and are thus effectively un-transplantable, unless measures such as splenectomy and plasmapheresis are used before transplantation.

DONORS

Living human donors (LD)

LD can contribute only a small proportion of the kidneys required for patients with renal failure. Most frequently, LD are relatives. In living related donor (LRD) transplantation, kidneys are usually transferred from parent to child or between siblings, including twins. Less frequently, children donate kidneys to parents.

Until recently, living unrelated individuals (LUD) were infrequent renal donors. This was because there is no immunological advantage for LUD over cadaveric donors and there are serious ethical considerations involved in the removal of an organ from a healthy individual to benefit another. However, the recent improvement in results of renal transplantation, principally because of improved immunosuppression, has led to increasing usage of LUD. Most groups prefer to restrict this donor source to those who have a special caring relationship with the recipient, especially spouses. Another occasional source of LUD kidneys is the rare normal kidney, removed from a patient for reasons other than sepsis or cancer, which is made available for transplantation.

In all LD transplantation, after blood grouping and tissue typing have confirmed suitability for transplantation, careful psychological assessment must be undertaken to see that the donor is well motivated and not under coercion. History, examination, bacteriological and renal function tests and intravenous pyelography should show the donor to be normotensive and free of renal infections or abnormalities and of unsuspected systemic disease or cancer. Aortography is required to show the renal arteries and that the kidney selected is suitable for transplantation while that remaining is normal. Kidneys with single renal arteries are usually selected for transplantation although the presence of multiple arteries is not an absolute contraindication. Some groups employ renal–donor-specific blood transfusions administered to the recipient prior to the operation to increase the likelihood of success. However this form of preparation is now usually restricted to recipients who are mismatched with the donor.

LRD transplantation has many advantages over cadaver donor transplantation besides increased graft compatibility. LD recipients have a limited time on dialysis and some receive transplants before dialysis is required. Operations can be planned for a time when the recipient is ideally prepared. Finally, the recipient receives a kidney damaged to the least possible extent by ischaemia so that good renal function is present from the time of transplantation.

Cadaveric donors

Patients who are 'brain dead', but with circulation and ventilation maintained, provide the great majority of all organs for transplantation. Any individual with normal kidneys before the terminal event can be considered as a possible renal donor. Younger donors are preferred but an upper age limit of 65 or 70 years is now usual. There should be no history of renal infection, diabetic nephropathy or cancer (excluding localized skin cancer and primary cerebral tumours). There should be no systemic or peritoneal infection and no recognized viral infection. Renal function tests and microscopy of the urine should be normal apart from variations related to the terminal illness. Tests for hepatitis B and C, as well as human immunodeficiency virus (HIV), must be negative while evidence of cytomegalovirus infection may help determine suitability for particular recipients. Personnel of the transplantation team should play no part in the terminal management of the patient and in many countries are excluded, by law, from making the diagnosis of brain death. The clinicians caring for the donor maintain normal fluid and electrolyte balance, as well as blood pressure, until permission from the relatives and coroner (when necessary) has been given and preparations for organ retrieval are completed.

Animal donors

In the mid-1960s, when clinical transplantation from human donors was becoming widespread, animals were used as donors on several occasions. Chimpanzees and baboons provided kidney, liver and heart xenografts, all in small numbers. However no transplantation from animal sources was successful. Such are the histocompatibility differences that rejection could not be controlled by the available immunosuppressive agents. Even so, some chimpanzee kidneys survived for up to 6 months in humans. Because of the continued shortage of donor organs and with the prospect of genetic manipulation, controlled breeding and increased understanding of the xenograft reaction and its modification, there is currently renewed interest in this source of donor organs.

RENAL PRESERVATION

The amount and reversibility of ischaemic damage which occurs when a kidney is transplanted depends on the duration of ischaemia caused by the interruption of blood flow and the temperature of the kidney. Cooling the organ greatly reduces the damage because the metabolic rate is markedly decreased. The period between cessation of renal circulation and cooling is the 'warm' ischaemia time, while the period during which the organ is maintained cold until revascularization in the recipient is the 'cold' ischaemia time. Warm times may be only a few minutes with LD transplantation, or near zero when kidneys are removed from 'brain-dead' cadaveric donors following in-situ cold perfusion before nephrectomy. Times up to one hour may occur when cadaveric donor death is determined by the cessation of the heart beat and some kidneys do not regain effective function after a warm time of one hour. Cold times are regularly of the order of 1 hour with LD transplantation but vary from 4–50 hours for cadaveric transplantation.

Cooling is achieved by perfusion of the kidneys via the renal arteries with chilled electrolyte solution. In cadaver transplantation this is usually undertaken in situ during organ retrieval. Immediately after removal the kidney(s) is/are immersed in ice slush solution. In the early years of organ transplantation the use of isotonic perfusate caused intracellular oedema, with increased leakage of intracellular ions and enzymes into the extracellular spaces and an associated incidence of poor function. Prevention of these effects by use of hypertonic solutions, or by the addition of agents with minimal permeability to cell membranes, has been shown to be important in organ preservation. A variety of such solutions, with electrolyte content broadly based on intracellular concentrations (Ross solution, Collins solution), are available, with the most recent development being the University of Wisconsin solution (UW). UW is based upon the impermeant trisaccharide raffinose and the lactobionate ion; it also contains hydroxyethyl starch, allopurinol, insulin, glutathione and co-trimoxazole. By the simple measures of cold perfusion and ice storage, allografts from suitable donors with short warm ischaemic intervals can be preserved satisfactorily for at least 30 hours. For safe preservation beyond 30 hours machine perfusion of kidneys is sometimes employed. Cold oxygenated plasma-like solution is pumped through the kidneys, resulting in safe preservation for periods of up to 50 hours.

OPERATIONS

Living donor nephrectomy

The surgical approach is via a loin incision. The kidney is prepared with minimum manipulation by division of all attachments except the renal artery, renal vein and ureter. After administration of heparin these structures are divided, and the kidney is removed and immediately placed in ice slush solution and perfused.

Cadaver donor nephrectomy

Until the late 1970s it was usual to await cessation of the heart beat after withdrawal of respiratory support before declaration of donor death and subsequent nephrectomy. Since then, however, the concept of cerebral death has been generally accepted, and donor respiration and circulation are maintained while donor nephrectomy proceeds.

Before or during the operation it is usual to administer a vasodilator drug and heparin, to maintain volume expansion with electrolyte solution and to establish a mannitol diuresis. In addition, some groups use cytotoxic drugs with a view to removing from the graft circulating nucleated cells which stimulate the immune re-

sponse in the recipient. However, several studies have failed to confirm the value of this treatment and subsequent work has shown that dendritic cells in the renal interstitium, rather than passenger leucocytes, are almost certainly the major provocateurs of the immune response.

Donor nephrectomy is now almost always part of multiorgan retrieval involving also the heart, liver and pancreas. The approach is transperitoneal. The lower abdominal aorta is cannulated and the aorta is occluded above the coeliac axis. In-situ perfusion of the abdominal organs (including the kidneys) then proceeds. If the heart is to be donated it is removed first, followed by the cooled abdominal organs. The liver and pancreas are usually removed first, and then the kidneys. The ureters on both sides are divided low in the pelvis, then dissected free, taking care to preserve the ureteric blood vessels. The kidneys may be removed individually or together, en bloc, with the inferior vena cava and aorta. Immediately after removal the kidneys are immersed in iced saline solution (see above). They are separated, secured in plastic bags surrounded by ice slush in sterile containers, and dispatched to the hospitals where the two recipient operations take place.

Recipient operation

The recipient is prepared for abdominal operation. Most groups administer antibiotics with the premedication but limit treatment to the first three postoperative days. Before the operation begins the allograft is inspected to establish that it is satisfactory for transplantation. Solitary cysts are not a matter for concern but polycystic kidneys should not be used. Manipulative damage to the kidney, vessels and ureter is assessed. If kidneys appear scarred or there is a history of hypertension or urinary infections, biopsies should be sent for immediate histological examination. Any unusual areas in the kidney should be assessed to avoid the possibility of transplantation of malignancy.

The allograft is placed in one or other iliac fossa (Fig. 24.5). An extraperitoneal approach is made to the iliac vessels. The transplant artery is anastomosed either to the internal iliac or to the external iliac artery. The transplant vein is joined

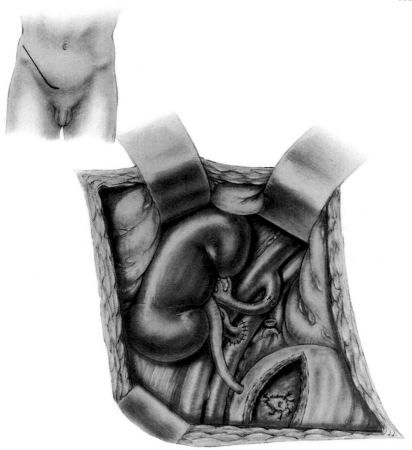

Fig. 24.5 Transplantation. The position of a left kidney transplanted into the right iliac fossa is shown. The operation is extraperitoneal. The renal artery is anastomosed end-to-end to the internal iliac artery and the renal vein end-to-side to the external iliac vein. The ureter is implanted in the bladder with construction of a submucosal tunnel. The skin incision used is shown in the inset.

to the external iliac vein. The ureter is usually implanted into the bladder with the construction of a submucosal tunnel aimed at preventing reflux of urine into the transplant ureter.

Immediate postoperative course

Allograft recipients are best managed in special units where exposure to exogenous infection is minimized and the nursing and ancillary staff become expert members of the transplantation team.

In the early postoperative period maintenance of normal circulation and of optimal fluid and electrolyte balance is critical. Frequent estimations of serum urea, creatinine and electrolyte levels are necessary. Some centres routinely use continuous electrocardiographic and central venous pressure monitors. The urinary catheter is checked frequently to ensure free drainage, and urine volume is measured hourly. Arteriovenous shunts or fistulae are protected carefully. Should electrolyte imbalance or fluid overload occur, haemodialysis may be required.

With LD transplantation, good early function of grafts can be expected and relatively few severe rejection episodes. With cadaveric transplantation, the average rate of good early function is about

70% and rejection episodes are common. Postoperative care is much easier in the presence of good allograft function as dialysis is not required, fluid and electrolyte balance is more easily achieved and rejection episodes can be diagnosed earlier and with more certainty. In the absence of complications, discharge form hospital is usually 2–3 weeks after operation.

In some patients massive diuresis occurs. This represents a degree of renal tubular damage. Patients may pass 20–30 litres of urine per day and are at extreme risk from dehydration and electrolyte imbalance. Hydration and electrolyte balance must be maintained by means of frequent electrolyte estimations and replenishment of fluid and electrolytes by administration of half-normal saline solution in volumes equivalent to urinary output. After 12–24 hours gradual restriction of fluid replacement together with recovery of tubular function usually halts the diuresis.

Oliguria or anuria in the postoperative period is usually due to varying degrees of renal tubular necrosis, but other causes must be considered and, as far as possible, excluded. These include cyclosporin nephrotoxicity, vascular thrombosis, irreparable ischaemic damage, allograft arterial stenosis, ureteric obstruction, urinary extravasation and severe acute rejection. Investigations which may be required include radioisotope scan, ultrasound examination, biopsy, angiography, intravenous pyelography and thin needle antegrade pyelography. Dialysis must be continued. Rejection is difficult to detect and repeated biopsies may be required. Renal tubular necrosis usually resolves within 2–3 weeks, but recovery may take up to 8 or 10 weeks. In the presence of poor graft function in the postoperative period most groups either do not use, or else severely restrict, cyclosporin.

Technical complications

Wound infections and abscesses can lead to loss of life or of the graft. Wound infections are predisposed to by preoperative infective states including urinary infections, by the usual requirement at operation for cystotomy and by postoperative immunosuppression. Their likelihood is enhanced in the presence of wound haematomas. While small haemotomas may require no active therapy, larger collections should be evacuated.

As soon as wound infections are diagnosed, active treatment should be initiated, including systemic antibiotics. In all but minor cases, exploration with lavage and debridement is required, together with irrigation with fluids containing appropriate antibiotics. Infection involving the arterial anastomosis and resulting in secondary haemorrhage requires graft removal, secure haemostasis, wound irrigation and vigorous systemic antibiotic therapy.

In the perioperative period a major complication is urinary extravasation, often with external fistula formation. Its reported incidence varies from 0.5–10% in different series. Extravasation may result from ischaemic necrosis of the terminal ureter, from leakage at the site of ureteric anastomosis, or from the cystotomy wound. It may also occur when infarction of a pole of the kidney transplant occurs, caused by polar vessel thrombosis or ligature. Urinary leakage can also occur as a late complication of severe rejection which causes ureteric necrosis. In all but minor cases early operation and urinary tract reconstruction is indicated.

Ureteric obstruction in the early postoperative period may be due to oedema, blood clot or technical error. The first two usually resolve, although cystoscopy and retrograde ureteric catheterization may be required. The last requires surgical correction. Later in the postoperative course, ureteric obstruction may occur in any part of the transplant ureter. It is commonly at the site of entry of the ureter into the bladder wall, and reimplantation into the bladder, either directly or by use of a bladder flap, is possible. Lesions of the proximal transplant ureter may have an ischaemic, immunological or cicatricial aetiology. Here the situation is more difficult and anastomosis of the native ureter to the transplant ureter or pelvis may be required.

Complications which relate to the vasculature include primary and secondary haemorrhage, arterial or venous thrombosis, arterial stenosis and pulmonary embolism. Primary and secondary haemorrhage require urgent operation. Arterial thrombosis, whether due to technical error or rejection, necessitates graft removal. Arterial stenosis detected soon after operation and sufficiently severe to interfere with function or produce severe hypertension should be corrected at operation. Renal artery stenosis detected months or years after operation may be caused in part by vascular rejection. Operation can be difficult and while results may be gratifying, sometimes little benefit ensues. The technique of endarterial dilation by means of an inflatable balloon inserted into the transplant renal artery under radiographic control via the femoral artery is a major advance for simplified relief of these lesions. Thrombosis of the transplant renal veins may follow technical error or result from iliac vein thrombosis. In the latter case, systemic heparinization may be successful. Pulmonary embolism is treated by systemic heparinization or thrombolytic agents.

Lymphatic collections, or lymphoceles, occur in from 3–20% in different series. They occur because of damage to the iliac lymphatic trunks during operation or because of unsecured lymph vessels from the allograft. When small and uncomplicated, lymphoceles require no treatment; larger collections can interfere with graft blood supply or cause obstruction of the graft ureter. They recur rapidly after aspiration and are best treated by operation with marsupialization into the peritoneal cavity.

GRAFT REJECTION

Hyperacute rejection

Irreversible hyperacute rejection is rare and due to preformed antibodies to donor antigens expressed on the vascular endothelium. These may lead to rapid destruction of the graft. The graft perfuses well initially but then turns from firm and pink to flabby and dusky blue. Biopsy reveals early polymorph invasion of the glomeruli, and thrombosis of the glomerular capillaries and parenchymal small vessels with accompanying severe interstitial haemorrhage. In the majority of cases, confirmed by frozen section, there is little option but to remove the graft. In rare instances the process can be reversed by plasmapheresis and immunosuppression. The incidence of hyperacute rejection is less than 1% with effective crossmatching, but some antibodies are not detected, either because they are directed at antigens expressed on vascular endothelium but not lymphocytes, or because they are not cytotoxic.

Acute rejection

Almost two thirds of recipients of cadaveric grafts and one third of recipients of LRD grafts experience one or more episodes of acute rejection in the early post-transplant weeks. Acute rejection episodes can occur as early as the first or second postoperative day in a sensitized patient, but more usually occur in the first or second week. They become much less frequent with passage of time, though they have been recorded as late as 12 years after transplantation.

The classic symptoms and signs of acute rejection are swelling and tenderness of the graft, reduction in urine volume, weight gain of the patient and elevation of the temperature. These obvious manifestations, common previously, are uncommon in patients receiving cyclosporin or high dose steroid immunosuppression. Many rejection episodes are clinically silent in their onset and are usually detected only by a rising serum creatinine level. Other less reliable indices are a rise in serum chloride concentration (hyperchloraemic acidosis), proteinuria, lysozymuria and microscopic haematuria. Every effort should be made to detect and treat rejection early. This is important because at this time much of the inflammatory damage is reversible whereas established rejection can swiftly become irreversible, particularly because of thromboses in blood vessels.

The diagnosis of rejection is often difficult, especially in patients with poor early graft function following transplantation. In the absence of clinical signs, biopsy is helpful to determine the presence or absence of rejection and the need for therapy. Biopsy may either use a conventional needle core technique which yields information on both the architecture of the graft and its cellular infiltrate, or fine needle aspiration cytology. The fine needle aspiration technique is more readily repeatable and carries a lower risk than the conventional needle core. When the predominant histological finding is cellular infiltration there is good correlation between the two, however rejection confined predominantly to the vascular endothelium may be missed by cytological analysis. The histological appearance of acute cellular rejection comprises interstitial oedema together with both focal and diffuse cortical infiltration by lymphocytes, lymphoblasts, plasma cells, eosinophils and macrophages, with invasion of tubules and vessels. In vascular rejection, the endothelium of peritubular capillaries, glomeruli and arterioles may be swollen with associated platelet aggregation and fibrin thrombi. More severe changes include fibrinoid necrosis of small arteries and arterioles, progressing to obliteration of the vascular bed and cortical necrosis. Interstitial haemorrhage and thrombosis of large vessels herald loss of the graft.

An infrequent complication of acute rejection is rupture of the allograft with haemorrhage. This may require urgent operation to achieve haemostasis and, when the rupture is extensive, allograft nephrectomy may be required.

Chronic rejection

Rejection can occur in a delayed or chronic form. Each year approximately 2% of patients surviving with cadaveric donor renal allografts suffer graft failure due to chronic rejection. It presents either as gradual worsening of renal function or as frequent episodes of acute rejection which only partially respond to usual therapy. The diagnosis is established by biopsy, which demonstrates interstitial fibrosis, tubular atrophy and obliterative vascular changes including concentric intimal fibroblastic thickening. Full investigations should be pursued to ensure that there is no remediable cause for worsening function such as renal arterial stenosis or ureteric obstruction. When the diagnosis of chronic rejection is confirmed little has been shown to affect insidious erosion of function.

IMMUNOSUPPRESSION

Transplantation is as successful as the immunosuppresive protocols used to prevent and treat allograft rejection. The balance is between too little immunosuppression, with associated graft loss, and too much, with death from infection and malignancy. Both the science and the art of clinical transplantation revolve around the narrow therapeutic margins available with current protocols.

There are three phases of immunosuppression for each patient: induction therapy in the first days or weeks, treatment of acute rejection, and long-term maintenance. The clinician currently has four drugs or classes of drug with which to treat each of these phases: cyclosporin, azathioprine, corticosteroids and antilymphocyte preparations. There are, in addition, drugs under investigation such as FK506, Rapamycin, RS61443, and a variety of monoclonal antibodies directed at different T lymphocyte surface molecules such as the interleukin 2 receptor.

Cyclosporin

Cyclosporin is now the mainstay of almost all immunosuppressive protocols in transplantation. The drug was first identified in the early 1970s as a fungal derivative which had weak antifungal and antimalarial activity. Powerful immunosuppressive properties were, however, demonstrated in vitro and then in experimental models of transplantation. It was first used in pilot clinical studies in clinical transplantation in 1978, and then in randomized controlled trials between 1978 and 1983. These studies showed unequivocally that there was a 15–20% improvement in graft survival when cyclosporin was used. It was thus widely adopted when it was marketed in 1983.

Cyclosporin is a highly lipophilic cyclic peptide with 11 amino acids, including one previously unknown. It is available for oral use, either as a solution or capsules, and as an intravenous preparaton. Soon after administration the drug is widely distributed in the body. In the blood, most is bound to either cells or lipoproteins. Elimination is almost entirely due to metabolism by the cytochrome P-450 system in liver and gut, but both the bioavailability and half-life of the parent drug are subject to very wide variation between individuals. Many metabolites are produced, some of which are immunosuppressive. Measurement of the trough blood level of the parent molecule is the most effective way of judging doses for an individual. A number of drugs affect cyclosporin metabolism, either increasing or decreasing the circulating cyclosporin level. Phenytoin, phenobarbitone, carbamazepine and rifampicin reduce cyclosporin levels. Erythromycin, ketoconazole and diltiazem all increase levels. Some centres make use of the interaction with diltiazem to allow a reduction in the prescribed dose of cyclosporin and thus lower the cost.

Cyclosporin's mechanism of action is probably mediated by binding to a cytosolic protein, and by interference with transcription of mRNA for IL-2 and other cytokines. This appears to interrupt T lymphocyte activation at a rate limiting step and thus suppresses one of the central processes in allograft rejection.

In clinical practice the drug has not proved easy to use because of its side effects. It is usually administered intravenously at 2–4 mg/kg/day in two divided doses for the first one or two postoperative days (if renal function is adequate). Oral administration commences at 8–10 mg/kg/day with gradual dose reduction over the ensuing months.

The most significant adverse effect of cyclosporin is nephrotoxicity, not only damaging the kidney but also causing diagnostic confusion whenever graft function deteriorates. This has placed greater reliance upon renal biopsy, which can distinguish whether or not rejection is present, some authorities claiming that changes characteristic of cyclosporin nephrotoxicity can also be of assistance in the differential diagnosis. There are two clearly distinguishable forms of nephrotoxity, one of which may be regarded as physiological in that renal function improves within a week of stopping cyclosporin and probably relates to its effects upon the renal vascular bed. The second form of nephrotoxicity is irreversible fibrosis which may appear in characteristic bands or stripes in biopsy specimens. Other side effects include generalized hair growth (hypertrichosis), gingival hypertrophy, fine tremor, increased propensity to gout, hyperkalaemia, hypercholesterolaemia and hypertension. A second group of side effects includes neurological seizures, haemolytic anaemia, intravascular coagulation, haemolytic–uraemic syndrome and hepatotoxicity which, though serious, are rare. The problems associated with the drug have led to attempts to lower the dose used and, in some centres, to conversion after 3–12 months to a regimen not including cyclosporin. In patients converted from cyclosporin there is a small but real risk of graft loss from rejection.

Azathioprine

The precursor of azathioprine in clinical transplant practice, in the early 1960s, was 6-mercaptopurine. Azathioprine, which is converted to 6-mercaptopurine and other active metabolites in the liver, was synthesized and tested in canine renal transplants in 1961 and came to clinical application in the same year. The drug inhibits DNA and RNA production by interfering with purine synthesis. It has also been shown to block interleukin 2 production in vitro. Metabolic breakdown of 6-mercaptopurine occurs through the xanthine oxidase pathway. This sequence is blocked by allopurinol. Simultaneous administration of azathioprine and allopurinol thus leads to potentially lethal accumulation of azathioprine and its active metabolites.

The oral dose is between 1 and 3 mg/kg/day as a single dose. Measurement of blood levels has proved ineffective and the dose is titrated against the commonest severe side effect, bone marrow depression. It is mandatory to monitor for leucopenia which occurs most commonly, thrombocytopenia which may be the earliest marker of toxicity, and anaemia. It is unusual to have depression of a single cell lineage and though azathioprine toxicity may be the cause of leucopenia, thought has always to be given to other marrow insults, such as cytomegalovirus infection. Macrocytosis is an almost inevitable consequence of the use of azathioprine, but may mask true iron, folate or vitamin B_{12} deficiency. Hair loss is the side effect that causes patients the most immediate concern, but hepatotoxicity and long-term increased risk of malignancy are of more importance.

Corticosteroids

The first drug to be used in an attempt to influence graft rejection in the 1950s was a corticosteroid. In isolation, steroids are not sufficient to prevent rejection; however, when combined with azathioprine they became the mainstay of clinical transplantation for 20 years. The mode of action of corticosteroids is complex and diverse, with mechanisms involving both the initiating and effector levels of the rejection process. The anti-inflammatory effects are clearly important, especially in the context of severe acute rejection, but it is probably post receptor interference with T cell activation and effects upon the interleukins that provide long-term efficacy.

The side effects of corticosteroids are well known and perhaps observed in their most extreme form in transplant recipients. Steroid facies, thin, fragile, easily bruised skin, central obesity, cataracts, osteoporosis and avascular bone necrosis characterize the long-term steroid-treated patient. Studies have shown that for renal transplantation high dose regimens cause more side effects with little gain in efficacy. It has thus proved possible to reduce the doses used for maintenance treatment, while alternatives to high dose intravenous steroids for the treatment of acute rejection have become progressively more effective. While it has been shown that almost one half of cadaver allograft recipients and 70% of living donor recipients can be weaned from maintenance steroids, there is a small proportion of graft failures which result, and most centres use continuous low dose prednisolone maintenance regimens.

Antithymocyte globulin

It has been known since the 1950s that lymphocytes were critical in graft rejection, and since the 1960s that the T lymphocyte was involved. The first antilymphocyte preparations came from repeated inoculation of animals with human lymphocytes. The antilymphocyte globulin was purified from the sera, tested for in-vitro cytotoxicity to separated lymphocytes, and absorbed with platelet and red cell suspensions. It was then available for injection into patients. There have been a number of variations upon the basic theme for production of anti T lymphocyte polyclonal antibodies. The immunizing cells may be separated lymphocytes, purified thymocytes or cultured cell lines. The immunized animal may be a horse, goat, rabbit or other animal. The absorbing cells may be random donor cells or specific cell lines. The strength and effectiveness of the various preparations vary, not only between different manufacturers but also from batch to batch.

Despite the problems associated with manufacture, the various preparations have proved highly effective, with a combination of azathioprine, prednisolone and antithymocyte globulin proving to be the most effective therapy for renal transplantation, before introduction of cyclosporin. There are a number of specific problems associated with use of a foreign antibody. The first and most serious is anaphylaxis in response to the injection, which may be predicted in some patients by injection of a small subcutaneous test dose. After a few days most patients develop antibodies to the injected immunoglobulin, which may limit the effectiveness of treatment. Pyrexial reactions and serum sickness occur and may both be attributed to such antibodies. As a result of the highly effective immunosuppression, both CMV infection and EBV-associated lymphoma have an appreciable incidence.

Despite introduction of cyclosporin and other agents, use of antithymocyte globulin continues in many centres, on the grounds of efficacy, cost and side-effect profile. Production difficulties and inconsistencies, however, continue to hamper its use.

OKT3

An alternative to a polyclonal anti T lymphocyte preparation became available with monoclonal antibody technology. It became possible to select a single clone, producing antibody to a particular cell surface molecule. The most successful of these was an antibody directed at the CD3 molecule on the surface of all T lymphocytes, and subsequently marketed as OKT3. The CD3 molecule is integrally involved with the T cell receptor and acts as the signal transducer for the receptor. A T lymphocyte without CD3 is not functional, thus the antibody OKT3 is directed at all functional T cells. Furthermore, the antibody, which leads to clearance of all circulating T lymphocytes initially, can effectively block the action of the T cell receptor without actually killing the cell. Indeed after the first few days of treatment, T lymphocytes reappear in the circulation, but they are without the CD3 molecule and T cell receptor, and thus functionally blind.

OKT3 is an effective prophylactic agent when used for the first 10–14 days after transplantation; it is also effective at reversing acute rejection. The studies comparing antithymocyte globulin with OKT3 suffer from the variability of the former, some showing equal efficacy and some less. Similarly there are conflicts over which provides the greatest number of serious side effects. Like the polyclonal preparations, OKT3 leads to a high incidence of CMV infection 5–10 days after treatment. The major difference is the 'first dose effect' of OKT3, probably due to rapid lysis of circulating T cells and release of tumour necrosis factor. Pyrexia, chills and malaise accompany the first dose in 80% of patients, but may extend to a more serious syndrome with hypotension and pulmonary oedema. Because of this syndrome it is vital to ensure that the patient is not fluid overloaded or in incipient pulmonary oedema before the dose is given.

New agents

There is a variety of new agents which are being assessed for their role in transplantation. There are, for example, a number of research strategies which centre around induction of donor-specific tolerance, including total lymphoid irradiation and simultaneous donor bone marrow transplantation. New monoclonal antibodies have been developed and are undergoing clinical trials, with specificities for molecules such as CD4, present on all helper T lymphocytes, or the interleukin 2 receptor. There are three drugs which appear to have significant immunosuppressive actions: FK506

and Rapamycin have mechanisms of action similar to cyclosporin; RS61443 on the other hand acts via inhibition of purine metabolism and thus lymphocyte proliferation. FK506 has been subjected to trial in the largest number of patients and appears to have many of the attributes and disadvantages of cyclosporin. While it may confer advantages in liver transplantation, the trials of FK506 in renal transplant recipients are currently being undertaken.

IMMUNOSUPPRESSIVE REGIMENS

The drugs that can be used to prevent and treat rejection of the kidney can be combined in many ways. The aim of treatment is to provide sufficient prophylactic immunosuppression to prevent graft loss, but without causing significant toxic side effects. To achieve this, most centres use an induction regimen during the first weeks or months after transplantation, followed by maintenance therapy with lower doses and often fewer drugs. In addition each centre has a method for treatment of acute rejection.

Induction

The combination of cyclosporin, azathioprine and prednisolone is currently used by most groups for initial therapy. The advantage of using the triple therapy is that, while the immunosuppressive effects of the individual drugs are additive, the side effects are markedly less because the drugs can be used at lower dosages. When used alone, cyclosporin requires a dosage of 17.5 mg/kg/day for effective immunosuppression, while in a triple therapy combination a dose of 8 mg/kg/day is more usual. Similarly, azathioprine was used at 2.5–3.0 mg/kg/day when combined only with steroids, while the dose is 1.0–1.5 mg/kg/day with triple therapy. Corticosteroids were once used in high doses, commencing at 60–120 mg/day, but it was shown that even in combination with azathioprine alone, a reduction of dose to 30 mg/day did not alter graft survival. There are some centres which rely on the combination of cyclosporin and azathioprine alone in order to avoid using corticosteroids. A difficulty with triple therapy is that when the graft suffers from acute tubular necrosis, cyclosporin delays recovery of function. For this reason some centres use a sequential therapy in which ATG or OKT3 is used for the first 10–14 days in conjunction with the other agents but with the omission or restriction of cyclosporin until graft function becomes adequate.

Maintenance

In the long term, the risks of malignancy and opportunistic infection relate to the amount of immunosuppression that the patient is given. The aim of long-term therapy is thus to reduce both the number of drugs and their doses. Stopping either cyclosporin, azathioprine or corticosteroids is practised in many centres. However the controlled trials of stopping one or another drug have yet to show convincing advantages. Most groups reduce doses of all three drugs after the first two to three months, but maintain triple therapy. In children and diabetics there is added impetus to avoid corticosteroids if possible. The long-term maintenance doses for most patients would be in the order of: cyclosporin 2–5 mg/kg/day, azathioprine 1–1.5 mg/ kg/day, and prednisolone 5–10 mg/day.

Acute rejection

Treatment of acute rejection is designed to provide a short intense period of immunosuppression during which the heightened rejection activity and the inflammatory mediators of graft damage are brought under control. The mainstay of treatment has been high dose intravenous corticosteroids, e.g methylprednisolone 500–1000 mg daily for 3–5 days. The penalty for use of such therapy is a high incidence of avascular necrosis affecting the hip or other susceptible sites. Both antithymocyte globulin and OKT3 offer effective alternatives, but their use is limited both by cost and by the fact that the patient's response to the first course may preclude subsequent courses. There is also reluctance to accept the high risk of cytomegalovirus, other opportunistic infections, and lymphoma. Most units reserve use of ATG or OKT3 for the situation of steroid-resistant rejection.

COMPLICATIONS OF RENAL TRANSPLANTATION AND IMMUNOSUPPRESSION

Infection

Infective complications are the commonest cause of morbidity and early mortality in transplant recipients. Infections include septicaemia and those affecting the lungs, urinary tract, transplant wound, central nervous system, shunt sites and sites of needle punctures. Susceptibility is greatest in the early postoperative weeks during the period of most intense immunosuppression. It may be heightened by the occurrence of drug-induced bone marrow suppression. This complication carries additional threats in that severe thrombocytopenia may develop.

The recipient is susceptible to organisms normally regarded as commensals and saprophytes, as well as to common bacterial infections. In addition, viral, fungal and protozoal infections may occur. While bacterial infections often respond dramatically to appropriate antibiotics, there is a danger that their successful eradication may be followed by viral or fungal overgrowth.

The type of infection to which patients are susceptible changes with the time after transplantation. In the first days and weeks, wound, intravenous line and chest infections provide the greatest risks. Infection must always be suspected in any febrile patient, though rejection is a common cause of pyrexia at this time. The principle of diagnosis, followed by treatment, has to be eschewed in favour of taking all appropriate bacteriological specimens followed by urgent broad spectrum treatment of the likely organisms, with subsequent refinement of antibiotic specificity when results become available.

A new series of risks develop after the immediate postoperative period. Pneumonia due either to conventional organisms such as *Haemophilus influenzae* or opportunistic organisms such as *Legionella* species may occur and progression can be rapid. Cytomegalovirus and *Pneumocystis carinii* infections are particular threats. The latter presents with progressive onset of dyspnoea, low blood oxygen saturations and diffuse 'ground glass' changes on the chest X-ray. The peak incidence is in the third postoperative month, in patients who have not received prophylaxis, but it must always be considered in transplant recipients with pneumonia. In patients with chest infections the specific diagnosis often requires cytological examination of bronchoalveolar lavage fluid. Systemic infections with listeria, aspergillus, candida and viral infections such as herpes simplex, varicella/zoster and Epstein–Barr may all cause threats to life. In the longer term, organisms such as toxoplasma, cryptococcus, atypical mycobacteria, hepatitis B and hepatitis C add to the list of potential concerns. Urinary tract infections are frequent and include graft and native kidney pyelonephritis. They can be diagnosed and monitored by regular midstream urine culture.

Cytomegalovirus

Cytomegalovirus (CMV) infection has become both a more frequent complication and less of a concern during the last few years. The incidence of CMV disease has increased with use of anti T lymphocyte preparations such as ATG and OKT3. Indeed CMV is almost entirely predictable 5–10 days after a second course of one of these agents. On the other hand, there is now effective treatment in the form of ganciclovir. Before this agent became available there was an appreciable mortality associated with the treatment of acute rejection.

Depending upon the age of the patient 60–80% will have evidence of previous infection by CMV. Donors have a similar incidence of past infection and transmit dormant virus with either blood transfusion or the kidney allograft. CMV becomes pathogenic in transplant recipients from primary infection or from reactivation of latent donor or recipient virus. Primary disease occurs in patients with no previous exposure and presents between 3 and 8 weeks after transplantation. Secondary disease commonly occurs either 8–12 weeks after transplantation or 10 days after OKT3 therapy.

Primary disease tends to be more aggressive than secondary, but both may involve bone marrow suppression, hepatitis, pneumonitis, retinitis and gastroenteritis. The classic clinical picture is of a patient with general malaise and a high swinging fever. The fever may resolve spontaneously over 1–2 weeks or the infection may progress to organ involvement. Serological diagnosis usually follows clinical certainty, though culture of the buffy coat of blood, with specific immunofluorescence detection, is becoming rapid enough to be useful. Treatment is with intravenous ganciclovir for 2–3 weeks at a dose appropriate to the level of the patient's renal function.

Prophylaxis

Prophylaxis in transplant recipients is directed at the prevention of wound infection, pneumocystis pneumonia, urinary tract infection and viral infections. In specific patients at risk of tuberculosis, prophylaxis also includes isoniazid.

General surgical measures and perioperative intravenous treatment with a broad spectrum antibiotic prevent most wound infections. The incidence of both *Pneumocystis carinii* and urinary tract infections can be greatly reduced by use of co-trimoxazole, the former requiring only one tablet daily for the first six months. Acyclovir has been used to reduce the incidence of herpes virus infections. While it is undoubtedly helpful in preventing herpes simplex and in high doses for treating both herpes simplex and varicella/zoster, its efficacy for prophylaxis of both varicella/zoster and CMV is in doubt.

Cardiovascular

Cardiovascular disease is the single largest cause of mortality in patients with renal failure. While infections are the most frequent cause of mortality in the early period after transplantation, death from myocardial infarction is the major long-term risk. Obesity, hypertension, hyperlipidaemia, hyperuricaemia and impaired glucose tolerance— well-known risk factors for cardiovascular disease —are all prevalent in transplant recipients. Preventive measures directed at these risk factors must therefore be pursued vigorously. Control of obesity is a difficult problem in patients on corticosteroid therapy, particularly for those recently released from the dietary restrictions of dialysis as a result of successful transplantation. Hypertension occurs in up to 90% of patients and requires aggressive drug treatment. There are difficulties with effective drug treatment for hyperlipidaemia because of a risk of interaction between HMG CoA reductase inhibitors and immunosuppressive drugs, and similarly for hyperuricaemia, because of the interaction between allopurinol and azathioprine.

Malignancy

Another concern is the increased occurrence of cancer in transplant recipients. Factors which may be involved in the aetiology of increased cancer risk include the effects of uraemia, decreased immune surveillance, oncogenic viruses, failure of feedback immunoregulation, chronic antigenic stimulation and a direct neoplastic action of immunosuppressive agents. The incidence of de novo cancer in allograft recipients has been reported to be 6%, which is approximately 100 times greater than in the age-matched general population. However, in patients surviving 15–20 years following transplantation, the proportion with malignancy other than of the skin rises to 20%.

Although, with time, most cancers common in the general population are being documented with increased frequency in transplant recipients, a common early malignancy is lymphoma. This may arise either as a discrete or multifocal lesion, or may be part of a more general post-transplant lymphoproliferative disorder. The malignant lymphomas constitute 12% of non-skin malignancies in transplant recipients and have an unusual tendency to involve the central nervous system. The most significant risk factor is intense immunosuppresion, particularly with ATG or OKT3. There is increasing evidence that viruses, particularly the Epstein–Barr virus, may be implicated in their aetiology. Kaposi sarcoma, a malignancy common in AIDS but rare in general populations other than South Africa, also occurs with greatly increased frequency, as do cancers of the vulva and vagina, liver and oesophagus. Viruses are thought to be implicated in all of these malignancies. Amongst the more usual cancers, those that affect the genitourinary tract are the most common. In general, malignancies occurring in transplant recipients behave in an aggressive fashion. In 'high risk' areas for skin cancer there is a special problem, as skin changes culminating in aggressive squamous cell carcinoma occur in up to 60% of long-term transplant survivors.

FOLLOW-UP AND REHABILITATION

Unlike other successful operations, long-term success requires careful follow-up of transplant recipients by their clinicians. They need continuing specialist review for life. After discharge from hospital, patients thus attend transplant clinics at least three times weekly for the first three months. At each visit the patient is examined carefully, and special attention is paid to the early detection of rejection or of urinary infection and the presence or absence of hypertension. The graft is examined for tenderness and swelling. Blood is taken for estimation of immunosuppressive drug (cyclosporin) levels, serum electrolytes, haemoglobin and haematocrit, and for differential white cell count and platelet count. Urine specimens are cultured and tested for blood, protein, glucose and bile. The urinary sediment is examined by microscopy. Results for each patient are entered on a 'flow sheet' which records all investigative and clinical parameters from the time of operation.

Patients are asked to keep a record of their temperatures, urine outputs, weights and drug therapies. They are advised to telephone or report to hospital if they feel unwell, develop a fever, or notice oliguria or sudden weight gain. The interval between out-patient attendances is gradually increased until eventually, when graft function is stable, patients can be reviewed every three months.

Within months of successful transplantation, well-motivated patients are usually fully rehabilitated to employment or household duties. Children show increased growth rate. Sexual drive returns in adult males and females become fertile.

Prednisolone, azathioprine and cyclosporin do not appear to be teratogenic in the doses used, and though many pregnancies are successful there is an increased risk of toxaemia, miscarriage and graft loss. This increased risk is largely related to hypertension and abnormal renal function. The overall aim of transplantation is, however, to return patients to a normal existence and lifestyle, an aim which can be realized in about 60% of patients.

RECOMMENDED READING

Brent L (ed) 1991 Transplantation. Current Opinion in Immunology 3: 707–751
Mathew T H 1991 Recurrent disease after renal transplantation. Transplantation Reviews 5: 31–45

Morris P J (ed) 1988 Kidney transplantation — principles and practice, 3rd ed. W B Saunders, Philadelphia

Miscellaneous

SECTION VII

Miscellaneous

25. The kidney in pregnancy

E. D. M. Gallery   M. A. Brown

INTRODUCTION

In this relatively brief review, we have summarized changes which occur in the anatomy and physiology of the urinary tract in normal pregnancy, and then considered separately the types of renal disease and hypertension most commonly found in association with pregnancy. The reader is referred to the attached bibliography for more detailed information about the pathophysiology and management of the diseases discussed.

RENAL PHYSIOLOGY

Many changes occur in both anatomy and function of the urinary tract in response to normal pregnancy. These changes must be taken into account in any consideration of renal disease.

In normal pregnancy the kidneys increase slightly in size, probably due to swelling rather than to true anatomical hypertrophy. There is dilatation of the renal pelvis and ureters, which may be considerable. This results in a marked increase in the urinary dead space and makes measurement of renal function somewhat more difficult than in the non-pregnant woman; in addition, it increases the risk of ascending infection in women with asymptomatic bacilluria.

There are significant changes in all aspects of renal function, the extent variable among subjects. Renal blood flow is increased by 20%–40%, glomerular filtration rate by 30%–60%. Tubular functions at all levels are also altered, with a rise in uric acid clearance, a concomitant fall in phenolsulfonphthalein (PSP) excretion, and significant diminution in maximal urinary concentrating abil-

ity. There is a dual disturbance in acid–base balance, with respiratory alkalosis counterbalanced by a metabolic acidosis, and the urinary acidification mechanisms resemble those seen in the chronically acid-loaded non-pregnant subject, probably reflecting maternal excretion of the end products of fetal metabolism.

Although these alterations in glomerular and tubular function all tend to cause sodium and water depletion (as does progesterone, secreted in great amounts in normal pregnancy), pregnancy is a condition characterized overall by salt and water retention, with significant increases in plasma and extracellular volumes and total body water. This is achieved predominantly by increased oestrogen secretion and physiological secondary hyperaldosteronism. There is relative hypotension due to progesterone-induced vasodilatation, and a compensatory rise in cardiac output. There is good evidence that women who have the greatest degree of salt and water retention have bigger babies and a lower incidence of premature labour and perinatal mortality.

PRE-ECLAMPSIA

The potential for previously normal pregnant women to develop hypertension, with or without proteinuria, has been recognized for many years. This syndrome has been known by many names, including toxaemia of pregnancy and pre-eclampsia; in line with recommendations by the Australian Society for the Study of Hypertension in Pregnancy, the term pre-eclampsia will be used throughout to refer to this specific hypertensive disorder of pregnancy. Although this is a common disorder, affecting 10–15% of women having their first baby and 2–5% of multigravid women, its ultimate cause (or causes) remains ill-defined.

There are many theories as to the cause of pre-eclampsia, the currently most popular being immunological, with vascular endothelial damage (either immunologically mediated or non-specific) resulting in the release of vasoactive substances, vasoconstriction, altered vascular permeability and secondary coagulation abnormalities. Whatever the original cause, the ultimate pathway leads to generalized vasoconstriction, plasma volume contraction and alterations in renal tubular function, followed in severe cases by a fall in total renal blood flow and glomerular filtration rate, with the appearance of proteinuria. In the severe syndrome there are also changes of variable degree in the function of other organs, including liver, heart, lungs and brain.

Most women at risk of developing pre-eclampsia can be identified by serial measurements of plasma volume and proximal renal tubular function (by PSP excretion, uric acid clearance, or even serum uric acid levels). These tests are of value in assessing the prognosis of the index pregnancy, as there is a good correlation with fetal outcome. Plasma volume contraction (haemoconcentration) and rapidly rising serum uric acid levels have been shown to be predictive of fetal death in utero. In clinical practice, serial measurements are made of (i) haematocrit to give a rough estimate of plasma volume changes, (ii) serum uric acid, and (iii) platelet count (a sensitive indicator of disseminated coagulation).

The major risks of pre-eclampsia to the fetus are the same as those of chronic hypertension, i.e. placental insufficiency and abruption, and spontaneous premature labour. The magnitude of the clinical problem is related to the stage of pregnancy at which it appears and the speed of progression of the underlying disease process. As its causation is still poorly understood, therapy is not entirely satisfactory. In mild forms of the syndrome, pregnancy can often be prolonged by treatment of the hypertension, but in the more rapidly progressive forms — characterized by severe hypertension, heavy proteinuria, gross hyperreflexia and vasospasm, and by deteriorating renal and hepatic function — early delivery may offer the compromised fetus the only chance of survival. The hypertension will endanger maternal welfare if rapidly progressive, so that early delivery may be necessary to protect the mother from the complications of malignant hypertension, as well as from the dangers of disseminated intravascular coagulation and its attendant multiorgan failure.

CHRONIC HYPERTENSION

A young woman's first contact with the medical profession may be during pregnancy and about 5% will be found to have hypertension (without renal functional abnormality). The majority of these women will have essential hypertension, but secondary causes (as outlined in Table 25.1) must be excluded, either during the index pregnancy or at its conclusion. Phaeochromocytoma is a rare cause of hypertension in pregnancy but, if undiagnosed, it carries a 50% risk of maternal mortality and a greater than 90% risk of perinatal mortality, particularly around the time of delivery, because of uncontrolled catecholamine secretion, resulting in life-threatening blood pressure instability. Fibromuscular dysplasia of the renal arteries, although a relatively uncommon cause of chronic hypertension in the population at large, is classically a disorder of young women. It has particular potential significance in pregnancy because of the potential for aneurysm formation (and rupture) in association with the post-stenotic dilatation which is a feature of significant degrees of stenosis. Because of these potentially catastrophic consequences, consideration should be given to these two diagnoses in all women with hypertension in pregnancy.

The majority of women with chronic essential hypertension have an uncomplicated pregnancy, with a fall in blood pressure in early and mid-pregnancy followed by a return to pre-pregnancy levels during the third trimester. A sizable minority (25–30%), however, do not follow this benign course and will require antihypertensive therapy for much of their pregnancy. A chronically hypertensive woman is at increased risk of developing accelerated hypertension during pregnancy, and her fetus is at increased risk from spontaneous

Table 25.1   Causes of hypertension in pregnancy

Diagnosis	Commonly found features/clues
Essential	Family history
	Investigations normal
Pre-eclampsia	Primigravid/late pregnancy
	S. uric acid/Proteinuria±
Renal disease	
Glomerular	Proteinuria
Tubulointerstitial	GFR
Vascular	Urinary casts
Renovascular (renal artery stenosis)	Bruit
Adrenal:	
Cushing's syndrome	Glucose intolerance/Cushingoid features
Conn's syndrome	Nocturia/hypokalaemia/PRA aldosterone
Phaeochromocytoma	Episodic hypertension/U. catecholamines
Ovarian:	
Stein–Leventhal syndrome	Hirsutism/irregular menstruation
Oral contraceptive induced	Relevant history

abortion, spontaneous premature labour and placental separation. Placental insufficiency with intrauterine fetal growth retardation is also common. There is no doubt, however, that these risks can be minimized by control of hypertension, which is mandatory at all stages of pregnancy.

Pregnant women with chronic essential hypertension experience the normal physiological alterations in renal function and salt and water balance if their blood pressure control is satisfactory. If it is uncontrolled, however, they will develop abnormalities similar to those of severe pre-eclampsia, with haemoconcentration, hyperuricaemia and coagulation disturbances. The same laboratory tests are therefore used to monitor their welfare during pregnancy.

A detailed discussion of the specific indications for therapy and of the most appropriate antihypertensives to use in pregnancy is outside the scope of this chapter and can be found elsewhere. Therapy is commenced at any time before the onset of labour if the sitting diastolic blood pressure remains above 90 mmHg on at least two occasions 24 hours apart. Antihypertensive therapy is adjusted as necessary to lower the blood pressure to 85 mmHg or below. Angiotensin-converting enzyme inhibitors and diuretics are avoided in most patients. Both maternal and fetal well-being are monitored closely, the former by frequent clinical examination and serial estima-

tions of haematocrit, platelet count and serum uric acid, the latter by fetal movement records, by serial ultrasonic evaluation of growth and by unstressed cardiotocography. The newer modality of umbilical venous waveform analysis is still at an experimental stage of development, and is not recommended for guidance of management decisions at the present time. Termination of the pregnancy may be recommended for either maternal or fetal indications and pregnancy is not continued beyond 40 weeks of gestation.

RENAL DISEASE

Primary renal disease and pregnancy have been known to coexist for most of this century. Undoubtedly, diseases such as chronic glomerulonephritis, brought to light by medical examination during pregnancy, have often been confused with severe PIH, because of their common manifestations of hypertension and proteinuria. No data are available for the prevalence of the various forms of chronic renal disease in pregnancy, and few authors have tried to classify the spectrum of renal disease which they have seen in association with pregnancy. Some such attempts are shown in Table 25.2, and even these suffer from their retrospective nature (which means that patients who have had problems during pregnancy will be over-represented) and from

Table 25.2 Primary diagnosis in patients with renal disease in pregnancy

Author	Year	Country	No. of patients	Percentage of patients with				
				GN	IN	HN	PCK	Other
Mackay	1963	Australia	150	50	22	17	3	8
Felding	1968	Sweden	511	25	48	0	2	25
Katz et al	1980	USA+UK	89	49	24	10	1	16

GN — glomerulonephritis; IN — interstitial nephritis; HN — hypertensive nephrosclerosis; PCK — polycystic kidneys.

differences in study design. The Swedish study listed, although large, has this defect, as patients were selected for a history of renal disease rather than hypertension, and emphasis was placed on records of radiographic examinations and urine cultures rather than renal biopsies, as was the case in the combined English and North American study.

The following areas will be considered in this section:

1. Chronic renal parenchymal disease
2. Urinary tract infection
3. Acute renal failure
4. Dialysis during pregnancy
5. Renal transplantation.

1. Chronic renal parenchymal disease

For many years the presence of any renal disease was seen as a contraindication to pregnancy or an indication for early termination. 'A patient with chronic glomerulonephritis, nephrosis, nephrosclerosis or with renal impairment should not become pregnant. If she is seen in the first half of pregnancy, an abortion should be performed and future pregnancies prevented' (Dieckmann 1941). It was generally believed not only that pregnancy would inevitably hasten the advance of maternal disease, but also that there was little, if any, chance of a successful outcome of pregnancy. Later authors challenged this view, and recent advances have allowed the selection of patients with renal disease who are at particularly high risk of fetal complications (e.g. spontaneous abortion, placental insufficiency, premature labour) and maternal complications (e.g. acceleration of the course of renal disease).

Glomerulonephritis

There are now reports dealing with fetal and maternal renal outcome from over 700 pregnancies in women with various forms of glomerulonephritis. These data are listed in Table 25.3. It is of note that in one third of those who were found to have a decline in glomerular filtration rate during pregnancy, this deterioration was irreversible. However, since most of the information reported has been gathered retrospectively, it is likely to represent the more severe end of the spectrum, with patients coming to notice because of the development of complications. Advice given to the pregnant woman with known glomerulonephritis therefore requires consideration of (i) the histological type of glomerulonephritis, (ii) the time of diagnosis and (iii) the presence of features known to have an adverse effect on pregnancy outcome.

Table 25.3 Pregnancy outcomes in renal parenchymal disease.
(Figures are estimates based on largely retrospective data.)

	GN %	RN %	DN %
Maternal complications			
Hypertension*	25–50	20	80
Proteinuria**	30–50	?	~100#
Fall in GFR	10–15	3	?
Fetal complications			
Spontaneous abortion	5	7	5
Fetal growth retardation	15–20	?	20
Perinatal mortality	10–15	6	6

GN — primary glomerulonephritis; RN — reflux nephropathy; DN — diabetic nephropathy; * — development of superimposed pre-eclampsia; ** — development or worsening of proteinuria during pregnancy, and may include development of superimposed pre-eclampsia; # — 75% of these women had nephrotic syndrome.

(i) Type of glomerulonephritis. There are limited data on this issue but it appears that diffuse mesangial proliferative glomerulonephritis with no immunoglobulin A (IgA) deposition carries a good prognosis for pregnancy while the reported outcome has been less successful in terms of both maternal and fetal welfare for membranous nephritis, focal and segmental glomerulosclerosis, and perhaps mesangiocapillary glomerulonephritis. Conflicting reports have been published for women with IgA nephropathy.

(ii) Time of diagnosis. As alluded to above, discovery of renal disease during or immediately after pregnancy is associated with a worse prognosis for the pregnancy, as these women are a selected population because of the development of complications such as accelerated hypertension. In women whose renal disease is diagnosed before pregnancy there is a much better fetal outcome, with reported perinatal mortality rates below 5%.

(iii) Presence of adverse features. The presence of hypertension (>140/90 mmHg), proteinuria or a serum creatinine above 0.13 mmol/l at conception is associated with a higher incidence of spontaneous abortion. Prematurity and perinatal mortality rates as high as 30–40% are reported, compared with 10–15% and 5% respectively for women with normal BP, no proteinuria and a serum creatinine below 0.13 mmol/l.

Reflux nephropathy

This disorder is much more common in females than in males. At least 70% are younger than 40 years of age at presentation and up to one third present due to a complication of pregnancy. Again, the data are largely retrospective, but some general principles have emerged (Table 25.3). The overall fetal loss rate is about 15%, the major determinants of fetal outcome being the serum creatinine at conception and the development of superimposed pre-eclampsia. In those whose initial serum creatinine is below 0.12 mmol/l, the fetal loss rate is marginally higher than that of normal pregnancy, but it is close to 20% in women whose initial serum creatinine is above 0.13 mmol/l, and more than 50% in those who start

pregnancy with a serum creatinine above 0.18 mmol/l.

Urinary tract infections occur in 30% of pregnant women with reflux nephropathy. While these require treatment to prevent pyelonephritis and worsening renal function, they do not appear to be associated with increased perinatal mortality provided that these complications can be prevented. About 3% of patients with reflux nephropathy will suffer a decline in their renal function, most commonly those with pre-existing impairment of renal function. Women with severe renal failure at conception may progress rapidly to end-stage renal failure, requiring dialysis post-partum. It is not possible to gauge accurately from published reports whether this represents the natural history of the disease in these women, or whether it is related specifically to the index pregnancy. It appears, however, that pregnancy is inadvisable in this group of patients, with progressive renal failure and a potentially limited life span.

Diabetic nephropathy

The hallmark of this disorder is proteinuria. As hypertension occurs in over half these women during pregnancy, it is often difficult to make an accurate distinction between diabetic nephropathy and proteinuric pre-eclampsia. Overall fetal survival is good in the patient with relative preservation of renal function (Table 25.3). Although small increments in maternal serum creatinine are common, pregnancy does not seem to cause acceleration of diabetic nephropathy. Hypertension and proteinuria usually settle to pre-conception values after delivery. There are few data concerning pregnancy in women with advanced renal failure due to diabetic nephropathy, but it is likely that all complications are increased in this situation.

Adult polycystic renal disease

It is uncommon for renal failure due to polycystic kidneys to be present in women of childbearing age, although hypertension is often well established at the time of conception. With appropriate treatment of hypertension, the pregnancy outlook is excellent and there is no evidence that pregnancy accelerates the rate of decline in renal function. Since it has an autosomal dominant pattern of inheritance, pre-conception counselling is essential for all patients with polycystic renal disease.

General management principles

It is clear that for all renal parenchymal diseases the factors present at conception which convey the worst prognosis are:

1. Elevated serum creatinine (probably above 0.12 mmol/l and certainly above 0.18 mmol/l)
2. Hypertension
3. Proteinuria.

Major risks developing during pregnancy are:

1. Superimposed pre-eclampsia
2. Urinary tract infection.

Management therefore requires:

a. Pre-conceptional counselling to alert prospective parents to the potential risks for the planned pregnancy, for long-term renal function and for the transmission of hereditary diseases (e.g. adult polycystic renal disease).

b. Close supervision during pregnancy, usually fortnightly up to about 32 weeks and weekly thereafter. In addition to a full history and thorough physical examination, tests at the first visit should include estimation of glomerular filtration rate (GFR) (endogenous creatinine clearance), serum electrolytes, albumin, uric acid and full blood count, and 24-hour urinary protein excretion if dipstick urinalysis is positive ($\geq 1+$). These tests should be repeated approximately every 6 weeks if the patient is well. After the initial visit, serum creatinine is a sufficient estimate of GFR, although it should be remembered that autoanalyser estimates of serum creatinine will show an increase in the last month of normal pregnancy, without any fall in GFR. Protein excretion is increased in most pregnancies in parallel with increased GFR, so that a 50% increase in pre-existing proteinuria from pre-conception values may not indicate worsening renal

disease. Monitoring of fetal well-being should include serial ultrasound estimation of growth and intermittent unstressed cardiotocography after 28 weeks' gestation. This area is dealt with in more detail elsewhere in this review.

c. Tight control of hypertension from early pregnancy. Should hypertension accelerate or develop de novo during pregnancy in women with primary renal disease, a careful clinical and laboratory search should be made for the presence of superimposed pre-eclampsia, as this conveys a worse prognosis for both mother and fetus. This distinction may not always be possible and the safest option is to assume its presence, treat hypertension aggressively and monitor mother and fetus accordingly.

2. Urinary tract infection

Asymptomatic bacteriuria occurs in 5–7% of pregnancies. Early studies reported that this was associated with intrauterine growth retardation, hypertension and premature labour, but this has not been confirmed by more recent reports. However, the 30–35% risk of acute pyelonephritis makes antibiotic treatment mandatory. Bacteriuria recurs in almost 30% of these women. If there are two recurrences despite adequate antibiotic therapy, then suppressive treatment is indicated for the remainder of the pregnancy (e.g. amoxycillin 250 mg nocte, or cephalexin 250 mg nocte).

Acute pyelonephritis occurs in about 1% of pregnancies, most commonly in the population with asymptomatic bacteriuria. *Esch. coli* remains the most common pathogen. Clinical features include loin pain, fever and rigors, but symptoms do not always localize the infection to the kidney. Transient worsening of renal function is common and bacteraemia occurs in 15–20%, but septic shock is rare.

Treatment with intravenous ampicillin or cephalosporin plus aminoglycoside may be necessary for the first 48 hours or longer, until the patient is afebrile. The potential of aminoglycosides for maternal and fetal ototoxicity is a concern and these should be withdrawn once the patient is afebrile. Oral antibiotics should be continued for 2–3 weeks after the initial response. Failure to respond within 72 hours should prompt a thorough search for anatomical renal abnormalities or stones. Oral quinolones (e.g. norfloxacin, ciprofloxacin) should be avoided during pregnancy.

3. Acute renal failure (ARF)

Thirty years ago, the incidence of ARF in pregnancy was 1/2000–1/5000, and 20% of all cases of ARF occurred in association with pregnancy. Many of these cases were due to septic abortion, but with altered abortion laws and better understanding of renal disease in pregnancy, its incidence has fallen to 1/10 000–1/35 000. Maternal mortality is less than 15%, considerably lower than that of ARF in non-obstetric settings.

ARF most commonly occurs in the third trimester as a result of pre-eclampsia, antepartum haemorrhage or, more rarely, acute pyelonephritis or fatty liver of pregnancy. Another important cause of obstetric renal failure is idiopathic post-partum ARF — part of the haemolytic–uraemic syndrome/thrombotic thrombocytopenic purpura spectrum of diseases. This condition is rare, but there is evidence suggestive of an increase in incidence. Typically it occurs in a multipara from 1–80 days post-partum, and may follow a 'flu-like illness. The patient has oliguric renal failure with microangiopathy, usually hypertension, and less commonly central nervous system abnormalities. Renal biopsy shows afferent arteriolar and capillary thrombi as well as endothelial cell swelling and a lucent subendothelial space which contains fibrin-like material. Blood vessels may show changes similar to scleroderma, and glomeruli may then exhibit ischaemic wrinkling.

Many cases of acute renal failure in pregnancy are preventable. The reduction in incidence over recent years is due to better understanding and control of precipitating events. This includes:

1. prompt and effective treatment of infection, particularly of the urinary tract;
2. adequate control of hypertension;
3. prompt and adequate replacement of blood loss;
4. avoidance of nephrotoxic agents; and
5. early and adequate replacement of electrolyte and fluid losses.

For patients with established acute renal failure during pregnancy, additional principles of management are:

1. Delivery of the fetus if fetal viability is likely. If ARF occurs too early in the pregnancy and there are no extra-renal manifestations which threaten the mother's safety, then dialysis may prolong pregnancy to a stage of fetal viability.
2. Administration of low-dose dopamine may be effective in some cases due to pre-eclampsia.
3. Plasma exchange and antiplatelet therapy (with or without prostacyclin infusions) may have a place in treatment of post-partum ARF, although there are as yet no evaluations of this treatment.

There is greater likelihood of the development of bilateral renal cortical necrosis when ARF occurs in pregnancy than in non-pregnant women, especially in multiparas following placental abruption. The diagnosis should be suspected if oliguria is prolonged, and can be confirmed by renal biopsy or selective renal angiography. The latter is preferred as the cortical necrosis is often 'patchy' in pregnancy. Renal function may recover slowly but incompletely for some months, and then deteriorate again, to require maintenance dialysis.

4. Dialysis during pregnancy

Dialysis has been used for the treatment of renal failure in pregnancy since the 1960s. There are many reports of successful pregnancy outcomes in women so treated, but these are of course skewed by the tendency to report only successful outcomes. Overall fetal survival is quoted at 20% but this includes women with residual renal function who later came off dialysis. There are two groups of women dialysed during pregnancy: those who conceive whilst already on dialysis (an uncommon event, because of the infertility which usually accompanies chronic renal failure), and those in whom dialysis becomes necessary after conception. The latter group has the better fetal outcome as well as the chance of recovering maternal renal function after the pregnancy.

Both haemodialysis and peritoneal dialysis, including CAPD, have been used successfully. Although never formally tested, it is usual practice to institute dialytic therapy at levels of blood urea about 15 mmol/l (i.e. much earlier than in the non-pregnant population), and aim to keep values at or below 10 mmol/l. The rationale is that fetal survival is only likely if the azotaemic 'milieu' is removed, though just which factors mediate the poor fetal outcome remain unknown. To achieve fetal survival daily dialysis may be required.

5. Renal transplantation

Successful renal transplantation restores fertility and 1 in 50 transplanted women of childbearing age will become pregnant. There are over 2000 such pregnancies reported. The spontaneous abortion rate of these women is no higher than that of the general population, although ectopic pregnancy may be slightly increased. Allograft function declines in about 15%, proteinuria may become severe in about 40%, and both these features are more likely to occur if pre-conception serum creatinine is above 0.18 mmol/l. Hypertension and/or pre-eclampsia occur in 30% of cases, but it is difficult to distinguish pre-eclampsia from declining allograft function, as usual markers such as proteinuria and hyperuricaemia may be present in either case. The main maternal worry is that of acute allograft rejection which occurs in about 9% of pregnancies. Overall, the pregnant woman has about a 50% chance of one of these complications occurring during pregnancy.

Fetal outcome is good — if complications occur after the 28th week then survival is above 90%, but earlier complications are associated with lower survival rates. About 50% of babies are born prematurely and 20% are small-for-dates. Despite immunosuppressive therapy during pregnancy, there does not appear to be an increased risk of congenital abnormality in offspring.

Thus, successful pregnancy can be achieved for mother and baby in women with a well-functioning renal allograft. The best outcomes are achieved if pre-conception serum creatinine is below 0.18 mmol/l, there is no or minimal proteinuria, blood pressure is well controlled, good general health has been maintained for two years post-transplant and immunosuppressant doses are minimal.

REFERENCES AND RECOMMENDED READING

Brown M A 1991 Pregnancy-induced hypertension: pathogenesis and management. Australian and New Zealand Journal of Medicine 21: 257–274
Davison J M 1987 Pregnancy in renal allograft recipients: prognosis and management. Bailliere's Clinical Obstetrics and Gynaecology 1: 1027–1045
Davidson J M 1987 Kidney function in pregnant women. American Journal of Kidney Diseases 9: 248–252
Felding C F 1968 Pregnancy following renal disease. Clinics in Obstetrics and Gynecology 11: 579–593
Gallery E D M, Boyce E S, Saunders D M, Gyory A Z 1991 Chronic hypertension in pregnancy. In: Cosmi EV, di Renzo GC (eds) hypertension in pregnancy — Proceedings of 7th World Congress of International Society for the Study of Hypertension in Pregnancy (Perugia, Italy, October 7–11, 1990). Monduzzi Editore, Bologna, pp 67–77
Hou S 1987 Pregnancy in women requiring dialysis for renal failure. American Journal of Kidney Diseases 9: 368–373

Katz A I, Davison J, Hayslett J P, Singson E, Lindheimer M D 1980 Pregnancy in women with kidney disease. Kidney International 18: 192–206
Lindheimer M D, Katz A I, Ganeval D, Grunfeld J P 1988 Acute renal failure in pregnancy. In: Brenner B M, Laazarus M J (eds) Acute renal failure. Churchill Livingstone, New York, pp 621–658
Mackay E V 1963 Pregnancy and renal disease: a ten year survey. Australian and New Zealand Journal of Obstetrics and Gynecology 3: 21–24
Packham D K, North R A, Fairley K F, Kloss M, Whitworth J A, Kincaid-Smith P 1989 Primary glomerulonephritis and pregnancy. Quarterly Journal of Medicine 71: 537–553
Pollak V E, Nettles J B 1960 The kidney in toxemia of pregnancy: a clinical and pathologic study based on renal biopsies. Medicine (Baltimore) 39: 469–526

26. Paediatric nephrology

L. P. Roy

INTRODUCTION

Apart from conditions which are uniformly lethal in the first few years of life, a physician dealing only with patients aged more than 14 years will occasionally be confronted by most, if not all, of the problems which confront the paediatric nephrologist.

This chapter will not deal comprehensively with all renal diseases affecting children. Conditions discussed in detail in other chapters (e.g. urinary tract infection, vesicoureteric reflux) are excluded, while those which mainly affect children and problems of growth and development are emphasized. Nevertheless it must be remembered that the natural history and incidence of diseases in children often differs from that in adults as well as from age group to age group throughout childhood.

ANTENATAL DIAGNOSIS OF URINARY TRACT ABNORMALITIES

Diagnostic ultrasonography has been used extensively in obstetric practice for some years, particularly for the estimation of gestational age and fetal growth. Enlarged fluid-filled spaces can also be demonstrated by this technique, in particular dilated urinary tracts associated with both obstructive and non-obstructive ureteric dilatation, and pelvi-ureteric junction obstruction. When the bladder is dilated but no neural tube defect is found or expected, and the baby can be shown to be male, a presumptive diagnosis of posterior urethral valves can be made and postnatal surgery may be facilitated. There is considerable contro-

versy about the use of intrauterine surgery for these problems. A number of ethical issues relating to the prognosis of the baby and the rights of the mother and the unborn child also require consideration.

Practical considerations

The major problem after diagnosis is the parental anxiety provoked by the knowledge that their baby probably has a renal abnormality, the severity of which may not be known until the baby is born. If the volume of amniotic fluid is normal, and the baby of normal size, the chances of satisfactory renal function are high. It may be possible to visualize a contralateral undilated system and this would make the prognosis more favourable. There is an increased risk of spontaneous premature delivery. If there is progressive bilateral dilatation, early delivery may be considered although the potential renal benefits, especially if there is major bilateral renal disease, must be balanced against the various problems of the premature baby.

Active prenatal intervention remains experimental. Vesicoamniotic shunting for posterior urethral valves has been done with favourable outcome but open fetal surgery still carries a high risk of early premature labour, and although satisfactory outcomes have been reported the relative risks and benefits remain to be determined. Where progressive bilateral dilatation and reduced amniotic fluid are observed, intervention or early delivery may be considered in an attempt to reduce renal morbidity and pulmonary hypoplasia. Hypotonic fetal urine (osmolality < 210 mosmol/l) and urine sodium < 100 mmol/l are additional adverse prognostic features. Other fetal anomalies should be excluded and fetal karyotype performed before intervention is considered.

In most instances the pregnancy can be allowed to proceed to term. Shortly after birth confirmatory ultrasound should be performed. Where an anomaly such as posterior urethral valves is confirmed plans for early surgical relief can be made.

Asymptomatic dilatation of the upper tracts is a common problem. If the baby is well and renal function normal there is benefit in delaying detailed investigation for 4–6 weeks. During that time considerable renal functional maturation occurs and obstruction may not be revealed. Prophylactic antibiotics should be commenced and continued until evaluation and definitive management are decided. Functional radionuclide assessment should be performed first (e.g. ^{99m}Tc-DTPA scan with induced diuresis) and if obstruction is excluded micturating cystogram completes an initial assessment.

THE NEWBORN

Development of renal function

Development of the definitive kidney begins at about the fifth week of gestation but is not complete until the end of the first 12–18 months of extrauterine life. Urine output commences at about the tenth week of gestation and by the 32nd week about 12 ml is produced per hour, increasing to about 28 ml per hour shortly before birth. Fetal urine is a major constituent of amniotic fluid and in the presence of markedly reduced renal function oligohydramnios can be expected.

The renal function of the fetus is not required for homeostasis as it is provided by the maternal kidney. Thus a neonate with bilateral renal agenesis whose mother has normal renal function will have a biochemistry pattern similar to that of the mother. The normal newborn infant often passes urine at delivery, but may not pass urine again for 48 hours, although most do. Strauss et al (1981) studied 17 healthy term babies and found that in the first three hours there was a rise, followed by a fall, in urine volumes, inulin clearance and p-aminohippuric

acid clearance. Urine osmolality tended to rise. At four hours, urine volume varied from 0.01–0.15 ml/min and urine osmolality from 240–520 mosmol/kg. From three days of age, the normal neonate has a urine output of 1–5 ml/kg per hour. The glomerular filtration rate (GFR) of the normal newborn at birth is 15–20 ml/min per 1.73 m^2, rising to 30–70 ml/min per 1.73 m^2 by the age of four weeks. Initial levels in premature babies are 10–20% lower but are equivalent by six weeks of age. Changes in GFR appear to be due to changes in renal vascular resistance and the maturation of the glomerulus, with rapidly increasing surface area and filtration coefficient. Serum creatinine levels depend on muscle mass and are thus lower in children than in adults. At birth the concentration reflects that of the mother. From the fifth day of life the value gradually declines to 30–40 μmol/l by day 14 and then rises progressively throughout childhood. Premature babies have higher levels and 80–100 μmol/l is not unusual in extremely premature (under 32 weeks) babies in the first few weeks of life in the absence of definable renal abnormalities. Although the intensely anabolic state of the neonate compensates to a certain degree for the relatively reduced excretory capacity the normal newborn resembles an older individual with moderate chronic renal failure. Therefore, when drugs are administered, adjustments in dosage and usage are required, in addition to those relating to body size and blood levels, and blood levels need to be monitored.

Acid–base control

The newborn baby has been said to have a physiological acidosis since the serum bicarbonate is normally 4–6 mmol/l lower than in older children or adults, where it is 20–25 mmol/l. The blood pH is 0.03–0.05 units less than in older children. Although there is a slight positive hydrogen ion balance, reduced buffering capacity is the important physiological corollary, and a sick baby (who may now be catabolic) becomes acidaemic faster and more profoundly than an older child. The ability to generate an acid urine pH is equivalent to that of older children, and the lower plasma bicarbonate is due to a lower renal threshold for bicarbonate, which is fixed at 20 mmol/l. In premature babies both the production of acid urine and net acid excretion are reduced in response to an ammonium chloride load, and they are at even greater risk of acidaemia and acidosis when stressed.

Salt and water

Newborn babies have a limited ability to conserve and excrete sodium chloride. Within the customary range (1–3 mmol/kg per day) normal neonates readily adapt. Higher sodium challenges (more than 10 mmol/kg per day), however, exceed the normal neonate's ability to excrete sodium, and hypernatraemia will ensue.

Infants of low birth weight may behave as salt-losers and, with no additional stress, develop marked hyponatraemic dehydration. The daily sodium requirements of such infants may be of the order of 10 mmol/kg and the 'salt-losing' phenomenon may persist for several weeks. Urinary tract infection and adrenogenital syndrome should be excluded, and an abdominal ultrasonographic examination should be considered.

The neonate is able to maximally dilute the urine by day five, but concentrating ability may not reach mature levels until 6–12 months of age. In the neonatal period maximal urine osmolality is 700–800 mosmol/kg. In relation to total water turnover of the baby, the water saved by increasing the concentration to 1200 mosmol/kg is not great, although it is of course significant. On the other hand, in spite of maximal diluting capacity, the neonate does not excrete a hypotonic load as rapidly as an adult, with the resultant risk of positive water balance and oedema. Plasma concentrations of renin, angiotensin and aldosterone are high in newborn infants and decrease during the first week of life, as does rate of synthesis of prostaglandins.

Clinical problems in the newborn

Abdominal mass

An abdominal mass which is not clearly due to an enlarged liver or spleen is most commonly due to an abnormality of the urinary tract. Mesenteric cysts and intestinal duplication are other possibilities.

The bladder

The bladder may be distended because of posterior urethral valves or because of a disturbance in nerve supply, e.g. in myelomeningocele. In the latter instance, urine can usually be expressed from the bladder. The neonatal bladder is an abdominal organ but its distension is sometimes not appreciated, as the baby's abdomen is often somewhat tense, especially in association with posterior urethral valves. Fullness of the lower abdomen is usually apparent and an area of dullness to percussion will be noted.

Posterior urethral valves

Not all children with posterior urethral valves present as neonates although up to one half present in the first three months of life. This sporadic condition is confined almost exclusively to males, although several cases have been described in girls. There is some difference of opinion as to incidence, as the commonest form is due to an apparent accentuation of the normal posterior urethral folds, and non-obstructive forms are included in some series. Three types have been described by Young. Type 1 valves, which pass from the verumontanum to the anterolateral urethral wall, are the commonest. Type 2 valves pass from the verumontanum towards the bladder neck, and type 3 are diaphragmatic valves located at the level of the verumontanum.

Initial presentation may be by antenatal ultrasonography. Infants present with urinary tract infections which are often severe, with sodium chloride depletion and renal insufficiency. There may be a history of a poor urinary stream. A lower abdominal mass may be noted and a poor urinary stream observed. In later infancy and early childhood intermittent dribbling may be the presentation, the bladder will usually be clearly distended and there may be growth failure if there is significant reduction in renal function failure.

The diagnosis is established by micturating cystourethrography and cystoscopy. At the time of cystoscopy, the valves are usually destroyed by diathermy. Critically ill babies require resuscitation, antibiotics and occasionally dialysis, with emergency relief of obstruction by nephrostomy and later elective destruction of the valves. Acute mortality has decreased dramatically in the past 15 years as a result of more effective antibiotics, improved surgical techniques and better resuscitation. The acute mortality is now less than 10% in those presenting in the first three months of life and considerably less in those presenting later. However, some of the children have other renal abnormalities (dysplasia or post-obstructive) which may lead to renal failure later. Most of these children have persisting urinary incontinence until puberty, when it tends to resolve with development of the prostate.

The kidney

Renal enlargement may be due to obstructive uropathy, cystic malformations, renal venous thrombosis or rarely tumour, and may be unilateral or bilateral. Grossly dilated ureters are sometimes palpable. Unilateral enlargement is usually due to pelvi-ureteric junction obstruction or multicystic dysplasia. Bilateral flank masses may be due to polycystic kidney disease (autosomal recessive 'infantile, or autosomal dominant 'adult'), bilateral pelvi-ureteric junction obstruction, bilateral multicystic dysplasia or renal venous thrombosis. Initial investigation by ultrasonography is followed by radionuclide imaging and functional studies and, if further investigation is required, by micturating cystourethrography, intravenous pyelography or computerized axial tomography.

Autosomal recessive (infantile) polycystic disease of the kidney. This condition may present in infancy or later in childhood. Those presenting in the neonatal period tend to have larger kidneys and a higher risk of early renal failure. However, many have satisfactory renal function and will continue well for years. In the newborn period, respiratory distress, pneumothorax and pulmonary interstitial emphysema occur with increased frequency. Salt wasting often impairs renal function during the first six to eight weeks of life. Hypertension is a frequent complication after the neonatal period. The kidneys are usually very large, but of normal shape. The cysts are small and due to dilatation of distal tubules and collecting ducts. Later there may be larger cysts and distortion of renal outline and the pelvicalyceal system. Most, if not all patients, have congenital hepatic fibrosis and older children may present with haematemesis due to bleeding varices. Cirrhosis and liver failure may develop, although this is said to be rare.

Although the severity varies significantly it tends to be similar among affected siblings.

Pelvi-ureteric junction obstruction. This may be of any degree and either unilateral or bilateral, although marked obstruction is usually unilateral and associated with fibrous constriction of the ureter. If differential renal scanning shows that the kidney provides more than 10% of total renal function, pyeloplasty may be considered, otherwise elective nephrectomy is preferred. The contralateral kidney is usually normal but, if it is affected, severe renal failure will be present.

Multicystic dysplasia. This is a sporadic condition which in 95% of cases is unilateral. When bilateral, it is incompatible with survival. The renal tissue is grossly malformed and there are no mature nephrons. Instead, primitive tubules, cysts of varying size, undifferentiated mesenchyme and multiple small arteries are seen. Stenosis or partial atresia of the associated ureter is common. The diagnosis is usually established by ultrasonography and radionuclide scans showing a cystic structure without function. Elective nephrectomy is the preferred treatment as the mass is usually very large.

Renal venous thrombosis. In neonates this usually occurs as a complication of severe hypoxia or sepsis. Renal venous thrombosis is more common in children of diabetic mothers. It often occurs in association with intravascular coagulation abnormalities and bleeding. Thrombocytopenia, often associated with a microangiopathic haemolytic anaemia, is an almost constant finding. When unilateral, the earliest signs are usually macroscopic haematuria and a large hard kidney. When bilateral, acute renal failure develops and, because of the resultant oliguria, haematuria may not be apparent. Ultrasonography showing a large kidney and increased parenchymal echoes with loss of

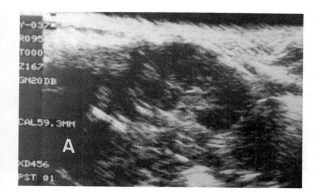
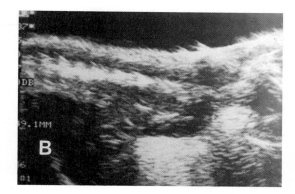
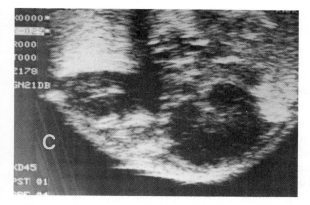
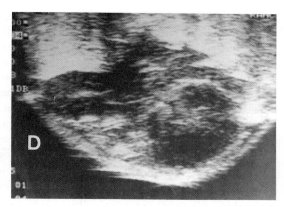

Fig. 26.1 Left renal venous thrombosis in a neonate. (**a**) Longitudinal section through the left kidney which is enlarged (6 cm). There is loss of definition of the corticomedullary junction. (**b**) Normal right kidney in longitudinal section. (**c** and **d**) Transverse views showing enlargement of the left kidney and change in echo pattern. (Reproduced by kind permission of Dr A Lam, Department of Radiology, Royal Alexandra Hospital for Children, Sydney.)

corticomedullary junction definition strongly supports the diagnosis (Fig. 26.1). Radionuclide scanning will show a non-functioning kidney. There is considerable controversy as to subsequent management. It is clear that the clotting mechanism begins in small veins in the parenchyma of the kidney and there is no evidence that anticoagulant, thrombolytic or surgical clot removal improves the prognosis. However, in over 50% of cases the vessels appear to recanalize, and spontaneous return to normal renal function may occur even after bilateral thrombosis. Therefore, management of the precipitating cause and supportive care is of paramount concern. The development of hypertension may be an indication for nephrectomy.

Acute renal failure (Table 26.1). Acute renal failure in the newborn is being increasingly recognized and better care facilities are now available for smaller babies. Problems secondary to renal hypoperfusion may not progress to oligo- and/or anuric renal failure, but salt wasting, further impairment of acid–base balance or increased fluid retention may complicate the baby's subsequent course. Acute renal failure should be suspected when urine output is less than 1 ml/kg per hour, and is confirmed by a rising serum creatinine. Much of neonatal renal failure is pre-renal and resolves with adequate resuscitation.

Renal failure due to hypoperfusion. This refers to the whole group of conditions leading to

Table 26.1 Aetiology of acute renal failure in the newborn

Pre-renal
  Maternal blood loss
  Feto–maternal transfusion
  Respiratory distress syndrome
  Asphyxia
  Sepsis
  Congenital heart disease, e.g. coarctation of the aorta,
  pulmonary atresia

Renal
  Congenital abnormalities, e.g. bilateral renal agenesis,
  bilateral multicystic kidney

Post-renal
  Posterior urethral valves
  Bilateral ureteric obstruction

Table 26.2 Differential diagnosis of pre-renal from intrinsic renal failure in the neonate

	Pre-renal	Intrinsic
Urine osmolarity mosmol/kg H_2O	> 400	< 400
Urine/plasma creatinine ratio	29 ± 16	10 ± 4
Fractional excretion sodium E Na %	< 2.5	> 2.5

hypotension or severe hypoxia. The neonatal kidney is prone to areas of cortical infarction following shock, and gross haematuria is not uncommon. Cortical infarction leads to permanent cortical scarring and a risk of early hypertension.

Bilateral renal agenesis (Potter's syndrome). This is a sporadic condition, occurring in about 1 per 5000 live births. The characteristic features are extreme oligohydramnios, typical physical appearance (see below) and early death from respiratory failure. These features are common to all babies with severe intrauterine renal functional impairment. They are often small and have a hyperflexed posture. The skin is redundant. The prominent facial features are a small mouth, medial canthic folds, a deep transverse cleft in the chin, and low-set or backward tilted ears which may be large but are flattened against the skull. The lungs are hypoplastic and dysplastic. The condition is incompatible with life.

Management of renal failure

The principles of management are essentially the same as for adults, with some additions. Resuscitation, correction of underlying abnormalities exclusion of obstruction and careful monitoring of weight, blood pressure, serum electrolytes, glucose and osmolality are of paramount important. In the differential diagnosis of pre-renal and intrinsic renal failure due to shock (Table 26.2), it must be remembered that sodium reabsorption and concentrating ability are already 'impaired'.

Ultrasonography, radionuclide scanning and micturating cystourethrography are important investigations. Intravenous pyelography is of limited value and gives the baby a substantial osmotic load.

Hypoglycaemia. Sick neonates are prone to hypoglycaemia and when fluid restriction becomes essential this may be the main indication for dialysis.

Fluid requirements. Insensible loss is about 200 ml/m^2 per day. Fluid should be given as 0.9% sodium chloride in 10% dextrose in the first instance. A variety of obligatory fluid inputs (e.g. arterial lines) can compromise fluid restriction.

Nutrition. This must be maintained orally or intravenously. Dialysis may be required to achieve adequate intake. The aim should be to provide 100 calories (420 kJ) and 1–2 g protein per kilogram body weight per day. For oral feeding, breast milk or a humanized milk formula should be used to provide the lowest solute load.

Dialysis. Peritoneal dialysis will be satisfactory in most instances. Haemodialysis, haemofiltration and continuous venovenous haemodiafiltration may be required where access to the peritoneal cavity is compromised. Most babies can tolerate 40–60 ml/kg body weight of dialysate in the peritoneal cavity, although very small premature babies may only tolerate much smaller volumes.

Triad syndrome (prune belly syndrome)

This syndrome (Fig. 26.2) is readily apparent at birth and may be diagnosed by antenatal ultrasonography. It is characterized by a variable degree of agenesis of the abdominal muscles, bilateral cryptorchidism and malformation of the urinary tract. Patients are usually male but a small number of female children with absent abdominal musculature, genital abnormalities and urinary

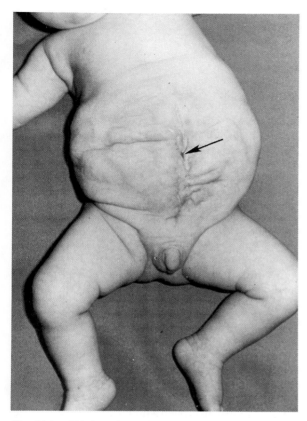

Fig. 26.2   Triad syndrome (prune belly syndrome) with the characteristic floppy wrinkled abdomen and hypoplastic scrotum. Note the patent urachus (arrow)

tract malformations have been described. The syndrome occurs sporadically. The skin of the abdominal wall is redundant and wrinkled and the abdominal viscera are readily palpable. The bladder is often distended. A few children have extremely poor renal function at birth but most have sufficient renal function for prolonged survival.

Pathology. The kidneys usually show some degree of dysplasia. The ureters tend to be dilated and tortuous. The bladder is large but non-trabeculated. A patent urachus may be present. The urethra may show stricture or atresia but usually has a dilated prostatic segment and a normal membranous portion, which may give the impression of a stricture or valve. Prostate tissue and pre-urethral muscle mass is reduced. The penis is often large.

Aetiology. There are three main theories of aetiology: (1) primary agenesis of the abdominal muscles, with passive bladder dilatation; (2) urethral obstruction in early gestation causing massive bladder dilatation with resultant atrophy of abdominal muscles; and (3) mesenchymal injury in the sixth to tenth week of gestation affecting the development of abdominal wall, kidneys, prostate and testes.

Management

If there is no frank obstruction, surgery is kept to a minimum. Prophylactic antibiotic therapy may be required if urine infection occurs. The lax abdomen often requires support once the child is walking. Surgical procedures to improve the musculature of the abdominal wall have had variable success. The testes are usually intra-abdominal. Normal puberty occurs but all patients have been infertile even after successful orchidopexy. End-stage renal failure may develop and the results of renal transplantation are equivalent to the general experience.

NEPHROTIC SYNDROME

Fifty years ago, a child with nephrotic syndrome had a less than 50% chance of surviving one year. Antibiotics and corticosteroids have altered this picture to the degree that most children with nephrotic syndrome now grow to be normal adults with normal renal function. Although some children with nephrotic syndrome have progressive glomerulopathies, about 85% have 'minimal glomerular pathology' (MGP) and most of these respond to prednisone treatment.

Nephrotic syndrome with minimal glomerular pathology

The annual incidence of this form of nephrotic syndrome is 2 per million population per year. The peak age at presentation is three years and the male-to-female ratio is 2:1. The aetiology is unknown but the constellation of problems related to T lymphocyte function suggests a role for the immune system. The relationship of this to the increased incidence of atopy in children with MGP is not clear. The identifiable changes are restricted largely to the glomerular epithelial cell, which loses its polyanionic coating and shows obliteration of foot processes.

Clinical features

The disease principally affects children aged 1–10 years with a peak incidence at age 3–4 years. The disease usually has an onset over 2–3 days, with morning facial oedema the first feature. There is often a prodromal acute febrile illness. At presentation, constitutional disturbance is unusual and oedema of the legs may be overlooked. Oliguria and increased thirst are often reported. There is heavy proteinuria and the serum albumin is often below 15 g/l. Less than 10% of patients have transient microscopic haematuria and/or mild hypertension lasting 2–3 days. Renal function and serum complement levels are typically normal.

Management

Corticosteroids remain the mainstay of therapy and there is a variety of empirical programmes. Most commence with a period of daily prednisone until remission is well established, followed by alternate day administration with gradually reducing dose over several months. Mean time to remission is 2–3 weeks. Steroid resistance is described as failure to respond to 60 mg/m^2 body surface area (BSA) per day given for six weeks.

A useful programme is prednisone 60 mg/m^2 per day for one month, then 60 mg on alternate days, reducing by 10 mg increments at monthly intervals, with a final month of 5 mg on alternate days. As over 90% of children respond within one month of commencing daily corticosteroids, a kidney biopsy should be considered at that stage if remission has not occurred. The continued management of those failing to respond to steroid therapy depends in part on the findings of the biopsy. The role of drugs such as alkylating agents and cyclosporin when the biopsy shows minimal change or focal and segmental glomerulonephritis is controversial. Some patients in this group appear to respond to additional

therapy but spontaneous remissions have also been described.

Frequent relapse

Most children with MGP follow a relapsing course. The aim of management is to reduce the frequency of relapses as far as possible, with minimal steroid side effects. The relapses often continue into adolescence. If relapses are so frequent as to interfere with general health, or if they are associated with steroid side effects such as growth retardation, treatment with alkylating agents (cyclophosphamide, chlorambucil) may be considered. Alkylating agents will produce a prolonged remission in 70% of patients, and 50% will remain relapse-free. This therapy is relatively contraindicated for children who have not had varicella or measles or have not received effective immunization as these diseases may be lethal if they occur during therapy. Bone marrow depression may occur and regular blood counts are essential. The therapy is usually limited to a single course of two to three months. The late potential side effects are sterility in boys and an increased risk of malignancy.

Cyclosporin has been shown to reduce relapse rates but the effect is usually lost when the drug is withdrawn. As the response can be achieved with small doses (3–4 mg/kg/day), thus limiting the side effects, this can be valuable for the child for whom alkylating agents are contraindicated.

The antihelminthic immunomodulating drug levamisole has been shown to reduce relapse rates and may prove to be valuable in these children. The effect may prove to be lost when the therapy is withdrawn. It appears to have a low incidence of side effects.

Supportive management

Diuretic therapy combined with albumin infusions may be very useful in reducing marked oedema. Infusion of the albumin should not commence until the diuretic response has become apparent. Salt and water restriction is of similar value.

Primary peritonitis caused by *Strep. pneumoniae*, Haemophilus or *Esch. coli* is an uncommon but potentially dangerous complication and the use of pneumococcal vaccine is recommended, especially for children with steroid resistant disease. The onset is usually marked by abdominal pain and distension, fever and vomiting. After culture of aspirated peritoneal fluid and blood, antibiotic therapy, e.g. with amoxycillin, should be instituted.

Prognosis

Although most children have relapsing disease over a number of years, more than 90% will reach adulthood with normal renal function. Women may experience late steroid-responsive relapses during pregnancy.

Congenital nephrotic syndrome

This rare condition is usually defined as nephrotic syndrome occurring in the first three months of life. Two clear forms are described: microcytic or Finnish, which is inherited as an autosomal recessive trait, and diffuse mesangial sclerosis. Both have a poor prognosis related to the massive urinary protein loss and renal failure. In recent years early intervention with intensive dialysis and nutritional support followed by bilateral nephrectomy and early transplantation has resulted in favourable outcomes.

The prognosis for children with similar diseases which do not meet all the criteria of the above two conditions is variable, and some remain well over many years. In assessing a child with congenital nephrotic syndrome a kidney biopsy is essential and congenital infections, including congenital syphilis, must be excluded.

HAEMOLYTIC–URAEMIC SYNDROME

The complex of microangiopathic haemolytic anaemia, thrombocytopenia and acute renal failure is referred to as haemolytic–uraemic syndrome (HUS). This syndrome clearly comprises more than one clinical variant and probably more than one disease. The incidence is 2 per million total population per year but geographical variation is observed. The disease has a peak incidence between the age of 1 and 2 years.

Presentation

Most children have a prodromal acute febrile illness, usually gastroenteritis. The diarrhoea may be bloody and occasionally appearances suggest ulcerative colitis. After several days, the child becomes pale and may become jaundiced. A few spontaneous bruises appear on the limbs. Oliguria is noted. In children presenting later in the illness, hypertensive encephalopathy or the features of renal failure may predominate. Half the patients are hypertensive at presentation. Laboratory investigations show anaemia with the characteristic bizarre distorted red cells (Fig. 26.3) and thrombocytopenia. The degree of renal failure varies, being mild in a small number. Coagulation studies usually reveal products of fibrin degradation and normal or elevated clotting factors. Less typical presentations are seen in older children in whom severe hypertension may be the predominant feature. This correlates to a degree with changes in histological appearance. A small group present with evidence of a more widespread disorder, often with major central nervous system manifestations.

Pathology

Several patterns are described. The predominant feature is endothelial damage with subendothelial and intraluminal fibrin deposition. The exact nature of the pathology depends on the degree of vascular obstruction, its site and extent. Symmetrical cortical necrosis may result in permanent renal failure. Glomerular disease is the most common form in children. The glomerular capillaries show varying degrees of occlusion and may appear distended with red cells. There may be some mesangial hypercellularity. The tubules may show changes consistent with acute tubular necrosis. Immunofluorescence reveals fibrin deposition in the capillary loops and electron microscopy subendothelial deposition of fibrin-like material. An arterial form is seen more often in older children in whom the vascular changes affect predominantly small arterioles, with distal ischaemic changes. Patients with this pathology often have severe hypertension.

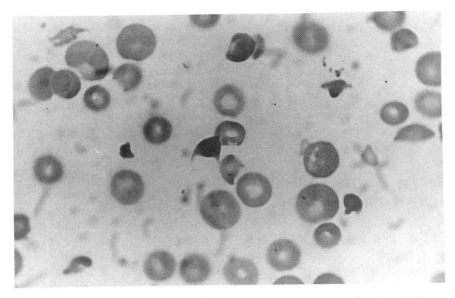

Fig 26.3   Blood film showing distorted red blood cells. (Original magnification × 400)

Aetiology

In the epidemic form of the disease there has been a high rate of recovery of verotoxin-producing bacteria from the stool. This toxin has similar properties to the Shiga toxin and may be responsible for the initial endothelial damage. Local intravascular coagulation subsequent to endothelial damage may be promoted by impairment of local fibrinolytic mechanisms and prostacyclin production. Rarer forms of the disease may be genetically determined or due to other acquired disturbances of endothelial function.

Management

This is mainly supportive. Early peritoneal dialysis — with avoidance of hyperkalaemia, salt and water overload and hypertension — has had a major impact on acute prognosis. For those with intractable hypertension, captopril and enalapril have proved of major benefit. Anticoagulants, fibrinolytic agents and agents which inhibit platelet adhesiveness have not been shown to influence acute mortality, although fibrinolytic therapy may favourably affect long-term prognosis. The results of controlled trials of therapy with fresh plasma have been contradictory but this therapy should be considered for the child with progressive disease or evidence of cerebral vascular involvement. Therapy with prostacyclin infusion and antioxidants such as vitamin E are undergoing clinical trials.

Prognosis

Acute mortality is about 5%. The incidence of residual damage has varied but about 25% have definite abnormalities at follow-up. A proportion eventually develop end-stage renal failure. The morbidity is adversely affected by hypertension, seizures, and prolonged (more than 14 days) anuria. Recurrences have been described and occurrence in more than one child in a family may be associated with an adverse prognosis.

HAEMATURIA AND PROTEINURIA

These features are increasingly detected as isolated findings, with no personal or family history of renal disease, normal physical examination, normal serum creatinine, negative assay for antinuclear antibodies and normal serum complement. The following statements refer to that situation.

Microscopic haematuria

Haematuria has a prevalence of about 1%, and in about 10% of these cases there is a urinary tract infection. Haematuria persists in about one third after six months and less than 10% of those have major anomalies on kidney biopsy. Renal ultrasound is a reasonable investigation, renal biopsy being reserved for those patients whose haematuria persists for several years or where clinical changes appear. The combination of microscopic haematuria and proteinuria renders significant glomerular pathology more likely but proteinuria should be quantified before considering a biopsy.

A proportion of children with isolated microscopic haematuria have hypercalciuria (> 6 mg/kg/24 h). These children have an increased incidence of renal calculus formation, and therapy designed to reduce urinary calcium excretion may be required. The phenomenon may be transient.

Proteinuria

Exclusion of orthostatic proteinuria has first priority, as this has a benign prognosis. Fixed proteinuria of more than 1 g/24 h is more likely to be associated with identifiable pathology. Analysis of the urinary proteins by polyacrylamide gel electrophoresis may assist in directing investigation. Glomerular disease, or renal scarring in association with vesicoureteric reflux or obstruction are possible causes.

HYPERTENSION

Children have very labile blood pressure and quite high levels may be seen transiently. Although the range of blood pressure in normal children in many parts of the world has been established, long-term studies on the significance of a child having a blood pressure in any particular percentile are not complete.

Measurement

Most studies have been done in a quiet environment but not under basal conditions. The cuff size is of major importance as a cuff that is too small will result in a falsely high level being obtained. The best cuff is the largest one which will comfortably fit the upper arm. The bladder should encircle the extremity without overlapping. It is recommended that Korotkoff sound IV (muffling) be used as the indicator of diastolic in children up to 13 years and thereafter Korotkoff V (disappearance). The blood pressure should be taken in the right arm and in all four limbs if the level is elevated. In infants, the preferred method is to use an electronic device using the Doppler principle although in many infants reliable auscultatory measurements can be made.

Expressed as 50th and 95th percentiles, systolic pressures rise from 70–90 mmHg in the neonate to 110–130 mmHg in 13 year olds. Diastolic pressures rise from 55–70 mmHg in the neonate to 60–80 mmHg in 13 year olds.

A child with a blood pressure persistently greater than the 95th percentile should be closely followed, and one whose blood pressure is greater than 130/90 mmHg should be investigated. The commonest cause of hypertension in children is renal disease (glomerulonephritis, reflux nephropathy, etc.). If there is no evidence of parenchymal renal disease, renal artery stenosis is the most common lesion followed by phaeochromocytoma. Essential hypertension has also been reported.

Renal artery stenosis

Renal artery stenosis may be due to a variety of pathological processes. Lesions are often multiple and confined to arterial branches. Levels of blood pressure in these children are often very high with few or no symptoms or signs. One common association is neurofibromatosis. Some stenoses can be dilated by percutaneous angioplasty and some are accessible to surgery, but occasionally blood pressure will be controlled with drug therapy.

Phaeochromocytoma

Most children with this tumour have symptoms suggestive of catecholamine excess, e.g. flushing, diarrhoea, agitation and syncope. Weight loss is common. Blood pressure is usually persistently elevated and urinary catecholamine excretion markedly elevated. The lesions are often multiple and may recur.

Investigation

In the absence of clinical or laboratory evidence of renal disease, renal ultrasonography, urinary catecholamine estimation, plasma adrenaline and noradrenaline, renal arteriography and computerized axial tomography are the most important investigations. The investigation of each child should be individualized.

Drug treatment

Apart from modification of doses for size, the principles of treatment are the same as those for adults. Compliance is enhanced by therapy with single daily dosage. Children, however, seem more prone to the soporific effects of centrally acting drugs than adults.

INHERITED RENAL DISEASE

There is a large and growing list of these disorders. Three will be briefly described.

Cystinosis

This is the commonest cause of a Fanconi syndrome in children. Inherited as an autosomal recessive trait, it is characterized by lysosomal storage of cystine, with frank crystallization in many tissues (reticulum cells, scleral conjunctiva, glomerular epithelial cells). The children usually present in the first two years with failure to thrive, polyuria, polydipsia and rickets. In early childhood, the problems relate to hypokalaemia, acidosis and hypophosphataemic rickets. The biochemical defect is inability to transport cystine across the lysosomal membrane. The diagnosis is established by demonstrating increased uptake of [35S]-labelled cystine by cultured fibroblasts. Antenatal diagnosis is possible using fibroblasts cultured from amniotic fluid or from chorionic villus samples. Therapy is by

mineral replacement and high dose vitamin D. Extremely poor linear growth is common. In the second five years, progressive renal failure develops and few reach 10 years without developing end-stage renal failure. Many develop hypothyroidism. The disease does not recur in a transplanted kidney. Cysteamine or phosphocysteamine, analogues of cysteine, are known to reduce intracellular cystine content. Given orally, these compounds appear to slow the rate of deterioration, at least in infants.

Photophobia is a major problem and appears to be due to corneal deposition of cystine crystals. Topical application of cysteamine reduces the degree of deposition and improves the symptom. Children with this disease are now reaching adult life with functioning transplants. Late involvement of other organ systems (oesophagus, pancreas, brain) has been described and long-term oral administration of cysteamine is recommended.

Familial juvenile nephronophthisis

This chronic renal disease is characterized by growth failure, polyuria, polydipsia and anaemia, and often little if any proteinuria or urinary sediment change. Half the children are hypertensive and most have reduced renal function at presentation. Some show eye changes with tapetoretinal degeneration (Senior–Loken syndrome). The kidney shows progressive tubular atrophy and interstitial fibrosis, with marked periglomerular fibrosis. Glomerular obsolescence is a late feature. The kidneys gradually shrink. Medullary cysts are common and cortical cysts may occur, but cystic changes are not constant. The treatment is supportive and patients gradually progress to renal failure. The disease is inherited as an autosomal recessive trait. A similar disease presenting in adults is said to be inherited in an autosomal dominant fashion.

Familial nephritis with sensorineural deafness (Alport syndrome)

This condition is most commonly inherited as an X-linked dominant trait. In most affected males

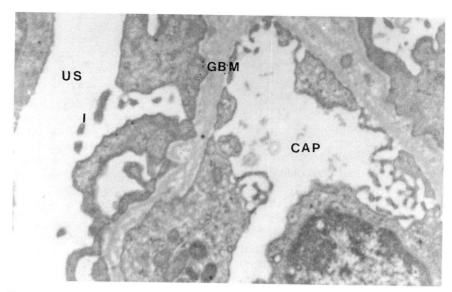

Fig. 26.4   Electron micrograph showing irregular thickness and fragmented appearance of the glomerular basement membrane (GBM). CAP — capillary lumen; US — urinary space. (Original magnification × 10 000.)

the Goodpasture antigen cannot be demonstrated in the glomerular basement membrane and there is evidence that there is a defect in assembly of glomerular basement membrane collagen. Most patients present with haematuria which, once developed, usually persists. Episodes of macroscopic haematuria may occur. Proteinuria is usually minimal early in the disease but may become more marked later, and nephrotic syndrome has been described. Hearing loss may be moderate or severe with predominantly high frequency loss. Both renal and auditory components tend to be more severe in males. Reduced severity in females may be due to early random inactivation of some X chromosomes carrying the defective gene. Expression may vary widely within a family. Haematuria may be detected in the first few years of life and although light microscopic renal changes may be minimal, characteristic changes in the basement membrane are seen on electron microscopy. These include areas of marked thinning, sometimes with breaks, and areas where the basement membrane shows a fragmented, splintered or foamy appearance (Fig. 26.4). Renal failure tends to develop late in the second or in the third decade.

CHRONIC RENAL FAILURE

The annual incidence of chronic renal failure in children under 14 years is 1.5 per million total population. Glomerulonephritis is the cause in about 25% (focal and segmental glomerulosclerosis being the most common), followed by reflux nephropathy, congenital dysplasia, juvenile nephronophthisis, posterior urethral valves, cystinosis, haemolytic–uraemic syndrome and others. The special problems of the child relate to growth failure, interference with psychosocial development and technical problems with dialysis and transplantation due to size and legal and ethical issues.

Growth

Growth retardation is a constant feature of chronic renal failure. Chronic acidosis, poor caloric (energy) intake, renal osteodystrophy and salt depletion are the major potential causes. Correction of these factors may improve, but will not usually normalize, growth rates. Caloric supplementation, especially combined with essential amino acids, keto acids or high biological value protein, has been shown to be benefical. There is evidence of impaired utilization of nutrients and every effort should be made to provide optimal caloric intake. Children with renal failure tend to have very poor dietary intake and while dietary protein restriction may reduce the rate of deterioration of renal failure this strategy carries the risk of compounding protein-calorie malnutrition. Dietary regimes should provide the equivalent of the recommended daily protein requirement which is greatest in infancy (Table 26.3). When dialysis has commenced it may be necessary to increase the protein intake. Provision of partial or total dietary supplementation orally, by nasogastric tube or by gastrostomy may be required. Control of serum phosphorus may be difficult in young children due to dependence on milk and milk products. Serum phosphorus levels are higher in early childhood than in adults (Table 26.4).

In spite of these measures many of these children have suboptimal growth and the use of recombinant human growth hormone can accelerate growth without significant side effects. Growth hormone is usually suspended after successful transplantation.

Table 26.3 Recommended daily allowances for protein by age

Age	g/kg body weight/day
6 months	1.8
12 months	1.5
5 years	1.1
10 years	1.0
Adult	0.7

Table 26.4 Normal values for serum phosphorus by age. (Derived from Clayton B, Jenkins P, Round B (eds) 1980 Pediatric chemical pathology, clinical tests and reference ranges. Blackwell Scientific Publications, Osney Mead, Oxford OX2 OEL.)

Age	Range (± 2 SD) mmol/l
1 month	1.4 – 2.25
6 months	1.2 – 2.1
12 months	1.1 – 1.9
5 years	1.0 – 1.7
10 years	1.0 – 1.6

Psychosocial problems

Illness in the first three years of life limits a child's opportunities for self-expression and enhances passivity. From the age of four to five years chronic illness may produce extreme guilt, with inhibition of initiative. From six to eleven years, interference with a sense of achievement may give rise to feelings of inferiority and inadequacy. Dependency needs must be fulfilled and increased gratification is desirable, but those caring for the child must be sensitive to indications that he or she wishes to act independently from time to time. In addition, excessive, dependent gratification from parents and staff may be an expression of guilt and should be confronted as it may retard rehabilitation. Restriction of activity may limit opportunities for play in which the child discharges tensions. Occupational therapists can often assist in developing programmes for the child which can be carried on by the parents. The above factors, together with short stature and delayed puberty, may result in excessive loss of time from school and impaired development of social skills, making independent life as an adult a difficult goal.

Dialysis and transplantation

Haemodialysis and peritoneal dialysis have been used successfully in the treatment of infants with renal failure.

Peritoneal dialysis (PD)

Either intermittent peritoneal dialysis or continuous ambulatory peritoneal dialysis (CAPD) may be used. In-dwelling Tenckhoff catheters are well tolerated. Initially an exchange volume of 30–50 ml/kg body weight is used. Larger volumes (40–60 ml/kg) can be used subsequently. CAPD is preferable, if small enough bags are available, and three exchanges a day are usually sufficient. Continuous cycled peritoneal dialysis (CCPD) used for 8–10 hours a night 5–6 days a week may be required, particularly if supplemental nutrition can only be given by gavage feeding at night.

Haemodialysis

Vascular access is difficult in small children. Although arteriovenous fistulas have been created in very small children, in-dwelling double or single-lumen cuffed catheters may be required for children under 10 kg. The paediatric dialyser should have low compliance and a low priming volume. The extracorporeal volume should not exceed 10% of the child's blood volume (e.g. for a 10 kg child the extracorporeal volume should not exceed approximately 75 ml). Blood flow rate should be adequate to achieve a urea clearance of 1.5 ml/kg/min for three 5-hour dialyses a week.

Transplantation

In terms of well-being, rehabilitation and freedom from dependency on a machine, transplantation is the choice for children. Adult donor kidneys can be successfully transplanted into children as small as 10 kg in weight and occasionally smaller. The orthotopic site may be chosen for the very small child. Parents are frequently very strongly motivated to donate a kidney, and living related donor transplantation is more common for children than for adults. Due in part to the lower incidence of other chronic illnesses, the results of transplantation in children are equal or superior to results for adults, with 5-year graft survivals of greater than 80%, and 5-year patient survivals greater than 90% in some reports.

Moral and ethical considerations

Dialysis and transplantation are established forms of treatment for end-stage renal failure (ESRF) in children of all ages. The multiply-handicapped child with ESRF poses major problems when any form of independent existence seems impossible. Whether dialysis and transplantation will provide effective treatment for such a child can be decided only on an individual basis.

The potential living related donor is always under some emotional pressure and the torment can be extreme for those who decide they are unable to be a donor. The potential donor must consider the procedure as non-curative and ex-amine the risks, possible loss of a job, family disruption, and the possibility of operative death. Although immature self-gratification is possible, most parents regard the procedure as one of the calculated risks they take when raising a family.

NON-ORGANIC BLADDER DISTURBANCE

Children with nocturnal and diurnal enuresis and urinary frequency may present difficult management problems with the result that they may be extensively and repeatedly investigated even when it is clear that no major organic disease exists.

Enuresis

Enuresis is the intermittent involuntary passage of urine. Diurnal enuresis refers to its occurrence in waking periods, and nocturnal to its occurrence during sleep. Primary nocturnal enuresis refers to children who have never had a period of being dry for more than six months, secondary nocturnal enuresis to children who have been dry for a significant period and then commence to wet again. More than 80% of those with nocturnal enuresis have primary enuresis. The time of acquisition of day and night dryness is very variable but by the age of two most children realize and report that they have dirtied their pants, and recognize the difference between urine and faeces. By three years of age, most children recognize the need to void and will go to the toilet by themselves. By the age of five they can usually initiate emptying of the bladder at any degree of fullness and 90% are dry during sleep. From then on, about 15% of those who are still wet at the end of each year will cease wetting spontaneously during the following 12 months. It has been estimated that, at the age of 20 years, approximately one person in a thousand has nocturnal enuresis. Normal children pass urine approximately 5–10 times a day.

Nocturnal enuresis

Nocturnal enuresis is a phenomenon which occurs during sleep and over which the child has no conscious control. There is an increased incidence in members of the same family. There is no increase in the incidence of organic abnormalities of the urinary tract but a small increase in the incidence of emotional disorders, although no consistent personality problem has emerged. A variety of explanations for the aetiology of enuresis have been proposed. Freud believed that it was a psychoneurotic disorder while others have proposed a small bladder, delay in maturation, or some relationship to allergy as the cause. More recently it has been suggested that the emergence of the normal behavioural pattern may be delayed in these children. The latter is based on observations that, in general, children with nocturnal enuresis have no significant emotional disorder and have no demonstrable abnormality of the urinary tract or the central nervous system. The sudden disappearance of the symptom also favours that hypothesis. It is not clear whether the familial tendency to nocturnal enuresis is the result of genetic or sociocultural factors but both appear to be involved. The condition is more frequent in lower socio-economic groups, but certainly not confined to them, and has been claimed to be more frequent in children who have been exposed to coercive toilet-training. Blunting of the nocturnal increase in vasopressin secretion has been reported but as nocturnal enuresis may be intermittent and may suddenly disappear the relationship to aetiology is not clear.

The phenomenon of nocturnal enuresis appears to occur during stage 1 or 2 sleep and any REM (rapid eye movement) sleep follows rather than precedes or accompanies the wetting episodes. The wetting episodes do not appear to depend on a full bladder and some observations have suggested that the urine is passed in a series of 'spurts' rather than in a single emptying of the bladder.

Many treatments have been tried over the centuries, e.g. 'lifting' or regularly waking the child at specific times during the night, deliberate dehydration by depriving the child of fluids from the late afternoon or early evening, and rewards and punishments. However, none of these seems to be associated with any greater rate of resolution than occurs naturally, although most have not been evaluated by any form of controlled study. Behaviour modification and hypnotherapy have also not

been exposed to controlled trial but are sometimes successful. Treatment with drugs such as imipramine, amitriptyline or nortriptyline is reported to be associated with a 30–40% remission rate, but the relapse rate is much higher than in the placebo-treated group and after withdrawal of the drug there is no difference in incidence of enuresis between the two groups. Treatment with synthetic vasopressin (desmopressin) is successful in about 60% of children but relapse on withdrawal is common.

The enuresis alarm. The enuresis alarm, or so-called 'conditioning equipment for the treatment of nocturnal enuresis' is effective in 80–90% of children who are motivated to lose the symptom and whose social situation allows the treatment to be undertaken. The equipment comprises a sensor which is placed beneath the child or otherwise close to the external urethral meatus and which activates a discontinuous noise of more than 85 decibels at 1 metre (Australian Standard 2394–1980). For optimal effect, the child should wish to lose the symptom and be able to take an active part in the use of the equipment. Children under 6 years of age are rarely able to use this treatment successfully. Equipment should be durable and make a sufficiently loud discontinuous noise to wake the child so that a pattern can be established in which the child wakes, turns off the alarm, gets out of bed and visits the toilet to complete voiding, and then returns to bed and switches the alarm back on.

It is usually necessary, at least for the first 4–5 nights, that an adult is available when the alarm is activated so that he or she can ensure that the child does wake during the noise and does turn off the alarm before completing the remainder of the procedure. In most instances, the child will assume responsibility for most of the treatment after about one week. All other treatment should be discontinued and the child be allowed to eat and drink normally.

Drug therapy is valuable for the child where temporary relief is required. Responsiveness can be determined by a short trial of a tricyclic antidepressant or desmopressin. A trial along the following lines should identify those children who are responsive to imipramine. A dose of 25 mg each night is given for one week and, if the child is still wet, the dose is increased to 50 mg, and then to 75 mg for a further week. If the child is still wet at the end of a week of 75 mg at night, the chance of subsequent response is extremely small. The treatment should be discontinued if there is a major change in the child's behaviour, if nightmares develop or if the child complains of dry mouth or blurred vision. The parents must be instructed in the possible toxic hazard to young children who may be in the house, and the drug should be kept in a locked cupboard. Desmopressin is usually given in a dose of 20 µg intranasally and is successful in responsive children within 2–3 nights.

Urge syndrome

Girls with the urge syndrome are often thought to be lazy because they seem unwilling to go to the toilet when the need arises. These girls have episodes of detrusor contraction during which they characteristically squat on their heels and sit very still. Any attempt to move leads to a wetting. The contraction lasts a few minutes before control is regained. For some the slightest bump will upset control. These girls should be allowed to control their problem in the way that is most convenient to them, but advised to go to the toilet as soon as the urge has passed. The syndrome usually subsides by about 10 years. The problem is exacerbated by coexistent urine infection.

Daytime incontinence

Children with intermittent wetting interspersed with long periods (several hours) of being dry who have no abnormality on physical examination are unlikely to have an organic abnormality. A urine culture is usually adequate investigation. The problem is commonest in girls aged 4–10 years who intermittently wet their pants, often without seeming aware of it. The problem tends to resolve with time. Practising holding their urine and interrupting the stream may be of some value. Some consider that formal behaviour modification techniques are useful. Drug therapy is not indicated.

Pollakiuria

Pollakiuria is the sudden onset of marked frequency in an apparently well child. The child may pass tiny amounts of urine every few minutes, but characteristically there is no dysuria. The phenomenon disappears when the child goes to sleep but may recur the next day. It rarely lasts more than a few days. It is more common in boys than girls. The cause is not known, although stress appears to play a major role. Urinary tract infection should be excluded.

REFERENCES

ANZDATA Report 1990 Disney APS (ed). Australia and New Zealand Dialysis and Transplant Registry, Adelaide, South Australia

Crombleholme T M, Harrison M R, Longacker M T, Langer J C 1988 Prenatal diagnosis and management of bilateral hydronephrosis. Pediatric Nephrology 2: 334–342

Jureidini K F, Hogg R J, van Renen M J et al 1990 Evaluation of long-term aggressive dietary management of chronic renal failure in children. Pediatric Nephrology 4: 1–10

Kaplan B S, Fay J, Shah V, Dillon M J, Barrett T M 1989 Autosomal recessive polycystic kidney disease. Pediatric Nephrology 3: 43–49

Kashtan C E, Kleppel M M, Butkowski R J, Michael A F, Fish A J 1990 Alport syndrome, basement membranes and collagen. Pediatric Nephrology 4: 523–532

Kolvin I, McKeith R C, Meadow S R 1973 Bladder control and enuresis. Heinemann Medical, London

Levin M, Walters M D, Barrett T M 1989 Hemolytic uremic syndrome. Advances in Pediatric Infectious Diseases 4: 51–81

Najarian J S, Frey D J, Matas A J et al 1990 Renal transplantation in infants. Annals of Surgery 212: 353–365

Potter E L 1972 Normal and abnormal development of the kidney. Year Book Medical Publishers, Chicago, Ch 2

Rudd P T, Hughes E A, Placzek M M, Hodes D T 1983 Reference ranges for plasma creatinine during the first month of life. Archives of Disease in Childhood 58: 212–215

Scharer K 1987 Hypertension in children and adolescents — 1986. Pediatric Nephrology 1: 50–58

Schneider J A, Katz B, Melles R B 1990 Update on nephropathic cystinosis. Pediatric Nephrology 4: 645–653

Shaffer S E, Norman M E 1989 Renal function and renal failure in the newborn. Clinics in Perinatology 16: 199–218

Strauss J, Daniel S S, James L S 1981 Postnatal adjustments in renal function. Pediatrics 68: 802–808

Task Force on Blood Pressure Control in Children 1987 Report of the second task force on blood pressure control in children — 1987. Pediatrics 79: 1–25

Tonshoff B, Mehls O, Heinrich U, Blum W F, Ranke M B, Schauer A 1990 Growth stimulating effects of recombinant human growth hormone in children with end-stage renal disease. Journal of Pediatrics 116: 561–566

Trompeter R S 1989 Immunosuppressive therapy in the nephrotic syndrome in children. Pediatric Nephrology 3: 194–200

Vehaskari V M, Rapola J, Koskimes O, Savilahti E, Vilska J, Hallmann N 1979 Microscopic haematuria in schoochildren. Journal of Pediatrics 95: 676–684

Warady B A, Alon U, Hellerstein S 1991 Primary nocturnal enuresis: current concepts about an old problem. Pediatric Annals 20: 246–251, 254–255

White R H R 1989 The investigation of haematuria. Archives of Disease in Childhood 64: 159–165

27. High blood pressure

G. J. Macdonald

INTRODUCTION

The term 'hypertension', as commonly used, means a systemic arterial pressure above a stated 'safe' level. The existence of such a disorder was inferred by Richard Bright in his descriptions of albuminuric nephropathy when he found increased left ventricular thickness and cardiac mass in patients dying of chronic renal disease, changes he attributed to increased resistance to flow through peripheral blood vessels. Our concepts of arterial hypertension owe much to his original observations. It was originally believed that diastolic pressure was the more important measure, representing a constant arterial stress. It has become apparent from large-scale epidemiological studies that systolic pressure more accurately predicts cardiovascular pathology, an observation which is altering our approach to the pathophysiology and treatment of high blood pressure.

Hypertension was regarded as a condition associated exclusively with renal disease until late in the nineteenth century when the studies of Mahomet, Albutt and von Basch showed that similar changes in the left ventricle and vessels could be demonstrated in people dying without evidence of severe renal disease. The development in the last decade of that century of sphygmomanometric measurement of systolic pressure by Riva-Rocci and the definition by Korotkow of brachial artery sounds during pressure release, made assessment of blood pressure in general, and diastolic pressures in particular, feasible for the first time in patients.

The term 'hypertension' is often criticized because it may be associated in the mind with ideas of stress and mental tension and also because it has come to be used by medical professionals as a diagnostic term like 'pneumonia' or 'thrombosis'. It is probably better to use the term 'high blood pressure', with the attendant suggestion that people with this condition fall into a statistically rather than pathologically definable group, whose position on the population frequency distribution curve for blood pressure puts them at higher risk of later pathological consequences. It also allows the possibility that the abnormality defined by sphygmomanometry or direct arterial pressure recording may be a single element of a wider spectrum of haemodynamic disorders and underlying cardiovascular structural abnormalities.

DEFINITION

The values for systolic and diastolic blood pressure which are accepted as 'normal' are derived from statistical analysis of large population groups. The usual method of measuring a variable in a large number of individuals and formulating a normal range on the basis of the mean or median plus or minus confidence limits is not reliable in such a common condition. The presence in a population of so many people who are 'abnormal' skews the definition of 'normal'. The contemporary method of assigning normal ranges for high blood pressure and other variables whose impact on health is not immediate (known as 'risk factors') is to observe a defined population for prolonged periods and assess the statistical contributions of values of suspect factors at the beginning of the study to later health outcomes. Such an assessment needs to be made with insight into the processes that underlie such outcomes. Normality is defined as values at which long-term risk of defined clinical or pathological events is not discernibly different from that of the population in the adjacent lower risk quantile for the value studied.

In the case of blood pressure, there appears to be no level at which a lower pressure is not associated with a lower cardiovascular risk than a higher one. High blood pressure has come to be defined as the level where the incidence of events begins to rise more sharply from the nearly horizontal regression line at lower pressures. From the deflection points of systolic and diastolic pressures have come the values of 135 and 83 mm of mercury respectively. These figures become very important in considering the economics of treating high blood pressure since they fall in the highest regions of frequency. Lowering target blood pressure by even one millimetre as a therapeutic goal markedly increases the population in need of treatment and the consequent expense. By definition, this is also the range of low attributable risk, and the calculated cost of preventing a stroke or myocardial infarction becomes very high indeed. In most countries, the threshold for treating blood pressure in people under the age of 50 is 140/90 mmHg.

CLASSIFICATION

High blood pressure is defined in two overlapping frameworks. The first is based on its severity — benign or malignant. Like the term 'hypertension', the word 'malignant' is not universally accepted, partly because of the implied association with neoplastic disease and also because it gives no insight into underlying processes. The term is appropriate in a prognostic sense since the outcome of this form is as poor as most neoplasms. Its failure to reflect processes has led to terms like 'necrotizing', indicating that in this condition arterial smooth muscle cells die rather than degenerate, or 'accelerated', consistent with its rapid downhill course.

The most commonly used classification is by cause (see Table 27.1) Essential hypertension

Table 27.1 Classification of high blood pressure

By Degree
  Benign
  Malignant (necrotizing, accelerated)

By cause
  Essential
  Secondary
    Renal
      (i)   Parenchymal:
              glomerulonephritis
              vesicoureteric reflux
              analgesic nephropathy
              diabetes mellitus
              polycystic kidneys
              (Virtually all parenchymal disease is
              associated with increased incidence of high
              blood pressure)
      (ii)   Vascular:
              renal artery stenosis
              polyarteritis nodosa
              arteriovenous malformations
              renal artery aneurysm
      (iii) Neoplastic:
              Wilm's tumour
              renin-secreting adenoma
              (haemangiopericytoma)
              (Most tumours are associated with high
              blood pressure, but tumours such as
              Grawitz tumours are believed to do this
              by distortion of renal blood vessels and
              intra-renal artery stenosis)
    Endocrine
      (i)   Adrenal cortex:
              Cushing's syndrome
              Conn's syndrome
              other mineralocorticoid excess
      (ii)   Adrenal medulla and splanchnic
              chain:
              phaeochromocytoma
      (iii) Others:
              acromegaly
              hyperparathyroidism
    Iatrogenic:
              oral contraceptives
              sympathomimetic amines (nasal
              decongestants)
              therapeutic corticosteroids
              non-steroidal anti-inflammatory drugs
              cyclosporin A
              tricyclic antidepressant drugs
              liquorice and liquorice-derived agents
  Pregnancy-associated hypertension
  Acute intermittent porphyria
  Carbon dioxide retention

accounts for at least 95% of patients with high blood pressure. Of the secondary causes, glomerulonephritis accounts for four out of five patients, with other causes being relatively uncommon. The major issue in initial diagnosis is therefore exclusion of nephritis.

PATHOGENESIS OF ESSENTIAL HIGH BLOOD PRESSURE

Normal blood pressure is controlled by the central nervous system via autonomic efferents acting on the heart and peripheral blood vessels to control cardiac output and peripheral vascular tone, and by renal control of extracellular volume, particularly the intravascular moiety. The interaction of these two groups of functions provides a simple physical analogy with pressure determination in a closed circuit pumping system.

High blood pressure has been attributed to abnormalities at all levels of regulation of this system. Continuing research has provided a picture of interdependent systems with body-wide distribution consistent with an abnormality which requires involvement of the heart and a major proportion of resistance vessels once established. While many types of secondary high blood pressure have evident causes, the mechanisms underlying the essential form remain elusive.

Genetically determined mechanisms

Essential high blood pressure has been shown to be strongly heritable. Identical twins have almost identical blood pressures, and first-degree relatives of hypertensive patients have significantly higher blood pressures than those of patients at unrelated hospital clinics and *their* first-degree relatives. Infants born to parents with high blood pressures have higher blood pressures than those born to normotensive parents, differences which some workers claim persist through to adulthood. The final expression of high blood pressure depends to varying degrees on accentuation by environmental factors.

Two major theories have been proposed for the genesis of essential high blood pressure. That elaborated by Guyton and co-workers posits renal sodium retention which leads to extracellular space expansion and thence to plasma volume expansion, increased cardiac output, increased arteriolar tone and high blood pressure which leads to sodium and water excretion by 'pressure' natriuresis and normalization of all elements except high blood pressure and peripheral resistance. All these elements have now been validated — a relative failure of sodium excretion by the proximal tubule has been found in man and rats with genetically determined high blood pressure; in young people, presumably early in the course of development of the condition, cardiac output rather than peripheral resistance is raised; increased cardiac output leads to increased peripheral arteriolar tone initially and later to fixed adaptive changes which perpetuate the increased peripheral resistance; high blood pressure leads to natriuresis. These changes have so far been shown to be mediated by the sympathetic nervous system, the renin–angiotensin–aldosterone system, which provides short- and long-term control over renal sodium handling, and as yet unknown renal mechanisms.

The other major theory also begins with reduced renal sodium excretion and extracellular space expansion, but arrives at high blood pressure by secretion of a hormone which causes arteriolar constriction and sodium excretion. There are many points at which both theories are congruent — the hormone may mediate the intrinsic (myogenic) arteriolar contractile response to increased cardiac output essential in the Guyton theory; natriuresis is a common endpoint. The hormone is believed to be a sodium–potassium ATPase inhibitor, probably related to the cardiac glycoside ouabain, and secreted by the hypothalamus or adrenal glands. It would also provide the conceptual basis for the link widely believed to exist between high dietary sodium intake and high blood pressure.

More recently, several workers have studied glucose homeostasis in people with high blood pressure and have shown hyperinsulinism with decreased sensitivity of non-oxidative glucose transport. While expected in obese individuals, the abnormality has been found equally in lean hypertensives. Insulin would raise blood pressure by its action on central nervous system receptors and on renal tubular receptors, causing increased sympathetic outflow and sodium retention respectively. In addition, such a defect is consistent with the impaired glucose homeostasis, hypercholesterolaemia and increased coronary artery disease strongly associated with high blood pressure.

There are many other factors in blood pressure regulation, abnormalities in whose production or function are suggested to play a part in the genesis of essential hypertension. The major ones are atrial natriuretic peptide (ANP, atriopeptin), the prostaglandins, endothelial factors — nitric oxide, endothelin, prostacyclin — smooth muscle second messenger systems mediated by adenylate and guanylate cyclases or the inositol phosphate pathways, and CNS centres and pathways utilizing as neurotransmitters serotonin, purine nucleotides and various peptides, particularly angiotensin II and neuropeptide Y. At the moment, their roles in the genesis of high blood pressure remain speculative although there is increasing evidence that inhibition of nitric oxide production produces stable high blood pressure in experimental animals.

Environmentally determined factors

Certain behavioural and dietary characteristics have been found to interact strongly with genetic predisposition to produce high blood pressure (see Table 27.2). Others have been proposed, such as high caffeine intake or western urban living; these either rest on dubious data or have not been adequately defined.

Obesity

Obesity is well established as a risk factor for high blood pressure and for cardiovascular morbidity in general. It accounts for 60% of essential hypertension in young Australian men and its correction is one of the most effective non-pharmacological methods of blood pressure reduction. The most likely mediating mechanism is insulin resistance (see above) which is present in virtually all obese people.

Dietary sodium

These is evidence that national and regional populations with high dietary sodium intakes have higher blood pressures and higher incidences of hypertension and stroke than those who consume

Table 27.2 Environmental factors in essential high blood pressure

Obesity
High dietary sodium
Alcohol intake
Sedentary lifestyle

less. In more formal studies, however, such associations are not as strong as originally thought and there is evidence that the chloride rather than sodium in sodium chloride may be responsible. The proposal rests more solidly on the efficacy of low salt diets in blood pressure reduction, although this too is debated. There appears to be a parallel aetiological role for low dietary potassium which occurs in conjunction with high dietary sodium in high protein western diets with relatively low vegetable consumption. High dietary sodium would act in conjunction with the abnormality in renal tubular sodium excretion which appears to be a heritable abnormality in families with essential high blood pressure.

Alcohol

High alcohol intake (over 20 g per day) is associated with proportional elevations in blood pressure. There may be a protective effect of moderate intake (10–20g daily), but this is uncertain. Alcohol probably raises blood pressure via increased sympathetic nervous system activity.

Sedentary living

Apart from contributing to obesity, a low exercise lifestyle appears to be associated with increased sympathetic outflow. It is hard to quantitate this risk factor but increasing exercise has been shown to reduce high blood pressure.

PATHOLOGICAL CHANGES IN HIGH BLOOD PRESSURE

Chronically elevated blood pressure produces recurrent stress on arteriolar walls with two types of effect. In the fine vessels of the cerebral circulation, weakening occurs in the media at bifurcations, with formation of Charcot-Bouchard microaneurysms. Chronic leakage or rupture of these lesions causes multiple foci of destruction of brain tissue. More commonly, here and throughout the rest of the circulation, there are hypertrophic and hyperplastic changes in all layers of arteriolar walls which result in generalized tissue ischaemia as lumina are reduced. The principal organs affected by this process are the brain, kidney and heart. Since the first two are major centres of blood pressure control, progressive ischaemia may be expected to contribute to continued or worsened blood pressure.

In the case of the left ventricle, occlusion of small vessels occurs in a ventricle wall undergoing progressive hypertrophy from the elevated blood pressure. The mechanism for this 'adaptive' ventricular growth is a focus of contemporary interest. By what afferent process does the heart receive the stimulus for cell enlargement? Is there a mechanism which calibrates the enlargement to the increase in peripheral resistance? If the answer

to the last question is 'no', can left ventricular hypertrophy become a sustaining factor in high blood pressure? Uncorrected, the combination of hypertrophy, increased nutrient and oxygen demands and diminished large and small vessel calibre predisposes to myocardial infarction and chronic ischaemic heart failure.

In benign hypertension, all arteriolar layers are involved with endothelial proliferation, reduplication and fracturing of the internal elastic lamina, and hyperplasia of smooth muscle with areas of glassy eosinophilic material known as hyaline degeneration (Fig. 27.1). The kidney, chronically affected by this process, shows wrinkling of the glomerular basement membrane (Fig. 27.2), believed to reflect reduced intracapillary pressure, and hyaline changes in the afferent arteriole leading long-term to glomerular sclerosis. The time course of these changes is prolonged, however, and it is doubtful if benign hypertension ever leads to end-stage renal failure except in African

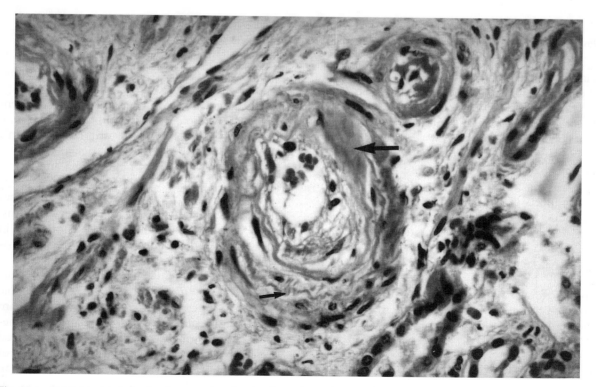

Fig. 27.1 Small arteriole in benign hypertension showing fracturing and reduplication of the internal elastic lamina (fine arrow) and hyaline degeneration of the media (thick arrow). (Haematoxylin and eosin.)

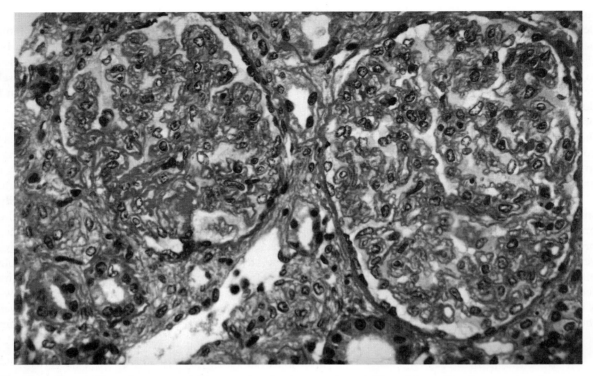

Fig. 27.2 Glomeruli in malignant essential hypertension showing extensive·wrinkling of the capillary basement membrane

black-derived races, although even in this group the epidemiological data are controversial.

Other ischaemic changes may be seen in the tubules with atrophy and interstitial inflammatory reaction leading to fibrosis. Macroscopically, there is a loss of renal substance with small subcapsular haemorrhages and fine cortical scarring. In malignant hypertension, arteriolar lesions are more pronounced with intimal proliferation frequently occluding the lumina, necrosis of the smooth muscle (fibrinoid necrosis) and adventitial fibrosis (Fig. 27.3). Glomeruli are destroyed by ischaemia and renal failure ensues rapidly. Malignant essential high blood pressure is a disease mainly of young adults; its incidence appears to have declined dramatically with the effective control of the benign form.

CLINICAL MANIFESTATIONS

High blood pressure was held to be asymptomatic but is now thought to cause vague constitutional symptoms, particularly bilateral early morning occipital headache, dizziness and fatigue. Symptoms of target organ damage are more prominent and often dramatic with acute focal cerebral pathology (haemorrhage or arterial occlusion), myocardial infarction or left ventricular failure.

The eye is also a major target organ and retinal arterial and venous occlusions are seen in malignant high blood pressure or when pressure rises rapidly over a short period. In less severe forms, retinal arterioles show the changes occurring in other vascular beds, with thickened media transforming a thin-walled column of blood into a reduced blood channel with a thicker refractile wall. This accounts for the milder fundoscopic changes — internal reflection of the light beam within the arteriolar wall produces the phenomenon of 'silver wiring' while the refraction produced where arterioles overlie veins gives the effect of arteriovenous 'nipping' ('nicking' in American texts). With more severe and prolonged hypertension, capillary endothelial damage permits the

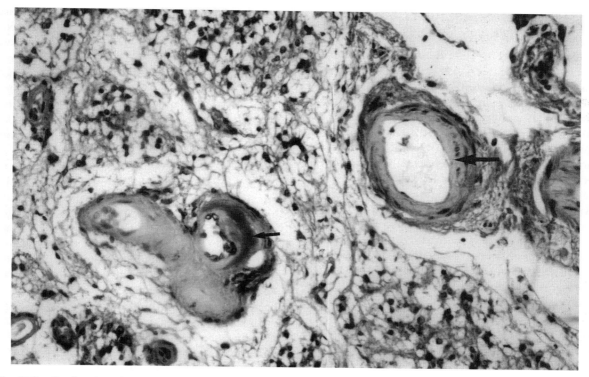

Fig. 27.3   Small and medium-sized renal arterioles in malignant (necrotizing) hypertension. The larger vessel shows extensive intimal thickening (large arrow) while the smaller shows fibrinoid necrosis (fine arrow). (Picro-Mallory stain.)

passage of plasma proteins and blood cells across the wall into the subhyaloid space, producing the soft white exudates and circumscribed haemorrhages of high blood pressure. In the most severe forms, reduction in arteriolar calibre results in ischaemia of the optic nerve head, producing swelling and blurring of the disc margins. This is known as anterior ischaemic optic neuropathy and, though distinguishable from papilloedema on full ophthalmological examination, it cannot be diagnosed on routine fundoscopy.

Chronic arteriolar disease with insidiously progressive loss of cerebral or cardiac function is equally common. More spectacular ischaemic lesions such as leg ulcers are now rarely seen as a result of high blood pressure alone although widespread vascular disease may affect the function of any organ. Renal arteriolar damage may result in proteinuria and haematuria. These may equally be due to primary renal parenchymal disease which is also raising blood pressure.

HIGH BLOOD PRESSURE AS A CARDIOVASCULAR RISK FACTOR

Epidemiology shows that while high blood pressure is a roughly equivalent risk factor for myocardial infarction and stroke, correction to normal range reduces the incidence of the later but has only reduced heart attacks significantly in one or two minor therapeutic studies. The most likely reason is that high blood pressure is strongly associated with hypercholesterolaemia, an even more crucial risk factor. Various workers have commented that the most useful thing one can do for a hypertensive patient is to stop him or her smoking, thereby removing a major risk factor which acts additively with high blood pressure (as do abnormalities of plasma lipids and glucose intolerance). Such data make it mandatory in the care of the hypertensive patient to seek all other risk factors and aim to reduce the total risk factor 'burden' rather than the blood pressure alone.

HIGH BLOOD PRESSURE AS A PUBLIC HEALTH ISSUE

Since high blood pressure is a major risk factor for the group of diseases which constitute the principal cause of untimely death and a major element in health care costs in western societies, it poses a problem of public and political importance. As modern therapy becomes increasingly expensive, governments and agencies which bear health costs are looking increasingly to preventive measures as economically preferable. However, while it is tempting to believe that lifestyle modification without costly intervention by health care professionals will remove cardiovascular diseases from the community, there is virtually no data on final disease outcome that bears this conviction out. Even if data supported the efficacy of educative measures, the time scale on which they operate seems considerably longer than the patience-span of governments or economists. Moves to reduce funding for treatment of and research into cardiac and vascular disease on the assumption that education will reduce its incidence in the short term are premature and compromise necessary medical care.

CLINICAL APPROACH TO THE HYPERTENSIVE PATIENT

Detection

Since most people with high blood pressure do not recognize symptoms, a major responsibility of all health care workers is to ensure that blood pressure is measured at least once a year in all patients with whom they come into professional contact. It is important to remember that measuring blood pressure raises it. If it is found to be high, blood pressure must be measured at least three times over at least a week to allow the patient to become accustomed to the measurer and the environment ('white coat' effect). Evidence of severe high blood pressure such as retinal changes, proteinuria or clinical heart failure cancels this policy and is an indication for rapid treatment. Blood pressures of over 180/110 call for a shortening of the confirmatory period to a day or for repeat measurement later the same day.

Variable (labile) blood pressure may require more continuous monitoring and some hypertension clinics provide 24-hour non-invasive measurement. Increasingly, home blood pressure measurement using portable electronic sphygmomanometry is being used to confirm the diagnosis. It is vital that the patient knows how to use the machine properly and that the doctor checks the patient's readings against his own, preferably using a mercury column sphygmomanometer, to ensure accuracy. Many people are first found to be hypertensive at community or worksite screening clinics or during medical examination for admission to the armed forces, public service or private employment or as part of assessment for life insurance coverage.

Error is common in blood pressure measurement. Observers tend to 'hunt' for the previous recorded reading or to avoid odd numbers. Both these errors are partly corrected by taking the reading before checking the previous one and recording pressures at the mark on the sphygmomanometer nearest to the relevant Korotkow sound. Other errors in BP measurement may be associated with the patient: 'white coat' effect or recent emotional upset, conflict situation or fright may raise it.

Blood pressure may be raised by sympathomimetic amines used to relieve upper respiratory tract obstruction from allergic or viral illness, either orally or by drops. Women may be taking oral contraceptive tablets, in which case it is necessary to withhold them for six months to confirm that they are the cause of the high blood pressure. Liquorice contains elements which mimic the effects of aldosterone and produce a mineralocorticoid hypertension with hypokalaemia, metabolic alkalosis and suppression of plasma renin. Plasma aldosterone, however, is also suppressed by the exogenous compound. (Most liquorice sweets are now made from by-products of sugar refining, with only minor amounts of active compounds.)

Measurement

In most clinics and doctors' offices, the mercury sphygmomanometer is the commonest method.

Aneroids may be used but most health workers concerned with accurate BP measurement use a mercury column — a simple system free of moving parts, whose values define blood pressure in its absolute units. The recommended use of the sphygmomanometer involves the following major points:

(i) A wider cuff than usual is needed in obese arms to avoid a falsely high reading. A general rule is that the largest cuff that fits on the arm should be used. There is little basis for the use of graded narrow cuffs in children to reduce the chance of a falsely low reading.

(ii) The cuff should be applied so as to fit closely without pressure with the centre of the inflatable bag over the brachial artery. The midline of the bag is often marked on new cuffs Recent WHO guidelines recommend that it be applied upside down with the air tubes facing up the arm so as not to interfere with auscultation at the elbow, a practice commonly used by hypertension specialists.

(iii) The cuff should be inflated as rapidly as possible and pressure released at 2 mm Hg per beat so as not to miss the first Korotkow sound which may be transient and followed by a silent period ('latent gap') before the first sustained pulsation is heard, the second Korotkow sound.

(iv) Systolic pressure is taken as the first appearance of sound and diastolic as the final disappearance (fifth phase). In people with wide pulse pressures such as in aortic incompetence, thyrotoxicosis and pregnancy, spontaneous sounds may be heard in the brachial artery and the fifth Korotkow phase will therefore not occur. In such cases it is usual to take the fourth phase (muffling) as diastolic. This should be marked in the patient's records. In pregnant women, the onset of high blood pressure often restores the fifth phase as diastolic pressure.

(v) It is recommended that the first time blood pressure is measured, it ought to be taken in both arms and the side reading higher (usually the dominant arm) used for future measurements. In patients on treatment it is useful to take the pressure lying and standing as a measure of compliance with agents known to cause a postural fall and to verify that symptoms of dizziness or lightheadedness correspond to a fall in pressure on standing. A marked fall from hypertensive to hypotensive levels without a rise in pulse rate may provide the first clue to dysautonomia.

Issues raised by discovery of high blood pressure

High blood pressure calls for the carer to look backward into possible underlying causes which may be amenable to surgery or require medical treatment apart from blood pressure reduction (steroids for glomerulonephritis, for example), and forward, to treatment with correction of concurrent coronary disease risk factors and attention to complicating pathology such as cerebrovascular and left ventricular disease. Treatment and investigation are integrated since failure to lower blood pressure is an important indication for investigation, and detection of left ventricular hypertrophy or dysfunction at an early stage influences the choice of treatment and the length of time over which planned blood pressure reduction will be achieved.

Since essential high blood pressure is so strongly heritable, it is advisable to draw this fact to the attention of the patient so that first-degree relatives may have their coronary risk status checked. The discovery of high blood pressure should lead to screening and correction of other cardiovascular risk factors, particularly cessation of smoking and reduction of high plasma LDL cholesterol.

The priorities in caring for the patient with high blood pressure are therefore:

1. Exclude severe high blood pressure with life-threatening complications or in a range where they will be likely to occur within the next 24 hours. (History of incipient left ventricular failure, chest pain, visual disturbances, haematuria, altered consciousness or motor or sensory symptoms. Clinical cardiomegaly, pulmonary congestion, evidence of aortic aneurysm formation, retinal haemorrhages, exudates or disc swelling. Laboratory evidence of renal failure, proteinuria,

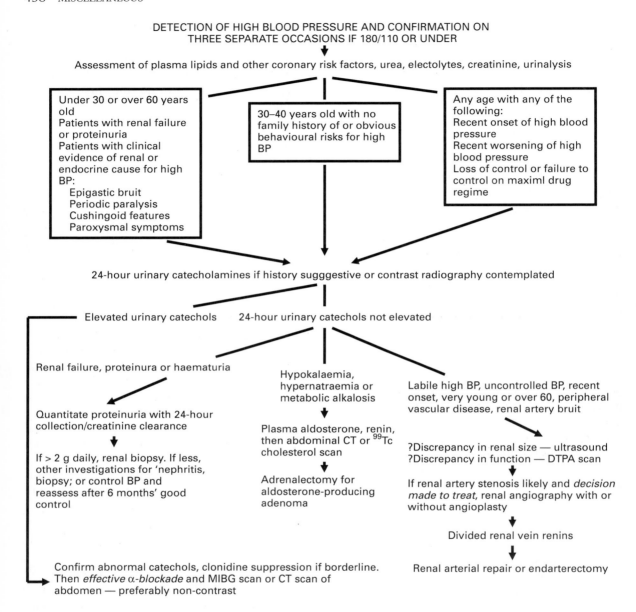

Fig. 27.4 Decisions to be made following detection of high blood pressure

increased left ventricular free wall thickness or concentric hypertrophy on echocardiography, aortic dilatation on X-ray or ultrasound.)

2. If none of the above is present and blood pressure is below 180/110, confirm high blood pressure with repeated measurements over two weeks.

3. All patients should have biochemical tests of renal function to detect renal failure or electrolyte abnormalities of secondary hypertension, an electrocardiograph and chest X-ray. There is a strong case for routine echocardiography but, at present, this seems inconsistent with an economically acceptable screening process.

Subsequent management is described in Figure 27.4.

INVESTIGATION OF HIGH BLOOD PRESSURE

This is summarized in Figure 27.4. If symptoms suggest phaeochromocytoma or contrast radiography is contemplated, measurement of urinary catecholamines should be done as an initial investigation since even intravenous contrast can trigger the release of large amounts of adrenaline or noradrenaline from a tumour.

Since many antihypertensive drugs can affect catechol release, it is advisable during this investigation to use agents without such an effect, such as debrisoquine or verapamil. Minor elevations in urinary free noradrenaline may result from anxiety and, if found, the collections should be repeated with neuronal noradrenaline release inhibited by several days of a low dose (75–100 µg daily) of clonidine.

The other essential investigation is plasma electrolytes, urea and creatinine, since any degree of renal failure is an indication for further investigation, and elevated plasma sodium, hypokalaemia or metabolic alkalosis may be the first suggestion of hyperaldosteronism. This may be secondary in renal artery stenosis or malignant hypertension or primary in Conn's syndrome. Urinalysis, part of the normal physical examination, may show proteinuria and initiate the search for glomerular disease. (It is fairly safe to conclude that this is absent if dipstick testing fails to show protein or blood in the urine of a patient with normal or mildly impaired renal function.)

TREATMENT OF HIGH BLOOD PRESSURE

It is customary to try non-pharmacological means in mild (160/105 or less) hypertension and retain these as background treatment if it becomes necessary to add pharmacological agents. The principal means are listed in Table 27.3 and may be combined to give greater efficacy. Even in more severe forms of high blood pressure, non-pharmacological measures may be an obvious choice in

Table 27.3 Non-pharmacological treatment of high blood pressure

Physical/consummative
  Weight loss
  Reduction in alcohol intake
  Physical exercise
  Low sodium (chloride?) intake
Metaphysical
  Progressive muscular relaxation
  Yoga
  Biofeedback
  Meditation

the obese, patients with high salt or alcohol intakes, or where it is felt that psychological techniques are likely to succeed. All pharmacological means are more effective in patients who lose weight or engage in an exercise programme.

Pharmacological treatment

Drugs ultimately become the means of treatment in the majority of patients. High blood pressure is a chronic disease with a high public health profile and the development and marketing of new antihypertensive agents is a major activity for the pharmaceutical industry. Clinical concepts relating to the use of antihypertensive agents have been strongly influenced by marketing demands.

Diuretics

Most of the diuretics used for reducing blood pressure are thiazides, sulphur-containing compounds related to sulphonamides, which are filtered by the glomerulus and act on the proximal and distal tubules to inhibit reabsorption of sodium. Their antihypertensive action is not totally related to reduction of the extracellular space, taking several months to reach its maximum effect at a time when extracellular volume is close to pretreatment levels.

Their use is decreasing because of a perceived lack of efficacy and a relatively high frequency of adverse effects (male impotence, rash, thrombocytopenia) and biochemical abnormalities (hyperglycaemia and insulin resistance, hyperuricaemia, hypokalaemia, hypertriglyceridaemia and diminished high density lipoprotein concentration, hypercalcaemia). They are used mainly in conjunction with angiotensin-converting enzyme inhibitors (ACEI) and β-adrenergic blockers, whose actions they enhance. They appear to have a specific application in patients of African black extraction and the elderly.

Thiazides are also presented in compound tablets with potassium-sparing diuretics (agents whose natriuretic action is on the late distal tubule and therefore avoid interaction with sodium–potassium exchange systems in cell membranes higher up the renal tubule). The agents available are amiloride and triamterene, and the tablets containing them in combination with hydrochlorothiazide (Moduretic and Dyazide respectively) are more potent than thiazides alone. In both preparations, the dose of hydrochlorothiazide is high (50 mg instead of the more usual 25) and hyponatraemia is quite common, especially in older patients, causing drowsiness, confusion and fitting.

Diuretics which act on the loop of Henle (frusemide, bumetanide and ethacrynic acid) are more potent but have little place in the management of benign high blood pressure. They find a place in more severe hypertension in combination with ACEI or minoxidil, or in patients with severely impaired renal function in whom water and sodium retention are major factors in the elevation of blood pressure.

Vasodilators

This heterogeneous group is seldom used, apart from minoxidil which is probably the most potent antihypertensive agent available. Hydralazine is most commonly used in hypertension of pregnancy. Diazoxide is virtually confined to its intravenous form in hypertensive emergencies (see below). The cellular mechanisms by which these compounds act are largely unknown and probably heterogeneous. Minoxidil opens potassium channels in cell membranes and blocks the formation of uridine monophosphate while diazoxide probably also impairs the function of ion pumps. The place of members of this group is largely as second or third line agents (given after maximum therapy

with one or two other agents has failed to lower blood pressure), combined with other types of drugs, particularly β-blockers.

Adverse effects are mainly extensions of pharmacological effect with headache and palpitations being prominent. Minoxidil causes oedema and hirsutism. Hydralazine is relatively frequently associated with lupus erythematosus, a dose-related phenomenon seen almost solely in slow acetylators who metabolize the drug more slowly than fast acetylators.

Centrally acting agents

This heterogeneous group includes clonidine, which stimulates CNS α-adrenergic receptors and thus reduces outgoing sympathetic nerve traffic, α-methyl DOPA which has similar actions and also appears to act as a false neurotransmitter in peripheral neurones, and guanabenz and guanfacine. Ketanserin, which blocks S_3 serotonin receptors in the CNS, is not usually grouped with the others. Adverse effects include drowsiness as a group effect, thirst in the case of clonidine, and depression and a range of autoimmune effects in the case of α-methyl DOPA (haemolytic anaemia, hepatic fibrosis).

Centrally acting agents are used less frequently since the advent of β-blockers. Clonidine is used in hypertension of pregnancy in some centres and α-methyl DOPA remains a standard treatment for this condition. Ketanserin has significant α-adrenergic blocking effects and is a useful substitute drug for patients who experience adverse effects from other agents.

α-Adrenergic blockers

At present, prazosin is the principal member of this group but longer-acting agents are becoming available including doxazosin, terazosin and trimazosin. Since they inhibit sympathetic venoconstrictor response to upright posture, allowing pooling of blood in capacitance vessels, postural hypotension is a predictable adverse effect. It has been shown in elderly patients, however, that these effects can be avoided by lower doses of prazosin. Postural syncope is potentially more dangerous in the elderly, in whom falls are more likely to be complicated by fractures of the neck of femur.

α-blockers are mildly anticholesterolaemic and may possess similar cell growth inhibiting effects to ACE inhibitors. They may thus be of benefit in patients with left ventricular hypertrophy or abnormal plasma lipids where they will at least not worsen the biochemical picture in a way likely to increase coronary risk.

Calcium channel blockers

There are three pharmacologically active chemical classes in this group: the benzalkylamines, related to morphine, with concurrent effects on slow sodium channels in the myocardium and conducting bundles leading to bradycardia and left ventricular inhibition; the benzothiodiazepines, with major coronary artery dilating properties; and the dihydropyridines, which are relatively specific peripheral vasodilators. The last group has become the principal type of calcium channel blocker used in high blood pressure. They act selectively on vascular smooth muscle to reduce peripheral resistance with expected unwanted effects of flushing, headache while blood pressure remains elevated, and 'wooziness'. They commonly cause oedema, due, it is thought, to dilatation of precapillary vessels exposing capillary blood to arteriolar pressure and causing transudation.

All three groups are now used for treating high blood pressure. Verapamil and diltiazem are not recommended for use with β-blockers because of their effects on the myocardium, and there is uncertainty about their synergy with diuretics. It is accepted that all three classes complement well the effects of ACEI, and the dihydropyridines those of β-blockers.

β-Adrenergic blockers

In the 1970s, these became the dominant antihypertensive medication but their adverse effects of fatigue and bronchoconstriction have led to their being superseded by the ACE inhibitors and calcium channel blockers. They remain in common use as sole agents and as adjuncts to dihydropyridines, α-blockers and vasodilators. Several effective compounds have been synthesized which combine β-blockade with other antihypertensive effects, such as labetalol (α-blockade) and celiprolol (smooth muscle relaxation). Some possess pharmacological properties which confer therapeutic advantage such as relative selectivity for the β-receptors or intrinsic sympathomimetic activity. Still, they can never be used in patients with obstructed airways in whom β_2-blockade results in bronchoconstriction, or peripheral vascular disease where unopposed α_2-adrenergic activity in small arteries exacerbates the ischaemia. They are also not indicated in diabetes where they unstabilize glucose homeostasis and mask symptoms of hypoglycaemia. They may precipitate cardiac failure in patients with left ventricular dilatation or dysfunction although they are used to correct the reduced diastolic filling associated with marked concentric hypertrophy of the ventricle (diastolic failure).

On the other hand, they are considered to have a mild anxiolytic effect which may be useful in some patients. Their proven benefits in angina and protective effects in patients who have had myocardial infarction are also useful. Although β-blockers have been shown to cause mild hypertriglyceridaemia and, in obese patients, hypercholesterolaemia, the hazards of this in terms of subsequent infarction have not been shown.

Angiotensin-converting enzyme inhibitors

ACEI are the dominant compounds in current use in terms of sales and scientific interest. Their actions may not depend solely on blockade of the renin–angiotensin system since ACE (originally classified as kininase II) degrades many small physiologically active peptides — including bradykinin, whose actions have been postulated to mediate many of the benefits of ACEI. It is said to inhibit tissue growth, platelet/endothelial interaction, toxic damage from reactive oxygen species and collagenosis of the myocardium. No physiological benefit has yet been ascribed to the other peptides whose ECF concentrations rise with ACE inhibition.

ACEI cause arteriolar dilatation, inhibit the synthesis of aldosterone and reduce α-adrenergic traffic to arterioles, proximal tubule sodium absorption and thirst. Since ACE is found in the medial layer of most of the arterial tree and many tissues, the action of inhibitors does not depend solely on circulating renin and pulmonary ACE. While the initial hypotensive effects depend on circulating renin and angiotensin II (ang II), the long-term effects do not. Whether the central nervous system renin–angiotensin system has a predominant role is unknown. It is of note that the major portion of this system is in the circumventricular organ, an area involved in vascular control and functionally outside the blood/brain barrier.

ACEI are very effective agents which act synergistically with most other classes although they are not usually added to β-blockers. Most adverse effects are extensions of pharmacological effect although neutropenia is a class effect seen most commonly in patients with renal impairment. Agents with sulphhydryl groups also cause penicillamine-like effects including proteinuria and membranous nephropathy. Unusual effects such as loss of taste or abnormal taste sensations and the 'scalded mouth' syndrome may be mediated by other peptides whose catabolism is inhibited such as substance P or capsaicin. Since ACEI reduce the effects of aldosterone, they are not usually given with potassium-sparing diuretics.

Their major adverse effect is cough, whose mechanism is ill-understood. It may occur in 15% of patients and its interaction with other cardiopulmonary disease can be severe. In patients who take these agents for severe heart failure, however, cough is said to be less common. Other major effects relate to the role of ang II in the maintenance of glomerular filtration. When preglomerular arteriolar pressure falls from renal artery stenosis, intra-renal vascular occlusion from high blood pressure or primary renal disease, or from cardiac pump failure, filtration pressure is maintained by increasing downstream resistance by efferent arteriolar constriction, a mechanism largely mediated on a nephron to nephron basis by locally formed ang II. ACE inhibition blocks this compensation and in patients with renal artery stenosis to a solitary kidney or bilateral renal artery stenosis, ACEI may cause acute renal failure. Similar changes occur less acutely in patients with severe heart failure. Acute renal failure is an indication for withdrawal of ACEI but in heart failure, mild stable renal failure may be an acceptable price to reduce the high risk of sudden death. As cardiac function improves, renal function often improves too. Although ACEI are the agents of choice in patients with peripheral vascular disease, for preservation of peripheral circulation, the probability of coexisting renal artery stenosis must always be borne in mind and such patients followed closely in the early stages to be sure renal function is not impaired.

The effects on efferent arteriolar tone are believed to account partly for the apparent specific benefit of ACEI in renal disease with proteinuria. Their role in diabetic nephropathy is controversial although they have the advantage of achieving blood pressures in the low normal range in a high percentage of patients, with minimum subjective adverse effects.

TREATMENT STRATEGIES

Where treatment is not urgent, patients ought to be given a trial of non-pharmacological treatment (Table 27.3), concentrating on obviously correctable factors where possible. This can be carried out during the early phase of medical contact and co-ordinated with the determination of basal blood pressure and basic investigations (see Fig. 27.4.)

The choice of a drug to start lowering blood pressure is controversial. Some researchers favour starting with the 'simplest' medication and working up to the most 'potent'. Simplicity and potency are difficult properties to define in antihypertensive drugs but are usually equated with cheapness and years of use on the one hand, and recent development and the concept of being effective in 'difficult' hypertensive patients on the other. This latter idea is particularly hard to put into a conceptual framework and the whole idea of 'stepped care' is now largely outdated although this approach is in effect what is used in most patients.

Modern selection of agents is now often referred to as 'tailored' to patients' individual needs. How this tailoring is done varies from nation to nation. In the United States, much has been made of dividing patients into 'low renin' and 'high renin' or 'salt-responsive' or non-responsive groups. In many countries, however, no such prior distinction is made and the choice of starting treatment is made on economic grounds, grounds of familiarity with particular agents or consideration of specific advantages of individual agents or combinations of agents. These may include concurrent treatment of associated disease (β-blockers in patients with angina pectoris or diuretics in patients with early left ventricular failure), avoidance of predictable complications (β-blockers in bronchial asthma or diabetes mellitus, diuretics in diabetes or gout) or the use of synergistic agents in lower doses to improve efficacy and give each agent in a dose likely to avoid adverse effects (β-blockers and calcium channel blockers or vasodilators, diuretics and ACE inhibitors).

On the whole it is a good idea for doctors to become familiar with a member of each major class of antihypertensive agent and confine treatment to these for the most part. First line treatment may be with agents of virtually any class although groups such as vasodilators are now mostly confined to severe high blood pressure as added agents and centrally acting agents are rarely used. Diuretics are not often used in young men because of the possibility of impotence, and rapidly acting dihydropyridine calcium channel blockers are avoided in patients with angina pectoris because they may precipitate symptoms by reflex tachycardia.

HYPERTENSIVE EMERGENCIES

These are vastly overdiagnosed and are conditions of emergency doctors rather than of patients. The term is most commonly applied to patients who attend casualty or a doctor's rooms with a blood pressure of 180/120 or above, usually with symptoms such as headache, dizziness, blurring of vision or nausea. The fundamental principle of management is that the blood pressure is unlikely to have reached that level over the last day or even the last week. This has two implications: first there

are almost certainly obstructive lesions in arteries and arterioles whose perfusion territories will be rendered ischaemic by an abrupt fall in blood pressure; second, the patient has been tolerating the elevated arterial pressure for so long that another 6–8 hours is most unlikely to cause significant extra harm.

The harmful effects of abrupt blood pressure reduction were observed with diazoxide, which caused an unacceptably high incidence of stroke and myocardial infarction when given as originally advised — 300 mg intravenously within 25 seconds. Similar results are reported for sublingual nifedipine.

True hypertensive crisis is confined to acute left ventricular failure and pulmonary oedema, hypertensive encephalopathy, intracranial haemorrhage, eclampsia of pregnancy, central retinal vascular occlusions or intraocular haemorrhage and the α-adrenergically mediated events associated with catecholamine release from a phaeochromocytoma or sympathetic nerve discharge in patients taking monoamine oxidase inhibitors who are exposed to catecholamine release stimuli such as ingestion of tyramine-containing foods like cheeses or meat products. In such cases rapid reduction by any means is indicated. The most effective means in patients unable to take oral medication are intravenous sodium nitroprusside infusion, intravenous diazoxide in 15 mg boluses at 1–5 minute intervals, sublingual nifedipine from a punctured capsule or sublingual captopril paediatric syrup. If oral medication is feasible, a 10 mg nifedipine capsule may be crushed in the mouth and swallowed. In acute left ventricular failure, intravenous glyceryl trinitrate is often used, reducing pre-load as well as afterload on the left ventricle. All these procedures are best carried out in an intensive care unit with central vascular pressure monitoring.

Mostly, however, more gradual blood pressure reduction is indicated. Useful agents are labetalol, 400 mg orally, a combination of a large dose of a β-blocker (100 mg atenolol or metoprolol or equivalent) with 20 mg prazosin, or a calcium channel blocker such as nifedipine, felodipine, amlodipine or isradipine. These regimes return blood pressure to acceptable levels in 6–8 hours and have a much lower complication rate.

SECONDARY HIGH BLOOD PRESSURE

Conn's syndrome — primary hyperaldosteronism

The production of excess aldosterone by adenomas or hyperplasia of the zona glomerulosa of the adrenal cortex results classically in hypokalaemia, metabolic alkalosis, with a plasma bicarbonate usually over 30 mmolar, and hypernatraemia. The clinical features are striking, with muscle weakness prominent, but the blood pressure is often only mildly elevated. There is now growing evidence that a significant proportion of such patients do not have florid abnormalities and this form of high blood pressure may require more sophisticated screening in the future using parameters such as plasma renin–aldosterone ratios and measurement of steroid responses to sodium loading and infused stimulatory hormones. The important issues are to establish the diagnosis with high blood pressure, elevated plasma aldosterone and suppressed plasma renin, to define the nature of the adrenal pathology — bilateral hyperplasia or tumour — and, if the latter, to localize it.

While various subtypes of Conn's syndrome have been described, their distinction is usually unnecessary. In a well-equipped metabolic ward, the sensitivity to sodium loading, ang II infusion or ACE inhibition can be explored. From these data, it is possible to construct a diagnostic algorithm to distinguish aldosterone-producing adenoma, bilateral adrenal hyperplasia, angiotensin-responsive adrenal hyperplasia and idiopathic hyperaldosteronism. It is recommended that adenomas and adrenals in angiotensin-responsive hyperaldosteronism are excised. While the hypertension of Conn's syndrome is rarely necrotizing in type, it is often malignant in course, with a high rate of stroke. There may be a case for bilateral adrenalectomy when both glands are involved, and steroid replacement is frequently more easily managed than the high blood pressure.

Phaeochromocytoma

Tumours of chromaffin cells of the sympathetic chain occur at all ages. In children, neuroblastomas and medulloblastomas produce severe high blood pressure and are highly malignant. In adults, phaeochromocytomas are rarely malignant in cell type but, if left untreated, have a sinister prognosis. Of particular importance is the sensitivity of such tumours to X-ray contrast and it is wise to exclude them by quantitation of urinary catecholamine excretion before embarking on tests using these compounds, especially renal or adrenal angiography. These are almost invariably lethal in patients with undiagnosed tumours who have not been given effective doses of α-adrenergic blockers (usually phenoxybenzamine, at least 100 mg daily). Localization of phaeochromocytoma is most commonly carried out by radionuclide scanning using meta-iodo benzguanine (MIBG). About 10% of phaeochromocytomas are malignant, multiple or extra-adrenal. The latter two groups are frequently associated with other endocrinological tumours in syndromes termed 'multiple endocrine neoplasia' (MEN).

Renal artery stenosis

The nature of renal artery stenosis in clinical practice has changed over the last 20 years. Originally the condition was sought in younger patients who were usually found to have non-atheromatous disease of the renal artery such as fibromuscular medial hyperplasia, intimal fibrous dysplasia in one of its forms, renal artery aneurysm or arteriovenous malformation. The most frequent form now seen is atheromatous in elderly patients and, since high blood pressure is at once a risk factor for this pathology and such a common complication of renal disease, there is an increased incidence in patients with pre-existing renal disease. Renal artery stenosis may be the only reversible element in a patient with multifactorial renal failure.

Renal artery stenosis should be suspected in any patient with documented recent onset or worsening of high blood pressure (Fig. 27.4). In patients with other renal disease, particularly analgesic nephropathy, worsening renal function should raise the possibility as should high blood pressure in people under 30 or occurring for the first time in people over 60 years of age. There is rarely any specific history to be obtained although loin pain or haematuria may occur. Nephrotic range proteinuria has been described and rapidly rising blood pressure may induce pressure diuresis through the opposite kidney.

The commonest physical finding is peripheral vascular disease, of which the renal artery stenosis is a manifestation. Renal artery bruits are helpful but rare. That described as characteristic of renal artery stenosis is heard in the epigastrium or over the origin of the renal artery, radiating towards the renal angle, smooth, high-pitched and prolonged through systole and diastole. Such a bruit is the strongest predictor of successful correction of the stenosis. Bruits heard on the right side are more reliable than on the left, where the long tortuous and unsupported splenic artery often generates bruits in normal people.

Intravenous pyelography shows delayed appearance of dye on the affected side, which is smaller than the opposite kidney, and delayed clearance with a persistent pyelogram. Rarely, the presence of dilated collateral vessels around the ureter causes indentations in the ureteric shadow. Pyelography is not used so much now and the usual course of action is to detect the discrepancy in renal size with ultrasound and to proceed to renal angiography with balloon dilatation. Radionuclide scanning with DTPA shows differences in renal perfusion and an ACEI (usually captopril) may be given to enhance this effect. Captopril may also be used in a screening test for renal artery stenosis. Plasma renin concentration is said to increase by a factor of more than 2.5 following 25 mg given orally. The definitive diagnosis is by renal angiography although some groups claim to be able to detect stenosis using pulsed doppler ultrasound in thinner people. Treatment is frequently by balloon angioplasty although it can be argued that surgery is to be preferred in atheromatous stenosis, particularly when it is bilateral.

HIGH BLOOD PRESSURE IN RENAL DISEASE

Virtually all renal diseases are associated with increased incidence of high blood pressure (see Table 27.1 — Renal causes). Since the kidney is also one of its principal targets, control of high blood pressure is a major facet of the treatment of renal disease and, in the case of some forms of glomerulonephritis and reflux nephropathy, may be the sole meaningful therapeutic goal. The transmission of elevated systemic pressure to the glomerulus is held to be a major element in the process of non-immune glomerular injury which leads inexorably, after the cessation of the primary pathological processes of glomerulonephritis, to end-stage renal failure.

Mechanisms in renal hypertension

Observation of the setting of renal hypertension shows us that there must be at least two basic groups of processes which link renal disease with high blood pressure. The first is active — action by the kidney which leads acutely or chronically to high blood pressure. Such a mechanism is the renin–angiotensin system. The second is the failure of the kidney to lower blood pressure — the so-called renoprival effect. This may be the failure to excrete water and sodium when nephron mass is reduced or the failure to produce significant amounts of vasodepressor substances such as prostaglandins or kinins.

Both mechanisms may be demonstrable in clinical or experimental renal hypertension. Plasma renin concentration is not often elevated in chronic renal disease, however, and the commonest setting for renal hypertension is chronic renal failure where functioning renal mass is drastically reduced and a renoprival mechanism is more logically invoked.

In other forms of renal disease, mechanisms of high blood pressure are more easily discernible. In the earlier stages of experimental renal artery stenosis, renin appears to be the prime mechanism. In established RAS, about 50% of patients have elevated plasma renin and many workers argue strongly that, in most of the others, renin acts in concert with other systems such as the sympathetic nervous system. Whatever the mediating system, renal artery distortion and intra-renal segmental stenosis have been held to be a major cause of high blood pressure in structural disorders such as

Grawitz tumour (renal cell carcinoma), polycystic kidneys and the scarring in reflux and analgesic nephropathies.

The renin–angiotensin system

Renin was originally described as a renal hormone and subsequently discovered to be an enzyme which acts on a fourteen amino acid moiety of a protein substrate to produce a ten amino acid chain (decapeptide) angiotensin I (ang 1). This in turn is degraded by a converting enzyme, mainly in the lung, to the active eight amino acid chain (octapeptide) ang II. It has since been shown that elision of amino acids from the N-terminal end of the molecule produces a family of angiotensins of which the first, ang III (des-aspartyl ang II), is almost equipotent with ang II and the rest show rapidly diminishing potency so that the C-terminal five acid chain is without activity.

Since 1975, it has become clear that our original concept of a renal hormonal system is in error. The components of the system (renin, substrate and converting enzyme) are found throughout the arterial and arteriolar system, apparently both synthesized in situ (the relevant messenger RNAs often being found) and carried there in blood. The large amounts found in the kidney are due to the presence there of highly specialized cells in the afferent glomerular arteriole, which are important in conditions such as renal artery stenosis where diminished perfusion pressure stimulates the production of renin, causing high blood pressure in a proportion of instances. The system may have a much wider role in essential hypertension where the response of the intra-arteriolar renin–angiotensin system to circulating and endothelially secreted pressor mechanisms may be of crucial importance.

Renin secretion is strongly stimulated by dietary sodium restriction, acute sodium loss by any route, or ECF contraction. Mostly, ECF state appears to be the dominant factor in blood pressure regulation — diuretic treatment reduces blood pressure by ECF contraction initially, in the face of rising renin concentration; patients with chronic renal failure often have high blood pressure with high ECF volume and normal or low renin. In some patients, this relationship is upset by unknown means so that renin becomes the dominant factor in blood pressure regulation. This is almost always associated with sodium-losing states, in particular analgesic nephropathy and malignant hypertension, a state termed 'hyponatraemic hypertension'. Paradoxically, diuretics raise blood pressure and plasma expansion with sodium chloride infusion lowers it. This state may reflect changed ang II-receptor characteristics, the stimulation of other pressor mechanisms or loss of depressor mechanisms. A parallel situation exists in toxaemia of pregnancy, a state of extracellular contraction where blood pressure may be lowered by ECF expansion with osmotic agents such as mannitol. There is now good evidence that this condition is associated with a marked increase in ang II-receptor numbers compared with normal pregnancy.

Endothelin

The cyclic peptide endothelin was first described in 1988 and, as its name suggests, was first isolated in arteriolar endothelial cells. Preliminary evidence suggests its actions (sustained vasoconstriction and vigorous platelet activation) may be involved in some forms of high blood pressure and of acute renal failure.

Prostaglandins

Prostaglandins are secreted by renal medullary interstitial cells where they may be seen on electron microscopy as osmiophilic secretory granules. The principal ones produced in the kidney are PGE_1 and $PGF_{2\alpha}$. They probably act locally, inhibiting reabsorption of sodium in the cortical diluting segment and late distal tubule, inhibiting the production of renin and dilating intra-renal arteries and arterioles. To date, failure of secretion has not been shown to be a major mechanism for renoprival hypertension.

Kinins

Kallikrein, the enzyme which degrades a substrate to produce bradykinin, is found in the medullary interstitium, and bradykinin is found in abundance in this region. It dilates intra-renal blood vessels, stimulates renin secretion and promotes natriuresis. It is doubtful if renally secreted bradykinin has systemic vascular effects or plays a part in renal hypertension.

Platelet-activating factor

Related to the prostanoids, this compound is secreted vigorously in the period following release of renal arterial constriction in the one kidney–one clip model of hypertension and may be a significant renal vasodepressor mechanism whose absence plays a part in high blood pressure associated with renal parenchymal disease.

Extracellular space expansion

Whatever other mechanisms may be in play, increased body sodium and water are the major and constant mechanisms for increasing blood pressure in parenchymal renal disease. The sensitivity of blood pressure to increases in ECFV induced by intravenous saline infusion and the almost total control of blood pressure in end-stage renal failure by removal of salt and water during dialysis reflect this.

INDICATIONS FOR INVESTIGATION

The overall indications are shown in the logic tree for the management of the hypertensive patient (Fig. 27.4). Part of the initial examination is urinalysis, which should include microscopy as well as dipstick testing and, if the protein strip is positive or multiple myeloma is suspected, boiling or treatment with salicylsulphonic acid. The presence of urinary abnormalities directs the clinician towards renal parenchymal disease, most commonly glomerulonephritis.

A common problem arises when subnephrotic proteinuria occurs. Up to 2 g of protein per day may be lost in the urine in hypertensive nephrosclerosis. While most patients with 0.5 g or more will have primary glomerular disease, it may be advisable with this degree of proteinuria, in the presence of normal renal function, to control the blood pressure scrupulously for six months while monitoring renal function, and to proceed to biopsy only if proteinuria persists. Studies of complement components and other non-invasive investigations for glomerular disease (ANCA, tests for systemic lupus erythematosus) will assist the decision.

Renal failure of any degree is an indication for further investigation, although clinical acumen often suggests that it results from hypertension and effective treatment is then instituted as a measure of the role of high blood pressure in its aetiology. Investigations in hypertensive patients with renal failure are as for any other patient with the condition.

CHRONIC RENAL FAILURE AND HIGH BLOOD PRESSURE

Blood pressure may be elevated from the renal disease which has led to impairment, and frequently requires pharmacological treatment to be continued until the institution of dialysis. Occasionally, blood pressure will be normal and rise as the capacity to excrete water and sodium declines. Before dialysis is needed, patients may respond to large doses of loop diuretics although recent evidence suggests that these may accelerate the rate of loss of residual renal function. Most patients are hypertensive by the time they require dialysis and blood pressure is best controlled in almost all by reduction of ECF by ultrafiltration. In about 1%, however, high blood pressure is associated with high circulating renin and does not fall with fluid removal or may even become worse. This was once an indication for bilateral nephrectomy but is now almost universally controlled by ACE inhibitors.

Where blood pressure cannot be controlled by ECF reduction, pharmacological agents will be necessary. Virtually all are used but the lipid-raising effects of β-blockers make them less useful. The ACE inhibitors available are excreted mainly by the kidney and doses must be reduced. Therapeutic concentrations of enalapril, for instance, are achieved by 5 mg given after two out of three dialyses weekly. Adverse affects of ACEI are commoner in renal failure. Patients on captopril need regular white cell counts since neutropenia and agranulocytosis are recognized hazards. Taste disturbances and 'scalded mouth' are also more common with all ACEI in patients with renal failure.

Chronic renal failure is also associated with other coronary risk factors, particularly elevated triglycerides, low HDL-cholesterol and, less commonly, high LDL. Not surprisingly, myocardial infarction and ischaemic loss of functioning myocardium are the commonest causes of death in patients on dialysis. Correction of lipid abnormalities is an important aspect of the management of patients on dialysis. Most agents available may be used and early studies suggest that newer agents such as the HMG Co-A reductase inhibitors may be particularly effective at lowering cholesterol, although no data regarding the coronary outcome of such treatment are yet available.

Where myocardial contractility is reduced, the left ventricle may be seen in a new light — as the buffer between systemic and pulmonary circulations. The degree to which fluctuations in ECF between and during dialysis are tolerated without pulmonary oedema on the one hand and postural hypotension on the other is a measure of left ventricular integrity.

HIGH BLOOD PRESSURE AFTER RENAL TRANSPLANTATION

The hypertension which occurred in many patients prior to transplantation may persist afterwards and require drug treatment where it was formerly controlled by dialysis alone. In addition, several factors lead to new hypertension and exacerbation of coronary risk factors which must be corrected.

Prednisolone

Corticosteroids remain an almost invariable facet of immunosuppression. As well as raising blood pressure, they cause hyperglycaemia and elevate plasma cholesterol, further predisposing to coro-

nary artery atheroma. Prednisolone can rarely be suspended but titrating other immunosuppression to allow early dose reduction, and alternate daily dosing have been found to reduce metabolic effects. Antihypertensive and cholesterol-lowering drugs are frequently needed all the same.

Cyclosporin A

Cyclosporin A raises blood pressure quite potently by a number of mechanisms. It causes renal water and sodium retention, stimulates sympathetic nerve traffic to limb circulations and causes specific renal changes which may, together with high blood pressure, lead to chronic failure. The last is more frequent with heart and liver transplantation where higher doses of cyclosporin A are administered. It has recently been claimed that this agent also raises plasma cholesterol.

Graft artery stenosis

Since donor kidneys are now usually taken en bloc with the related segment of aorta, giving an arterial cuff to perform end-to-side (rather than end-to-end) anastomosis to the recipient internal iliac artery, this has become rare. It should be considered in any transplanted patient in whom blood pressure rises and renal function deteriorates at the same time (although cyclosporin toxicity will result in a similar clinical course). Arterial stenosis is frequently discovered when an ACE inhibitor is given for rapidly rising blood pressure and causes oligo-anuric renal failure. Histology of the stenotic segment often shows changes of rejection rather than atheroma.

SPECIAL GROUPS WITH HIGH BLOOD PRESSURE

Hypertension in pregnancy
See Chapter 25.

High blood pressure in the elderly

Blood pressure rises with age in most European societies, a phenomenon apparently associated with high dietary sodium intake. Only recently has it been shown that this results in early cardiovascular events and that lowering blood pressure reduces their incidence. Most pharmacological agents may be used although the major trial data are based on diuretics, β-blockers, α-methyl DOPA and hydralazine. ACE inhibitors are effective but the possibility of renal artery stenosis in elderly patients with vascular disease must be borne in mind. Similarly, β-blockers are contra-indicated in people with vascular disease, airflow limitation or any degree of systolic left ventricular failure. Whatever agent is used, it must be remembered that baroreceptor buffering of postural falls in blood pressure is slow. It is essential to begin with very low doses and increase them slowly — the period of 18 months is cited as a reasonable time to spend reducing blood pressure in this group.

FURTHER READING

Collins R, Peto R, MacMahon S et al 1990 Blood pressure, stroke and coronary heart disease. Part 2, short term reductions in blood pressure: overview of randomised drug trial in their epidemiological context. Lancet 335: 827–838

Dickinson C J 1990 Reappraisal of the Cushing reflex: the most powerful neural blood pressure stabilising system. Clinical Science 79: 543–550

Folkow B 1982 Physiological aspects of primary hypertension. Physiological Reviews 62: 347–504

Intersalt Cooperative Research Group 1988 Intersalt: an international study of electrolyte excretion and blood pressure. Results for 24 hour urinary sodium and potassium excretion. British Medical Journal 297: 319–328

MacMahon S, Peto R, Cutler J et al 1990 Blood pressure, stroke and coronary heart disease. Part 1, prolonged difference in blood pressure, prospective observational studies corrected for regression dilution bias. Lancet 335: 765–774

O'Brien E, O'Malley K 1991 Blood pressure measurement. Part 14 in: Reid J L, Birkenhager W M (eds) Handbook of hypertension. Elsevier, Amsterdam

Williams R R, Hunt S C, Hasstedt S J et al 1988 Definition of genetic factors in hypertension: a search for major genes, polygenes and homogeneous subtypes. Journal of Cardiovascular Pharmacology 12 (Suppl 3): S7–S20

28. Urology

V. R. Marshall

It is not possible in a single chapter to encompass all aspects of urology. As in the previous edition of this book, the focus has been placed on areas where there have been recent changes in investigation or management and, also, where there is a significant interface between nephrology and urology.

Diagnostic techniques

In spite of the many new modalities that have been introduced, urine microscopy and culture, as well as intravenous urography (IVU) and cystoscopy, still remain important diagnostic tools in the evaluation of individuals with urological complaints. There is, however, no doubt that ultrasound, CT and MRI scanning, ureteroscopy and urodynamics are playing an increasingly important role in the diagnosis of urological disorders. With the introduction of these modalities, there is undoubtedly scope for duplication and the introduction of unnecessary steps in the diagnostic process. Particularly when one is assessing individuals with disorders of micturition, in particular the control of micturition, the need to take a thorough and detailed history cannot be overemphasized before resorting to the use of some of these newer diagnostic techniques. However, in spite of the introduction of many of these new techniques, one of the major weaknesses that still exist is our lack of ability to detect lymph node involvement when we are attempting to stage urinary tract malignancies.

RENAL–UROTHELIAL–PROSTATIC MALIGNANCIES

In the investigation of patients presenting with symptoms from these carcinomas, the investigations need to fill two roles: diagnostic and staging.

Renal cell carcinomas

In the past, patients with renal cell carcinomas usually presented for further evaluation because of haematuria, loin pain or a mass. Fever, metastatic disease or endocrine abnormalities were rare reasons for the initiation of investigation. This has now changed quite dramatically, as the most common presentation of a renal carcinoma is as a coincidental finding as a result of an ultrasound examination or a CT scan.

An intravenous urogram is still the most appropriate initial investigation if the patient presents with haematuria. However, if there is a suspicion of a mass or persistent loin pain, a CT scan with contrast enhancement is potentially the most appropriate investigation. If the intravenous urogram suggests a mass then a CT scan will still be necessary to establish the diagnosis of a renal cell carcinoma. In the case of renal cell carcinomas, a CT scan has a diagnostic accuracy of between 92–95%, however it is important to note that the staging accuracy of this investigation is approximately 80%. This is superior at the present time to most other diagnostic modalities, but it does mean that it is not always possible to establish pre-operatively whether a tumour is still confined to the kidney or has spread to the surrounding structures. This observation is particularly important; the outcome of surgery is much less favourable once the tumour has involved other structures as there is then little chance of cure.

Fine needle aspiration performed with either ultrasound or CT control has been used to confirm the presence of renal tumours, but its accuracy is similar to that of a CT scan. Therefore it would appear that this investigation is best reserved for tumours where diagnostic doubts exist after the CT scan has been performed or if surgery is not planned.

Treatment

The treatment of choice for a renal cell carcinoma is still nephrectomy. The only exceptions are stage 4 tumours which have extensive local organ involvement or where there is a small relatively asymptomatic primary tumour with extensive metastases. At the present time, initial studies examining the use of laparoscopic nephrectomy in the case of small primary tumours have been undertaken, but it is too early to say that a laparoscopic approach will supplant the more traditional forms of open surgery, particularly in the case of a large tumour. Other forms of therapy have been disappointing: radiotherapy pre- and post-operatively, and single and multiple agent chemotherapy appear to have little effect on survival. There have been some reports of the use of interferon in the management of patients with metastatic disease, however the primary needs to be removed and even in these individuals, dramatic response rates and significant prolongation of life have not been reported.

Radiotherapy can be useful for palliation of local disease, particularly the management of osteolytic bone secondaries. However, patient survival still depends to a large degree on the stage and grade of tumour at the time of diagnosis, hence increased detection of coincidental renal cell carcinomas may inadvertently lead to superior outcomes.

TRANSITIONAL CELL CARCINOMAS

Renal pelvis, ureter and bladder

Although these tumours are almost all transitional cell carcinomas, it is more convenient to group the pelvic and ureteric tumours together and to consider them separately from bladder tumours.

Renal pelvis and ureteric tumours

Although transitional cell carcinomas are undoubtedly the most common tumour type, both squamous cell carcinomas and adenocarcinomas have been reported. The importance of analgesic abuse in the aetiology of these tumours is now well recognized, but since the relevant drug combinations were removed from sale, the relevance of the agents to the incidence of this disease has reduced markedly. However, the fact that it has been possible to identify a number of agents which do have carcinogenic potential for the epithelium makes it important to document the drug and occupational history of any individual with these tumours.

Presentation

Haematuria is the usual reason for presentation, but occasionally the only symptom is loin pain due to obstruction.

Investigation

In at least two thirds of patients an intravenous urogram will confirm the diagnosis; a high false negative rate (40–50%) makes urine cytology a poor screening test, but it may be of value if uncertainty exists after intravenous urography. In the remaining one third, retrograde ureterography, ureteric washings or brushings, or ureteroscopy may be necessary to establish a diagnosis.

The conditions that are most difficult to distinguish from a transitional cell carcinoma in the pelvis are non-opaque stones, blood clot, a sloughed renal papilla and rarely tuberculosis or (in immunosuppressed patients) fungal balls. However, in the case of nonopaque stones, the introduction of renal ultrasound or CT scanning has made it much easier to demonstrate the presence of a stone. With regard to the other lesions, the availability of flexible ureteroscopes has the potential to enhance pre-operative diagnostic accuracy.

Treatment

The treatment of choice is nephroureterectomy; however, such an approach is only appropriate if it has been possible to establish that the tumour is confined to the urinary tract. Since the development of a new tumour involving other parts of the urothelium is always possible, all patients need to be followed up regularly with cystoscopies and intravenous urography. In rare instances, for example in a patient with a low grade tumour in a solitary kidney, local removal by percutaneous techniques may be appropriate. It is possible with greater experience in this form of management that these techniques, which allow the preservation of renal function, may be more widely used. However, the risk is that in attempting to preserve renal function one may jeopardize the eradication of the tumour.

Radiotherapy and chemotherapy have, to date, failed to affect significantly the course of metastatic disease, but they do have a role as palliative agents. Therefore, as with renal cell carcinomas, the patient's survival depends largely on the stage and histological grade of the tumour at the time of diagnosis.

Bladder cancer

Transitional cell carcinomas account for over 90% of primary bladder tumours; the remainder are either squamous cell carcinomas, adenocarcinomas or sarcomas. Although the aetiological factors for all bladder cancers have not been established, it has been known for a long time that there is a definite link between 2-naphthylamine, benzidine and bladder cancer. Epidemiological studies have also implicated tobacco and coffee in the development of these tumours and animal experiments have identified saccharin and cyclamates as possible aetiological factors.

Presentation

Most patients with bladder cancer present with haematuria and occasionally with symptoms of a urinary tract infection. It is important to note that even with large bladder tumours, haematuria may be episodic and microscopic in a significant proportion of cases.

Routine ward testing of urine can also give false positive results; if a urine test is positive for blood, it is essential to confirm this finding by microscopic examination of the same sample. Failure to do this may lead to a chain of unnecessary investigations being initiated by this one false positive result.

Staging

Since patient survival and management depend to a very great extent on tumour stage and histological grade, it is important that both of these parameters are accurately determined at the time of diagnosis. While many staging classifications have been proposed, that based on the TNM (primary tumour/lymph nodes/metastases) system has gained widest acceptance.

Investigation

In all cases urine needs to be sent for microscopic examination and culture. However, because of the episodic nature of the haematuria, if, on the basis of the history, the clinician is convinced that there has been significant bleeding, then the failure to demonstrate blood in a particular urine sample should not discourage further investigation. While cytology may be of value in difficult diagnostic cases, it is not sufficiently accurate to warrant routine use. Intravenous urography is an integral part of the investigation, but failure to demonstrate a filling defect in the bladder films by no means excludes a tumour. Even in the absence of a filling defect, all patients require cystoscopy which is the only way to reliably exclude bladder lesions. If possible, the tumour should be completely resected with some bladder muscle at the time of cystoscopy; if this is not possible, an adequate biopsy, including muscle, should be taken. Recently, random mucosal biopsies have also been advocated in order to assess field changes, as areas of carcinoma in situ may coexist with bladder tumours and these areas may not appear particularly remarkable at the time of cystoscopy. Although such an approach allows accurate histological grading, there is very good evidence that there is a strong tendency to under-stage tumours clinically.

Ultrasound, CT and MRI scanning have been used in an attempt to improve the accuracy of assessing the T (primary tumour) component, but to date it does not seem that these techniques are superior to bimanual examination. The other disadvantage is that if staging is attempted with these modalities after local resection, then the resultant reaction to the resection may make interpretation of the scans difficult. Information regarding the status of the draining lymph nodes is often vital to patient management — if nodes are involved then radical surgery will not achieve a cure. Accurate information regarding node involvement is difficult to obtain. While lymphangiography was used initially, it has high false negative and positive rates, making it insufficiently reliable for clinical use. Likewise, CT scanning and MRI scanning have both been used, but often with disappointing results. With the introduction of laparoscopic surgery, this may well be an appropriate way to establish the status of the lymph nodes without embarking on a formal laparotomy with lymph node dissection and frozen section.

Management

Tumours that are superficial (involving only the mucosa or superficial muscle) can be treated by endoscopic resection. Intravesical instillation of agents such as ethoglucid (Epodyl) and thiotepa have been reported to eradicate small tumours, but the most valuable role for these agents is to minimize recurrence once the bladder has been cleared of tumour by endoscopic resection. However, the efficacy of these substances as preventive agents has by no means been unequivocally established.

The agent which has had the greatest reported success in the control of recurrence has been BCG (bacillus Calmette–Guérin). Instillation of BCG bacilli into the bladder at weekly intervals for six weeks has been shown to eradicate recurrences in between 60 and 80% of patients. It has also been shown to be particularly effective in the management of patients with widespread in-situ transitional cell carcinoma which would otherwise require a total cystectomy to control the problem. If the patient is not suitable for major surgery or the tumour has spread beyond the bladder, relatively few options are available. Radiotherapy can be effective, however response rates are unpredictable.

High grade T2 and T3 tumours require a more radical approach and, if the patient's general condition allows, the treatment of choice is total cystectomy and urinary diversion. However, in the case of young patients, there has been a trend away from a conduit-type diversion to a continent reservoir system.

Continent reservoir system

The options for urinary diversion are now considerable, with the introduction of orthotopic urinary diversion in appropriate circumstances.

Continent reservoirs can be constructed from detubularized colon, ileum or a combination of ileum and colon. These reservoirs can be constructed so that they can either open on to the abdominal wall where continent stomas can be fashioned and be emptied by intermittent catheterization or, if it is possible to safely retain the urethra, they may be anastomosed to the urethra with preservation of essentially normal voiding. In some instances, it is possible to remove the urethra completely, construct a urethra from the appendix and to implant an artificial sphincter, once again providing a reservoir which is continent. However, relatively few patients are suitable for this type of extensive surgery.

A wide range of chemotherapeutic agents have been trialled in the management of this condition. Recent studies using a regimen which incorporated methotrexate, vinblastine, doxorubicin and cisplatin (the MVAC regimen) appeared to confirm a significant survival advantage over cisplatin alone in the management of metastatic disease. At the present time, there are a number of international and national randomized trials under way which compare multi-agent chemotherapy with standard treatment. Until the outcome of these trials is available, it is difficult to determine which of the potential regimens are going to be most efficacious.

Follow-up is required in all cases of transitional carcinoma. However, its frequency and diligence are usually determined by the grade of tumour, recurrence rate and general health of the patient. It is also important to point out that patients who have had continent urinary diversions, because of the absorptive nature of the intestinal reservoir, have the potential to develop metabolic disturbances, particularly a metabolic acidosis. Concern has also been raised about the possible development of new malignancies in these reservoirs.

CARCINOMA OF THE PROSTATE

In the last decade there have been very substantial changes in our attitudes to the management of adenocarcinomas of the prostate. Whilst transitional cell carcinomas, squamous cell carcinomas and sarcomas can arise in the prostate, to all intents and purposes it is only the adenocarcinoma which presents a significant clinical problem. The increased interest in adenocarcinoma of the prostate has, to some extent, been driven by the fact that it is now the most commonly diagnosed cancer in American men and is likely to become the most common cause of cancer death in men. The other important feature is that, even in the 1990s, the majority of men will still have this disease diagnosed when it is at an advanced stage. It is also evident that at present it is not possible to cure advanced carcinoma of the prostate, but cure is possible if it is confined to the prostate. Therefore, it has been proposed that screening programmes may be one way of overcoming this problem because screening may allow detection of disease while it is confined to the prostate. However, at the present time, considerable uncertainty about the value of screening programmes still exists. One problem is that there is a high prevalence of

'histological' cancers and this may result in over-diagnosis. Another difficulty is that the natural history of prostate cancer is quite long; the likelihood that early intervention will significantly alter the outcome has not been established by any means. The other factor that needs to be determined is whether the proposed screening tests will in fact provide the early diagnosis that is required. It therefore seems unlikely at the moment that expensive screening programmes will be introduced generally, however a number of large studies have been established to determine whether screening will be particularly valuable. It may take 10–15 years before this question can be answered. With the rising incidence and concern about prostate cancer, more men with urinary symptoms are seeking to be reassured that they do not have prostate cancer, thus leading almost to a de facto screening process.

Presentation

The presenting urinary symptoms are usually identical to those of benign prostatic hypertrophy, and diagnosis is still reliant on digital rectal examination (DRE); the major change has been the addition of serum prostatic-specific antigen (PSA) estimations. A normal rectal examination and PSA estimation indicates a very low probability of prostate cancer — less than 2%. However, if the patient has an abnormal rectal examination and a PSA level in excess of 10 ng/ml then he has an approximately 80% chance of having cancer of the prostate. In individuals who have a normal DRE but a PSA in excess of 10 ng/ml, we also know that there will be a high incidence of prostate cancer, probably around 60%, and in this group further evaluation is necessary.

The advent of transrectal ultrasound has been particularly useful in this group of patients, as it has the ability to identify abnormal regions in the prostate; as well as allowing multiple random biopsies of each lobe of the prostate to be performed. In the case of patients who have a normal rectal examination but a PSA level between 4 and 10 ng/ml, precise management has not been established. Some authors would suggest it is reasonable to watch these patients and repeat the

PSA in three months, whereas others have suggested that it is appropriate to proceed to a transrectal ultrasound and multiple biopsies. The clinical benefit of this more aggressive approach still needs to be established. However, there is little doubt at the present time that DRE, serum PSA and transrectal ultrasound guided biopsy of the prostate have now become integral parts of the diagnostic process. In particular, PSA measurements have probably made the greatest impact. With greater experience it is likely that PSA measurements will have greater clinical influence, particularly using serial measurements to detect small rises and also in monitoring responses to treatment. However, it is important to note that PSA is not cancer-specific and that it will be elevated in the presence of large glands and if the prostate is infected.

Staging

The staging of prostate carcinoma, as with all tumours, takes into account local extent; increasingly, transrectal ultrasound is being used to determine whether the malignancy is localized to the prostate. For example, transrectal ultrasound has the ability to detect seminal vesicle involvement and capsular extension, and is more accurate than DRE. An elevated PSA level above 30 ng/ml also suggests that there is metastatic disease, however at the present time there is no absolute correlation between PSA levels in this range and spread beyond the gland. The other important modality in staging is, of course, the bone scan, however this is not particularly sensitive and will not detect early spread. Once again, attempts to define the status of the lymph nodes by either CT scans or MRI have been disappointing and in a number of centres the nodal status is being determined prior to radical surgery by laparoscopic means.

Management

At the present time, there has been a strong swing towards radical prostatectomy for the management of localized disease, particularly in fit men under the age of 70 where there is a life expectancy of between 10 and 15 years. It does appear from the literature that under those circumstances, radical prostatectomy does offer the most favourable outcome, however these results are not dramatically better than those described for radiotherapy. Thus, there is still support for radiotherapy as the primary treatment for localized disease, particularly in patients with major medical problems. Unfortunately, it is likely to be some time before it is possible to establish on the basis of randomized controlled trials that surgery is significantly better than radiotherapy as the primary treatment and which patients will obtain the greatest benefit.

In patients with disseminated disease, the treatment of choice is androgen suppression. It can either be achieved by orchidectomy or with the use of LH RH analogues, or anti-androgens such as cyproterone acetate. Unfortunately, particularly in patients with disseminated disease (D2), the median survival after diagnosis of this stage is approximately two years, even with androgen ablation. Initial reports with the use of total androgen blockade, in which both androgens from testicular and adrenal origin were blocked, suggested a more favourable outcome, however subsequent studies have suggested that the advantages are not enormous and that the benefit is only noted if there is minimal metastatic disease. If patients do escape from androgen ablation there is not a great deal to offer. Chemotherapy has been disappointing and there does not, at the moment, seem to be any place for the routine use of chemotherapy in the management of disseminated prostate cancer; it seems that chemotherapy should be restricted to randomized clinical trials until it is possible to establish that a particular regime is effective.

URINARY TRACT OBSTRUCTION

Upper urinary tract obstruction

Obstruction to urine flow invariably leads to disastrous consequences for the urinary system, and in general should be overcome as soon as possible. A combination of obstruction and infection represents an even more urgent clinical problem, and, as a corollary, infection must be excluded in any patient in whom obstruction is suspected. Obstruction to the urinary tract, irrespective of the nature or the level, will result in dilatation of the system and back pressure on the kidney. It is this back pressure which will result in permanent impairment of renal function. The extent of back pressure is not necessarily reflected by the degree of dilatation. Acute complete obstruction of the ureter may be associated with minimal calyceal dilatation.

Some of the pressure effects that follow acute urinary tract obstruction are reduced as a result of pyelotubular and pyelolymphatic backflow, but neither mechanism affords long-term protection. After ureteric ligation in animals it has been found that renal blood flow falls within 4 hours, and after 7 days of complete obstruction glomerular filtration is permanently reduced to 70% of pre-obstructed levels, thus necessitating rapid relief of obstruction.

Diagnosis of obstruction

It is usually clear, for example from an intravenous pyelogram, when a stone is causing obstruction. However, during the last decade it has become apparent that dilatation seen on intravenous urography does not necessarily indicate an obstructed high pressure system. In the case of megaureters there can be gross dilatation without obstruction, in which case corrective surgery would not be required.

Having accepted that dilatation does not necessarily indicate an obstructed system, it is now more difficult for the clinician to decide which patients require surgery for presumed obstruction. A typical problem is the patient who presents with mild loin pain and whose intravenous urogram shows the renal pelvis to have a configuration consistent with pelvi-ureteric junction obstruction. Whitaker proposed that obstruction could be confirmed by puncturing the urinary tract and then perfusing it with saline at a rate of 10 ml/min. This rate is well above the normal rate of urine production, and a rise in pressure in excess of 15 cm of water was taken to indicate obstruction. The main disadvantages of this approach are that it is invasive, it may provide an unphysiological flow, and it assumes that the obstruction is constant. More recently diuresis renography and urography have been used instead of the Whitaker technique and both appear to provide reliable diagnostic information. They are also non-invasive and can thus be easily repeated. They appear to provide the greatest diagnostic information if performed while the patient has symptoms.

Management of upper urinary tract obstruction

There are many causes of upper urinary tract obstruction and an equally wide variety of surgical methods for overcoming them. If the patient is unfit for surgery or there is doubt as to the diagnosis or the level of obstruction, temporary stabilization of the problem may be achieved by percutaneous nephrostomy. This is a simple procedure which can be performed under local anaesthesia and either radiological or ultrasonic control. A small catheter can be introduced into the renal pelvis and the kidney drained until definitive surgery can be undertaken. By relieving the obstruction it is also possible to determine whether the function of the kidney will improve. Differential renal function studies frequently underestimate the function of an obstructed kidney. By allowing a period of free drainage it is easier to determine whether a grossly damaged kidney has significant function and is worth preserving. The placement of a nephrostomy is only a temporary measure and often difficult for the patient to manage, hence the need to ensure that it is practical to relieve the obstruction in the long term.

Lower urinary tract obstruction

Lower urinary tract obstruction is seen primarily in males and is virtually synonymous with bladder neck or prostatic obstruction. Although such obstruction is common, and often seemingly straightforward, the clinical diagnosis may be difficult to confirm by any of the currently available tests. For many years, a residual urine, bladder diverticula and trabeculation seen on the intravenous urogram were considered to be the hallmarks of obstruction. However, the recognition that they are by no means completely reliable indicators of obstruction has led to the use of voiding pressure measurements and urine flow rates in an attempt to improve the accuracy of diagnosis. The main disadvantage of these tests is that the presence of the catheter required to measure the voiding pressure affects the flow and that this artefact will in turn significantly affect the categorization of patients. Thus, in patients with outflow obstruction there is no simple test that will establish the diagnosis. A diagnosis of obstruction still requires careful evaluation of the patient's history, radiological investigation and, if available, the results of the urodynamic studies. In most instances, it has been believed that acceptable diagnostic accuracy can be achieved by careful clinical assessment without the need to resort to urodynamic studies. However, recent Scandinavian studies have argued that there is a significant number of men who will be diagnosed as being obstructed using these criteria, but this is not confirmed by urodynamic studies and, more importantly, their symptoms are not relieved by surgery to overcome the obstruction.

Benign prostatic hyperplasia

Benign prostatic hypertrophy is an extremely common disease in older men worldwide. The prevalence rate of this disease can rise to approximately 80% in men over the age of 70, and at least 30% of men who reach the age of 80 can expect to undergo a prostatectomy. In the United States it is the second most common operation performed on men over the age of 65, the most common being a cataract extraction. The precise aetiology of benign prostatic hyperplasia has not been established, however it is now evident that the prostate will not develop unless dihydrotestosterone is present. The precise role of dihydrotestosterone and other growth factors is yet to be established. As already indicated, the diagnosis of outflow obstruction secondary to benign prostatic hyperplasia has usually been made on clinical grounds, but there have been strong proposals that more invasive investigations should be performed as a routine. It has often been difficult to assess the criteria that were used to determine the need for surgery; recently an international conference was held on benign prostatic hyperplasia to try to establish diagnostic criteria. This consensus committee recommended that there should be a prostate symptom score and a quality of life assessment as part of the process. The recommendation was that there should be, as well as the quantification of symptoms, the recording of an adequate medical history, a focussed physical examination, dipstick urine analysis and the measurement of serum creatinine. The other basic standard evaluations recommended were urine flow rate estimations and the measurement of a residual urine, however these were considered optional. Optional studies proposed were ultrasonography or intravenous urography, PSA and endoscopic evaluation of the urinary tract. In summary, the committee agreed that the symptom score evaluation was the most important point in the evaluation of patients with bladder outlet obstruction due to BPH and that, to a large extent, the other investigations that could be used were optional and would be best tailored to the individual patient.

Treatment

As far as the treatment of BPH is concerned, there are several possible options. The simplest is 'watchful waiting' and this may well be appropriate in men with minimal symptoms. Medical therapy, another option, has to a large extent been based on two approaches: to reduce either the tone or the bulk of the gland. α-Adrenergic blocking agents are clearly the most appropriate if one wishes to reduce the tone of the gland, however, on the available information, it seems that these drugs are likely to be effective only for short-term treatment. In the case of agents aimed at reducing the bulk of the gland, the most active seem to be the 5α-reductase inhibitors. These inhibitors block the effect of the enzyme 5α-reductase which converts testosterone to dihydrotestosterone, which is the active androgen for the prostate. Initial studies with this drug have shown an improvement in flow rate, symptom score and a reduction in size of the prostate. However, the drug is clearly not effective in all males, and undoubtedly further evaluation of such agents will be necessary.

If medical therapy is not used, then the standard surgical treatment is still transurethral resection of the prostate. However, hyperthermia, thermal therapy, laser ablation of the prostate, stents and coils are all currently being evaluated. Many of these have considerable attraction in that they have lower morbidity and require shorter hospitalization than transurethral resection of the prostate, however the long-term efficacy and safety of these alternative treatments still need to be established. At the present time there are a number of randomized trials comparing, in particular, laser treatment with transurethral prostatectomy, and it is only by this means that these alternative treatments should be allowed to gain wide application.

What, perhaps, is important to note is that this interest in other modalities, both medical and surgical, has been born out of the results of a number of recent studies that have shown that the outcome of transurethral resection of the prostate is not without problems — significant patient dissatisfaction occurs in approximately 25% of cases.

VESICOURETERIC REFLUX

The diagnosis and classification of vesicoureteric reflux are discussed in Chapter 15. The major area of contention surrounding this condition is its management. Reflux can be satisfactorily corrected surgically in over 90% of cases. While traditionally open surgery with reimplantation of the ureter has been the procedure of choice, sub-trigonal injection of Teflon has also been used to prevent reflux. This technique is simple and effective, but concern exists about the potential long-term problems associated with the injection of this agent.

From a purely technical standpoint, therefore, it would seem preferable to liberalize rather than restrict the criteria for operation. However, it has become increasingly obvious that not all reflux is harmful and that in many instances it will disappear with age. This has meant that in spite of excellent surgical results the frequency of anti-reflux operations has tended to diminish as the understanding of the natural history of this condition has improved.

In children, the primary indications for operation are intra-renal reflux, a short or non-existent submucosal ureteric tunnel, recurrent urinary tract infections despite appropriate antibiotic treatment, and the development of renal scars. These indications are by no means unquestionably established, and the therapeutic dilemmas that still exist in the treatment of this condition have been clearly indicated by a recent prospective international study in children. If a non-operative course is to be pursued, the child should stay under surveillance until fully grown.

In adults it has been shown that correction of reflux does not arrest the scarring or deterioration of renal function, but if infection cannot be controlled by long-term antibiotics and no other cause for the infection can be found, it would seem reasonable to correct the reflux in an attempt to eradicate the infections.

URINARY INCONTINENCE

Urinary incontinence is one of the major urological problems affecting women. It may be divided into four main types on the basis of the patient's history: stress, urge, total or overflow. Stress incontinence is almost invariably seen in females and may be defined as the involuntary loss of urine due to an increase in the intra-abdominal pressure for any reason. It results from incompetence of the bladder neck mechanism.

Urge incontinence differs from stress incontinence in that it results from detrusor abnormality and the bladder neck mechanism is normal. However, some patients may have both stress and urge incontinence.

Total incontinence is due to damage to the sphincters so that urine continually leaks from the bladder. Overflow incontinence occurs as a result of chronic obstruction, either from the prostate or from a neurological cause.

Bladder innervation and continence

In order to understand the different approaches to the investigation and management of incontinence it is necessary to understand the innervation of the bladder. A detailed account of the neuroanatomy of the bladder is beyond the scope of this chapter. In essence, the bladder is controlled by the autonomic nervous system, but is brought under conscious control by connections between the autonomic nervous system and centres in the cerebral hemispheres. The detrusor muscle is supplied by parasympathetic fibres arising from the second, third and fourth sacral segments. These provide the motor supply. The detrusor muscle is richly supplied with cholinergic receptors. The sympathetic supply arises from the lower two thoracic and upper two lumbar segments which pass to the bladder via the superior hypogastric plexus. The sympathetic fibres are responsible for the contraction of the bladder neck smooth muscle fibres, and in this region α-adrenergic receptors predominate. Therefore micturition requires stimulation of the detrusor by parasympathetic fibres and relaxation of the bladder neck fibres which are under sympathetic control. While acetylcholine and noradrenaline have been long considered to be the principal neurotransmitters, it is evident that neuropeptides such as neuropeptide Y (NPY) or vasoactive intestinal peptide (VIP) may play a significant role in modulating detrusor contraction. Further evaluation of the role of neuropeptides and other neurotransmitters such as nitric oxide may have a significant effect on our understanding of the control of micturition.

Investigation of urinary incontinence

A major advance in the management of incontinence has been the introduction of cystometry. The ability of this technique to demonstrate uninhibited detrusor contractions without any detectable neurological abnormalities has led to the diagnosis of the so-called 'unstable bladder'. The reason for this instability is unclear, but in the past women with this form of detrusor abnormality were often subjected to surgery in the mistaken belief that their symptoms were due to bladder neck incompetence. Clearly, not all women with urinary incontinence require cystometry. This investigation should be reserved for those with urgency, urge incontinence or severe nocturia, i.e. the clinical hallmarks of an unstable bladder.

Women with the urethral syndrome may also have frequency and severe urgency, sometimes bordering on urge incontinence, but in this situation a cystometrogram will show a stable bladder, indicating that these woman have sensory urgency.

Other methods of assessing incontinence, particularly the urethral pressure profile, have been disappointing in clinical practice. No correlation has been observed between symptomatic improvement and changes in the urethral closure pressure. However, further research in this area is important as a better understanding of the function of the bladder neck mechanism and the development of techniques to diagnose functional abnormalities are vital if the management of incontinence is to improve.

Treatment of urinary incontinence

Stress incontinence. In women with stress incontinence conservative treatment is only of value if symptoms are minimal. If the woman needs to wear pads it is unlikely that pelvic floor exercises will significantly improve the situation. Most women with stress incontinence will therefore need some form of surgery, either vaginal or retropubic, if their symptoms are to be relieved. Because of the cause-and-effect relationship between childbirth and incontinence, it is unwise to recommend any form or surgery until the woman has completed her family. Occasionally, in women, stress incontinence may be confused with 'urethral failure' — a situation where the urethra, often after surgery, may become almost inert. In this instance, either peri-urethral contigen injection or an artificial sphincter will be the only means of achieving acceptable continence.

Urge incontinence. In patients with urge incontinence in whom it has been possible to demonstrate an unstable bladder, symptomatic improvement can often be achieved by the use of anticholinergic drugs such as propantheline bromide. But before treating any patient as a case of primary detrusor instability, it is important to exclude conditions such as infection, carcinoma and outflow obstruction, all of which can produce an unstable bladder.

Patients with a combination of stress and urge incontinence obviously require careful assessment and may need a combination of surgery and anticholinergic therapy. In women who have only sensory urgency and no incontinence, bladder training programmes offer the best prospect of overcoming this distressing problem.

Total incontinence. This is almost invariably due to sphincteric damage and requires either an artificial sphincter or, if this is not possible, urinary diversion or an indwelling catheter.

Overflow incontinence. As overflow incontinence is almost always due to chronic obstruction, it can usually be readily corrected by the relief of obstruction.

REFERENCES AND RECOMMENDED READING

Barry M J 1990 Medical outcomes research and benign prostatic hyperplasia. Prostate 3: 61–65

Carter H B, Coffey D S 1990 The prostate: an increasing medical problem. Prostate 16: 39–48

Chisholm G D, Fair W R (eds) 1990 Scientific Foundations of Urology, 3rd edn. Heinemann Medical, Oxford

Cockett ATK, Aso Y, Chatelain C, Denis L, Griffiths K, Khoury S, Murphy G (eds) 1991 The International Consultation on Benign Prostatic Hyperplasia (BPH), Paris, June 1991

Hinman F Jr 1991 Screening for prostate carcinoma. Journal of Urology 145: 126–130

Koch M O, McDougal W S, Leddy P K, Lange P H 1991 Metabolic alterations following continent urinary diversion through colonic segments. Journal of Urology 145: 270–275

Mostofi F K, Sobin L H, Torloni H 1973 Histological typing of urinary bladder tumours. International histological classification of tumours, No. 10. World Health Organisation, Geneva

Osterling J E, 1991 Prostatic specific antigen: a critical assessment of the most useful markers for adenocarcinomas of the prostate. Journal of Urology 145: 907–923

Paulson D F, Monck J W, Walther P J 1990 Radical prostatectomy for clinical stage T1-2 NoMo prostatic adenocarcinoma: long term results. Journal of Urology 144: 180–184

Pfister R C, Nevhouse J H, Hendren W H 1982 Percutaneous pyeloureteral urodynamics. Urological Clinics of North America 9: 41–49

Raghavan D, Shipley W U, Garwick M B, Russell P J, Richie J P 1990 Biology and management of bladder cancer. New England Journal of Medicine 322: 1129–1138

Report of the International Reflux Study Committee 1981 Medical versus surgical treatment of primary vesicoureteral reflux: a prospective international reflux study in children. Journal of Urology 125: 277–283

Ryall R L, Marshall V R 1982 The effect of urethral catheter on the measurement of maximum urinary flow rate. Journal of Urology 128(2): 429–432

29. Fluid and electrolyte disorders

W. R. Adam

BODY FLUIDS AND SODIUM

Total body water (TBW) is distributed in the following compartments (Fig. 29.1):

1. Intracellular
2. Extracellular
   a. intravascular
   b. extravascular.

Changes in total body water are reflected by changes in plasma osmolality or plasma sodium, as sodium and its anions are the major osmotic constituents of the extracellular fluid, the sample for these determinations.

Changes in total body water are best described by the terms overhydration and dehydration.

Because of the osmotic equilibrium across the cell membrane, water cannot be shifted from the intracellular to the extracellular compartment (or vice versa) without a change in the osmotic content of one of the spaces. Similarly, a change in osmotic content in one of the spaces (e.g. as a result of sodium removal from the extracellular space) will lead to a change in volume of that space (in this case contraction) without a change in the osmotic equilibrium between the two spaces.

Changes in sodium content of the body lead to changes in the volume of the extracellular space (because of the relative localization of sodium to that space) without a corresponding change in the volume of the intracellular space (Fig. 29.1). These changes are best described as (extracellular) volume excess and volume depletion and not as dehydration or overhydration.

The extracellular space is further divided into intravascular and extravascular compartments.

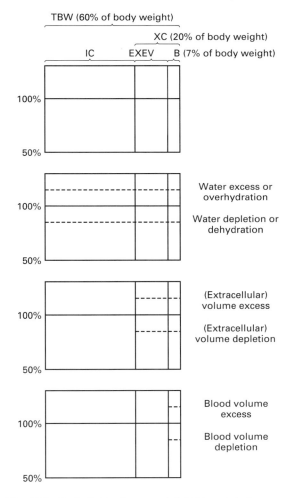

Fig. 29.1 Body fluid volumes and definition of their disturbances. TBW — total body water; XC — extracellular fluid volume; ECEV — extracellular extravascular fluid volume; B — extracellular intravascular (or blood) volume; IC — intracellular water

Fluid distribution between these intravascular and extravascular spaces depends on hydrostatic pressure gradients (which tend to move fluid from the intra- to the extravascular compartment) and oncotic pressure gradients (which tend to move fluid from the extra- to the intravascular compartment). Disturbances of these pressure gradients can lead to a maldistribution of fluid between these two compartments (the commonest example being associated with hypoproteinaemia).

When there is intravascular volume depletion with extravascular volume excess, this is best described as blood (or plasma) volume depletion and its opposite as blood volume excess (see Fig. 29.1).

CHANGES IN EXTRACELLULAR FLUID VOLUME AND SODIUM STATUS

Sodium status and extracellular fluid volume are closely interrelated. Changes in sodium status are usually associated with, or lead to, changes in extracellular fluid status by the following mechanisms:

1. Changes in sodium status cause changes in osmolality which tend to be corrected by changes in water intake and excretion, thus leading to changes in fluid volume.
2. Sodium loss usually occurs in association with fluid loss (e.g. diarrhoea).

Therefore, under most circumstances changes in sodium status are assessed and managed as changes in extracellular fluid volumes. The major extracellular fluid volumes are: (a) blood volume, and (b) extravascular extracellular volume.

While these volumes often change in parallel there can be a maldistribution between blood volume and extravascular extracellular volume (e.g. hypoproteinaemia, local causes for oedema such as incompetent valves of deep veins in the legs).

The following discussion groups the changes in extracellular fluid volume into two broad categories:

1. Blood volume depletion
2. Extracellular fluid volume excess.

Assessment of extracellular fluid volume and sodium status

History and physical examination

As mentioned above, changes in sodium status are usually associated with changes in fluid status, thus minimizing the effect on plasma osmolality (and plasma sodium). Therefore sodium status cannot be assessed by plasma sodium concentration or other routinely available biochemical tests. The history and physical examination are the most important methods by which sodium status and extracellular fluid volume are assessed.

Volume depletion. The term 'volume depletion' as commonly used refers to a decrease in blood volume. The signs and symptoms of volume depletion relate to decreased cardiac output and are thus non-specific: they may reflect primary cardiac disease rather than volume depletion. As most symptoms of volume depletion are due to a decreased cardiac output, the severity of symptoms produced by a given degree of volume depletion will be influenced by the cardiac response of the patients, the healthy heart coping with a greater degree of volume depletion than the diseased heart. Mild volume depletion may give non-specific symptoms (tiredness, weakness, a feeling of being cold) and the earliest signs may be tachycardia and a drop in blood pressure on standing; more severe postural hypotension produces dizziness and fainting and the patient may complain of thirst. Severe volume depletion results in sustained hypotension and can lead to shock, with cold, clammy, cyanosed extremities and oliguria. The degree of volume depletion can be estimated from the severity of clinical signs (Table 29.1). It is unusual to find volume depletion due to excessive loss of sodium from the body without symptoms such as diarrhoea and/or polyuria. A history of such fluid loss is important in assessing both the extent and the aetiology of volume depletion.

Extracellular fluid volume excess. The cardinal sign of volume excess is oedema, i.e. the accumulation of fluid in the extracellular space. This may be due to local factors such as inflammation, injury, incompetent valves of leg veins or lymphatic obstruction, or it may be generalized.

Table 29.1 Estimation of the degree of volume depletion* from clinical signs, assuming that extracellular volume is approximately 20% of body weight and blood volume approximately 7% of body weight.

Clinical signs	Degree of volume depletion	Estimated volume depletion (in litres) Intravascular (as in blood loss or with decreased serum albumin)	Extravascular (as in sodium and water depletion)
JVP ↓	Mild	0.5	1.0
Standing blood pressure ↓	Moderate	1.0	2.5
Lying blood pressure ↓, oliguria	Severe	1.5	4.0

* Values given are for a 70 kg man.
JVP — jugular venous pressure.

Localized pulmonary oedema reflects left heart abnormalities. Oedema not solely related to local factors is called generalized oedema, although it may be more obvious in dependent areas (or in the peritoneal space with portal hypertension).

Generalized oedema always represents an abnormal excess of sodium. Oedema is usually due to abnormal urinary sodium retention rather than abnormal sodium ingestion. However, given a propensity for sodium retention, the degree of oedema can be increased by increased sodium intake.

Virtually all cases of generalized oedema can be subdivided into two groups:

1. Oedema associated with a decreased plasma volume which, at least in part, is due to decreased intravascular oncotic pressure from hypoalbuminaemia, which allows fluid to transfer to the extravascular space. The decreased plasma volume also leads to impaired renal perfusion and renal sodium retention.

2. Oedema associated with an increased plasma volume is due to renal retention of sodium and water (from whatever cause) with a normal plasma albumin and a normal plasma oncotic pressure. The jugular venous pressure may be raised.

Mild oedema (just detectable) usually signifies an excess of extracellular volume of at least 15% (about 2–3 litres in a 70 kg man) whereas severe generalized oedema may represent an increase of more than 100% (14 litres in a 70 kg man).

There are no other bedside tests of volume status but since short-term changes in body weight reflect mainly changes in fluid status they are of help in assessing progress of a volume abnormality.

Laboratory investigation

As mentioned above, measurements of plasma sodium concentration are of little help in assessing sodium or extracellular fluid status. While hyponatraemia may occur with sodium depletion, this is a measure of the associated abnormality in water metabolism. Nevertheless, unexplained hyponatraemia should lead to consideration of volume status.

Estimations of urinary sodium excretion are of value in assessing sodium status. A low urinary sodium excretion implies active reabsorption of sodium, which may relate to sodium depletion or decreased renal perfusion from volume-related or cardiac causes. The combination of a concentrated urine (high specific gravity, high osmolality, high creatinine concentration) and a low urine sodium concentration is even more supportive of a diagnosis of volume depletion.

In the absence of renal disease or diuretics a high urinary sodium makes the diagnosis of sodium depletion unlikely.

Direct measurement of total body sodium (by exchangeable sodium) or extracellular volume (e.g. by $^{35}SO_4^{2-}$ space) is not always possible but can be helpful in some situations (management of fluid volume in patients with renal and cardiac failure).

Plasma renin activity correlates indirectly with renal perfusion and will be high when there is volume depletion, leading to decreased renal perfusion, and low with volume excess. Normal volumes for plasma renin activity vary greatly from laboratory to laboratory and need to be established prior to interpretation of results.

Causes of blood volume depletion

Blood volume depletion has four main causes:

Causes of blood volume depletion
1. Blood loss (acute, chronic)
2. Hypoalbuminaemia
   Liver disease
   Nephrotic syndrome
   Protein-losing enteropathy
   Malnutrition
3. Sodium depletion
   Gastrointestinal loss
      Diarrhoea
      Vomiting
   Renal loss
      Diuretics
      Some forms of renal failure
      Osmotic diuretics (diabetes mellitus)
      Addison's disease
4. Septicaemia — third space

---

1. Blood loss, either acute or chronic. This may be obvious but in some cases it is only discernible by a falling haematocrit (packed cell volume) or haemoglobin value.

2. Hypoalbuminaemia, with a decreased plasma oncotic pressure and transfer of fluid from the intravascular to the extravascular space. In this situation, unlike in sodium depletion (see below), intravascular volume depletion may be associated with an extracellular sodium excess manifested by oedema (see earlier).

3. Sodium depletion. Loss of sodium is usually associated with loss of fluid, which minimizes changes in plasma sodium. The effect on plasma sodium is further reduced by the sensitivity of the body's osmostats to lowered osmolality, leading to inhibition of antidiuretic hormone and water diuresis. The sodium and water depletion produce a decrease in extracellular (including intravascular) fluid volume. Because of the associated water loss, there is usually no change in plasma sodium with sodium depletion. In prolonged severe volume depletion, stimulation by perfusion-dependent mechanisms can lead to osmotically inappropriate thirst and antidiuretic hormone release. This leads to a degree of water retention and thus hyponatraemia. Although osmotically inappropriate, the response is an appropriate defence of extracellular fluid volume. It should be noted that the hyponatraemia is not due to sodium loss alone but rather to the alteration in water handling. The diagnosis of sodium depletion depends on a history of sodium and/or fluid loss and the symptoms and signs of volume depletion outlined above. Sodium depletion is rarely caused by a low sodium intake, yet a low sodium intake will exacerbate the problem of sodium depletion due to sodium loss. The major sources of sodium loss are the gastrointestinal tract and the kidney. Sweating rarely produces sufficient sodium loss to cause volume depletion.

A history of sodium-containing fluid loss is common and is an important feature of the diagnosis of sodium depletion.

4. Septicaemia and the third space. Septicaemia can reduce the blood pressure by direct myocardial toxicity and also by fluid loss. In the absence of obvious fluid loss, hypotension may be correctable by fluid replacement, suggesting a loss of fluid from the circulatory system into an unknown third space. This may reflect occult gastrointestinal accumulation of fluid and/or dilatation of the capacitance vessels of the circulation.

Causes of extracellular volume excess

Causes of extracellular volume excess
Associated with decreased blood volume
Hypoalbuminaemia
   Liver disease
   Nephrotic syndrome
   Protein-losing enteropathy
   Malnutrition
Associated with increased blood volume
Renal retention of sodium and water
   Congestive cardiac failure
   Renal failure
   Mineralocorticoid excess
   Drugs (corticosteroids, non-steroidal anti-inflammatory agents, vasodilators)
   Idiopathic (periodic) oedema

Extracellular volume excess with blood volume depletion

Hypoalbuminaemia may be due to decreased production (e.g. malnutrition and liver disease, both usually obvious) or increased loss, due either to renal loss of protein (e.g. nephrotic syndrome, when the patient may give a history of frothy urine) or, more rarely, to bowel loss of protein (these patients usually give a history of diarrhoea). The nephrotic syndrome due to glomerulonephritis, one of the causes of hypoalbuminaemia, may also be caused by a direct renal effect of retaining sodium, which will contribute to oedema. The dual mechanism of sodium retention explains the lack of a good correlation between the degree of hypoalbuminaemia and to the extent of the oedema in this condition.

Extracellular and intravascular volume excess

Oedema associated with an increased intravascular volume is always due to renal retention of sodium and water. Renal failure is an obvious cause but the kidney will also conserve sodium when underperfused, when stimulated by sodium-retaining hormones (aldosterone), or in response to neural input and to certain drugs. Both neural and hormonal factors are probably important in sodium retention in cardiac failure.

Isolated cardiac failure is usually diagnosed by the history and clinical examination (cardiac dilatation, raised jugular venous pressure, pulmonary oedema) and renal failure by assessment of renal function (urine output, plasma creatinine, creatinine clearance). However, when there is evidence of both cardiac and renal failure it can be difficult to differentiate the primary factors responsible for the oedema, as retention of sodium and water due to renal disease can lead to signs of cardiac failure. Similarly, severe cardiac failure can lead to signs and symptoms of renal failure. The evidence of cardiac and/or renal failure may diminish with treatment of the oedema.

Oedema is rarely due solely to an increase in mineralocorticoid production (e.g. Conn's syndrome and Cushing's syndrome are rarely associated with oedema) because of an escape mechanism which, after a certain degree of sodium retention, prevents further retention. However, ectopic production of ACTH by tumours is quite often associated with oedema, and drugs acting through the aldosterone receptor (fludrocortisone, prednisolone, carbenoxolone) may cause oedema. Other drugs, such as non-steroidal anti-inflammatory drugs (e.g. indomethacin) and vasodilators (e.g. felodipine and diazoxide), can also cause sodium retention and oedema (through as yet unknown mechanisms). Idiopathic (periodic) oedema occurs predominantly but not exclusively in women of reproductive age. It is usually intermittent and sometimes difficult to distinguish from the secondary effect of discontinuation of self-administered potent diuretics. Its cause is still unclear.

Treatment

Blood volume depletion

This requires replacement by appropriate fluids, e.g. blood, protein (albumin or stable plasma protein solution), saline (150 mmol/l) or Hartman's solution. The urgency of replacement depends on the severity of cardiovascular effects. Sustained hypotension requires urgent repletion and thus close monitoring.

Extracellular fluid excess

Diuretics to enhance urinary sodium excretion are effective in most patients. A combination of diuretics that act at different nephron sites (e.g. frusemide with either thiazides and/or amiloride and/or spironolactone) is generally more effective than massive doses of frusemide alone. Reduction in sodium intake will facilitate control of extracellular volume in resistant cases. In severe renal failure, removal of sodium requires dialysis.

DISTURBANCES OF PLASMA OSMOLALITY AND PLASMA SODIUM

Plasma osmolality and plasma sodium usually rise and fall in parallel so that changes in plasma sodium levels tend to be a reliable marker of changes in plasma osmolality. There are, however, two exceptions:

1. Hyperosmolality without hypernatraemia may occur when there are other osmotically active particles, such as urea or glucose (both of which are usually evident because of the clinical situation or following basic biochemical tests).

2. Hyponatraemia without hypo-osmolality may be artefactual, i.e. due to gross hyperlipid-aemia or hyperproteinaemia. Correction of plasma volume for the lipid or protein content will then give a normal plasma sodium concentration. Hyponatraemia without hypo-osmolality may also occur in the presence of other osmotically active particles. These may be obvious (diabetes with hyperglycaemia, renal failure with uraemia) or they may be ill-defined substances extruded from cells in sick patients. This sick-cell syndrome may explain some of the mild hyponatraemia seen in sick patients.

As stated earlier, an abnormal plasma sodium rarely reflects parallel changes in total body sodium because of the body's efficient response to osmotic disturbances, which, by adjusting intake or excretion of water to the altered sodium status, will maintain a normal plasma sodium. Therefore an abnormal plasma sodium usually reflects an abnormality of water handling and is a convenient and common way of defining a disturbance in osmolality.

Laboratory investigations

Abnormalities of plasma osmolality and sodium define the syndrome(s). Urine concentration or osmolality often corresponds to the plasma abnormality (e.g. increased concentration with hyper-osmolality and dilution with hypo-osmolality). Inappropriate urine concentration or osmolality is of help in diagnosing the mechanism of the plasma disturbance. For example, dilute urine in the presence of hyperosmolality suggests diabetes insipidus (either pituitary or nephrogenic) while concentrated urine in the presence of hypo-osmolality suggests inappropriate plasma levels of antidiuretic hormone (ADH).

HYPEROSMOLALITY AND HYPERNATRAEMIA

Causes of hyperosmolality and hypernatraemia

Causes of hyperosmolality and hypernatraemia
Water loss in excess of sodium
Absence of antidiuretic hormone (diabetes insipidus)
Inability of the kidney to respond to ADH
   Nephrogenic diabetes insipidus
   Primary or drug-induced
   Hypokalaemia
   Hypercalcaemia
Solute diuresis (diabetes)
Renal impairment
Impaired water ingestion
Coma
Lesion of thirst centre (hypothalamic tumours, post-traumatic)

The commonest cause of a deficit in water intake is coma, as thirst (stimulated by hyperosmolality) is a very potent stimulus to drinking. Rarely, impaired thirst sensation can occur with hypothalamic tumours or after head injury. Water loss in excess of sodium loss may be due to:

1. absence of ADH (diabetes insipidus);
2. inability of the kidney to respond to ADH (e.g. nephrogenic diabetes insipidus) — this may be familial, drug-induced (lithium carbonate, demeclocycline) or metabolic (e.g. hypokalaemia and hypercalcaemia);
3. solute diuresis — glycosuria (as in diabetes) and high urinary urea (secondary to increased urea production following a hypercatabolic state or major trauma) both remove water in excess of sodium;
4. renal impairment — this is due partly to the inability of the diseased kidney to respond to ADH and partly to urea producing a solute diuresis.

Hyperosmolality without hypernatraemia may be caused by glucose (in hyperosmotic diabetic states) or by urea (in renal failure).

History and physical examination

Hyperosmolality and hypernatraemia. These patients usually have a history of decreased fluid intake (due to unavailability or coma) or polyuria (diabetes mellitus, diabetes insipidus). If renal function is normal they invariably have oliguria although this is not diagnostic of hyperosmolality. There may be reduced tissue turgor and decreased orbital tension but these are often difficult to assess (particularly in the elderly) and non-specific, as they also may occur in extracellular volume depletion.

The differential diagnosis of diabetes insipidus from compulsive water drinking should be relatively easy if plasma antidiuretic hormone levels can be measured. If not, the diagnosis depends on the response of plasma and urine osmolality to water deprivation. Water deprivation is potentially dangerous in patients with diabetes insipidus and great care should be taken. Figure 29.2 summarizes the diagnostic process in the investigation of hypernatraemia and hyperosmolality.

Treatment of hyperosmolality and hypernatraemia

The treatment of hyperosmolality and hypernatraemia consists of water replacement and treatment of the underlying disease. The deficit (or excess) of water can be calculated from the total body water (60% of body weight) multiplied by the deficit (or excess) of plasma sodium concentration (or osmolality) and divided by the normal plasma sodium concentration (or osmolality). For example, in a 70 kg man with a plasma sodium concentration of 160 mmol/l the deficit of water is

$$40 \times \frac{20}{140} = 5.7 \text{ litres}$$

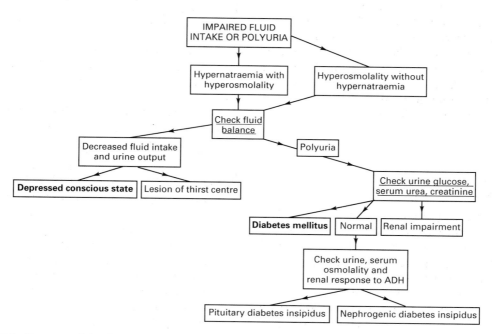

Fig. 29.2 Summary of the diagnostic process which may be used in the investigation of hypernatraemia and hyperosmolality. (Common diagnostic steps are shown underlined and common end diagnoses in bold type.) In many situations the diagnostic process will not be required, as the end diagnosis (e.g. uncontrolled diabetes mellitus) will lead to a search for the biochemical abnormality (hyperosmolality)

Synthetic analogues of antidiuretic hormone (e.g. diamino-D-arginine vasopressin) may be used in pituitary diabetes insipidus.

In idiopathic nephrogenic diabetes insipidus the urine volume can be decreased by decreasing the ability to generate free water. This is done by giving diuretics which cause volume depletion and enhance proximal tubular reabsorption of sodium.

HYPO-OSMOLALITY AND HYPONATRAEMIA

Causes of hypo-osmolality and hyponatraemia

Causes of hypo-osmolality and hyponatraemia
Without signs of blood volume depletion
Inappropriate ADH secretion
   Cancer of the lung, other tumours
   Intracranial pathology
   Tuberculosis, pneumonia
      Drugs
      Chlorpropamide
      Vincristine
      Clofibrate
      Carbamazepine
Other causes of impaired free water excretion
   Hypopituitarism (glucocorticoid deficiency)
   Hypothyroidism
   Renal failure
Free water overload
   Compulsive water drinking (rare to give a decrease in sodium)
   Intravenous dextrose
With signs of blood volume depletion
Addison's disease
Diuretics
Uncontrolled diabetes
Other causes of volume depletion
With signs of blood volume depletion and oedema
Hypoalbuminaemia
With signs of blood volume excess
Congestive cardiac failure
Artefactual
Hyperlipidaemia
Hyperproteinaemia

Hyponatraemia with hypo-osmolality is rarely caused by excess water intake alone, as normal kidneys can excrete up to about 20 litres of free water a day. However, excess water intake may well exacerbate hypo-osmolality when water excretion is impaired. Hyponatraemia is usually caused by decreased water excretion.

History and examination

Hypo-osmolality and hyponatraemia. Frequently there is nothing in the history or examination to suggest hypo-osmolality or hyponatraemia. There may be a transient oliguria despite adequate fluid intake, but this is often unnoticed. Hyponatraemia may be suspected in patients with known causes (e.g. carcinoma of the lung) who develop disturbances of the central nervous system, but these again are non-specific symptoms.

Impaired water excretion may be due to: excess ADH or an enhanced response to ADH; impaired free water excretion by the kidney due either to impaired delivery of fluid to the diluting segment (thick ascending limb) of the kidney or to impaired activity of the segment (the possible cause of impaired dilution in glucocorticoid deficiency); or to other, as yet undefined, causes.

Excess ADH

Excess ADH may be due to any of the following:

1. Inappropriate non-regulated production by tumours (e.g. carcinoma of the lung).

2. Inappropriate production by the hypothalamus due to local damage or stress (e.g. head injury, tumour, cerebral infarction, stroke, etc.).

3. Stimulation of volume receptors in the vascular system. Volume depletion from any cause leads to a stimulation of ADH secretion that can override osmotic inhibition of ADH secretion. This causes osmotically inappropriate ADH secretion and water retention. Thus sodium depletion, as a cause of volume depletion, can result in hyponatraemia. This is not a primary effect of the sodium depletion but rather a secondary defect in water handling. The increased water retention helps to correct the volume depletion and is thus volume-appropriate, but osmotically inappropri-

ate. Aberrant stimulation of volume receptors may also occur with intrathoracic pathology such as tuberculosis or pneumonia, thus causing inappropriate ADH secretion.

4. Stimulation of ADH secretion by drugs, e.g. nicotine, clofibrate, vincristine.

5. Peripheral enhancement of the effect of ADH, possibly by chlorpropamide.

Non-regulated production of ADH (e.g. 1, 2 and 4 above) usually produces more severe and less stable hyponatraemia than those conditions in which ADH is still subject to some regulation, although at lower osmolality (e.g. 3).

Impaired delivery of sodium

Impaired delivery of sodium to the distal diluting segment, and thus impaired free water excretion, occurs with:

1. Decreased glomerular filtration rate (chronic renal failure).

2. Enhanced proximal reabsorption of sodium due to blood volume depletion, either real or perceived as such by the kidney (e.g. the decreased effective arterial volume of cardiac failure); thus hyponatraemia can occur in the presence of oedema and a total body sodium excess.

3. Possibly glucocorticoid deficiency (e.g. hypopituitarism, Addison's disease). Thus, in Addison's disease, mineralocorticoid deficiency can produce blood volume depletion due to sodium loss and thus a secondary increase in ADH. The glucocorticoid deficiency may also cause hyponatraemia because of decreased urinary dilution due to both decreased distal fluid delivery and decreased tubular removal of sodium.

Other causes

Hyponatraemia with hypo-osmolality may also occur in hypothyroidism. The exact mechanism is unclear. The suggestion that it may be due to inappropriate secretion of ADH has not been substantiated.

Hyponatraemia with a lesser degree of, or without, hypo-osmolality may occur in severely ill patients — the sick-cell syndrome. This is thought to be due to extrusion of osmotically active particles from the intracellular to extracellular space, but is usually by itself only responsible for mild hyponatraemia (plasma sodium more than 130 mmol/l).

Hyponatraemia and hypo-osmolality in congestive cardiac failure

This is an excellent example of the multifactorial mechanisms which may be involved in the production of hyponatraemia. These include:

1. increased thirst due to stimulation of volume receptors by the decreased effective arterial volume;
2. inappropriate ADH secretion secondary to volume receptor stimulation; and
3. decreased ability to clear free water because of enhanced proximal sodium reabsorption.

The diagnostic process for the investigation of hypo-osmolality and hyponatraemia is summarized in Figure 29.3.

Treatment of hypo-osmolality and hyponatraemia

Hyponatraemia in itself is not an absolute indication for treatment. Cerebral manifestations of hyponatraemia such as confusion and coma or a plasma sodium below 120 mmol/l are indications, for urgent but cautious treatment with sodium, e.g. 3% NaCl intravenously (usually combined with diuretic treatment to avoid pulmonary oedema). Too rapid, or over-correction of plasma sodium may also lead to central nervous system damage so the plan should be to raise the plasma sodium by 1 mmol/hour and not to fully correct the plasma sodium but, rather, to correct the symptoms. Increasing the plasma sodium to about 120 mmol/l or raising it by 10 mmol/l is usually sufficient. To acutely raise the plasma sodium concentration by 10 mmol/l (or osmolality by 20 mmol/kg) in a patient with profound hyponatraemia (say 110 mmol/l) the required dose of NaCl (in mmol) is calculated, roughly, as total body water (in litres) multiplied by the increase required (10 mmol/l), i.e. 10. Since total body water (60% of body weight) in a 70 kg man is approximately 40 litres,

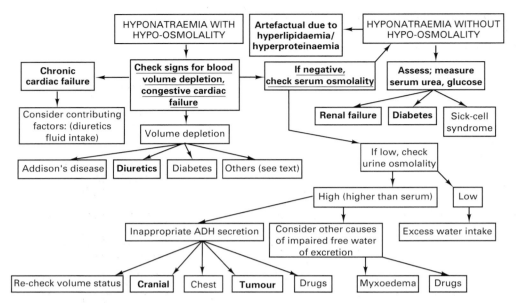

Fig. 29.3 Summary of the diagnostic process which may be used in the investigation of hyponatraemia and hypo-osmolality. (Common diagnostic steps are shown underlined and common end diagnoses in bold type.) In many situations this diagnostic process will not be required, as the end diagnosis (e.g. carcinoma of the lung) will lead to a search for the biochemical abnormality (hypo-osmolality).

the required dose of sodium is 40 × 10 = 400 mmol. Concentrated NaCl is usually supplied in a strength of 3% (i.e. 500 mmol/l) so that 0.8 litres would provide 400 mmol. Obviously, continuing urinary loss of sodium will require more NaCl to be given. It should be noted that the 'cost' of correcting plasma sodium by this method is an expansion of the extracellular fluid volume of about 2.5 litres (the remaining fluid coming from the intracellular space, thereby increasing intracellular osmolality), which may cause problems such as pulmonary oedema.

If there are no cerebral signs, intravenous treatment is not required unless the sodium concentration is below 120 mmol/l. The basis of conservative treatment is water restriction (500 ml/day). Despite the best of efforts adequate water restriction is sometimes not achievable. Urea 10 g t.d.s., in cordial or fruit juice, can provide a predictable, if unpalatable, water diuresis. Less predictable, and potentially dangerous treatments are drugs which inhibit the action of ADH in the kidney (e.g. demeclocycline).

POTASSIUM

Assessment of potassium status

Both hyperkalaemia and hypokalaemia are often unsuspected. Symptoms of hyperkalaemia only occur when it is severe (more than 6 mmol/l) and are due to heart block (producing fainting, Stokes–Adams attacks) and generalized weakness. Terminal events may be either asystole or ventricular fibrillation. The history may suggest the possibility of hyperkalaemia (e.g. increased potassium ingestion, potassium-retaining diuretics, renal failure) but the diagnosis can only be confirmed by measuring the plasma potassium. Electrocardiographic changes of peaked T waves with or without heart block are also suggestive of hyperkalaemia but again the diagnosis needs confirmation by direct measurement.

Similarly, symptoms of hypokalaemia also usually occur only when it is severe (less than 2.5 mmol/l) and are due to muscle weakness and cardiac arrhythmias. A history of either abnormal fluid losses (e.g. diuretic therapy, vomiting, diarrhoea) or ingestion of excess alkali (e.g. sodium bicarbonate for dyspepsia) may suggest the possibility of hypokalaemia but the diagnosis will only be established by measuring the plasma potassium.

Laboratory investigations

Plasma potassium concentration is the most useful guide to potassium status. It clearly shows alterations in distribution of potassium between extracellular and intracellular fluid (Fig. 29.4). After correction for factors which can influence potassium distribution, the then notional plasma potassium is also a reasonable guide to total body potassium (see below). As an alteration in acid–base status is the commonest cause of altered potassium distribution in the body, this should be either excluded or corrected before using plasma potassium estimations to assess total body potassium.

A quantitative assessment of potassium status must take into account total body potassium and the effects of alkalosis and acidosis on plasma potassium concentration.

1. Total body potassium. This relates to muscle mass and is about 45 mmol/kg body weight in muscular young men and about 20 mmol/kg in weak fat elderly ladies (these being the extremes of the normal range).

2. Correction of alkalosis. An increase in pH value of 0.1 (e.g. from 7.45 to 7.55) produces an approximate decrease in plasma potassium of 0.6 mmol/l (say from 3.7 to 3.1 mmol/l). Therefore, for each 0.1 pH unit above normal, 0.6 mmol/l should be added to the measured plasma potassium. If this brings the (now notional) plasma potassium value within the normal range (3.5–5.0) the total body potassium is probably normal. If not, a decrease in plasma potassium of 1 mmol/l after correction for alkalosis, represents an approximate total body potassium deficit of about 10% (i.e. 10% of total body potassium content as calculated from weight and likely potassium content — see above).

3. Correction for acidosis. A decrease in pH value of 0.1 (e.g. from 7.4 to 7.3) produces an approximate increase in plasma potassium of

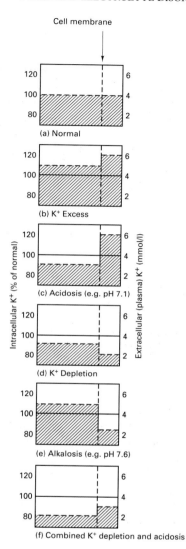

Fig. 29.4 The relationship between intracellular and extracellular potassium. Intracellular potassium accounts for more than 97% of total body potassium and is shown here as the percentage of normal because of the wide range in normal potassium content/kg body weight (see text). Extracellular potassium constitutes less than 3% of total body potassium and is shown as the measurable component, plasma potassium. An increase in plasma potassium is associated with an increase in total body potassium in K⁺ excess (example b) but with a decrease in a total body potassium in acidosis (c). A decrease in plasma potassium is associated with a decrease in total body potassium in K⁺ depletion (d) but an increase in total body potassium in uncomplicated alkalosis (e). A mixed disorder, e.g. acidosis coexisting with K⁺ depletion, may appear to diminish the degree of total body potassium deficit by shifting K⁺ from the intracellular to the extracellular space (f)

0.7 mmol/l (say from 4.5 to 5.2 mmol/l)*. Therefore, for each 0.1 pH unit below normal, 0.7 mmol/l should be subtracted from the measured plasma potassium. If this correction makes the notional plasma potassium less than 5.0 mmol/l then total potassium is probably normal and correction of the acidosis should normalize the serum potassium. If, after correction for acidosis and exclusion of other causes of an intra- to extracellular shift, the plasma potassium is still raised, an increase of 1 mmol/l represents an approximate total body potassium excess of about 6% (6% of total body potassium content calculated from weight and likely potassium content — see above).

The measurement of urinary potassium is most helpful in distinguishing between gastrointestinal and renal losses of potassium as a cause of decreased total body potassium and hypokalaemia. In the presence of hypokalaemia (less than 3.5 mmol/l) a urinary potassium excretion of more than 30 mmol/24 h suggests renal potassium wasting, whereas less than 20 mmol/24 h suggests gastrointestinal potassium wasting or dietary potassium deficiency.

Measurements of plasma renin activity and plasma or urinary aldosterone levels are available and are useful in understanding disorders of potassium homeostasis but do require some skill in interpretation (see below).

Causes of hyperkalaemia

Redistribution of potassium

Once hyperkalaemia has been established, and shown not to be artefactual (haemolysed blood), it is essential to determine the contribution from changes in potassium distribution (from intracellular to extracellular fluid) as opposed to an increase in total body potassium (usually due to a failure of urinary excretion). This is not always possible to ascertain from the history, as factors which can cause a failure of potassium excretion (e.g. renal failure or decreased mineralocorticoid

secretion) can also cause a metabolic acidosis, the major factor responsible for a redistribution of potassium from intracellular and extracellular fluid. Therefore hyperkalaemia should not be interpreted unless data on acid–base status are also available.

If a metabolic acidosis is present, the plasma potassium should be corrected for this abnormality (see above). If after correction the (then notional) plasma potassium is still raised (more than 5.0 mml/l) then other causes for a shift of potassium from intracellular to extracellular fluid should be considered. These include: severe insulin lack, as in insulin-dependent diabetes; hypoaldosteronism; impaired β-agonist activity (e.g. with β-blockers) and in the interesting but rare condition, familial hyperkalaemic periodic paralysis.

Compared to acidosis, these factors alone have a lesser effect on potassium distribution, but exacerbate hyperkalaemia in combination with other factors.

Causes of hyperkalaemia

Causes of hyperkalaemia
Shift from intracellular to extracellular fluid
Acidosis
Severe hypoaldosteronism
Insulin deficiency
β-blockers (mild effect only)
Familial hyperkalaemic periodic paralysis (rare)
Increase in total body potassium
Decreased renal excretion of potassium
  Renal failure
  Hypoaldosteronism
    Addison's disease
    Hyporeninaemic hypoaldosteronism
    ACE inhibitors
Drugs inhibiting distal tubule transport of potassium
    Spironolactone
    Amiloride
    Triamterene
Decreased sodium delivery to the distal tubule
  Volume depletion, cardiac failure
Acidosis
Increased potassium intake — produces hyperkalaemia only in association with decreased renal excretion of potassium (see above)

---

* The degree of shift of potassium with acidosis also depends on the associated anion; inorganic acidosis produces a greater shift than organic.

Increased total body potassium

If the hyperkalaemia cannot be explained by a shift of potassium from the intracellular to the extracellular space then total body potassium is probably increased. Total body potassium is controlled by dietary intake and urinary excretion, gastrointestinal excretion usually contributing little to homeostasis. In most cases urinary excretion, and not dietary intake, is the major factor determining total body potassium.

The following factors limit urinary excretion of potassium:

1. Renal failure. Hyperkalaemia is a major problem in acute renal failure, particularly in the presence of increased tissue breakdown due to trauma or infection. There is specific adaptation in potassium excretion in chronic renal failure,

and hyperkalaemia is usually only a problem if kidney function is severely impaired (creatinine clearance less than 0.15 ml/s) or if there are other causes of decreased potassium excretion (see 2–4 below).

2. Specific problems in renal potassium excretion. Hypoaldosteronism, either primary, as in Addison's disease (the diagnosis may be suggested by the history and the examination), or secondary to, either a low plasma renin (associated with diabetes, ageing, chronic volume expansion) or angiotensin-converting enzyme inhibiting drugs. Other important causes of hyperkalaemia are drugs known to inhibit renal transport of potassium (e.g. spironolactone, amiloride, triamterene).

3. Decreased sodium delivery to the distal tubule (as in volume depletion).

4. Acidosis.

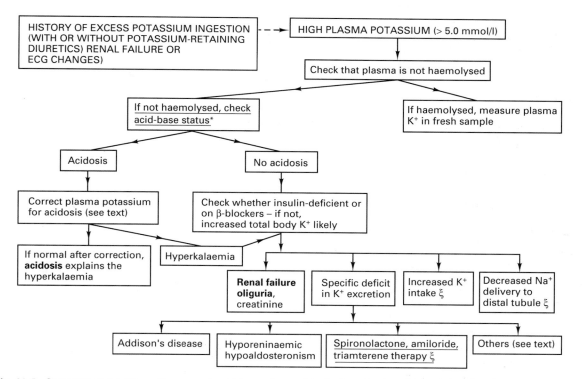

Fig. 29.5 Summary of the diagnostic approach which may be used in the investigation of hyperkalaemia. (Common diagnostic steps are shown underlined and common end diagnoses in bold type.) In many situations the diagnostic process will not be required, as the end diagnosis (e.g. renal failure) will lead to a search for the biochemical abnormality (hyperkalaemia).
* Acid–base status may be measured directly (arterial pH) or estimated from plasma bicarbonate concentration and assessment of respiratory function (see text).
ξ Rarely causes hyperkalaemia when sole abnormality but contributes to its development when associated with other abnormality (or abnormalities)

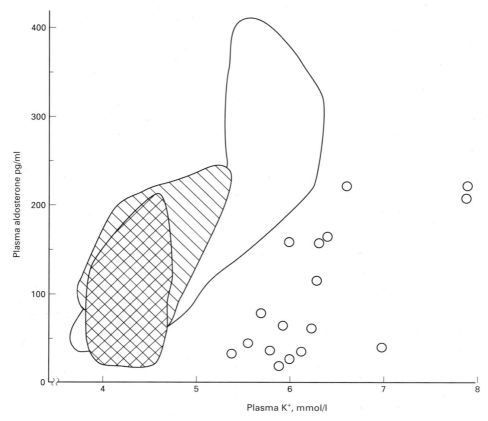

Fig. 29.6   The relationship between plasma potassium and plasma aldosterone derived from data of Dulhy et al (1972) (23 samples from 5 patients on a 200 Na⁺, 40 K⁺ diet plus KCl infusion ◯), Barnes et al (1985) (48 samples from 8 patients with hypertension plus a KCl infusion ⬿) and ourselves (14 samples from 14 patients with a low normal plasma renin level and normal renal function ⬿). The lines encompass all data points from the different groups. Patients with hyperkalaemia which we attributed to a relative hypoaldosteronism are illustrated by the small circles and represent 9 samples from 4 patients collected by us (unpublished), 5 patients abstracted from the paper of Schambelan et al (1981), 3 patients from Isenring et al (1992) and one patient from Lee et al (1979). The results illustrate the distinct nature of the hyperkalaemic group despite the 'normal', or even high, plasma aldosterone level

Hypoaldosteronism and decreased distal sodium delivery rarely cause hyperkalaemia by themselves, but in combination with or in the presence of an increased potassium intake potassium-retaining drugs [e.g. amiloride], mild renal impairment may produce symptomatic hyperkalaemia.

The diagnostic steps in the investigation of hyperkalaemia are summarized in Figure 29.5. One particular problem in deciding the cause of hyperkalaemia is the interpretation of plasma aldosterone levels. The normal range for plasma aldosterone is broad enough to encompass the variability of plasma renin activity and plasma potassium, the major factors controlling aldosterone secretion. Attempts have been made to relate the aldosterone secretion to plasma potassium concentration and sodium status. Figure 29.6 relates plasma potassium to plasma aldosterone in the presence of sodium repletion and helps define whether the level of aldosterone is appropriate for the potassium concentration. While the data is limited it does provide some guidance. If, for example, a patient has a plasma potassium of 5.5 mmol/l and a plasma aldosterone of 70 pg/ml then the patient has a defect in aldosterone secretion contributing to the high plasma potassium, despite a plasma level of aldosterone in the 'normal' range (10–160 pg/ml).

Treatment of hyperkalaemia

Urgent treatment of hyperkalaemia is required when there are electrocardiographic changes and/or the plasma potassium exceeds 6.5 mmol/l. The first priority is not to correct the hyperkalaemia but to inhibit its cardiotoxic effect by administration of calcium gluconate (i.v.). Treatment of hyperkalaemia due to a shift of potassium from intra- to extracellular space is most effective when directed at the underlying cause, e.g. acidosis should be treated with sodium bicarbonate and insulin deficiency with insulin and/or glucose. There is no place for attempting to remove potassium from the body in these situations.

Treatment of a total body excess of potassium is also best directed at the cause, e.g. by reversal of renal failure; fludrocortisone (an aldosterone agonist) in patients with hypoaldosteronism; cessation of potassium-retaining drugs; decreasing potassium intake; or increasing sodium delivery to the distal tubule (sodium-loading or diuretics).

However, in non-correctable or urgent situations other methods may need to be used, e.g. removal of potassium by cation exchange resins (Resonium A) given either orally or by enema; administration of glucose and insulin to increase potassium uptake into the cells as a temporary respite; or dialysis.

Causes of hypokalaemia

Redistribution of potassium

Once hypokalaemia has been established it is essential to determine the contribution of changes in potassium distribution (from extracellular to intracellular fluid) as opposed to changes in total body potassium. This is not always possible from the history alone, as factors which cause potassium loss can also cause alkalosis, the major factor responsible for a redistribution of potassium from extra- to intracellular fluid. Further complicating

---

Causes of hypokalaemia

Shift from intracellular to extracellular fluid
Alkalosis
Insulin excess
Mineralocorticoid excess
β-agonist - salbutamol
Hypokalaemic periodic paralysis (rare)
Decrease in total body potassium
Loss of potassium from the gastrointestinal tract
  Diarrhoea
  Purgatives
  Villous adenoma of the rectum
  Fistulae
  Vomiting
Loss of potassium in urine
  Diuretics
  Alkalosis
  Hyperaldosteronism
    Primary (Conn's syndrome)
    Secondary (nephrotic syndrome, liver failure, chronic cardiac failure, renal artery stenosis, malignant hypertension, renin-secreting tumour)
  Cushing's syndrome (especially due to ectopic ACTH production)
  Exogenous mineralocorticoids
    Fludrocortisone
    Carbenoxolone
    Liquorice
  Increased sodium delivery to distal tubule
    Increased sodium ingestion
    Diuretics
  Unreabsorbable anion in large quantities
    e.g. carbenicillin sulphate
  Hypomagnesaemia
  Renal loss due to type I renal tubular acidosis
  Bartter's syndrome
  Liddle's syndrome (very rare)

---

factors are alkalosis, which increases urinary potassium loss so that a decreased total body potassium may be secondary to the alkalosis, and potassium deficiency which can cause alkalosis (see earlier).

Thus, a change in plasma potassium should not be interpreted without reference to the patient's acid–base status. If there is evidence of alkalosis, the plasma potassium should be corrected for this abnormality (see above). If after correction the (then notional) plasma potassium is still low (less than 3.5 mmol/l) a deficit in total body potassium is likely.

If there is no alkalosis other factors affecting potassium distribution should be considered, including exogenous or endogenous mineralocorticoid excess; insulin excess; β-agonist excess (such as salbutamol usage) and hypokalaemic periodic paralysis.

Decreased total body potassium

Hypokalaemia associated with a decreased total body potassium is rarely due to decreased potassium intake alone because of the ubiquity of potassium in foods. Complete starvation rarely causes hypokalaemia because of the endogenous potassium load from tissue breakdown. Dietary idiosyncrasies leading to consumption solely of processed foods with a low potassium content can lead to hypokalaemia but other nutritional deficiencies would also be expected.

Hypokalaemia associated with a decreased total body potassium is usually due to potassium loss, either gastrointestinal or urinary. Gastrointestinal loss is often obvious from the history (diarrhoea, vomiting) but surreptitious vomiting is often difficult to diagnose. A low urinary chloride strongly suggests gastrointestinal loss of chloride by vomiting, and is thus a useful test in this difficult group of patients.

A hypokalaemic patient should normally conserve potassium. A potassium excretion of more than 30 mmol/day in the presence of a plasma potassium concentration of less than 3.5 mmol/l is inappropriately high and indicates increased urinary potassium loss as a cause for the hypokalaemia. Urinary potassium wasting may be due to any of the following:

1. Alkalosis.
2. Increased levels of aldosterone, either primary (as in Conn's syndrome) or secondary to a high renin state (e.g. heart failure, diuretic-induced volume depletion, Bartter's syndrome). Exogenous mineralocorticoids (e.g. fludrocortisone, carbenoxolone, liquorice) can also cause potassium wasting.

3. Cushing's syndrome may be associated with sufficient mineralocorticoid excess to produce hypokalaemia, particularly when due to ectopic ACTH production.
4. Increased sodium delivery to the distal tubule (increased sodium ingestion, diuretics) enhances distal potassium excretion.
5. Unreabsorbable anions in the large quantities associated with pharmacological administration (e.g. carbenicillin sulphate) also enhance distal potassium excretion.
6. Specific non-mineralocorticoid-dependent renal potassium wasting, Bartter's syndrome and a few other uncommon specific renal diseases (e.g. Liddle's syndrome) are associated with renal potassium wasting. Type I renal tubular acidosis is occasionally associated with non-steroid-dependent renal potassium wasting.
7. Hypomagnesaemia.

The combination of two or more of these factors (e.g. the increased distal sodium delivery and increased aldosterone levels occurring with diuretic treatment) produces a more potent mechanism for increasing potassium excretion and, when combined with alkalosis (secondary to volume depletion, hyperaldosteronism), is often associated with hypokalaemia.

The diagnostic steps in the investigation of patients with hypokalaemia are summarized in Figure 29.7. One particular problem in deciding the cause of hypokalaemia is the interpretation of aldosterone status, the normal range for plasma aldosterone being broad enough to encompass the variability of renin activity and plasma potassium, the major factors controlling aldosterone secretion.

Attempts have been made to define appropriate aldosterone levels in the presence of hypokalaemia. There is no useful guide except to say that a low plasma potassium should suppress plasma aldosterone levels; thus 'normal' levels of aldosterone, in the presence of hypokalaemia, may reflect hyperaldosteronism. Patients should be reassessed after potassium repletion, when any hyperaldosteronism will become more obvious. The appropriateness of aldosterone levels for the level of plasma potassium may also help define the

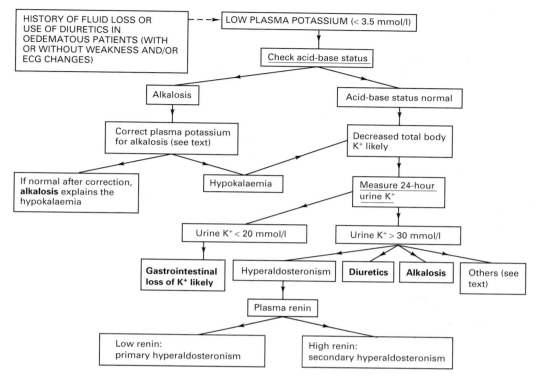

Fig. 29.7 Summary of the diagnostic approach which may be used in the investigation of hypokalaemia. (Common diagnostic steps are shown underlined and common end diagnoses in bold type.) In many situations the diagnostic process will not be required, as the end diagnosis (e.g. gastrointestinal loss) will lead to a search for the biochemical abnormality (hypokalaemia)

presence of exogenous kaliuretic factors (Adam 1986).

Treatment of hypokalaemia

Treatment of hypokalaemia due to alkalosis requires correction of the alkalosis, usually by potassium chloride supplementation to replenish chloride depletion, and cessation of alkali ingestion. Only rarely is the administration of acid salts (NH_4Cl) required (see below).

Treatment of total body potassium depletion almost always requires potassium chloride if the cause cannot be readily corrected. The use of potassium citrate or tartrate is not recommended, other than in the presence of coexisting acidosis, as these latter anions exacerbate alkalosis and urinary potassium wasting with consequent effects on plasma potassium. Any quantitative assessment of potassium depletion must take into account total body content (calculated from body weight and likely potassium content) and alkalosis (see below).

ACIDOSIS AND ALKALOSIS

Acidosis and alkalosis are defined as abnormal increases or decreases in the free hydrogen ion concentration ($[H^+]$) in plasma. The plasma $[H^+]$ is generally representative of total body status.

Free hydrogen ions in the plasma are in equilibrium with plasma bicarbonate, carbonic acid and carbon dioxide:

$$H_2O + CO_2 \rightleftharpoons H_2CO_3 \rightleftharpoons H^+ + HCO_3^-$$

Alkalosis (a decrease in hydrogen ion concentration) may be produced by:

1. removal of H^+ (metabolic alkalosis); or

2. driving the reaction to the left by
   a. increasing HCO_3^- (metabolic alkalosis)
   b. removing CO_2 through overbreathing (respiratory alkalosis).

Respiratory alkalosis is associated with a low bicarbonate concentration. By contrast, metabolic alkalosis, from any cause, is associated with a high bicarbonate concentration.

Acidosis (an increase in hydrogen ion concentration) may be produced by:

1. addition to H^+ (metabolic acidosis); or
2. driving the reaction to the right by
   a. lowering HCO_3^- (metabolic acidosis)
   b. increasing (retention of) CO_2 (respiratory acidosis).

Respiratory acidosis is associated with a high bicarbonate concentration, whereas metabolic acidosis from any cause is associated with a low bicarbonate concentration.

In many clinical situations the first indication of an acid–base disturbance is the finding of an abnormal plasma bicarbonate concentration. Since, as shown above, a high plasma bicarbonate may be due to either respiratory acidosis or metabolic alkalosis, and a low plasma bicarbonate to either metabolic acidosis or respiratory alkalosis, it is possible to assess acid–base status on plasma bicarbonate concentration alone.

Ideally, the plasma pH should be measured. However, if a clinical assessment can be made of the likely P_{CO_2} then the pH can be calculated from this and the plasma bicarbonate concentration. According to the Henderson–Hasselbalch equation:

$$pH = pKHCO_3^- + \log \frac{[HCO_3^-]}{[H_2CO_3]}$$

If the HCO_3^- concentration (in mmol/l) and P_{CO_2} (in mmHg) are known, the hydrogen ion concentration, and thus pH, can be calculated from the following formula:

$$pH = 6.1 + \log \frac{[HCO_3^-]}{0.03 \times Pa_{CO_2}}$$

Assuming normal respiratory compensation for metabolic acidosis there is also a simple empirical method for determining pH from the plasma bicarbonate concentration, which is fairly accurate for concentration ranges of H^+ from 8 to 44 nmol/l and pH ranges from 7.2 to 7.5. The first two digits after the decimal point are calculated by the addition of 15 to the bicarbonate concentration (in mmol/l). For example, at a bicarbonate concentration of 13 mmol/l, pH = 7 (15 + 13) = 7.28.

If plasma CO_2 is normal, then a low HCO_3^- always reflects a metabolic acidosis and a high HCO_3^- always a metabolic alkalosis. Respiratory compensation for a metabolic acidosis (by lowering hydrogen ion concentration) will also lower P_{CO_2} and further reduce bicarbonate, but this will not completely restore the pH to normal. Attempting to raise the hydrogen ion concentration by respiratory compensation for a metabolic alkalosis will also raise P_{CO_2} and bicarbonate concentration, but this mechanism is limited by the need for oxygen and is thus far less effective than respiratory compensation for metabolic acidosis. Respiratory compensation may be limited by intrinsic pulmonary disease or factors inhibiting respiration (e.g. coma, muscle weakness, obstruction, opiates).

The absence of respiratory compensation for metabolic acidosis leads to profoundly different outcomes in terms of pH and HCO_3 or $PaCO_2$. Figure 29.8 gives a nomogram for interpreting mixed acid–base disorders but does not deal with mixed primary acid–base disorders (see Brenner & Stein 1978 b or Narins & Gardiner 1981 for further clarification).

Unlike the respiratory compensation for metabolic disturbance, which can be immediate, the renal compensation for respiratory acid–base disturbance is by varying bicarbonate reabsorption, which takes time. Therefore chronic respiratory acidosis and alkalosis are readily differentiated from their acute precursors (Fig. 29.8).

Metabolic acidosis is commonly produced by increased generation of hydrogen ions from both volatile acids (organic acids that can be degraded to CO_2 and water) and non-volatile acids (acids that are degraded to sulphuric or phosphoric acid). The volatile acid production exceeds

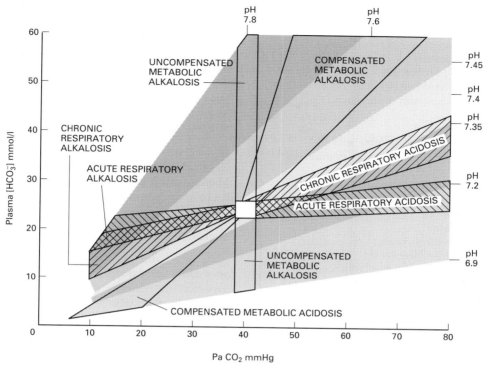

Fig. 29.8 An acid–base nomogram for clinical use showing the relationship between plasma $[HCO_3^-]$ and $PaCO_2$ at different plasma pH levels. The shaded areas help define a normal pM (7.35–7.45) from moderate and severe acidosis and alkalosis. Development of a chronic respiratory acid–base disturbance leads to compensatory metabolic changes to modify the relationship between $[HCO_3^-]$, $PaCO_2$ and thereby the resultant pH. Development of a metabolic acid–base disturbance is usually, but not always, associated with respiratory compensation which profoundly modifies $PaCO_2$, HCO_3^-, or pH. The nomogram is derived from that of Kaehny (1980).

13 000 mmol/day, compared to only about 60 mmol/day for non-volatile acids. Therefore an intact mechanism for both degrading volatile acids to CO_2 and water, and subsequently excreting CO_2 via the respiratory system, is essential for acid–base homeostasis.

Because of the rate of production of hydrogen ions, disturbances in volatile acid excretion (e.g. lactic acidosis, respiratory failure) can rapidly produce an overwhelming acidosis that is often fatal. By contrast, disturbances in excretion of non-volatile acids produce a much slower onset of acidosis because the body can buffer the increased hydrogen ion load for some time. For example, with an approximate body buffer capacity of 600 mmol, a deficit in hydrogen ion excretion of 60 mmol/day would produce severe acidosis only after 5–10 days.

Alkalosis (Box falls on next page)

Causes of alkalosis

Respiratory alkalosis. Respiratory alkalosis is caused by overbreathing, which may be due to:

1. anxiety
2. septicaemia
3. acidosis (partial compensation only)
4. acetylsalicylic acid overdose (direct stimulation of the respiratory centre produces a respiratory alkalosis offset by the metabolic acidosis induced by acetylsalicylic acid)
5. impaired oxygen exchange in the lungs (e.g. pulmonary fibrosis, pulmonary oedema).

Overbreathing is often obvious but may be ignored or difficult to detect. Measurement of respiratory rate is therefore helpful in diagnosis.

Causes of alkalosis

With low bicarbonate
Respiratory alkalosis — hyperventilation
    Secondary to anxiety
    Gram-negative septicaemia
    Acetylsalicylic acid overdose
    Central nervous system disturbance
    Hypoxaemia
With high bicarbonate
Ingestion of excess alkali (soluble antacids)
Loss of H^+ and/or Cl^- from the gastrointestinal tract
    Vomiting (e.g. pyloric stenosis)
    Gastric suction
    Chloride diarrhoea
Loss of H^+ in urine
    Hyperaldosteronism (primary or secondary)
    Exogenous mineralocorticoids
Extracellular volume depletion (enhanced bicarbonate reabsorption)
    Diuretics
    Other causes of volume depletion
Potassium depletion

Metabolic alkalosis. Metabolic alkalosis can be caused by any of the following:

1. Ingestion of excess alkali (e.g. antacids). With normal renal function the kidney can usually excrete large amounts of bicarbonate and thus only a mild alkalosis develops.

2. Loss of hydrogen ion from the gastrointestinal tract and in the urine. Loss from the gastrointestinal tract can occur with gastric suction or vomiting and is usually obvious. Surreptitious vomiters are a difficult diagnostic problem. A low urinary chloride excretion (less than 10 mmol/day) strongly suggests gastrointestinal loss of chloride (and H^+) and is a useful test in this group of patients. Loss in the urine may be due to excess aldosterone which stimulates hydrogen ion excretion and may produce a mild alkalosis. The presence of non-absorbable anions in the distal tubule facilitates both potassium and hydrogen ion excretion and can lead to alkalosis. Carbenicillin and penicillin are examples of these anions.

3. Extracellular volume depletion, especially associated with a disproportionate loss of chloride compared to bicarbonate (e. g. with gastrointestinal loss or diuretics). Both extracellular volume depletion and chloride depletion lead to enhanced bicarbonate reabsorption and thus metabolic alkalosis.

4. Potassium depletion. This enhances bicarbonate reabsorption and thus produces a metabolic alkalosis. Since alkalosis can cause hypokalaemia, the plasma potassium needs to be corrected for the degree of alkalosis before potassium depletion can be diagnosed (see above).

The diagnostic steps in the investigation of patients with a low bicarbonate concentration, or alkalosis, are summarized in Figure 29.9.

Diagnosis

History and physical examination and laboratory investigations. Alkalosis may be suspected in patients taking large quantities of antacids, in those who are likely to have potassium depletion (see above) and in those with a history of prolonged vomiting. Alkalosis is usually asymptomatic. Paraesthesia or tetany, due to a reduction in ionized calcium, may occur, particularly with the rapidly induced respiratory alkalosis seen with overbreathing. The hypokalaemia induced by alkalosis can also produce symptoms of muscle weakness and cardiac arrhythmias.

Measurement of arterial plasma pH is the most accurate means of assessing disturbances in hydrogen ion concentration. However, determination of plasma bicarbonate concentration is usually adequate to categorize an abnormality of hydrogen ion concentration, provided the $P\text{co}_2$ is likely to be normal on the basis of the respiratory examination.

Assessment of $P\text{CO}_2$ is particularly important with overbreathing as it is the cause of respiratory alkalosis.

Treatment

As most patients with alkalosis are asymptomatic, management of both respiratory and metabolic alkalosis should be directed at the primary cause (e.g. potassium chloride or volume replacement, cessation of alkali ingestion). Respiratory alkalosis due to overbreathing may be treated by persuading

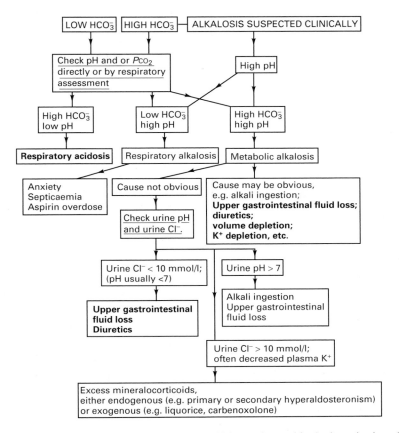

Fig. 29.9 Summary of the diagnostic process which may be used in the investigation of the alkalosis and/or a high plasma bicarbonate concentration. (Common diagnostic steps are shown underlined and common end diagnoses in bold type.) In many situations the diagnostic process will not be required, as the end diagnosis (e.g. upper gastrointestinal fluid loss) will lead to a search for the biochemical abnormality (e.g. alkalosis)

the patient to rebreathe in a paper bag in order to raise the P_{CO_2} and hydrogen ion concentration. Mild to moderate metabolic alkalosis (pH below 7.6) often requires only correction of the precipitating factors. Severe metabolic alkalosis (pH above 7.6) may lead to serious cardiac arrhythmias (secondary to disturbance in potassium and calcium) and requires more urgent treatment. Intravenous infusion of HCl or NH_4Cl may be used, but HCl should be given only if NH_4Cl would aggravate hyperammonaemia (hepatic failure) or uraemia. HCl is given as an 0.1– molar solution, by a central venous line, at no more than 20 mmol/h. A safe recommendation is to base the calculation on bicarbonate excess and

extracellular fluid volume. For example, to lower plasma bicarbonate by 10 mmol/l, the extracellular fluid volume (20% of body weight, i.e. 14 litres in a 70 kg man) is multiplied by this desired drop in concentration (i.e. 10) to give the required amount (140 mmol). This estimate is very conservative and approximate, and pH (or bicarbonate concentration) should be checked repeatedly during therapy.

Acidosis (Box on next page)

Causes of acidosis

Respiratory acidosis. Respiratory acidosis is caused by impaired CO_2 exchange. Pulmonary

---

Cause of acidosis

With high bicarbonate (respiratory)
Respiratory acidosis (hypoventilation)
With low bicarbonate (metabolic)
With high anion gap
   Diabetic ketoacidosis
   Renal failure
   Lactic acidosis
   Acetylsalicylic acid poisoning
   Methanol
With normal anion gap
   Renal tubular acidosis
   Diarrhoea (or other alkaline gastrointestinal fluid
     loss such as ileal conduits)
   Ingestion of HCl or NH_4Cl
   Carbonic anhydrase inhibitors (acetazolamide)
   Hypoaldosteronism

---

oedema rarely causes CO_2 retention. Inadequate respiration (coma, opiates, obstruction) or pulmonary disease leading to a decreased alveolar area or permeability (to CO_2) is usually responsible for a high $P\text{CO}_2$.

Metabolic acidosis. Metabolic acidosis can be produced by:

1. introducing excess hydrogen ions (e.g. acetylsalicylic acid overdose);
2. excess hydrogen ion production within the body (i.e. lactic acidosis, diabetic ketoacidosis);
3. failure of renal excretion of hydrogen ions (e.g. renal failure, renal tubular acidosis and, to a lesser extent, hypoaldosteronism); and
4. loss of alkaline (bicarbonate-rich) fluid (e.g. gastrointestinal loss in diarrhoea or renal loss).

Laboratory investigation

Urinary acid excretion (e.g. the relatively high urine pH in renal tubular acidosis) may help in diagnosing the aetiology of a pH disturbance.

The plasma anion gap ($[Na^+]$ — $[Cl^-]$ — $[HCO_3^-]$) gives a measure of other anions.

The normal anion gap is about 7–15 (mmol/l) and the unmeasured anions in this gap include phosphate, sulphate and proteins. A high anion gap implies unmeasured anions which may relate to the hydrogen ions contributing to the coexistent acidosis.

Acidosis with a low plasma chloride and a large anion gap may be due to:

1. Increased amounts of non-volatile acids (sulphuric and phosphoric), the usual cause of acidosis in renal failure.
2. Ingested non-volatile acids such as acetylsalicylic acid.
3. Unmetabolized volatile acids, e.g. butyric acid and keto acids in diabetic ketoacidosis and lactic acidosis. Lactic acidosis may arise from increased production in peripheral tissues due to anoxia or decreased metabolism by the liver (e.g. related to biguanide treatment).

Acidosis with a high plasma chloride and a normal anion gap, hyperchloraemia acidosis, is usually due to one of the following:

1. Renal tubular acidosis where the kidney either leaks bicarbonate ion (type I), or has a selective deficit in hydrogen ion excretion (type II) which may be due to aldosterone deficiency (type IV) (see Ch. 17). A urine pH of more than 5.4 in the presence of systemic acidosis confirms the diagnosis but a lower urine pH does not exclude it (see Ch. 17).
2. Gastrointestinal loss of alkaline fluid. This may be due to intrinsic bowel disease but also occurs with urinary–intestinal fistulae (e.g. ileal bladder). Surreptitious purgative users are a difficult problem, but melanosis coli on sigmoidoscopy may suggest the diagnosis.
3. Ingestion of hydrochloric acid or its precursor, ammonium chloride.

Diagnosis

History and physical examination. Acidosis may be suspected in patients with an obvious cause such as uncontrolled diabetes, renal failure or diarrhoea. Symptoms of metabolic acidosis are non-existent or non-specific (e.g. failure to thrive in children, malaise), but deep respiration due to hydrogen ion stimulation of the respiratory centre is very suggestive, especially if the history and signs are consistent with a cause for the acidosis.

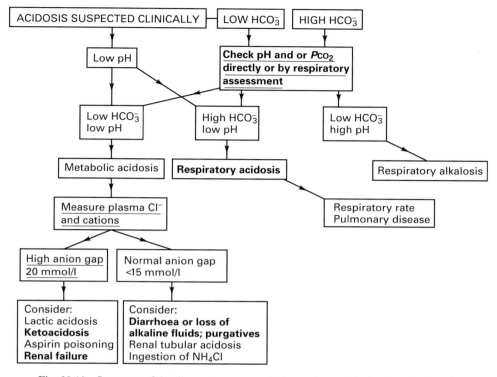

Fig. 29.10 Summary of the diagnostic process which may be used in the investigation of the acidosis and/or a low plasma bicarbonate concentration. (Common diagnostic steps are shown underlined and common end diagnoses in bold type.) In many situations the diagnostic process will not be required, as the end diagnosis (e.g. diabetic ketoacidosis) will lead to a search for the biochemical abnormality (e.g. metabolic acidosis)

Again, examination of the respiratory system is of critical importance as a guide to the likely PCO_2 and thus interpretation of the plasma bicarbonate concentration.

The diagnostic steps in the investigation of patients with a low bicarbonate concentration and acidosis are summarized in Figure 29.10.

Treatment

Treatment of the underlying cause is essential for acidosis due to volatile acids, because the massive production rates that can be achieved (up to 13 000 mmol/day) can rapidly lead to fatal acidosis (pH less than 6.8). Correction of respiratory difficulties (e.g. obstruction) rapidly relieves respiratory acidosis, and improvement in the peripheral circulation can improve lactic acidosis.

In acidosis due to non-volatile acids the primary cause should be treated but management often depends on alkali administration. Administration of bicarbonate is certainly justified in severe acidosis (pH below 7.2) from any cause but rapid correction of pH may cause cardiac problems due to redistribution of potassium (hypokalaemia) and lowering of ionized calcium by increased protein binding. Acidosis due to a bicarbonate leak requires large amounts of bicarbonate to maintain a normal pH. In a steady state the amount of bicarbonate or lactate required to correct the acidosis can be calculated from the bicarbonate deficit. For example, at a plasma bicarbonate of 10 mmol/l the plasma deficit is 15 mmol/l. The total body deficit is then calculated as total body water (taken as 60% of body weight) multiplied by this deficit. For a 70 kg man this would be 40 litres $\times$ 15 mmol/l = 600 mmol. This estimation is only approximate,

and pH (or bicarbonate concentration) should be checked repeatedly during therapy.

RECOMMENDED READING AND REFERENCES

Adam W R 1986 A simple method for definition of incomplete suppression of aldosterone and its association with hypertension and hypokalaemia in man. Clinical Sciences 71: 375–383

Ayus J C, Olivero J J, Frommer J P 1982 Rapid correction of severe hyponatremia with intravenous hypertonic saline solution. American Journal of Medicine 72: 43–48

Barnes J N, Drew P J T, Furniss S S, Holly J M P, Knight A R, Skehan J D, Goodwin F J 1985 Effect of angiotensin converting-enzyme inhibition on potassium-mediated aldosterone secretion in essential hypertension. Clinical Science 68: 625–630

Bichet D. Szatalowicz V, Chaimovitz C, Schrier R W 1982 Role of vasopressin in abnormal water excretion in cirrhotic patients. Annals of Internal Medicine 96: 413–417

Brenner B M, Stein J H (eds) 1978a Contemporary issues in nephrology. Sodium and water homeostasis. Churchill Livingstone, New York

Brenner B M, Stein J H (eds) 1978b Contemporary issues in nephrology. Acid-base and potassium homeostasis, Churchill Livingstone, New York

Dluhy R G, Axelrod L, Underwood R H, Williams G H 1972 Studies of the control of plasma aldosterone concentration in normal man. Journal of Clinical Investigation 51: 1950–1957

Edwards O M, Bayliss R I S 1976 Idiopathic oedema of women. Quarterly Journal of Medicine 45: 125–144

Emmett M, Narins R G 1977 Clinical use of the anion gap. Medicine 56: 38–54

Flear C T G, Gill G V, Burn J 1981 Hyponatraemia: mechanisms and management. Lancet 2: 26–31

Halperin M L, Goldstein M B 1988 Fluid, electrolyte and acid-base emergencies. W B Saunders, Philadelphia

Isenring P, Lebel M, Grose J H 1992 Endocrine sodium and volume regulation in familial hyperkalemia with hypertension. Hypertension 19: 371–377

Kaehny W D 1980 In Schrier R W (ed) Renal and electrolyte disorders, 2nd edn. Little Brown, Boston, p. 172

Lee M R, Ball S G, Thomas T H, Morgan D B 1979 Hypertension and hyperkalaemia responding to Bendrofluazide. Quarterly Journal of Medicine 190: 245–258

MacGregor G A, Tasker P R W, de Wardener H E 1975 Diuretic induced oedema. Lancet 1: 481–492

Narins R G, Gardiner L B 1981 Simple acid-base disturbances. Medical Clinics of North America 65: 321–346

Robertson G L, Aycinena P, Zerbe R L 1982 Neurogenic disorders of osmoregulation. American Journal of Medicine 72: 339–353

Schambelan M, Sebastian A, Rector F C Jr 1981 Mineralocorticoid-resistant renal hyperkalemia without salt wasting (type II pseudohypoaldosteronism): role of increased renal chloride reabsorption. Kidney International 19: 716–727

Smith K 1980 Fluids and electrolytes. A conceptual approach. Churchill Livingstone, New York

Zerber R L, Robertson G L 1981 A comparison of plasma vasopressin measurements with a standard indirect test in the differential diagnosis of polyuria. New England Journal of Medicine 305: 1539–1546

Index